Behavioral Neurology: Clinical Frontiers and Functions

Behavioral Neurology: Clinical Frontiers and Functions

Edited by Catelyn Wilkerson

hayle medical
New York

Hayle Medical,
750 Third Avenue, 9th Floor,
New York, NY 10017, USA

Visit us on the World Wide Web at:
www.haylemedical.com

ISBN: 978-1-63241-671-1

The publisher's policy is to use permanent paper from mills that operate a sustainable forestry policy. Furthermore, the publisher ensures that the text paper and cover boards used have met acceptable environmental accreditation standards.

Printed in China.

Cataloging-in-Publication Data

Behavioral neurology : clinical frontiers and functions / edited by Catelyn Wilkerson.
p. cm.
Includes bibliographical references and index.
ISBN 978-1-63241-671-1
1. Clinical neuropsychology. 2. Brain--Diseases--Complications. 3. Neuropsychology.
4. Neuropsychiatry. I. Wilkerson, Catelyn.
RC341 .B44 2019
612.8--dc23

Table of Contents

Preface

Behavioral neurology is a specialization of neurology that is focused on the pathological and clinical aspects of neural processes that are associated with cognitive function, mental activity, emotional states and social behavior. Some of the domains of interest in this field are the understanding of memory, attention, high-order perceptual processing, language, problem-solving operations, etc. Advancements in the field of cognitive neuroscience brought about by brain imaging techniques, experimental cognitive neuropsychology and electrophysiological methods have led to the growth and evolution of behavioral neurology. This book is a valuable compilation of topics, ranging from the basic to the most complex advancements in the field of behavioral neurology. It presents this complex subject in the most comprehensible language. For someone with an interest and eye for detail, it covers the most significant dermatologic treatments.

This book is a comprehensive compilation of works of different researchers from varied parts of the world. It includes valuable experiences of the researchers with the sole objective of providing the readers (learners) with a proper knowledge of the concerned field. This book will be beneficial in evoking inspiration and enhancing the knowledge of the interested readers.

In the end, I would like to extend my heartiest thanks to the authors who worked with great determination on their chapters. I also appreciate the publisher's support in the course of the book. I would also like to deeply acknowledge my family who stood by me as a source of inspiration during the project.

Editor

1

Stroke Survivor and Caregiver Perspectives on Post-Stroke Visual Concerns and Long-Term Consequences

Theresa M. Smith,[1] **Monique R. Pappadis**,[2,3] **Shilpa Krishnan**,[4] **and Timothy A. Reistetter**[2,3,5]

[1]*Department of Occupational Therapy, Texas Woman's University, 6700 Fannin Street, Houston, TX 77030, USA*
[2]*Division of Rehabilitation Sciences, School of Health Professions, University of Texas Medical Branch, 301 University Blvd, Galveston, TX 77555, USA*
[3]*Sealy Center on Aging, University of Texas Medical Branch, 301 University Blvd, Galveston, TX 77555, USA*
[4]*Department of Rehabilitation Medicine, Division of Physical Therapy, Emory University, School of Medicine, 1462 Clifton Road, Atlanta, GA 30322, USA*
[5]*Department of Occupational Therapy, School of Health Professions, University of Texas Medical Branch, Galveston, 301 University Blvd, Galveston, TX 77555, USA*

Correspondence should be addressed to Timothy A. Reistetter; tareiste@utmb.edu

Academic Editor: Carolyn Baum

Approximately 800,000 people in the United States have a stroke annually. Up to two thirds of stroke survivors have some visual problems, which result in disability and can affect survivors' overall rehabilitation outcomes. Although some post-stroke visual impairments can be corrected and respond well to intervention, ocular signs can be subtle and may not be recognized or reported by the stroke survivor but rather by a vigilant caregiver. The purpose of this study was to explore the post-stroke visual concerns and consequences expressed by stroke survivors and caregivers. This study employed a qualitative design using semistructured interviews conducted with a convenience sample of stroke survivors and caregivers recruited from either a community support group or skilled nursing and long-term care facilities. Interviews were recorded and transcribed verbatim. Comparative content analysis was used to identify vision-related themes by two independent coders. All research team members completed quality checking of coding. Twenty participants (11 stroke survivors and 9 caregivers) expressed visual concerns or consequences following stroke: (1) eye movement problems, (2) perceptual issues, and (3) consequences of vision problems or issues, which affected their daily life/quality of life. Stroke survivors and caregivers reported receiving vision care from (1) eye doctors, (2) occupational therapists, and (3) other healthcare professionals. All vision care providers need to be observant of potential post-stroke visual concerns. Stroke survivors should have a thorough vision evaluation to optimize their independence in everyday activities and quality of life.

1. Introduction

Approximately 800,000 people in the United States have a stroke annually [1]. With the rising population of older adults, the incidence of stroke is expected to increase and survival rates of stroke continue to rise [2]. Up to two thirds of stroke survivors have some visual problems that result in disability [3]. A wide range of visual impairments can occur following stroke including low vision, eye movement and visual field abnormalities, and visual perceptual difficulties [4, 5]. These impairments invariably affect survivors' independence in daily living and quality of life, negatively influencing their ability to drive, work, and their confidence and familial relationships [6].

Stroke survivors reported low vision acuity for near and distance vision [4]. Nearly 20–60% of stroke survivors have permanent or resolving visual field deficits usually homonymous hemianopia or quadrantanopia, and 70% may be affected by eye movement disorders [7]. Eye movement disorders can result in a loss of depth perception, reduced eye-hand coordination, problems with scanning, and difficulties reading [7]. Strabismus, a misalignment of the eyes, can affect stroke survivors with resulting complaints of diplopia [8]. Visuospatial inattention, also termed visual neglect or hemispatial neglect, can occur following right hemisphere stroke [9]. Other post-stroke visual concerns pertain to eye-hand coordination deficits. These deficits have been shown to result in reduced independence and quality of life [10]. Other conditions that can lead to decreased visual acuity such as glaucoma, cataract, retinal diseases, macular degeneration, and refractive errors [10].

Visual impairments are not as evident as motor or speech impairment [11] and without thorough screening subtle visual complications may go undiagnosed. In the United States, visual acuity is commonly assessed with a Snellen chart [12, 13] and visual fields by the Humphrey visual field [14]. Visual field deficits may be screened using a confrontation test. Most eye movement disorders can be detected during a clinical evaluation [15]. Paper and pencil tasks are used routinely to assess visual perceptual symptoms of visual inattention even though they may not detect symptoms in a chronic stage [16].

Prior studies have identified patients with significant vision impairments, many of whom did not have proper corrective lens following a stroke. One study found that individuals admitted for rehabilitation following stroke usually do not have their glasses with them or have glasses that were not in acceptable condition [17]. Even among those with existing glasses, some still had impaired vision.

Ninety-two percent of stroke survivors with suspected visual problems have been determined to have low vision, eye movement deficit, visual field impairment, and/or visual perceptual deficits such as visual inattention [4]. It is important to treat visual problems that can adversely affect rehabilitation outcomes of stroke survivors [5, 17, 18]. Treatment for eye movement disorders could be restorative, compensative, substitutive, pharmacological, or assessment and screening interventions [19]. Visual fields deficits may improve, but maximal improvement generally occurs within a month [18]. Treatment for visual field deficits involves training in compensatory eye movements, and some patients have prisms in their glasses. Visual inattention is commonly treated by training the patient to scan to the neglected side. Increasing more complex tasks is completed to increase attention [20]. Other treatments for visual inattention include video feedback during treatment, training in visual imagery, diplopia, and vestibular, somatosensory, and optokinetic stimulation. Prisms may also be used [18]. With rehabilitation, partial to full recovery is possible for some visual disorders secondary to stroke [11, 18, 21].

Many of these visual impairments can be corrected and respond well to intervention [18]. However, some visual impairments can be subtle and may not be recognized or reported by the patient but rather by a vigilant caregiver [5]. Some visual problems resulting from stroke such as visual field deficits can be chronic [18] or resistant to treatment. The consensus in the literature is that a thorough vision evaluation in the rehabilitation setting and targeted rehabilitation are critical to maximize patient functional performance [4, 5, 11, 18, 21]. It is important for healthcare providers to understand how stroke survivors and their caregivers experience visual concerns after stroke to ensure that care is focused on areas that matter most to those affected by stroke. Hence, the purpose of this study was to identify the vision concerns of stroke survivors and the consequences of visual impairments as perceived by stroke survivors and caregivers.

2. Methods

2.1. Research Design. In the current qualitative study, interviews of stroke survivors and caregivers were only included if they discussed aspects related to vision. This cross-sectional study is a part of a larger patient-centered outcomes research study that collected data on stroke survivors and caregivers on their preferences and needs following stroke [22]. The University's Institutional Review Board approved this study.

2.2. Participants and Recruitment. Participants were recruited using convenience sampling techniques from local stroke support groups as well as skilled nursing and long-term care facilities in the Houston and Galveston area in Texas. The stroke survivors were included if they were 18 years and older, self-identified with a previous diagnosis of stroke, and communicated in English. The caregivers were recruited into the study if a survivor identified them as their primary caregiver. Not all caregivers agreed to participate, and in some cases, the caregivers identified by the stroke survivors participated even if the stroke survivors themselves did not participate. The eligible participants were identified and enrolled into this study by a research coordinator with a background in psychology.

2.3. Data Collection. After obtaining the participant's written consent to participate, semistructured, in-person interviews were conducted. Separate, independent interviews were conducted for stroke survivors and caregivers at their preferred location [23–25]. The interview guide was developed by a multidisciplinary team involving an occupational therapist (TR) with expertise in health services and outcomes research and a social scientist with over 30 years of experience in qualitative research [25, 26]. The semistructured interview guide included the following content: description of the stroke event and consequences following stroke, therapy and services received, goals in rehabilitation, and what was most important. The interview guide for caregivers included similar content, in addition to content related to their role in the decision-making process, need for information, and advice for other caregivers. All participants were probed for clarification and additional information [27]. The interview guide did not include specific vision-related questions; however, it did include general questions to identify all perceived stroke-related symptoms or concerns.

Male and female licensed occupational (TR) and physical therapists (SK) conducted the interviews. The interviewers had prior experience in conducting semistructured interviews, qualitative methods, and rehabilitating individuals with stroke. In addition, the interviewers had no current or previous connection with any participants recruited in this study. The interviewers revealed their existing affiliations and the purpose of the study to the participants. On an average, each interview lasted for 30 minutes (range: 20–60 minutes). These interviews were audio-recorded and transcribed using professional transcription services. The participants were compensated with a $25 gift card for their time and contribution to this study.

2.4. Data Analysis. We used a combination of thematic and content analysis approaches to code the transcripts (Bernard and Ryan [25]). We started with open coding (i.e., identifying initial codes and categories) and then continued with axial coding (i.e., identifying relationships between the initial codes), and then proceeding with selective coding (i.e., coding any data associated with our core vision-related themes). The transcripts of the stroke survivors were read and coded independently by MP and TR for themes and subthemes related to voluntarily disclosed vision concerns and quality-checked by SK and TS for relevance and consistency. The transcripts for the caregiver interviews were read and coded independently by SK and TR and quality-checked for consistency and relevance by MP and TS. Constant comparison was done within and across transcripts to enhance trustworthiness of the coding process.

For the current study, only themes related to vision were coded and discussed. Of the 65 interviews (41 stroke survivors and 24 caregivers) from the larger study, 20 participants (11 stroke survivors and 9 caregivers) expressed themes or concepts related to vision. Any disagreements in codes were resolved by discussion with the entire research team. The benefits of utilizing multiple coders with multidisciplinary backgrounds including occupational therapy, low vision rehabilitation, physical therapy, social work, expertise in qualitative methods and analyses, and expertise treating individuals with neurological impairments helped us refine our themes from multiple perspectives and limited specific biases [25, 28]. All members of the research team had their primary appointment in an academic university with a medical center during the time of this study.

The final codebook was created, and the refined themes and subthemes were entered into a qualitative analysis software, NVivo 10 [29]. We also performed text search queries in NVivo 10 with words and concepts related to vision, including but not limited to "see," "vision," "read," "eye," "glasses," and "perception" to make sure all concepts related to vision were coded from all interviews. Text queries also identified words with the same stem or synonyms. For example, when we queried *see*, we obtained text related to *seeing*, *read*, and *saw*. In addition, NVivo helped us organize and synthetize our themes.

The final set of themes and subthemes was formed after combining relevant subthemes and was agreed upon by all members in the research team. The themes were grouped into relevant categories to align in a consistent manner with the rehabilitation process along with supportive quotations. To ensure quality control of the data [30], we used triangulation methods for clarification and to better understand vision concerns if mentioned by both the caregiver and the stroke survivor. In addition, all members of the research team have been sufficiently engaged with stroke survivors and caregivers due to their clinical experience. Lastly, we maintained an audit trail by keeping records regarding code/theme development and team decisions regarding the analysis and interpretation of the data.

3. Results

During the qualitative interviews of a larger study including 65 participants, which included 40 stroke survivors and 25 caregivers, 11 stroke survivors and 9 caregivers reported visual concerns. There were four female and seven male survivors ranging in age from 42–74 years of age (mean age = 62.1, SD = 9.4). Five of the survivors were Caucasian, five were African-American, and one was Hispanic. Five survivors had inpatient rehabilitation, one of which also had home health, three had outpatient therapy, one survivor's rehabilitation was unknown, one had "other therapy," and one had no rehabilitation. The majority of stroke survivors were 1–2 years post-stroke ($n = 8$), while the others were 3–5 years post-stroke. There were eight female caregivers and one male caregiver who ranged in age from 24 to 89 years (mean age = 66.7, SD = 18.6). Eight of the caregivers were Caucasians, and one was African American. Half of the caregivers were caring for a stroke survivor who was 1–2 years post-stroke, whereas the others were 3–5 years post-stroke. A formal caregiver cared for a number of patients; therefore, it is unclear how long post-stroke they were.

The qualitative data results are presented below. The results are based on the two main themes derived from the data, which are the visual concerns and consequences mentioned by the stroke survivors and caregivers and the vision care providers to which they attributed their care.

3.1. Visual Concerns and Consequences. Three subthemes of visual concerns emerged from the data including eye movement problems, perceptual issues, and consequences of these problems or issues (see Table 1). Codes representing the eye movement problems subtheme included double vision, eyes cannot focus, eyes jumping around, and eyelid does not close. Codes demonstrating the perceptual issues subtheme consisted of trouble distinguishing colors, loss of depth perception and peripheral vision, left neglect, and impaired visual processing. The third subtheme of visual concerns and consequences encompassed the following codes: reading, impaired balance and falls, incapacity to drive, and inability to work.

3.2. Vision Care Providers. The stroke survivors and caregivers discussed which vision care providers they saw for these visual concerns and interventions they received from the different vision care providers (see Table 2). The three named vision care providers were eye doctors, occupational therapists, and other healthcare professionals. Participants related that eye doctors were seen for examination, magnifiers, glasses, and eye patch. Occupational therapists addressed visual concerns with scanning, gaming, and eye-hand coordination activities. Other healthcare professionals included

Table 1: Subthemes and codes for the theme: visual concerns and consequences.

Subthemes	Code frequency	Prototypical quotations
		Eye movement problems
Double vision	1 ss; 3 c	"I got up to go to the bathroom and the double vision was so bad I could not make it from the bathroom to the bed." (ss24, 68, M, IRF) "She was now having real visual problems. She was seeing double and things were happening." (c17, 74, M, acute rehab only)
Eyes do not focus	1 ss	"Well, worse problem I have is with my eyes. They do not focus together." (ss5, 71,M, no rehab)
Eyes jumping around	1 c	"The one thing that I do regret is that I did not jump on them more about his eye and even Dr. *** and them ... I mean finally after we'd been there all through intensive care obviously they know his eyes are jumping around." (c1, 65, F, IRF)
Eyelid does not close	1 c	"...and the idea of his eye not staying shut is one big thing. And had I known more about it I would have insisted they get somebody in there to close that eye so that it would not get hurt, the cornea." (c1, 65, F, IRF)
		Perceptual issues
Trouble distinguishing colors	1 ss	"I can see colors, all kinds of colors but if you have a pink and close to a pink, I can't distinguish, or a white and a yellow. Like, if it's a light yellow, I'm using that as a for instance. I can't distinguish that anymore." (ss23, 74, F, IRF)
Loss of depth perception	1 ss; 1 c	"My depth perception is real off." (ss7, 57, F, acute rehab) "We lay things out and his eyes still are a problem because he cannot see the depth perception." (c1, 65, F, IRF)
Lost peripheral vision	4 ss; 2 c	"It's my eyes. I can't see out of the peripheral..." (ss42, 67, F, IRF) "He did have peripheral vision on the right side was lost, and we noticed that weeks later we were driving down 610 and there's a Derek Hotel... he said, "What is a Derek Hot?" He didn't get the last part of it, the E-L, hotel." (c20, 76, F, outpatient rehab)
Left neglect	3 ss; 2 c	"I was determined to have left neglect as well. If you're not familiar with that, it's a pretty bizarre condition. Someone came from behind me and startled me. I kind of was spooked, so I, "Whoa," by the person coming around." (ss19, 55, M, acute care rehab only) "His perception is pretty off, he has left side of negligence." (c11, 73, F, home health)
Impaired visual processing	2 ss; 2 c	"I can see things all around me. No problem that way but when it comes to them together, I can put them together but I have to really concentrate." (ss23, 74, F, IRF) "And a problem she has today is that she can see something but it doesn't...it happened too quickly for her to digest." (c17,74, M, acute rehab only)
		Consequences of vision problems or issues
Decreased eye-hand coordination	3 c	"But the hand-eye, those that have had visual issues and coordination issues" (c17,74, acute rehab only)
Difficulty reading	3 c	"He did teach himself to read, though. He worked about five hours a day on the computer and reading." (c20, 76, F, outpatient)
Impaired balance and falls	2 ss; 2 c	"Balance and vision? Yea...that's my main complaints." (ss7, 57, F, acute rehab only) "You are going to fall or something else is going to happen to you if we do not get you to the doctor and get your eyes examined." (c4, 76, F, NR)
Incapacity to drive	1 ss	"He said that I had lost peripheral vision in my left eye... I do not drive my car anymore." (ss37, 63, M, NR)
Inability to work	1 c	"For the longest time, all he wanted to do was go back to work and he began to realize that he couldn't read properly." (c11, 73, F, home health)

ss = stroke survivor; c = caregiver; IRF = inpatient rehabilitation facility; F = female; M = male; NR = not reported.

TABLE 2: Subthemes and codes for the theme: vision care providers.

Subthemes	Code frequency	Prototypical quotations
	Eye doctor	
Examination	2 c	"She's actually a[n] ophthalmologist. The exam that she performed was very thorough." (c17,74, M, home health)
Magnifiers	1 c	"The VA gave ** one of these magnifiers for reading, he used it for probably a year, and then... didn't need it anymore." (c11, 73, F, home health)
Glasses	3 ss; 1 c	"I also received prism glasses from a neuro ophthalmologist in California which was very helpful." (ss19, 55, M, outpatient) "*** can either come and have prism lenses or do some exercises for the eyes." (c2, 54, F, no rehab)
Eye patch	1 c	"An ophthalmologist...had us tape the eye shut...he did say if you were staying I think I would go ahead and stitch that eye up." (c1, 65, F, IRF)
	Occupational therapist	
Scanning	1 ss	"Occupational therapists showed me some techniques to ... to improve on my visual scanning." (ss36, 44, M, IRF)
Gaming	1 ss	"They [occupational therapists] gave me aids, such as apps and also games to play or something that will help with that." (ss36, 44, M, IRF)
Eye-hand coordination	2 c	"I guess the occupational therapy focused more on the hand-eye coordination kind of stuff." (c14, 24, F, IRF)
	Others	
Compensation	2 ss	"They had to turn my bed so I actually look to the left" (ss19, 55, M, outpatient)
Therapy	1 ss; 1 c	"A lot of therapies...for my vision." (ss41, 69, M, IRF & home health) "We didn't have occupational therapy because...vision comes out of our physical therapy budget, according to Medicare." (c17,74, M, home health)

ss = stroke survivors; C = caregivers; IRF = inpatient rehabilitation facility; M = male; F = female; rehab = rehabilitation.

unidentified professionals who provided compensation techniques and therapy.

4. Discussion

The purpose of this study was to explore voluntarily disclosed visual concerns from the perspectives of the stroke survivors and caregivers. Persons with stroke and caregivers expressed how the consequences of eye movement problems and perception issues led to a decrease in occupational performance of daily activities, such as eye-hand coordination, reading, maintaining balance, driving, and working. Conjugate eye deviations and neglect commonly occur together and reduce fast eye movements needed for reading, mobility, and visual exploration [11], and visual field deficits negatively affects one's ability to drive [31].

The emergence of visual concerns from survivors and caregivers within our study is substantiated by the findings of another research study that employed similar qualitative methodologies [7]. One of the top five priorities of stroke survivors and caregivers was to learn the best ways to treat visual problems after stroke [7]. Participants in our study described specific consequences of visual problems and perceptual issues, such as difficulty reading, impaired balance and falls, incapacity to drive, and inability to work. Other researchers have studied how visual problems can affect balance and contribute to fear of falling and falls [6]. Visuospatial neglect was associated with risk for falls, but the correlation of visual field deficit and falls is less clear [32]. Postural stability is also related among other factors to visual condition of stroke survivors, and decreased visual acuity increases the risk for falls [33]. Driving is a complicated occupation requiring many skills, but sufficient visual function is fundamental as it is for work.

Both stroke survivors and caregivers conveyed the importance of specialized care for visual concerns and named specific interventions used by vision care providers. Further, they expressed frustration when they were unable to access vision care providers or felt vision concerns were overlooked. Stroke survivors in a study by Rowe also communicated that visual concerns were overlooked by medical staff members as their attention was directed to other disabilities from the stroke [6]. Caregivers as well as survivors lamented that survivors were not referred for vision rehabilitation when it was needed following stroke.

I guess I am wishing and hoping something can be done about my eyesight ... I wish I would have pushed harder on my primary care doctor to look into the eye problem, but I didn't and we just kept passing that over.

Some participants discussed their issues with misdiagnosis of their visual impairments that resulted in them not receiving timely eye care. This misinformation frustrated the patients and their caregivers. For instance, a caregiver stated:

First we went to the Ophthalmology ... ... .and we saw doctor and he said this was probably a neurological issue for the visions so he sent us to the Neuro-Ophthalmologist doctor downtown ... [the] doctor was looking for horses before zebras, so he tested [him] for myasthenia gravis and thyroid malfunction cause he felt those could be an explanation for [his] vision problems, which also included some double vision, and of course, those test came back negative. [The] doctor wanted to see his CAT scan and everything from immediately after the stroke. Unbelievably, he just saw those on the last couple of weeks even though our report was back in July ... I just spoke from someone from their office today and [the doctor] said he can either come and have prism lenses and/or do some exercises for the eyes. It's taken from July 25th to literally today (December 4th) to find that out.

Accurate diagnosis for visual impairments must be conducted by utilizing reliable and valid outcome tools so that these individuals are referred to appropriate rehabilitation services. Healthcare providers must discuss these concerns in their multidisciplinary team meetings which can augment the diagnosis of vision-related impairments following stroke [34]. Our data suggest that stroke survivors who received inpatient rehabilitation (IRF) were more likely to be seen by occupational therapists. Prototypical quotations stating that occupational therapy was received were attributed to two caregivers and two stroke survivors. These stroke survivors received occupational therapy in an IRF.

The emerging themes from this study illuminate a number of implications for vision care providers. Stroke rehabilitation programs may not address stroke-related vision problems unless stroke survivors report difficulty and survivors thereby go untreated [35]. To date, no standardized vision screen to accurately assess all post-stroke visual impairment exists [36]. In a recent systematic review, the authors identify two vision screening tools purported to screen for vision problems post-stroke [36]. Due to varying levels of sensitivity when administered, we argue first that all stroke survivors should be screened using a standardized performance-based functional vision screen. At the Royal London Hospital, all stroke survivors are administered a functional vision screen by occupational therapists to assess convergence, smooth pursuits, saccades, visual field deficits, and visual inattention [5] before being referred to an orthoptist for a full evaluation, including acuity testing. When compared to orthoptist findings, outcomes of the occupational therapy functional vision screen of stroke survivors were 68% analogous [5]. Routine use of a standardized vision screening tool could lead to targeted referrals to other vision care specialists and for appropriate interventions [36].

Second, it is vital that persons post-stroke be evaluated for refractive error correction or prisms as needed. All stroke survivors and caregivers strongly suggest the need for more thorough assessment of eye movement problems (i.e., double vision, eyes do not focus, eyes jumping around, and eyelid does not close) as well as perceptual issues (i.e., trouble distinguishing colors, loss of depth perception, loss of peripheral vision, left neglect, and impaired visual processing). Studies have shown that a significant number of visual deficits from stroke are undetected [4, 18].

Third, it would be advantageous for stroke survivors and caregivers to understand the behaviors or signs and symptoms that may be indicative of a visual problem and/or visual concerns. Vision care providers at all levels of care should provide education on post-stroke visual concerns to stroke survivors and caregivers that may require treatment. If these visual concerns cannot be remediated, then stroke survivors and caregivers would benefit by education on coping strategies [11].

Fourth, a straightforward linkage of diagnosed visual impairment to targeted interventions is needed [37]. Vision care providers need to know how to use evidenced-based practice to assess and treat eye movement problems and perception issues at all levels on the continuum of care to prevent and/or lessen their consequences [38]. Barriers to use of evidence-based practice for visual inattention by occupational therapists have been shown to be their lack of basic knowledge in accessing and using the evidence [39]. It is the ethical responsibility of vision care providers to ensure timely referral to other providers as indicated such as ophthalmologists, neurologists, optometrists, orthoptists, physiatrists, occupational therapists, physical therapists, low vision therapists, orientation and mobility specialists, or social workers. Last, all providers need to advocate for stroke survivors and their caregivers to receive much needed services throughout the care continuum and not be limited to IRFs.

4.1. Limitations of the Study. There are a number of limitations in the study. The original interview guide in the larger study did not include any direct questions on vision problems. Rather, stroke survivors and caregivers were asked to describe their post-stroke experiences. Only 20 of them discussed noticeable vision changes following stroke. This could have resulted in selection bias occurring with those 20 reporting vision problems possibly being more sensitive to vision problems, and their concerns may not be representative of other stroke survivors and caregivers. Conversely, those who did not mention vision problems may have focused on other stroke sequelae, lacked awareness of vision-related changes, or did not ultimately have vision problems. Although participants were queried on post-stroke experiences, they may not have taken into consideration premorbid visual problems or other diagnoses, such as diabetes or thyroid dysfunction, adversely affecting vision. Although vision-related questions were not probed, a large number of participants discussed these consequences—justifying the importance of the analysis conducted for this study.

Further, we did not have participants' baseline visual function and there was no optometrist or ophthalmologist involved in this study or in the assessment of the stroke survivor's visual complains. However, the first author is a certified low-vision occupational therapist with extensive experience with stroke-related vision problems. Since the majority of our participants were recruited from the community, we did not have access to clinical indicators (e.g., stroke location, type, and severity), which may confound the results and conclusions of this study. Future research is needed to explore how such clinical factors influence the development of vision-related concerns following stroke. However, our sample was diverse, and the results may guide future research and programs to address the vision-related needs of persons following stroke.

5. Conclusion

Findings from this study indicate that visual concerns of stroke survivors and caregivers may not be addressed sufficiently, thereby adversely affecting survivors' independence in everyday activities and quality of life. All vision care providers need to be vigilant of these unmet visual concerns and complement their care accordingly, including referring to other appropriate eye care providers. A thorough post-stroke vision evaluation is imperative to assess visual acuity, eye motility, visual fields, and visual perception. Evidence-based assessments and targeted treatments to address visual concerns are needed across the continuum of care, not limited to IRFs. Future research should focus on barriers to adhering to best practice in detecting and treating post-stroke visual concerns.

Disclosure

The content is solely the responsibility of the authors and does not necessarily represent the official views of the AHRQ, NIA, or NIDILRR, and you should not assume endorsement by the Federal Government.

Acknowledgments

This work was supported by the Agency for Healthcare Research and Quality (AHRQ) (R24HS022134 and R01HS024711); National Institute on Disability, Independent Living, and Rehabilitation Research (NIDILRR) (90SFGE0002 and 90AR5009), a center within the Administration for Community Living, Department of Health and Human Services; UTMB Claude D. Pepper Older Americans Independence Center (5P30-AG024832) funded by the National Institute on Aging (NIA); and UTMB Institute for Translational Sciences supported by the National Institutes of Health (NIH) Clinical Translational Science Award (CTSA) (UL1TR001439, KL2TR000072). The content is solely the responsibility of the authors and does not necessarily represent the official views of the AHRQ, NIDILRR, NIA, or NIH, and you should not assume endorsement by the Federal Government.

References

[1] D. Mozaffarian, E. J. Benjamin, A. S. Go et al., "Heart disease and stroke statistics—2015 update: a report from the American Heart Association," *Circulation*, vol. 131, no. 4, pp. e29–e322, 2015.

[2] A. S. Go, D. Mozaffarian, V. L. Roger et al., "Executive summary: heart disease and stroke statistics—2014 update: a report from the American Heart Association," *Circulation*, vol. 129, no. 3, pp. 399–410, 2014.

[3] Stroke Association, *Visual Problems after Stroke*, Stroke Association, London, UK, 2012.

[4] F. Rowe, D. Brand, C. A. Jackson et al., "Visual impairment following stroke: do stroke patients require vision assessment?," *Age and Ageing*, vol. 38, no. 2, pp. 188–193, 2009.

[5] Z. Naeem, "The prevalence of visual problems in stroke patients and the effectiveness of the current screening tool used," *British and Irish Orthoptic Journal*, vol. 9, pp. 55–58, 2015.

[6] F. J. Rowe, "Stroke survivors' views and experiences on impact of visual impairment," *Brain and Behavior*, vol. 7, no. 9, article e00778, 2017.

[7] A. Pollock, B. St George, M. Fenton, and L. Firkins, "Top 10 research priorities relating to life after stroke – consensus from stroke survivors, caregivers, and health professionals," *International Journal of Stroke*, vol. 9, no. 3, pp. 313–320, 2014.

[8] F. Rowe and VIS group UK3, "The profile of strabismus in stroke survivors," *Eye*, vol. 24, no. 4, pp. 682–685, 2010.

[9] S. P. Stone, P. Patel, R. J. Greenwood, and P. W. Halligan, "Measuring visual neglect in acute stroke and predicting its recovery: the visual neglect recovery index," *Journal of Neurology, Neurosurgery & Psychiatry*, vol. 55, no. 6, pp. 431–436, 1992.

[10] Y. Shen, P. W. Gu, S. K. Ong, and A. Y. C. Nee, "A novel approach in rehabilitation of hand-eye coordination and finger dexterity," *Virtual Reality*, vol. 16, no. 2, pp. 161–171, 2012.

[11] K. M. Sand, A. Midelfart, L. Thomassen, A. Melms, H. Wilhelm, and J. M. Hoff, "Visual impairment in stroke patients – a review," *Acta Neurologica Scandinavica*, vol. 127, no. 196, pp. 52–56, 2013.

[12] J. H. Levenson and A. Kozarsky, "Visual acuity change," in *Clinical Methods: The History, Physical, and Laboratory Examinations*, H. K. Walker, W. D. Hall, and J. W. Hurst, Eds., pp. 553–555, Butterworths, Boston, MA, USA, 1990.

[13] S. Sue, "Test distance vision using a Snellen chart," *Community Eye Health*, vol. 20, no. 63, pp. 52–52, 2007.

[14] M. K. Birch, P. K. Wishart, and N. P. O'Donnell, "Determining progressive visual field loss in serial Humphrey visual fields," *Ophthalmology*, vol. 102, no. 8, pp. 1227–1235, 1995.

[15] C. Danchaivijitr and C. Kennard, "Diplopia and eye movement disorders," *Journal of Neurology, Neurosurgery & Psychiatry*, vol. 75, Supplement 4, pp. iv24–iv31, 2004.

[16] E. Pedroli, S. Serino, P. Cipresso, F. Pallavicini, and G. Riva, "Assessment and rehabilitation of neglect using virtual reality: a systematic review," *Frontiers in Behavioral Neuroscience*, vol. 9, p. 226, 2015.

[17] A. J. Lotery, M. I. Wiggam, A. J. Jackson et al., "Correctable visual impairment in stroke rehabilitation patients," *Age and Ageing*, vol. 29, no. 3, pp. 221-222, 2000.

[18] S. A. Jones and R. A. Shinton, "Improving outcome in stroke patients with visual problems," *Age and Ageing*, vol. 35, no. 6, pp. 560–565, 2006.

[19] A. Pollock, C. Hazelton, C. A. Henderson et al., "Interventions for disorders of eye movement in patients with stroke," *Cochrane Database of Systematic Reviews*, no. 10, article CD008389, 2011.

[20] P. T. Diamond, "Rehabilitative management of post-stroke visuospatial inattention," *Disability and Rehabilitation*, vol. 23, no. 10, pp. 407–412, 2001.

[21] K. M. Sand, G. Wilhelmsen, H. Naess, A. Midelfart, L. Thomassen, and J. M. Hoff, "Vision problems in ischaemic stroke patients: effects on life quality and disability," *European Journal of Neurology*, vol. 23, no. S1, pp. 1–7, 2016.

[22] S. Krishnan, M. R. Pappadis, S. C. Weller, S. R. Fisher, C. C. Hay, and T. A. Reistetter, "Patient-centered mobility outcome preferences according to individuals with stroke and caregivers: a qualitative analysis," *Disability and Rehabilitation*, vol. 40, no. 12, pp. 1401–1409, 2018.

[23] M. B. Miles, A. M. Huberman, and J. Saldaña, *Qualitative Data Analysis: a Methods Sourcebook*, SAGE Publications, Inc, 2013.

[24] S. J. Taylor, R. Bogdan, and M. DeVault, *Introduction to Qualitative Research Methods: A Guidebook and Resource*, John Wiley & Sons, 2015.

[25] H. R. Bernard and G. W. Ryan, *Analyzing Qualitative Data: Systematic Approaches*, SAGE Publications, Inc, 2009.

[26] W. C. Adams, "Conducting semi-structured interviews," in *Handbook of Practical Program Evaluation*, p. 365, Jossey-Bass, 2010.

[27] M. Brod, L. E. Tesler, and T. L. Christensen, "Qualitative research and content validity: developing best practices based on science and experience," *Quality of Life Research*, vol. 18, no. 9, pp. 1263–1278, 2009.

[28] L. Berends and J. Johnston, "Using multiple coders to enhance qualitative analysis: the case of interviews with consumers of drug treatment," *Addiction Research & Theory*, vol. 13, no. 4, pp. 373–381, 2005.

[29] QSR International Pty Ltd, *NVivo Qualitative Data Analysis Software (Version 10)*, QSR International Pty Ltd, Doncaster, VIC, Australia, 2012.

[30] D. K. Padgett, *Qualitative Methods in Social Work Research*, SAGE Publications, Inc, 2016.

[31] J. S. Gilhotra, P. Mitchell, P. R. Healey, R. G. Cumming, and J. Currie, "Homonymous visual field defects and stroke in an older population," *Stroke*, vol. 33, no. 10, pp. 2417–2420, 2002.

[32] G. B. Campbell and J. T. Matthews, "An integrative review of factors associated with falls during post-stroke rehabilitation," *Journal of Nursing Scholarship*, vol. 42, no. 4, pp. 395–404, 2010.

[33] H. Corriveau, R. Hébert, M. Raîche, and F. Prince, "Evaluation of postural stability in the elderly with stroke," *Archives of Physical Medicine and Rehabilitation*, vol. 85, no. 7, pp. 1095–1101, 2004.

[34] F. J. Rowe, "The importance of accurate visual assessment after stroke," *Expert Review of Ophthalmology*, vol. 6, no. 2, pp. 133–136, 2011.

[35] K. H. Siong, G. C. Woo, D. Y. L. Chan et al., "Prevalence of visual problems among stroke survivors in Hong Kong Chinese," *Clinical and Experimental Optometry*, vol. 97, no. 5, pp. 433–441, 2014.

[36] K. L. Hanna, L. R. Hepworth, and F. Rowe, "Screening methods for post-stroke visual impairment: a systematic review," *Disability and Rehabilitation*, vol. 39, no. 25, pp. 2531–2543, 2017.

[37] A. M. Barrett, L. J. Buxbaum, H. B. Coslett et al., "Cognitive rehabilitation interventions for neglect and related disorders: moving from bench to bedside in stroke patients," *Journal of Cognitive Neuroscience*, vol. 18, no. 7, pp. 1223–1236, 2006.

[38] S. Trauzettel-Klosinski, "Current methods of visual rehabilitation," *Deutsches Ärzteblatt International*, vol. 108, no. 51-52, pp. 871–878, 2011.

[39] A. Petzold, N. Korner-Bitensky, N. M. Salbach, S. Ahmed, A. Menon, and T. Ogourtsova, "Determining the barriers and facilitators to adopting best practices in the management of poststroke unilateral spatial neglect: results of a qualitative study," *Topics in Stroke Rehabilitation*, vol. 21, no. 3, pp. 228–236, 2014.

2

Scoping Review: The Trajectory of Recovery of Participation Outcomes following Stroke

Batya Engel-Yeger[1] **Tamara Tse**[2,3,4] **Naomi Josman,**[1] **Carolyn Baum**[5] **and Leeanne M. Carey**[2,3]

[1]*Department of Occupational Therapy, Faculty of Social Welfare and Health Sciences, University of Haifa, Haifa, Israel*
[2]*Occupational Therapy, Department of Community and Clinical Allied Health, School of Allied Health, La Trobe University, Melbourne, VIC, Australia*
[3]*Neurorehabilitation and Recovery, Stroke Division, The Florey Institute of Neuroscience and Mental Health, Heidelberg, VIC, Australia*
[4]*Occupational Therapy Department, St Vincent's Hospital Melbourne, Fitzroy, VIC, Australia*
[5]*Program in Occupational Therapy, Washington University School of Medicine, St Louis, MO, USA*

Correspondence should be addressed to Batya Engel-Yeger; bengel@univ.haifa.ac.il

Academic Editor: Norbert Kovács

Participation is a central concept in health and well-being and healthcare, yet operationalizing this concept has been difficult. Its definition, uses in healthcare, and impacts on recovery require ongoing research. Our review question goes like this: from the longitudinal evidence investigating participation among stroke survivors, what are the patterns of participation recovery in stroke survivors over time, and what interventions are used to improve participation? To fully understand these questions, we also ask, how is participation defined in the stroke literature, and what are the measures of participation used in the stroke literature? A systematic scoping review was undertaken using the search terms "stroke," "longitudinal," "participation," and "outcome" in seven databases. Articles included were published until April 2017, written in English, and had at least two longitudinal assessments of participation. Fifty-nine articles met the inclusion criteria. The International Classification of Functioning, Disability and Health was the most frequent definition of participation used (34%). There were 22 different measures of participation. Eight of ten studies demonstrated significant improvements in participation up to 12 months poststroke. Efficacy of interventions and their impact on participation varied. The various definitions, measures, and intervention efficacies of participation highlight the need for further research worldwide into achieving meaningful participation and quality of life among stroke survivors. Future practice should include participation as a main outcome measure.

1. Introduction

Stroke is the leading cause of adult disability worldwide [1]. Stroke remains a major global health concern, and its significance is likely to increase in the future due to ongoing demographic changes including the aging of the population and health transitions [2, 3].

Participation is considered a major outcome of successful rehabilitation [4–6] and an essential component of rehabilitation science [7]. Previous findings suggest that participation is a concern for stroke survivors [4], is considered an unmet need [8], is influenced by the environment [9], and may be affected by age, acceptance of stroke, body functions (including upper limb function, depression, and other comorbidities [10, 11]), cognition [12], skills like walking, and stroke severity [13].

Stroke is a chronic condition for survivors, with long-term implications such as loss of control over their bodies, valued activities, meaningful skills, and social roles [14, 15] which may disrupt their daily life, relationships, and expectations of the future [16]. These multiple losses may further influence one's ability to participate in everyday life activities across their lifespan, thus highlighting the importance of investigating participation outcomes among stroke survivors over an extended period of time [17]. While task-specific and learning-based approaches to rehabilitation have the strongest evidence base [18], evidence regarding participation after stroke and intervention programs for enhancing participation in the long term is lacking [19]. Moreover, rehabilitation studies do not often include participation outcomes [19], and studies that do refer to participation do not often use a conceptual framework nor a clear definition of participation. This lack of consensus surrounding the conceptualization of participation has led to difficulties operationalizing participation [20–23]. These difficulties may result from the diverse definitions and interpretations of participation as a concept and from the wide variety of tools purporting to measure participation [24], making participation evaluation variable, challenging, and difficult to interpret.

In summary, participation is a central concept in healthcare and in disciplines such as occupational therapy [25]. Yet its definition and inclusion in health outcomes and its impacts on recovery over time are relatively limited to date and require ongoing research [7]. The rising prevalence of stroke and its significant consequences, in particular, the fact that participation is a significant factor that affects people's functioning [26], emphasize that it is essential to better understand the recovery of participation as an outcome and how participation may be a targeted outcome in interventions for stroke survivors. This directed investigation may contribute to the conceptualization of participation and its application in health theory and practice [25].

1.1. Objective of the Scoping Review. To the best of our knowledge, a scoping review of the literature investigating the recovery of participation outcomes after stroke has not been conducted. The aim of this scoping review was to critically review the evidence investigating recovery of participation outcomes following stroke. The main questions guiding our review evaluation and evidence synthesis of the longitudinal studies investigating participation after stroke: (i) what are the patterns of recovery in participation outcomes in stroke survivors over time and (ii) what interventions are used to improve participation? To fully understand these questions, we also ask, how is participation defined, and what are the measures of participation used in the stroke literature?

2. Materials and Methods

This scoping review was based on the methods outlined by Arksey and O'Malley [27], which include six iterative steps: (1) identifying the research question; (2) searching for relevant studies; (3) selecting the studies; (4) charting the data; (5) collating, summarizing, and reporting the results; and (6) consulting with stakeholders to inform or validate findings. A scoping review methodology was selected because it can include broad questions and a range of research approaches surrounding a topic of interest. This methodology assists to identify the gaps in the current knowledge base to help guide future research in the field. Step 6, consultation with stakeholders is optional. We did not directly consult stroke stakeholders. However, ongoing consultation by the authors as the key stakeholders occurred throughout the review process.

The research question and the search terms were developed in consultation amongst the authors. The search terms were related to the study population, the intervention, the comparison or outcome, and the types of study design to include in the review. Seven databases were searched: EMBASE, PubMed, Web of Science, CINAHL, CINAHL Plus, Medline, and PsycINFO using the search terms "stroke," "longitudinal," "participation," and "outcome." Synonyms, wildcards, and Boolean operators were used in the search strategy (Table 1). Study designs included were longitudinal cohort, case control, pre-post test, and case series and case report studies with or without intervention. Included studies were written in English, published up to April 2017, and had at least two participation evaluation time points in the same sample, and with the same participation instrument, as defined by the authors of the study under review. Studies investigating paediatric stroke and severe comorbidities such as Alzheimer's, diabetes, and cancer were excluded.

2.1. Data Extraction. Three reviewers worked together to evaluate all articles for this review using Covidence online systematic review platform [28]. Each article was independently reviewed following a systematic process according to the inclusion and exclusion criteria. Any disagreements between reviewers were resolved by consensus.

3. Results

The flow of studies through the process is shown in Figure 1. The final number of studies included in this scoping review was 59. The summary of data extracted from each of the articles is provided in Table 2. Most of the studies included an assessment of participation in a community setting (85%); four of the 59 studies (7%) included assessments of participation only in an inpatient setting; and three studies did not state the setting location. Sixteen studies did not describe the assessor; of the remaining studies, the majority (81%) of assessors were physiotherapists and occupational therapists. When grouped into continents, the majority of the studies were based in North America (47%), followed by Europe (32%), Australasia (15%), Africa (3%), mixed countries (3%), and South America (2%). Interestingly, the earliest study in our scoping review was in 2001.

3.1. Patterns of Participation Recovery after Stroke. Of the 59 studies, all included two time points, 38 had a third measurement time of participation, 18 had a fourth, and 18 had a fifth measurement time. The terminology used to describe when participation was measured varied across the studies. Thirty-four of the studies (58%) called the first measure a baseline measure; the remaining studies described the measure in terms of a time point poststroke (37%) or postintervention/discharge (5%). The most frequent measurements of participation poststroke were 6 months, then 3 months, and then 12 months (see Table 3 for details).

Table 1: Search terms.

cerebrovascular accident.sh. OR stroke.ti. OR stroke.ab. OR cerebro vascular accident.ti. OR cerebro vascular accident.ab. OR cerebral vascular accident.ti. OR cerebral vascular accident.ab. OR brain ischaemic attack.ti. OR brain ischaemic attack.ab. OR brain ischemic attack.ti. OR brain ischemic attack.ab. OR brain vascular accident.ti. OR brain vascular accident.ab. OR CVA.ti. OR CVA.ab. OR ischaemic cerebral attack.ti. OR ischaemic cerebral attack.ab. OR ischemic cerebral attack.ti. OR ischemic cerebral attack.ab.	and	participation.sh. OR participation.ti. OR participation.ab. OR patient participation.sh. OR social participation.sh. OR patient involvement.ti. OR patient invovlement.ab. OR community participation.ti. OR community participation.ab. OR community integration.ab. OR community integration.ti. OR client participation.ab OR client participation.ti. OR social integration.ab. OR social integration.ti. OR community involvement.ab OR community invovlement.ti. OR activity participation.ab OR activity participation.ti	and	longitudinal study.sh. OR longitudinal stud*.ti. OR longitudinal stud*.ab. OR longitudinal eval*.ti. OR longitudinal eval*.ab. OR longitudinal survey.ti. OR longitudinal survey.ab. OR prospective stud*.ti. OR prospective stud*.ab. OR follow up.sh. OR follow* up.ti. OR follow* up.ab. OR follow up stud*.ti. OR follow up stud*.ab.	and	outcome assessment.sh. OR outcome measurement.sh. OR patient outcome assessment.sh. OR treatment outcome.sh. OR outcome*.ti. OR outcome*.ab. OR measure*.ti. OR measure*.ab. OR asses*.ti. OR asses*.ab. OR eval*.ti. OR eval*.ab.

Following an intervention (35 of the 59 studies), the most frequent time to measure participation was immediately after the intervention (32%). The interventions ranged in duration (e.g., 30 hours of therapy to 4 months of therapy). The next most frequent time point to measure participation following an intervention was 6 months, followed by 3 months postintervention. Four studies measured participation following a period after discharge from a hospital/rehabilitation unit or physiotherapy. One study did not specify whether the 12-month follow-up was 12 months after baseline, intervention, or poststroke.

Although all 59 studies reported at least two measurement times of participation after stroke, only 10 studies statistically tested for change during the natural recovery of participation over time. Of these 10 studies, 8 demonstrated a significant improvement in participation over time. These eight studies included the following time points: stroke to 3 months; stroke to 6 months; 2-3 months to 6 months; and 6 months to 12 months. The two studies that did not find a significant change included one study that tested participation at a mean time poststroke of 6 years poststroke and then measured participation again 3 months later following intervention. The other study did not show a significant improvement from 3 months to 6 months poststroke.

3.2. Intervention Efficacy and Impact on Participation. There were 17 randomized control trials included in this review, as detailed in Table 4. Of the 12 studies, 8 demonstrated a significant association with participation. Three of these studies used a form of supervised exercise program, compared to usual care, to improve participation, and measured using the Participation domain of the Stroke Impact Scale (SIS-P). One study demonstrated the use of a leisure therapy program on improved participation, measured in minutes engaged in leisure activities and the number of leisure activities compared to controls. One study showed that the use of therapist-supervised repetitive task practice (RTP) had a greater effect on participation than RTP combined with robotic-assisted therapy at 2 months follow-up. Three studies found that participation improved over time regardless of the intervention (cognitive behavioral therapy versus computerized cognitive training, aerobic exercise versus no therapy, and patient education program versus placebo group).

The four studies that did not demonstrate a significant relationship with participation included three interventions focusing on the use of specific physical therapy interventions (foot drop stimulator versus standard ankle foot orthosis, body weight–supported exercise compared to overground walking training, and community-based fitness and mobility exercise protocol versus usual care) and one intervention focusing on a client-centred activities of daily living (ADL) program versus usual care.

3.3. Measuring Participation. There were 22 different measures of participation used in the included studies. The SIS-P was the tool used by 24 of 59 studies (46%) included in this review, as detailed in Table 5. Of the 24 studies that used the SIS-P, 9 used the ICF definition of participation, 13 used an operational definition, four used "meaningful activities/

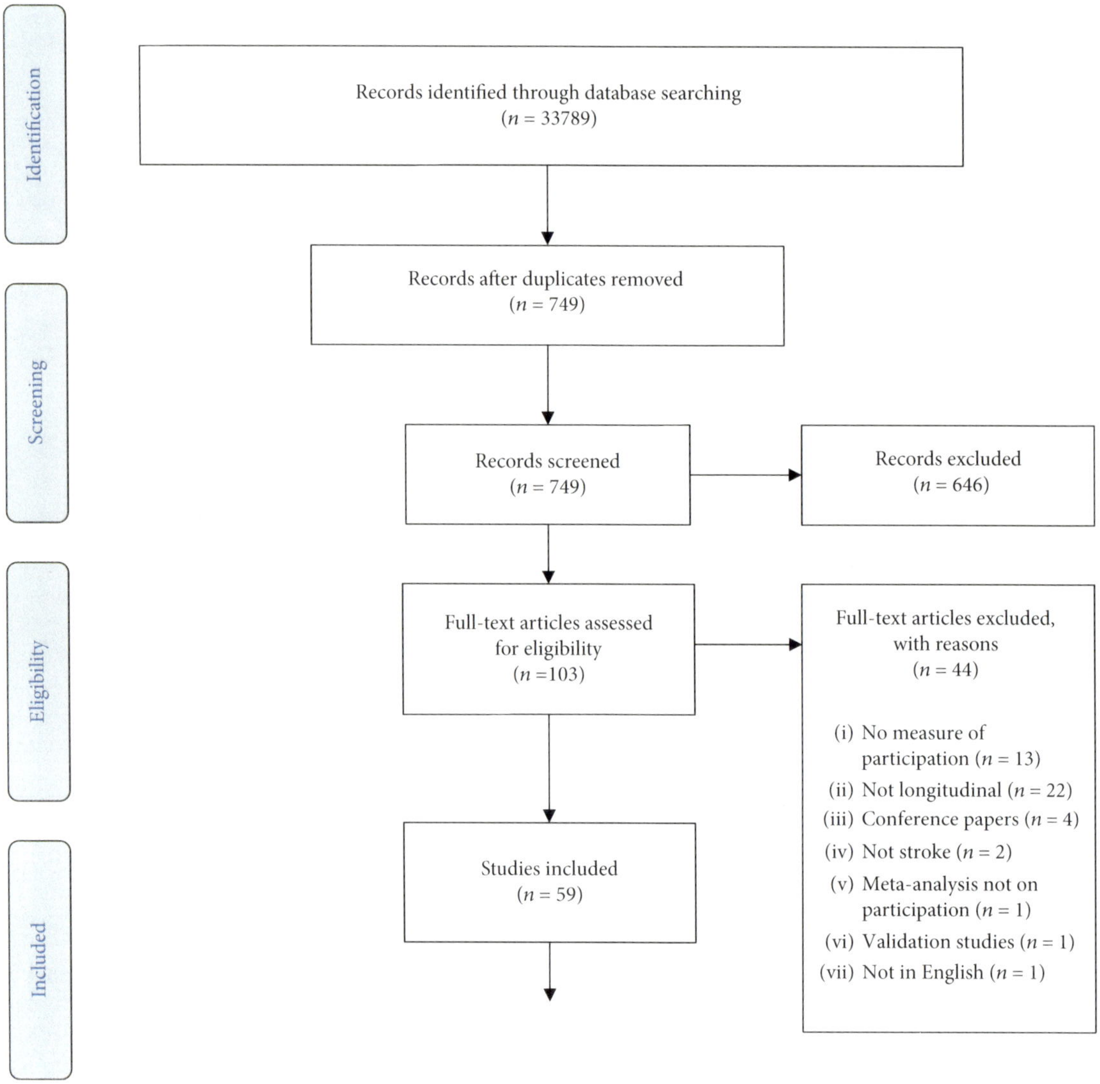

FIGURE 1: PRISMA 2009 flow diagram.

occupations," two used "community participation," and one used the term "social participation." The next most frequent measure of participation was the LIFE-H. All studies using the LIFE-H ($n = 5$) used the Disability Creation Process conceptual framework definition. Four studies used the London Handicap Scale; of these, three used the International Classification of Functioning, Disability and Health (ICF) definition of participation, and the other used an operational definition. Three studies used the Utrecht Scale for Evaluation of Rehabilitation-Participation; of these, all used an operational definition of participation. Three studies used the Short Form Health Survey (SF-36); of these, two used the operational definition, and the other used the term "role participation."

3.4. Definitions of Participation. Of the 59 studies included in this review, many did not provide a definition of participation (41%), instead only describing the tool used in the study as measuring participation (e.g., "participation was measured using the Stroke Impact Scale"). This was categorized as an operational definition. Of the remaining studies, the most frequent definition of participation was the ICF definition (34%), "i.e. involvement in a life situation." The remaining definitions used by two or fewer studies are reported in Table 6.

When we compared the definition of participation used in the study as a proportion of the studies from each of the continents, we found that operational definitions and the ICF definition were widely used across all continents (see Table 7).

4. Discussion

This scoping review aimed to critically review the evidence regarding patterns of recovery of participation outcomes among stroke survivors and to summarize the patterns of recovery and intervention efficacy on participation outcomes over time. The earliest publication included in this scoping review was in 2001, when the World Health Organization (WHO) endorsed the ICF, of which participation is a core

TABLE 2: Extracted data from studies included in the scoping review on longitudinal participation outcomes after stroke.

Author	Year	Country	Setting	Study design	Measure	Sample size	1st measure	2nd measure	3rd measure	4th measure	Assessors	Age (*yr*) mean (SD), median (IQR)	Define participation
Altman et al. [46]	2013	USA	Community	Retrospective cohort of completers and noncompleters	MPAI-4	Completers $n = 738$, noncompleters $n = 150$	Baseline	Discharge	Postdischarge (3 months)	Postdischarge (12 months)	Not described	Completers 51.10 (11.46), noncompleters 52.96 (52.96)	Operational
Awad et al. [47]	2014	USA	Research laboratory	Case series pretest-posttest	SIS-P	$n = 13$	Baseline	Postbaseline (12 weeks)			PT	61 (8.31)	Self-perceived participation
Beaudoin et al. [48]	2013	Canada	Community	Prospective cohort study	LIFE-H	$n = 57$	Baseline	Postbaseline (6 months)	Postbaseline (9 months)		Not described	76.9 (8.1)	DCP
Bertilsson et al. [49]	2016	Sweden	Inpatient and community	Multicentre cluster RCT	SIS-P OGQ	Client-centred $n = 88$, usual $n = 95$	Baseline	Postbaseline (3 months)	12 months		OT	Client-centred 74.1 (9.5), usual 71.3 (10.1)	ICF, meaningful activities/ occupation
Brown et al. [50]	2014	Canada	Community	Prospective cohort study, with intervention and interrupted time series	PASIPD	$n = 61$	Baseline	Postbaseline (2 months)	Postbaseline (4 months)		PT	Intervention 65 (13), control 66 (13)	Operational
Butler et al. [51]	2006	USA	Community	Case study: pre-post test	SIS-P	$n = 1$	Baseline	Postbaseline (4 weeks)	Postintervention (8 weeks)	Postintervention (3 months)	OT	44	ICF
Chou et al. [52]	2015	Taiwan	Inpatient and community	Prospective cohort study	SIS-P	Baseline $n = 263$	Baseline	Postbaseline (2 weeks)			OT	59.8 (13.0)	Operational
Combs-Miller et al. [53]	2014	USA	Research laboratory and community	RCT	IMPACT-P	$n = 20$	Baseline	Postintervention	Postbaseline (3 months)		PT	Body weight-supported 56.20 (7.61), overground walking 65.50 (6.17)	ICF
Demetrios et al. [54]	2014	Australia	Community	Nonrandomized controlled study	GAS	High-intensity program $n = 28$, usual care $n = 31$	Baseline	Postintervention (6 weeks)	Postintervention (12 weeks)	Postintervention (24 weeks)	Not described	High-intensity 60.6 (48.6–65.9), usual care 61.4 (47.8–68.6)	ICF
Desrosiers et al. [55]	2006	Canada	Community	Prospective cohort study	LIFE-H	T1 $n = 102$, T2 $n = 66$	Poststroke (6 months)	Poststroke (2–4 years)			OT	T1 68.1 (14.1), T2 67.6 (13.7)	DCP
Desrosiers et al. [56]	2007	Canada	Community	RCT	Minutes	Experimental $n = 29$, control $n = 27$	Baseline	Postintervention			OT	Experimental 70.0 (10.2), control 70.0 (12.0)	DCP
Desrosiers et al. [57]	2006	Canada	Community	Prospective cohort study	LIFE-H	T1 $n = 102$, T2 $n = 66$	Postdischarge (6 months)	Poststroke (2–4 years)			OT	T1 68.1 (14.1), T2 67.6 (13.7)	DCP
Egan et al. [58]	2014	Canada	Community	Prospective cohort study	RNL	$n = 67$	Poststroke (6 months)	Poststroke (9 months)	Poststroke (12 months)	Poststroke (18 months)	Not described	64.8 (13.3)	ICF
Egan et al. [59]	2015	Canada	Community	Prospective cohort study	RNL	$n = 67$	Poststroke (6 months)	Poststroke (9 months)	Poststroke (12 months)	Poststroke (18 months)	Not described	64.8 (13.3)	ICF
Evan et al. [60]	2012	USA	Community	Case study pre-post test	GPS	$n = 1$	Baseline	Postbaseline (4 weeks)	Postbaseline (8 weeks)	Postdischarge (6 and 12 months)	PT	56	ICF
Flansbjer et al. [61]	2012	Sweden	Community	Prospective cohort study follow-up from RCT	SIS-P	$n = 18$	Baseline	Postintervention	Postintervention (5 months)	Postintervention (4 years)	PT	4 years 66 (4)	ICF
Flansbjer et al. [62]	2008	Sweden	Community	RCT	SIS-P	$n = 24$	Baseline	Postintervention	Postintervention (5 months)		PT	Intervention 61 (5), control 60 (5)	ICF

Table 2: Continued.

Author	Year	Country	Setting	Study design	Measure	Sample size	1st measure	2nd measure	3rd measure	4th measure	Assessors	Age (*yr*) mean (SD), median (IQR)	Define participation
Guidetti et al. [63]	2015	Stockholm, Uppsala, and Gävleborg County, Sweden	Community	RCT	SIS-P	$n = 280$	Poststroke (3 months)	Poststroke (6 months)	Poststroke (12 months)		OT	CADL 74 (10), UADL 71 (11)	Operational
Guidetti et al. [64]*	2014	Stockholm, Sweden	Community	Comparative study no controls	SIS-P	$n = 349$	Poststroke (3 months)	Poststroke (12 months)			OT, PT	74 (14)	Operational
Hamzat and Peters [65]*	2009	Nigeria	Community	Longitudinal descriptive study	LHS	$n = 20$	Poststroke (1 month)	Poststroke (2 months)	Poststroke (3 months)	Poststroke (4 months)	PT	Not reported	ICF
Horgan et al. [66]*	2009	Ireland	Community	Comparative study no controls	FAI	$n = 23$	Poststroke (2 weeks)	Poststroke (6 months)	Poststroke (12 months)		PT	69.7 (11.3)	Operational
Ilse et al. [67]	2008	Belgium	Community	Comparative study no controls	NEADL, mRS	$n = 90$	Poststroke (2 months)	Poststroke (4 months)	Poststroke (6 months)		PT	67.3 (11.2)	Operational
Baert et al. [68]	2012	Belgium	Inpatient	Case series pretest, posttest	SIS-P, NEADL	$n = 50$	Baseline	Poststroke (2 months)	Poststroke (6 months)	Poststroke (12 months)	PT	57.2 (11.4)	ICF
Jalayondeja et al. [69]	2011	Thailand	Community	Prospective cohort study	SIS-P	$n = 98$	Poststroke (1 month)	Poststroke (3 months)	Poststroke (6 months)		Researcher/ research assistant	61.9 (11.02)	Operational
Jalayondeja et al. [70]*	2014	Thailand	Community	Prospective cohort study	SIS-P	$n = 98$	Poststroke (1 month)	Poststroke (3 months)	Poststroke (6 months)		Researcher/ research assistant	Fallers 65.4 (10.2), nonfallers 60.7 (11.2)	Community participation
Kluding et al. [71]	2013	USA	Community	RCT	SIS-P	$n = 197$	Baseline	Postintervention (6 weeks)	Postintervention (12 weeks)	Postintervention (30 weeks)	PT	Interventions 60.7 (12.2), control 61.6 (11.0)	Operational
Kootker et al. [72]	2017	Netherlands	Community	RCT	USER-P	$n = 61$	Baseline	Postintervention	Postintervention (4 months)	Postintervention (8 months)	Health psychologist	CBT 61 (45–79), CCT 61 (25–76)	Operational
Kutner et al. [73]	2010	USA	Inpatient and community	RCT	SIS-P	RTP $n = 7$, combined therapy group $n = 10$	Baseline	Postintervention	Postintervention (2 months)		OT, PT	RTP 51.0 (11.3), combined therapy group 61.9 (13.4)	Operational
Kwok et al. [74]*	2011	Hong Kong	Inpatient	Observational cohort study	LHS	Baseline $n = 594$, 3 months $n = 500$, 12 months $n = 433$	Poststroke (3 months)	Poststroke (12 months)			Not described	72 (65–77)	ICF
Laufer et al. [75]	2009	Israel	Research laboratory and community	Time series no control	SIS-P	$n = 24$	Baseline	Postintervention (8 weeks)	Postintervention (12 months)		PT	Study group 55.0 (14.6)	Meaningful activities/ occupation
Lennon et al. [76]	2006	Ireland	Inpatient and community	Pre-post test	LHS	$n = 9$	Poststroke (6 weeks)	Discharge from physiotherapy				64.3 (9.6)	Operational
Levin et al. [77]	2012	Canada + Israel	Research laboratory and community	Case series pre-post test	MAL	VR $n = 8$, conventional $n = 6$	Baseline	Postbaseline (1 week)	Postintervention	Postintervention (1 month)	OT	VR 58.1 (14.6), conventional 59.8 (15.1)	ICF
Lund et al. [78]	2012	Norway	Community	RCT	SF-36	Intervention $n = 39$, control $n = 47$	Poststroke (3 months)	Poststroke (9 months)			Researcher/ research assistant	Intervention 75 (7.2), control 79 (6.5)	Operational
Mayer and Reid [79]*	2004	Canada	Community	Prospective longitudinal cohort study	IPA	$n = 18$	Poststroke (3 months)	Poststroke (6 months)			OT	67.4 (13.4)	ICF

TABLE 2: Continued.

Author	Year	Country	Setting	Study design	Measure	Sample size	1st measure	2nd measure	3rd measure	4th measure	Assessors	Age (yr) mean (SD), median (IQR)	Define participation
Mayo et al. [80]	2009	Canada and England	Inpatient and community	Longitudinal cohort study	SIS-P	$n = 408$	Poststroke (1 month)	Poststroke (3 months)	Poststroke (6 months)	Poststroke (12 months)	Not described	66.5 (14.6)	Operational
Mayo et al. [81]	2011	Canada	Community	Reanalysis of RCT	SF-36	Nurse case-manager group $n = 96$, usual care group $n = 94$	Postintervention	Postintervention (6 months)			Not described	Nurse case-manager 70 (14), usual care 72 (13)	Role participation
Mayo et al. [82]	2013	Canada	Community	RCT	SIS-P, RAND-36	Cycle group $n = 43$, exercise group $n = 44$	Baseline	Postbaseline (12 months)			PT	Cycle 67.7 (14.4) ,exercise 67.8 (12.3)	ICF, role participation
Mercer et al. [83]	2009	USA	Inpatient and research laboratory	Prospective cohort study	SIS-P	$n = 33$	Poststroke (1 month)	Poststroke (3 months)	Poststroke (6 months)		Not described	58.7 (17.3)	ICF
Nijenhuis et al. [84]	2015	Netherlands	Community	Comparison within subjects, longitudinal	SIS-P	$n = 24$	Baseline	Postintervention (6 weeks)			Biomechanical engineering	59 (13)	Operational
Page et al. [85]	2015	USA	Research laboratory and community	Comparison within subjects longitudinal no control	SIS-P	$n = 5$	Baseline	Postintervention			OT	43.7 (6.43)	Meaningful activities/ occupation
Pang et al. [86]	2005	Canada	Community	RCT	PASIPD	$n = 63$	Baseline	Postintervention			OT, PT	Intervention group 65.8 (9.1), control 64.7 (8.4)	Operational
Parker et al. [87]	2001	UK	Community	RCT	NLQ	$n = 466$	Postintervention (6 months)	Postintervention (12 months)			OT	Leisure 72 (65–79), ADL 71 (66–78), control 72 (65–78)	Operational
Penney et al. [88]	2007	Canada	Not stated	Single case study	IPA, 6-minute walk test	$n = 1$	Poststroke (3 months)	Poststroke (12 months)			PT	62	ICF
Pundik et al. [89]	2012	USA	Not stated	Pre-post test with interrupted time series no control	SIS-P	$n = 44$	Baseline	Postintervention	Postintervention (3 months)		Not described	60 (16.8)	ICF
Raghavan et al. [90]	2016	USA	Community	Mixed-method pre-post design with 1 year follow-up	SIS-P	$n = 13$	Baseline	Postintervention	Postintervention (12 months)		OT	52 (14)	Operational
Rochette et al. [91]	2013	Canada	Inpatient and community	RCT	LIFE-H	$n = 186$	Baseline	Postbaseline (6 months)	Postintervention (12 months)		OT, PT	YOU CALL 63.2 (12.4), WE CALL 61.7 (12.7)	DCP
Sabariego et al. [92]	2013	Germany	Inpatient and community	RCT	SIS-P	$n = 260$	Baseline	Postintervention (1 week)	Postintervention (6 months)		Not described	Experimental 55.3 (12.6), control 59.3 (12.7)	ICF
Sandberg et al. [93]	2016	Sweden	Community	RCT	SIS-P	$n = 56$	Baseline	Postintervention (3 months)			Not described	Intervention 71.3 (7.0), control 70.4 (8.1)	Social participation
Segura et al. [94]	2006	Brazil	Research laboratory and community	Prospective, comparative, no control	SIS-P	$n = 18$	Baseline	Postintervention (3 months)			PT	52.9	Operational
Singam et al. [95]	2015	Sweden	Inpatient	Prospective, longitudinal study	FAI	$n = 349$	Poststroke (5 days)	Poststroke (3 months)	Poststroke (6 months)	Poststroke (12 months)	OT, PT	69.4 (13.8)	ICF
Stuart et al. [96]	2009	Italy	Not stated	Nonrandomized control trial	SIS-P	Intervention $n = 40$, control $n = 38$	Baseline	Postintervention (6 months)			Not described	Intervention 66.8 (1.4), control 70.0 (1.7)	Operational

Table 2: Continued.

Author	Year	Country	Setting	Study design	Measure	Sample size	1st measure	2nd measure	3rd measure	4th measure	Assessors	Age (yr) mean (SD), median (IQR)	Define participation
Studenski et al. [97]	2005	USA	Community	RCT	SIS-P	Intervention $n = 44$, usual care $n = 49$	Baseline	Postintervention	Postintervention (6 months)		Blinded assessor	Intervention 68.5 (9.0), usual care 70.4 (11.3)	Operational
Teoh et al. [98]*	2009	Australia	Community	Longitudinal cohort study	SIS-P	$n = 135$	Baseline	Postbaseline (10 weeks)	Postbaseline (6 months)		Not described	67.5 (14.3)	Social participation
Tielemans et al. [99]	2015	Netherlands	Community	RCT	USER-P	$n = 113$	Baseline	Postintervention	Postintervention (3 months)	Postintervention (9 months)	Researcher/ research assistant	Self-management 55.2 (8.9), education 58.8 (8.7)	Operational
van Mierlo et al. [100]*	2016	Netherlands	Community	Longitudinal cohort study	USER-P	$n = 368$	Poststroke (2 months)	Poststroke (6 months)	Poststroke (12 months)	Poststroke (24 months)	Researcher/ research assistant	66.8 (12.3)	Operational
Vincent-Onabajo et al. [101]	2014	Nigeria	Research laboratory and community	Case series	LHS	$n = 83$	Poststroke (1 month)	Poststroke (3 months)	Poststroke (6 months)	Poststroke (9 months and 12 months)	Not described	Male 60.7 (12.4), female 58.1 (12.6)	ICF
Viscogliosi et al. [102]*	2011	Canada	Inpatient and community	Comparative study no controls	LIFE-H	$n = 197$	Poststroke (3 months)	Poststroke (6 months)	Poststroke (9 months)		OT	76.9 (7.0)	DCP
Worrall et al. [103]	2017	Australia	Inpatient and community	Prospective longitudinal cohort study	ALA	$n = 58$	Poststroke (3 months)	Poststroke (6 months)	Poststroke (9 months)	Poststroke (12 months)	Not described	66.1 (13.6)	ICF
Yang and Kong [104]*	2013	Singapore	Inpatient	Prospective observational cohort study	SF-36	$n = 122$	Baseline	Predischarge			OT, PT	58.2 (10.5)	Operational

Note: ADL: activity of daily living; ALA: assessment for living with aphasia; DCP: disability creation process; FAI: Frenchay activity index; GAS: goal attainment scale; GPS: global positioning system; ICF: International Classification of Functioning, Disability and Health; IMPACT-P: participation subsection of the ICF measure of participation and activities; IPA: impact on participation and autonomy; LHS: London handicap scale; LIFE-H: assessment of life habits; MAL: motor activity log; MPAI-4: Mayo-Portland adaptability inventory; mRS: modified ranking scale; NEADL: Nottingham extended activities of daily living; NLQ: Nottingham leisure questionnaire; OGQ: occupational gaps questionnaire; PASIPD: physical activity scale for individuals with physical disabilities; RAND-36: physical function index of the medical outcomes study RND-36 item health survey; RCT: randomized control trial; RNL: reintegration of normal living; RTP: repetitive task practice; SF-36: short form 36; SIS-P: stroke impact scale participation domain; USER-P: Utrecht scale for evaluation of rehabilitation-participation; VR: virtual reality. *Cohort studies that statistically tested for changes in participation.

TABLE 3: Time point of participation measurement by authors measuring participation longitudinally after stroke.

Poststroke	Poststroke	Postintervention	Postbaseline	Postdischarge
At baseline			34	
Pre/at discharge				3
Immediately		14		
5 days	1			
1 week		1	1	
2 weeks	1		1	
1 month	6	1	2	
6 weeks	1	3		
2 months	4	3	2	
10 weeks			1	
3 months	15	6	4	1
4 months	2	1	1	
5 months		2		
6 months	18	7	3	2
30 weeks		1		
8 months		1		
9 months	6		1	
12 months	13	4	1	2
18 months	2			
24 months	1			
2–4 years	2			

component, suggesting that the use of the term "participation" is related to the release of the ICF by the WHO. The impact of the ICF on participation may also be reflected by the origin of the included publications. Our scoping review revealed that the majority of the studies were conducted in North America—the origin of conceptual frameworks including participation such as the Person-Environment-Occupation-Performance (PEOP) and ICF [29]. Interestingly, this scoping review also included studies performed in many other counties and continents (e.g., Europe, Australasia, Africa, and South America), supporting the perception that participation is a major outcome measure of intervention and recovery and is accepted worldwide.

4.1. Patterns of Participation Recovery Outcomes over Time. The findings from this scoping review revealed that participation is most often measured 6 months poststroke, followed by 3 months poststroke, and 12 months poststroke. These findings may lead us to suggest that participation recovery occurs at these time points. However, this may not be the true trajectory of recovery of participation. Rather, we are limited by the measurement tools and time points under which they occurred. Nonetheless, previous studies have suggested that, among stroke survivors, progressive and significant functional recovery in participation outcomes may occur during the first 6 months [30]. The findings from our scoping review extends this knowledge, highlighting that improvements in participation does occur over time and up to 12 months poststroke. However, the percentage of the studies that performed these longer follow-ups to 12 months is low. There were even fewer studies conducting follow-up beyond 12 months. This may be due to the difficulties of a cohort study, such as the financial cost of conducting long-term studies, participant drop-outs, difficulties following up participants in rural and remote settings, and educational background of the population (the ability to read and write) [30].

4.2. Intervention Efficacy on Participation and Recovery. Findings of intervention efficacy and impact on participation were not consistent in the studies included in this scoping review—only some studies found improvement in participation resulting from posttreatment recovery. Some reported improvement in participation due to spontaneous recovery. Other studies did not find a relationship between intervention and participation.

The studies that found improvement in participation used varying intervention strategies, such as supervised exercise programs, leisure therapy programs, and repetitive task practice. The studies that did not find a relationship between intervention and participation applied specific techniques such as cognitive behavior therapy or focused on improving specific body functions, mainly motor functions (using, for example, foot drop stimulator, body weight support, or walking training). These results raise questions regarding the literature claiming that intervention should aim to improve one daily activity, such as walking, to enhance participation. As previous research has stressed [30], improvements in participation levels of patients with stroke require particular attention to situations demanding community, social, and civic involvement. Further, in this scoping review, several of

TABLE 4: Summary of randomized control trial data in this review on longitudinal participation outcomes after stroke.

Author	Year	Country	Setting	Intervention	Age (*yr*) mean (SD), median (IQR)	Sex (% male)	Time poststroke (*months*) mean (SD) or median [range]	Association on participation
Bertilsson et al. [49]	2016	Sweden	Inpatient and community	Client-centred ADL intervention specifically guided by client needs and expressed desires, focused on enabling the person with stroke to become an active agent in daily activities and participation in everyday life, and the caregivers were invited to participate in rehabilitation as much as they wanted.	Client-centred 74.1 (9.5), usual 71.3 (10.1)	Client-centred 53%, usual care 62%	Not described	There was no significant difference between those receiving client-centred ADL intervention and usual care in terms of participation at 12 months.
Combs-Miller et al. [53]	2014	USA	Research laboratory and community	Comparison of two types of walking training: body weight-supported and overground.	Body weight-supported 56.20 (7.61), overground walking 65.50 (6.17)	Body weight-supported 40%, overground walking 70%	Body weight-supported 62.3 (48.6), overground walking 60.0 (51.7)	No evidence found to support this type of intervention (body weight-supported or overground walking training) on improving participation.
Desrosiers et al. [56]	2007	Canada	Community	Leisure education program at home once a week for 8–12 weeks. Control participants ($n = 29$) were visited at home at a similar frequency.	Intervention 61 (5), control 60 (5)	Intervention 16 (57.1), control 12 (42.9)	Months: experimental 24.5 (25.7), control 32.7 (37.8)	Some evidence to support the use of this leisure education program for improving the number of minutes of leisure and number of leisure activities participated in compared to control group.
Flansbjer et al. [62]	2008	Sweden	Community	Progressive resistance training on muscle strength, muscle tone, gait performance, and perceived participation after stroke.	Intervention 61 (5), control 60 (5)	Intervention 60%, control 56%	Baseline: intervention 18.9 (7.9), control 20 (11.6)	Some evidence to support this type of intervention (supervised progressive resistance training of the knee extensors and flexors) compared to usual care on improving participation after the intervention and maintained at 5 months.
Guidetti et al. [64]	2015	Sweden	Community	The CADL intervention was conducted within a client-centred context. The UADL interventions varied in extent and methods according to the knowledge	CADL 74 (10), UADL 71 (11)	CADL 57%, UADL 63%	CADL 25 [6–96], UADL 28 [3–115]	There were no differences between the groups regarding changes in perceived participation, independence in ADL, or life satisfaction during the

Table 4: Continued.

Author	Year	Country	Setting	Intervention	Age (*yr*) mean (SD), median (IQR)	Sex (% male)	Time poststroke (*months*) mean (SD) or median [range]	Association on participation
				and clinical experience of the individual OT and according to the routines and praxis of the participating rehabilitation units.				first 12 months. There was a trend towards a clinically meaningful positive change in perceived participation that favoured client-centred ADL intervention. Good design.
Kluding et al. [71]	2013	USA	Community	Standard treatment versus electric stimulation therapy to improve foot drop.	Interventions 60.7 (12.2), control 61.6 (11.0)	Intervention 56.8%, control 43.2%	Intervention 4.8 (5.3) *yrs*, control 4.3 (4.1) *yrs*	No difference in participation between the intervention of 30 weeks of either foot drop stimulator or a standard ankle foot orthosis.
Kootker et al. [72]	2017	Netherlands	Community	Individually tailored CBT for reducing depressive symptoms.	CBT 61 (45–79), CCT 61 (25–76)	CBT 61.3%, CCT 63.3%	CBT 26 [2–243], CCT 21.5 [2–138]	Some evidence to support the use of both CBT and CCT to improve participation at this level of intervention.
Kutner et al. [73]	2010	USA	Inpatient and community	This preliminary study explored change in patient-reported, health-related quality of life associated with robotic-assisted therapy combined with reduced therapist-supervised training. Sixty hours of therapist-supervised repetitive task practice (RTP) was compared with 30 hours of RTP combined with 30 hours of robotic-assisted therapy.	RTP 51.0 (11.3), combined therapy group 61.9 (13.4)	Total 59%, RTP 71%, combined therapy group 50%	Total *days* 234.4 (121.8), RTP *days* 184.1 (126.5), combined therapy group *days* 269.6 (111.1)	Significant differences in participation pre- and postintervention for RTP group at 2 months follow-up but not for combined therapy group.
Lund et al. [78]	2011	Norway	Community	A lifestyle course in combination with physical activity (intervention group) compared with physical activity alone (control group). Both programmes were held once a week for nine months.	Intervention 75 (7.2), control 79 (6.5)	Intervention, control 43%	Intervention 161 (178) *days*, control 137 (124) *days*	No statistically significant differences between the groups at the nine-month follow-up.

Table 4: Continued.

Author	Year	Country	Setting	Intervention	Age (*yr*) mean (SD), median (IQR)	Sex (% male)	Time poststroke (*months*) mean (SD) or median [range]	Association on participation
Mayo et al. [82]	2013	Canada	Community	Two dose-equivalent interventions, one involving stationary cycling and the other disability-targeted intervention, were tested. Both protocols required daily moderate intensity exercise at home building up to 30 minutes per day. One group exercised on a stationary bicycle; the second group carried out mobility exercises and brisk walking. An observer-blinded, randomized, pragmatic, trial with repeated measures. At baseline and after 1, 6, and 12 months of exercise and home-based assessments at 3 and 9 months.	Cycle 67.7 (14.4), exercise 67.8 (12.3)	Cycle 80%, exercise 59%	Cycle *days* 265.4 (131.8), exercise *days* 252.0 (165.3)	A significant effect for role participation was found in the exercise group for cycling versus exercise.
Pang et al. [86]	2005	Canada	Community	19 weeks (1-hour sessions, 3 sessions per week). Intervention included the Fitness and Mobility Exercise (FAME) program 10 minutes initially, with increment of 5 minutes every week, up to 30 minutes of continuous exercise as tolerated.	Intervention group 65.8 (9.1), control 64.7 (8.4)	79%	Intervention *yrs* 5.2 (5.0), control *yrs* 5.1 (3.6)	There was no significant time × group interaction on participation.
Parker et al. [87]	2001	United Kingdom	Community	Occupational therapy interventions at home for up to six months after recruitment, minimum of 10 sessions lasting not less than 30 minutes each. The treatment goals set in the ADL group were in terms of improving independence in self-care tasks, and	Leisure 72 (65–79), ADL 71 (66–78), control 72 (65–78)	Leisure 58%, ADL 62%, control 54%	Not described	At six months and compared to the control group, those allocated to leisure therapy had nonsignificantly better leisure participation scores. Those allocated to the ADL group had nonsignificantly worse leisure scores compared to controls. The

Table 4: Continued.

Author	Year	Country	Setting	Intervention	Age (*yr*) mean (SD), median (IQR)	Sex (% male)	Time poststroke (*months*) mean (SD) or median [range]	Association on participation
				therefore, treatment involved practicing these tasks (such as preparing a meal or walking outdoors). For the leisure group, goals were set in terms of leisure activity, and so, interventions included practicing the leisure tasks as well as any ADL tasks necessary to achieve the leisure objective.				results were similar at 12 months.
Rochette et al. [91]	2013	Canada	Community	YOU CALL participants were provided with the name and phone number of a trained healthcare professional whom they were free to contact should they feel the need. WE CALL participants received a multimodal support intervention including new or ongoing issues, family functioning, and individualized risk factors. Call frequency was weekly for the first 2 months, biweekly during the third month, and monthly for the past 3 months and included support material and referrals as needed.	YOU CALL 63.2 (12.4), WE CALL 61.7 (12.7)	YOU CALL 53.2%, WE CALL 62%	Not described	No significant differences were seen between groups at 6 months. Significant improvements in social participation for both groups from 6 to 1 year. No significance between group differences.
Sabariego et al. [92]	2013	Germany	Inpatient and community	ICF-based patient-education programme. The programme was performed by a psychologist in 1-hr sessions over 5 days. The group size was four participants, and it was a closed group.	Intervention 55.3 (12.6), control 59.3 (12.7)	Intervention 63%, control 45%	Intervention *days* 151.1 (399.3), control *days* 149.5 (634.7)	Participation improved for both groups, but no between-group difference was found. Large study, good design. Exploratory post hoc model identified life satisfaction, self-efficacy, memory, and mood as significant factors for change with SIS-P as dependent variable.

Table 4: Continued.

Author	Year	Country	Setting	Intervention	Age (*yr*) mean (SD), median (IQR)	Sex (% male)	Time poststroke (*months*) mean (SD) or median [range]	Association on participation
Sandberg et al. [93]	2016	Sweden	Community	Sixty minutes of group aerobic exercise, including 2 sets of 8 minutes of exercise with intensity up to exertion level 14 or 15 of 20 on the Borg rating of perceived exertion scale, twice weekly for 12 weeks.	Intervention 71.3 (7.0), control 70.4 (8.1)	50%	Intervention *days* 4.9 (5.8), control *days* 6.3 (7.3)	Significant change in SIS-P from preintervention to postintervention (aerobic exercise versus no therapy); also, significant time effect within groups but nonsignificant group × time effect and nonsignificant between-subjects' effects.
Studenski et al. [97]	2005	USA	Community	The 36-session, 12-week, home-based exercise program, supervised by an occupational or physical therapist, targeted strength (major muscle groups of the upper and lower extremity using elastic bands and body weight), balance, and endurance (using an exercise bicycle) and encouraged use of the affected upper extremity. There were structured protocols for the exercise tasks, criteria for progression, and guidelines for reintroducing therapy after intercurrent illness. After completing the intervention, participants received written guidelines for continued exercise.	Intervention 68.5 (9.0), usual care 70.4 (11.3)	53%	Intervention *days* 77.5 (28.7), usual care *days* 74.1 (27.2)	Support for this intervention (home-based exercise program) compared to usual care immediately after the intervention but not at 6-month follow-up.
Tielemans et al. [99]	2015	Netherlands	Community	The 10-week self-management intervention consisted of 7 sessions, 6 × 2 h sessions in the first 6 weeks and 1 × 2 h booster session in week 10. It was provided to groups of 4–8 participants by 2 rehabilitation professionals	Self-management 55.2 (8.9), education 58.8 (8.7)	Self-management 54.8%, education 60%	Self-management 15.6 (20.9), education 21.9 (34.1)	No significant differences between self-management and education intervention, on either primary or secondary outcome measures, but there were trends towards a difference in participation restriction at follow-up.

Table 4: Continued.

Author	Year	Country	Setting	Intervention	Age (*yr*) mean (SD), median (IQR)	Sex (% male)	Time poststroke (*months*) mean (SD) or median [range]	Association on participation
				(e.g., psychologist or occupational therapist) at hospitals and rehabilitation centre outpatient facilities. The intervention aimed to teach proactive action planning strategies within 4 themes: "handling negative emotions," "social relations and support," "participation in society," and "less visible stroke consequences." The 10-week education intervention consisted of 3×1 h sessions in the first 6 weeks and 1×1 h booster session in week 10. It was provided in groups of 4–8 participants by one rehabilitation professional at hospital and rehabilitation centre outpatient facilities.				

Note. ADL: activity of daily living; CBT: client-centred therapy; CBT: cognitive behavioral therapy; ICF: International Classification of Functioning, Disability and Health; RTP: repetitive task practice.

Table 5: Tools measuring participation longitudinally after stroke.

Participation measure	Frequency of participation measures
SIS-P	24
LIFE-H	5
LHS	4
USER-P	3
SF-36	3
RNL	2
FAI	2
MPAI-4	1
SIS-P, NEADL	1
GPS	1
ALA	1
Number of minutes	1
NLQ	1
SIS-P, OGQ	1
SIS-P, RAND	1
NEADL, mRS	1
GAS	1
PASIPD	2
FAI, 6-minute walk test	1
IMPACT-P	1
IPA	1
MAL	1
Grand total	59

Note. ALA: assessment for living with aphasia; FAI: Frenchay activity index; GAS: goal attainment scale; GPS: global positioning system; IMPACT-P: participation subsection of the ICF measure of participation and activities; IPA: impact on participation and autonomy; LHS: London handicap scale; LIFE-H: assessment of life habits; MAL: motor activity log; MPAI-4: Mayo-Portland adaptability inventory; mRS: modified ranking scale; NEADL: Nottingham extended activities of daily living; NLQ: Nottingham leisure questionnaire; OGQ: occupational gaps questionnaire; PASIPD: physical activity scale for individuals with physical disabilities; RAND-36: physical function index of the medical outcomes study RND-36 item health survey; RNL: reintegration of normal living; SF-36: short form 36; SIS-P: stroke impact scale participation domain; USER-P: Utrecht scale for evaluation of rehabilitation-participation.

the outcomes on participation referred to mobility, fitness, and other aspects of physical/motor function. It may be assumed that because these studies were performed by physiotherapists, special attention was given to this area. This supports Kjellberg et al. [31], who stated that participation in the physical field is highly represented in the literature of stroke survivors. To fully utilize and apply these findings in health theory and practice, they should be interpreted in relation to how the measurement of participation was conceptualized and measured by the studies in this scoping review.

4.3. Measuring Participation. This scoping review found various measures of participation that were used across studies. The most prevalent measures found in this scoping review were the SIS-P, followed by the LIFE-H. Previous studies investigating these tools and other tools purporting to measure participation have highlighted that the different tools measure different domains of participation (e.g., Community, Social and Civic Life, Domestic Life, and Activities of Daily Living) and different aspects of participation (i.e., frequency, restrictions, satisfaction); the administration and response formats are different (e.g., self-report, interviewer-administered), and the psychometric properties varied [24, 32–34]. For example, in the study by Tse et al. [24], the Participation domain of the SIS covered four of the nine Activities and Participation domains of the ICF, whereas the LIFE-H covered seven of the nine domains. Further, each tool covered each domain of the ICF to varying degrees: the SIS-P contained three items in the Community, Social and Civic Life domain of the ICF, whereas the LIFE-H contained nine. These differences in how participation is measured impacts on our future understanding and conceptualization of participation. For example, Kossi et al. [35], who measured participation using the Participation Measurement Scale (PM-Scale) that covers all nine ICF domains, found that some participation domains are affected by stroke more than others: participation in community, social, and civic life; interpersonal interactions and relationships; and domestic life [35]. Similarly, Heinemann et al. [36] stressed that greater restrictions in participation among stroke survivors are related to community, social, and civic life.

Table 6: Definitions of participation reported by authors measuring participation longitudinally after stroke.

Definition of participation	Frequency
Operational definitions	24
ICF	20
LIFE-H	6
Meaningful activities/occupations	2
Social participation	2
ICF and role participation	1
Self-perceived participation	1
ICF and meaningful activities/occupations	1
Community participation (role contribution)	1
Role participation	1
Total	59

Note. ICF: International Classification of Functioning, Disability and Health; LIFE-H: assessment of life habits.

Further, it has been shown that the different aspects of participation are only partially correlated [37]. Blomer et al. [37] compared the association between participation frequency, participation restriction, and participation satisfaction using the Utrecht Scale for Evaluation of Rehabilitation-Participation. They found that the strongest independent association was between participation restriction and participation frequency in vocational activities. Participation frequency in leisure and social activities was not independently associated with participation restriction, nor was participation frequency in leisure and social activities associated with participation satisfaction. This finding suggests the need for measures of participation to cover the varying aspects of participation in discrete scores and not measures that combine aspects of participation into one overall score. We suggest that, because the SIS-P covers a

TABLE 7: Definitions of participation relative to the proportion of studies from each continent in this review on longitudinal participation outcomes after stroke.

	North America	Europe	Australasia	South America	Africa	Mixed
Operational definitions	7	12	3	1		1
ICF	9	5	3		2	1
LIFE-H	6					
Meaningful activities/occupations	1		1			
Social participation	1		1			
Community participation (role contribution)	1					
Role participation	1					
ICF and role participation	1					
Self-perceived participation		1				
ICF and meaningful activities/occupations			1			
Total	26	19	9	1	2	2

Note. ICF: International Classification of Functioning, Disability and Health; LIFE-H: assessment of life habits.

brief range of domains in Activities and Participation section of the ICF and it combines different aspects of participation into one score, it is best described as a screening tool of participation.

4.4. Definitions of Participation. Since the publication of the ICF in 2001, the concept of participation has become central in discussions across rehabilitation science [5]. Yet this scoping review found that many publications did not provide a definition of participation but rather described the tool used in the study to measure participation (such as the SIS). The studies that used a definition of participation used varying definitions, such as role participation, community participation, social participation, participation as reflected in meaningful activities/occupations, or life habits. Nevertheless, the most frequently used definition was that of the ICF, which emphasizes that health is broader than a purely medical or biological conceptualization of dysfunction and must consider the influence of the environment and other contextual factors on functioning. Participation is defined by the ICF as an individual's involvement in life situations [26]. It represents the societal perspective of functioning. According to the ICF, functioning is the interaction of individuals with their physical, social, and environment. More concretely, emphasis is on the individual's ability to perform activities and to participate in real-life, everyday situations [26]. Indeed, since the publication of the ICF in 2001, the concept of participation has become central in discussions across rehabilitation science and practice.

Although the ICF conceptualization of participation is widely used, there are other conceptualizations of participation used within the health rehabilitation literature. The Person-Environment-Occupation-Performance (PEOP) is a model stemming from occupational therapy [29]. In the PEOP model, participation is defined as active engagement in daily life, families, work, and communities. In this model, occupational performance and participation are a result of the interaction between factors related to the person, the environment, and one's chosen activity or occupation. According to the PEOP model, occupational performance reflects the doing, and participation reflects the active engagement in life. The conceptual framework on participation by Hammel and colleagues' emphasizes the importance of participation choice, control, and engagement [38].

Using conceptual frameworks such as the ICF and the PEOP assist to develop theory and provide the rationale and guide the application of theory into practice [39]. The studies in this review conducted in Africa used only the ICF definition of participation, while those originating from other countries out of Africa (as seen in Table 7) used a variety of definitions of participation. Indeed, participation, specifically meaningful participation in everyday occupations, is a complex phenomenon to conceptualize and measure [40]. The reason for choosing one definition over another requires further study—is it because conceptual frameworks such as the ICF and the PEOP are not applied in specific geographic areas? Does it result from cultural reasons, from practical reasons such as the setting, or is it linked with existing evaluations of participation that cover definitions such as that of the ICF? Is it easier/more practical to measure participation in that specific definition? Are there financial reasons? Answers to these questions may help in establishing future studies and in turn better outcomes for stroke survivors.

Another finding is that the number of publications per year has not increased linearly. Considering that participation is an important outcome measure of intervention, it would be expected that the number of publications should rise. Research and practice should elucidate factors that may lead to an increase in participation outcomes: for example, what may enhance the conduct of studies investigating participation in stroke survivors and longitudinal studies relating to intervention efficacy on participation? This information may contribute to evidence-based practice for the benefit of stroke survivors expressed in better engagement in real-life settings, meaningful participation, and better quality of life.

To summarize, participation is a critical factor that should be considered in intervention programs for stroke survivors. The various definitions of participation, the assessments, and the limited information about intervention efficacy in meanings of participation highlight that further studies should be performed worldwide and contribute to a coherent and consistent discussion targeted at achieving meaningful participation among stroke survivors.

Considering the challenges that stroke survivors face and that participation is a critical outcome measure of intervention, evaluations of participation should reflect meaningful participation—the subjective experience of the individual's performance of activities [41], the enjoyment from participating in the activity [42–44], the context where the participation takes place, and also the activities desired by the individual.

4.5. Implications for Stroke Rehabilitation. Participation as a main outcome measure of intervention should continue to receive special attention in rehabilitation programs for stroke survivors. For example, occupational therapy intervention programs for participation should include clinical reasoning, in which therapists profile the individual's challenges, map problem priorities, and, together with the individual, set meaningful goals to enhance participation in real-life context to achieve the optimal rehabilitation experience. As such, therapists should combine self-reports with observations, use an elaborated point of view to understand factors that influence participation (including personal and environmental factors), and use conceptual models such as the PEOP alongside theoretical frameworks such as the ICF to accurately understand these complicated relationships [45] and focus interventions accordingly. Therapists must also consider the measurement tool used to assess participation. Different tools assess different domains and aspects of participation [24]. Consistent use of the most appropriate participation measure will assist to meet stroke survivor's specific participation needs.

4.6. Implications for Research. In general, further studies are needed in order to (1) profile participation among stroke survivors as an outcome measure of recovery and/or intervention and (2) expand the body of knowledge about study designs, sensitive assessments, and time points of evaluations that may provide data about occupation-based interventions and their effectiveness in terms of participation and well-being.

More studies should be performed by disciplines where participation is the focus, such as occupational therapy, and we must extend beyond the emphasis found today on motor function and mobility; provide more data about the interaction between body function, performance, and participation; illuminate the interaction between personal and environmental factors; and consider contextual factors such as sociocultural background to find optimal strategies that meet patients' specific needs and interests.

4.6.1. Strengths and Limitations. Strengths of this review include using recommended and rigorous methods widely accepted in the conduct of scoping reviews and using broad search terms across a range of databases in order to maximize the likelihood of capturing the available research in the recovery of participation outcomes following a stroke. Limitations of this scoping review result from the variability in studies' designs and methods, their definitions of participation, the relatively small number of studies that examine intervention impacts on participation in stroke survivors, and the multiple assessments, assessors, and interventions, which make it difficult to profile the effects of specific intervention tools and strategies on participation. Many studies focused on symptom management and on activities of daily living. Participation evaluation mainly referred to type of activities and did not use an elaborated perspective about where and with whom does the individual participate and how much they enjoy engaging in the activity. Further studies focussing on participation outcomes may contribute to filling this gap in research.

5. Conclusion

Stroke rehabilitation research and practice regarding stroke survivors should refer to participation as a major outcome measure of recovery and intervention effectiveness. Assessments should be used that include a broad perspective on participation domains. However, tools measuring participation must not combine the different aspects of participation into one overall score. This will assist us to better understand which interventions have a better impact on participation and recovery.

Further research should be performed to support occupation-based intervention effectiveness for providing stroke survivors optimal intervention, meaningful participation, and meaningful life.

Authors' Contributions

Batya Engel-Yeger and Tamara Tse are joint first authors. Batya Engel-Yeger, Tamara Tse, and Leeanne M. Carey codesigned the study. Batya Engel-Yeger and Tamara Tse collected the data, analysed the data, interpreted the findings, and cowrote the paper. Naomi Josman, Carolyn Baum, and Leeanne M. Carey contributed to the interpretation of the results and review of the manuscript.

Acknowledgments

This scoping review was supported by the James S. McDonnell Foundation 21st Century Science Initiative in Cognitive Rehabilitation-Collaborative Award (# 220020413) and the Neurorehabilitation Science Collaborative, a consortium of rehabilitation scientists and neuroscientists formed with the mission to use our collective knowledge and diverse science perspectives to advance the science of neurorehabilitation.

References

[1] V. L. Roger, A. S. Go, D. M. Lloyd-Jones et al., "Heart disease and stroke statistics–2011 update: a report from the American

Heart Association," *Circulation*, vol. 123, no. 4, pp. e18–e209, 2011.

[2] V. L. Feigin, M. H. Forouzanfar, R. Krishnamurthi et al., "Global and regional burden of stroke during 1990-2010: findings from the global burden of disease study 2010," *Lancet*, vol. 383, no. 9913, pp. 245–255, 2014.

[3] G. A. Roth, M. H. Forouzanfar, A. E. Moran et al., "Demographic and epidemiologic drivers of global cardiovascular mortality," *The New England Journal of Medicine*, vol. 372, no. 14, pp. 1333–1341, 2015.

[4] A. Bergstrom, S. Guidetti, K. Tham, and G. Eriksson, "Association between satisfaction and participation in everyday occupations after stroke," *Scandinavian Journal of Occupational Therapy*, vol. 24, no. 5, pp. 339–448, 2017.

[5] J. Desrosiers, "Muriel driver memorial lecture. Participation and occupation," *Canadian Journal of Occupational Therapy*, vol. 72, no. 4, pp. 195–203, 2005.

[6] B. Engel-Yeger and S. Hamed-Daher, "Comparing participation in out of school activities between children with visual impairments, children with hearing impairments and typical peers," *Research in Developmental Disabilities*, vol. 34, no. 10, pp. 3124–3132, 2013.

[7] C. M. Baum, "Fulfilling the promise: supporting participation in daily life," *Archives of Physical Medicine and Rehabilitation*, vol. 92, no. 2, pp. 169–175, 2011.

[8] N. E. Andrew, M. Kilkenny, R. Naylor et al., "Understanding long-term unmet needs in Australian survivors of stroke," *International Journal of Stroke*, vol. 9, no. SA100, pp. 106–112, 2014.

[9] S. Jellema, R. van der Sande, S. van Hees, J. Zajec, E. M. Steultjens, and M. W. Nijhuis-van der Sanden, "Role of environmental factors on resuming valued activities post-stroke: a systematic review of qualitative and quantitative findings," *Archives of Physical Medicine and Rehabilitation*, vol. 97, no. 6, pp. 991–1002.e1, 2016.

[10] J. Desrosiers, L. Demers, L. Robichaud et al., "Short-term changes in and predictors of participation of older adults after stroke following acute care or rehabilitation," *Neurorehabilitation and Neural Repair*, vol. 22, no. 3, pp. 288–297, 2008.

[11] A. Rochette, J. Desrosiers, G. Bravo, D. St-Cyr-Tribble, and A. Bourget, "Changes in participation after a mild stroke: quantitative and qualitative perspectives," *Topics in Stroke Rehabilitation*, vol. 14, no. 3, pp. 59–68, 2007.

[12] J. Spitzer, T. Tse, C. M. Baum, and L. M. Carey, "Mild impairment of cognition impacts on activity participation after stroke in a community-dwelling Australian cohort," *OTJR: Occupation, Participation and Health*, vol. 31, Supplement 1, pp. S8–S15, 2011.

[13] T. K. Hamzat and A. Kobiri, "Effects of walking with a cane on balance and social participation among community-dwelling post-stroke individuals," *European Journal of Physical and Rehabilitation Medicine*, vol. 44, no. 2, pp. 121–126, 2008.

[14] N. Nasr, S. Mawson, P. Wright, J. Parker, and G. Mountain, "Exploring the experiences of living with stroke through narrative: stroke survivors' perspectives," *Global Qualitative Nursing Research*, vol. 3, article 233339361664651, 2016.

[15] J. Robison, R. Wiles, C. Ellis-Hill, K. McPherson, D. Hyndman, and A. Ashburn, "Resuming previously valued activities post-stroke: who or what helps?," *Disability and Rehabilitation*, vol. 31, no. 19, pp. 1555–1566, 2009.

[16] I. Wallenbert and H. Jonsson, "Waiting to get better: A dilemma regarding habits in daily occupations after stroke," *American Journal of Occupational Therapy*, vol. 59, no. 2, pp. 218–224, 2005.

[17] C. Arntzen, T. Borg, and T. Hamran, "Long-term recovery trajectory after stroke: an ongoing negotiation between body, participation and self," *Disability and Rehabilitation*, vol. 37, no. 18, pp. 1626–1634, 2015.

[18] L. M. Carey, *Stroke Rehabilitation: Insights from Neuroscience and Imaging*, Oxford University Press, New York, 2012.

[19] R. Teasell, S. Mehta, S. Pereira et al., "Time to rethink long-term rehabilitation management of stroke patients," *Topics in Stroke Rehabilitation*, vol. 19, no. 6, pp. 457–462, 2012.

[20] M. P. Dijkers, "Issues in the conceptualization and measurement of participation: an overview," *Archives of Physical Medicine and Rehabilitation*, vol. 91, no. 9, pp. S5–S16, 2010.

[21] M. Rybski, *Structural Relationship between Stroke Indicators from the International Classification of Functioning, Disability and Health and Stroke Variables from the National Health Interview Survey*, The Ohio State University, Ohio, USA, 2009.

[22] K. Salter, J. W. Jutai, R. Teasell, N. C. Foley, J. Bitensky, and M. Bayley, "Issues for selection of outcome measures in stroke rehabilitation: ICF activity," *Disability and Rehabilitation*, vol. 27, no. 6, pp. 315–340, 2005.

[23] G. G. Whiteneck, "Issues affecting the selection of participation measurement in outcomes research and clinical trials," *Archives of Physical Medicine and Rehabilitation*, vol. 91, no. 9, pp. S54–S59, 2010.

[24] T. Tse, J. Douglas, P. Lentin, and L. Carey, "Measuring participation after stroke: a review of frequently used tools," *Archives of Physical Medicine and Rehabilitation*, vol. 94, no. 1, pp. 177–192, 2013.

[25] K. Vessby and A. Kjellberg, "Participation in occupational therapy research: a literature review," *British Journal of Occupational Therapy*, vol. 73, no. 7, pp. 319–326, 2010.

[26] World Health Organization (WHO), *International Classification of Functioning, Disability and Health (ICF)*, WHO, Geneva, 2001.

[27] H. Arksey and L. O'Malley, "Scoping studies: towards a methodological framework," *International Journal of Social Research Methodology*, vol. 8, no. 1, pp. 19–32, 2005.

[28] *Covidence Systematic Review Software*, Veritas Health Innovation, Melbourne, Australia, June 2017, http://www.covidence.org/.

[29] J. D. Bass, C. M. Baum, and C. H. Christiansen, "Welcome to occupational therapy: performance, participation, and well-being, fourth edition," in *Occupational Therapy: Performance, Participation, and Well-Being*, C. H. Christiansen, J. D. Bass, and C. M. Baum, Eds., pp. 1–9, Slack Incorporated, Thorofare, United States, 4th edition, 2014.

[30] O. Kossi, C. S. Batcho, T. Adoukonou, and J. L. Thonnard, "Functional recovery after stroke in Benin: a six-month follow-up study," *Journal of Rehabilitation Medicine*, vol. 48, no. 8, pp. 671–675, 2016.

[31] A. Kjellberg, I. Kahlin, L. Haglund, and R. R. Taylor, "The myth of participation in occupational therapy: reconceptualizing a client-centred approach," *Scandinavian Journal of Occupational Therapy*, vol. 19, no. 5, pp. 421–427, 2012.

[32] I. C. Eyssen, M. P. Steultjens, J. Dekker, and C. B. Terwee, "A systematic review of instruments assessing participation: challenges in defining participation," *Archives of Physical Medicine and Rehabilitation*, vol. 92, no. 6, pp. 983–997, 2011.

[33] S. Magasi and M. W. Post, "A comparative review of contemporary participation measures' psychometric properties and content coverage," *Archives of Physical Medicine and Rehabilitation*, vol. 91, no. 9, pp. S17–S28, 2010.

[34] C. Brandenburg, L. Worrall, A. Rodriguez, and K. Bagraith, "Crosswalk of participation self-report measures for aphasia to the ICF: what content is being measured?," *Disability and Rehabilitation*, vol. 37, no. 13, pp. 1113–1124, 2015.

[35] O. Kossi, F. Nindorera, C. S. Batcho, T. Adoukonou, M. Penta, and J. L. Thonnard, "Measuring participation after stroke in Africa: development of the participation measurement scale," *Archives of Physical Medicine and Rehabilitation*, vol. 99, no. 4, pp. 652–659, 2018.

[36] A. W. Heinemann, S. Magasi, R. K. Bode et al., "Measuring enfranchisement: importance of and control over participation by people with disabilities," *Archives of Physical Medicine and Rehabilitation*, vol. 94, no. 11, pp. 2157–2165, 2013.

[37] A. M. V. Blomer, M. L. van Mierlo, J. M. Visser-Meily, C. M. van Heugten, and M. W. Post, "Does the frequency of participation change after stroke and is this change associated with the subjective experience of participation?," *Archives of Physical Medicine and Rehabilitation*, vol. 96, no. 3, pp. 456–463, 2015.

[38] J. Hammel, S. Magasi, A. Heinemann et al., "Environmental barriers and supports to everyday participation: a qualitative insider perspective from people with disabilities," *Archives of Physical Medicine and Rehabilitation*, vol. 96, no. 4, pp. 578–588, 2015.

[39] G. Kielhofner, *Conceptual Foundations of Occupational Therapy*, I. NetLibrary, Ed., F.A. Davis Co., Philadelphia, Pennsylvania, 3rd edition, 2004.

[40] M. Law, B. Cooper, S. Strong, D. Stewart, P. Rigby, and L. Letts, "The person-environment-occupation model: a transactive approach to occupational performance," *Canadian Journal of Occupational Therapy*, vol. 63, no. 1, pp. 9–23, 1996.

[41] J. Hammel, S. Magasi, A. Heinemann, G. Whiteneck, J. Bogner, and E. Rodriguez, "What does participation mean? An insider perspective from people with disabilities," *Disability and Rehabilitation*, vol. 30, no. 19, pp. 1445–1460, 2008.

[42] A. L. Bergstrom, G. Eriksson, E. Asaba, A. Erikson, and K. Tham, "Complex negotiations: the lived experience of enacting agency after a stroke," *Scandinavian Journal of Occupational Therapy*, vol. 22, no. 1, pp. 43–53, 2015.

[43] M. Law, "Participation in the occupations of everyday life," *The American Journal of Occupational Therapy*, vol. 56, no. 6, pp. 640–649, 2002.

[44] T. Mallinson and J. Hammel, "Measurement of participation: intersecting person, task, and environment," *Archives of Physical Medicine and Rehabilitation*, vol. 91, no. 9, pp. S29–S33, 2010.

[45] T. W. Kang and H. S. Cynn, "Progressive intervention strategy for the gait of sub-acute stroke patient using the International Classification of Functioning, Disability, and Health tool," *NeuroRehabilitation*, vol. 40, no. 4, pp. 473–481, 2017.

[46] I. M. Altman, S. Swick, and J. F. Malec, "Effectiveness of home- and community-based rehabilitation in a large cohort of patients disabled by cerebrovascular accident: evidence of a dose-response relationship," *Archives of Physical Medicine and Rehabilitation*, vol. 94, no. 9, pp. 1837–1841, 2013.

[47] L. N. Awad, D. S. Reisman, T. M. Kesar, and S. A. Binder-Macleod, "Targeting paretic propulsion to improve post-stroke walking function: a preliminary study," *Archives of Physical Medicine and Rehabilitation*, vol. 95, no. 5, pp. 840–848, 2014.

[48] A. J. Beaudoin, B. Fournier, L. Julien-Caron et al., "Visuoperceptual deficits and participation in older adults after stroke," *Australian Occupational Therapy Journal*, vol. 60, no. 4, pp. 260–266, 2013.

[49] A. S. Bertilsson, G. Eriksson, L. Ekstam et al., "A cluster randomized controlled trial of a client-centred, activities of daily living intervention for people with stroke: one year follow-up of caregivers," *Clinical Rehabilitation*, vol. 30, no. 8, pp. 765–775, 2016.

[50] C. Brown, J. E. Fraser, E. L. Inness et al., "Does participation in standardized aerobic fitness training during inpatient stroke rehabilitation promote engagement in aerobic exercise after discharge? A cohort study," *Topics in Stroke Rehabilitation*, vol. 21, Supplement 1, pp. S42–S51, 2015.

[51] A. J. Butler, S. Blanton, V. T. Rowe, and S. L. Wolf, "Attempting to improve function and quality of life using the FTM protocol: case report," *Journal of Neurologic Physical Therapy*, vol. 30, no. 3, pp. 148–156, 2006.

[52] C. Y. Chou, Y. C. Ou, and T. R. Chiang, "Psychometric comparisons of four disease-specific health-related quality of life measures for stroke survivors," *Clinical Rehabilitation*, vol. 29, no. 8, pp. 816–829, 2014.

[53] S. A. Combs-Miller, A. Kalpathi Parameswaran, D. Colburn et al., "Body weight-supported treadmill training vs. overground walking training for persons with chronic stroke: a pilot randomized controlled trial," *Clinical Rehabilitation*, vol. 28, no. 9, pp. 873–884, 2014.

[54] M. Demetrios, A. Gorelik, J. Louie, C. Brand, I. J. Baguley, and F. Khan, "Outcomes of ambulatory rehabilitation programmes following botulinum toxin for spasticity in adults with stroke," *Journal of Rehabilitation Medicine*, vol. 46, no. 8, pp. 730–737, 2014.

[55] J. Desrosiers, L. Noreau, A. Rochette, D. Bourbonnais, G. Bravo, and A. Bourget, "Predictors of long-term participation after stroke," *Disability and Rehabilitation*, vol. 28, no. 4, pp. 221–230, 2006.

[56] J. Desrosiers, L. Noreau, A. Rochette et al., "Effect of a home leisure education program after stroke: a randomized controlled trial," *Archives of Physical Medicine and Rehabilitation*, vol. 88, no. 9, pp. 1095–1100, 2007.

[57] J. Desrosiers, A. Rochette, L. Noreau, D. Bourbonnais, G. Bravo, and A. Bourget, "Long-term changes in participation after stroke," *Topics in Stroke Rehabilitation*, vol. 13, no. 4, pp. 86–96, 2006.

[58] M. Egan, C. G. Davis, C. J. Dubouloz, D. Kessler, and L. A. Kubina, "Participation and well-being poststroke: evidence of reciprocal effects," *Archives of Physical Medicine and Rehabilitation*, vol. 95, no. 2, pp. 262–268, 2014.

[59] M. Egan, L. A. Kubina, C. J. Dubouloz, D. Kessler, E. Kristjansson, and M. Sawada, "Very low neighbourhood income limits participation post stroke: preliminary evidence

from a cohort study," *BMC Public Health*, vol. 15, no. 1, p. 528, 2015.

[60] C. C. Evans, T. A. Hanke, D. Zielke, S. Keller, and K. Ruroede, "Monitoring community mobility with global positioning system technology after a stroke: a case study," *Journal of Neurologic Physical Therapy*, vol. 36, no. 2, pp. 68–78, 2012.

[61] U. B. Flansbjer, J. Lexell, and C. Brogardh, "Long-term benefits of progressive resistance training in chronic stroke: a 4-year follow-up," *Journal of Rehabilitation Medicine*, vol. 44, no. 3, pp. 218–221, 2012.

[62] U. B. Flansbjer, M. Miller, D. Downham, and J. Lexell, "Progressive resistance training after stroke: effects on muscle strength, muscle tone, gait performance and perceived participation," *Journal of Rehabilitation Medicine*, vol. 40, no. 1, pp. 42–48, 2008.

[63] S. Guidetti, M. Ranner, K. Tham, M. Andersson, C. Ytterberg, and L. Koch, "A "client-centred activities of daily living" intervention for persons with stroke: one-year follow-up of a randomized controlled trial," *Journal of Rehabilitation Medicine*, vol. 47, no. 7, pp. 605–611, 2015.

[64] S. Guidetti, C. Ytterberg, L. Ekstam, U. Johansson, and G. Eriksson, "Changes in the impact of stroke between 3 and 12 months post-stroke, assessed with the Stroke Impact Scale," *Journal of Rehabilitation Medicine*, vol. 46, no. 10, pp. 963–968, 2014.

[65] T. K. Hamzat and G. O. Peters, "Motor function and participation among Nigerian stroke survivors: 6-month follow-up study," *NeuroRehabilitation*, vol. 25, no. 2, pp. 137–142, 2009.

[66] N. F. Horgan, M. O'Regan, C. J. Cunningham, and A. M. Finn, "Recovery after stroke: a 1-year profile," *Disability and Rehabilitation*, vol. 31, no. 10, pp. 831–839, 2009.

[67] I. B. Ilse, H. Feys, L. de Wit, K. Putman, and W. de Weerdt, "Stroke caregivers' strain: prevalence and determinants in the first six months after stroke," *Disability and Rehabilitation*, vol. 30, no. 7, pp. 523–530, 2008.

[68] I. Baert, Y. Vanlandewijck, H. Feys, L. Vanhees, H. Beyens, and D. Daly, "Determinants of cardiorespiratory fitness at 3, 6 and 12 months poststroke," *Disability and Rehabilitation*, vol. 34, no. 21, pp. 1835–1842, 2012.

[69] C. Jalayondeja, J. Kaewkungwal, P. E. Sullivan, S. Nidhinandana, S. Pichaiyongwongdee, and S. Jareinpituk, "Factors related to community participation by stroke victims six month post-stroke," *The Southeast Asian Journal of Tropical Medicine and Public Health*, vol. 42, no. 4, pp. 1005–1013, 2011.

[70] C. Jalayondeja, P. E. Sullivan, and S. Pichaiyongwongdee, "Six-month prospective study of fall risk factors identification in patients post-stroke," *Geriatrics & Gerontology International*, vol. 14, no. 4, pp. 778–785, 2014.

[71] P. M. Kluding, K. Dunning, M. W. O'Dell et al., "Foot drop stimulation versus ankle foot orthosis after stroke: 30-week outcomes," *Stroke*, vol. 44, no. 6, pp. 1660–1669, 2013.

[72] J. A. Kootker, S. M. C. Rasquin, F. C. Lem, C. M. van Heugten, L. Fasotti, and A. C. H. Geurts, "Augmented cognitive behavioral therapy for poststroke depressive symptoms: a randomized controlled trial," *Archives of Physical Medicine and Rehabilitation*, vol. 98, no. 4, pp. 687–694, 2017.

[73] N. G. Kutner, R. Zhang, A. J. Butler, S. L. Wolf, and J. L. Alberts, "Quality-of-life change associated with robotic-assisted therapy to improve hand motor function in patients with subacute stroke: a randomized clinical trial," *Physical Therapy*, vol. 90, no. 4, pp. 493–504, 2010.

[74] T. Kwok, J. H. Pan, R. Lo, and X. Song, "The influence of participation on health-related quality of life in stroke patients," *Disability and Rehabilitation*, vol. 33, no. 21-22, pp. 1990–1996, 2011.

[75] Y. Laufer, J. M. Hausdorff, and H. Ring, "Effects of a foot drop neuroprosthesis on functional abilities, social participation, and gait velocity," *American Journal of Physical Medicine & Rehabilitation*, vol. 88, no. 1, pp. 14–20, 2009.

[76] S. Lennon, A. Ashburn, and D. Baxter, "Gait outcome following outpatient physiotherapy based on the Bobath concept in people post stroke," *Disability and Rehabilitation*, vol. 28, no. 13-14, pp. 873–881, 2006.

[77] M. F. Levin, O. Snir, D. G. Liebermann, H. Weingarden, and P. L. Weiss, "Virtual reality versus conventional treatment of reaching ability in chronic stroke: clinical feasibility study," *Neurology and Therapy*, vol. 1, no. 1, p. 3, 2012.

[78] A. Lund, M. Michelet, L. Sandvik, T. Wyller, and U. Sveen, "A lifestyle intervention as supplement to a physical activity programme in rehabilitation after stroke: a randomized controlled trial," *Clinical Rehabilitation*, vol. 26, no. 6, pp. 502–512, 2012.

[79] R. Mayer and D. Reid, "Changes in autonomy and participation in seniors after stroke: a pilot study," *Activities, Adaptation, & Aging*, vol. 28, no. 3, pp. 49–70, 2004.

[80] N. E. Mayo, L. K. Fellows, S. C. Scott, J. Cameron, and S. Wood-Dauphinee, "A longitudinal view of apathy and its impact after stroke," *Stroke*, vol. 40, no. 10, pp. 3299–3307, 2009.

[81] N. E. Mayo and S. Scott, "Evaluating a complex intervention with a single outcome may not be a good idea: an example from a randomised trial of stroke case management," *Age and Ageing*, vol. 40, no. 6, pp. 718–724, 2011.

[82] N. E. Mayo, M. J. MacKay-Lyons, S. C. Scott, C. Moriello, and J. Brophy, "A randomized trial of two home-based exercise programmes to improve functional walking post-stroke," *Clinical Rehabilitation*, vol. 27, no. 7, pp. 659–671, 2013.

[83] V. S. Mercer, J. K. Freburger, S. H. Chang, and J. L. Purser, "Step test scores are related to measures of activity and participation in the first 6 months after stroke," *Physical Therapy*, vol. 89, no. 10, pp. 1061–1071, 2009.

[84] S. M. Nijenhuis, G. B. Prange, F. Amirabdollahian et al., "Feasibility study into self-administered training at home using an arm and hand device with motivational gaming environment in chronic stroke," *Journal of Neuroengineering and Rehabilitation*, vol. 12, no. 1, p. 89, 2015.

[85] S. J. Page, P. Levine, and V. Hill, "Mental practice-triggered electrical stimulation in chronic, moderate, upper-extremity hemiparesis after stroke," *American Journal of Occupational Therapy*, vol. 69, no. 1, pp. 6901290050p1–6901290050p8, 2015.

[86] M. Y. C. Pang, J. J. Eng, A. S. Dawson, H. A. McKay, and J. E. Harris, "A community-based fitness and mobility exercise program for older adults with chronic stroke: a randomized, controlled trial," *Journal of the American Geriatrics Society*, vol. 53, no. 10, pp. 1667–1674, 2005.

[87] C. J. Parker, J. R. F. Gladman, A. E. R. Drummond et al., "A multicentre randomized controlled trial of leisure therapy and conventional occupational therapy after stroke," *Clinical Rehabilitation*, vol. 15, no. 1, pp. 42–52, 2016.

[88] J. Penney, M. J. MacKay-Lyons, and A. McDonald, "Evidence-based stroke rehabilitation: case analysis using the International Classification of Functioning, Disability and Health framework," *Physiotherapy Canada*, vol. 59, no. 1, pp. 22–36, 2007.

[89] S. Pundik, J. Holcomb, J. McCabe, and J. J. Daly, "Enhanced life-role participation in response to comprehensive gait training in chronic-stroke survivors," *Disability and Rehabilitation*, vol. 34, no. 18, pp. 1535–1539, 2012.

[90] P. Raghavan, D. Geller, N. Guerrero et al., "Music upper limb therapy-integrated: an enriched collaborative approach for stroke rehabilitation," *Frontiers in Human Neuroscience*, vol. 10, p. 498, 2016.

[91] A. Rochette, N. Korner-Bitensky, D. Bishop et al., "The YOU CALL-WE CALL randomized clinical trial: impact of a multimodal support intervention after a mild stroke," *Circulation. Cardiovascular Quality and Outcomes*, vol. 6, no. 6, pp. 674–679, 2013.

[92] C. Sabariego, A. E. Barrera, S. Neubert, M. Stier-Jarmer, C. Bostan, and A. Cieza, "Evaluation of an ICF-based patient education programme for stroke patients: a randomized, single-blinded, controlled, multicentre trial of the effects on self-efficacy, life satisfaction and functioning," *British Journal of Health Psychology*, vol. 18, no. 4, pp. 707–728, 2013.

[93] K. Sandberg, M. Kleist, L. Falk, and P. Enthoven, "Effects of twice-weekly intense aerobic exercise in early subacute stroke: a randomized controlled trial," *Archives of Physical Medicine and Rehabilitation*, vol. 97, no. 8, pp. 1244–1253, 2016.

[94] A. P. C. Segura, S. V. Fontes, M. M. Fukujima, and S. L. de Andrade Matas, "The impact evaluation of physical therapy on the quality of life of cerebrovascular stroke patients," *International Journal of Rehabilitation Research*, vol. 29, no. 3, pp. 243–246, 2006.

[95] A. Singam, C. Ytterberg, K. Tham, and L. von Koch, "Participation in complex and social everyday activities six years after stroke: predictors for return to pre-stroke level," *PLoS One*, vol. 10, no. 12, article e0144344, 2015.

[96] M. Stuart, F. Benvenuti, R. Macko et al., "Community-based adaptive physical activity program for chronic stroke: feasibility, safety, and efficacy of the Empoli model," *Neurorehabilitation and Neural Repair*, vol. 23, no. 7, pp. 726–734, 2009.

[97] S. Studenski, P. W. Duncan, S. Perera, D. Reker, S. M. Lai, and L. Richards, "Daily functioning and quality of life in a randomized controlled trial of therapeutic exercise for subacute stroke survivors," *Stroke*, vol. 36, no. 8, pp. 1764–1770, 2005.

[98] V. Teoh, J. Sims, and J. Milgrom, "Psychosocial predictors of quality of life in a sample of community-dwelling stroke survivors: a longitudinal study," *Topics in Stroke Rehabilitation*, vol. 16, no. 2, pp. 157–166, 2009.

[99] N. S. Tielemans, J. M. A. Visser-Meily, V. P. M. Schepers et al., "Effectiveness of the Restore4Stroke self-management intervention "Plan ahead!": a randomized controlled trial in stroke patients and partners," *Journal of Rehabilitation Medicine*, vol. 47, no. 10, pp. 901–909, 2015.

[100] M. L. van Mierlo, C. M. van Heugten, M. W. Post, T. R. Hajos, L. J. Kappelle, and J. M. Visser-Meily, "Quality of life during the first two years post stroke: the Restore4Stroke cohort study," *Cerebrovascular Diseases*, vol. 41, no. 1-2, pp. 19–26, 2016.

[101] G. O. Vincent-Onabajo, T. K. Hamzat, and M. O. Owolabi, "Are there gender differences in longitudinal patterns of functioning in Nigerian stroke survivors during the first year after stroke?," *NeuroRehabilitation*, vol. 34, no. 2, pp. 297–304, 2014.

[102] C. Viscogliosi, S. Belleville, J. Desrosiers, C. D. Caron, B. Ska, and BRAD Group, "Participation after a stroke: changes over time as a function of cognitive deficits," *Archives of Gerontology and Geriatrics*, vol. 52, no. 3, pp. 336–343, 2011.

[103] L. E. Worrall, K. Hudson, A. Khan, B. Ryan, and N. Simmons-Mackie, "Determinants of living well with aphasia in the first year poststroke: a prospective cohort study," *Archives of Physical Medicine and Rehabilitation*, vol. 98, no. 2, pp. 235–240, 2017.

[104] S. Y. Yang and K. H. Kong, "Level and predictors of participation in patients with stroke undergoing inpatient rehabilitation," *Singapore Medical Journal*, vol. 54, no. 10, pp. 564–568, 2013.

3

Indication of Disrupted Temporal Structure in the Case of Thought Blocks in Schizophrenia: The Role of the Metastable Balance

Elias Koutsoukos [1,2] **and Elias Angelopoulos** [1,2]

[1] *Medical School, 1st Psychiatric Department, Eginition Hospital, Athens University, 72-74 Vas. Sofias Ave., 115 28 Athens, Greece*
[2] *Signal Processing Laboratory, University Mental Health Research Institute, 2 Soranou Efessiou, 115 27 Athens, Greece*

Correspondence should be addressed to Elias Koutsoukos; eliaskoutsoukos@gmail.com

Academic Editor: Jesus Pastor

This study is aimed at investigating probable disruption of the metastable balance relevant to a disruption of the mental processes observed in the neurophenomenal level. This disruption was found to occur under dense auditory verbal hallucinations (AVHs) which are accompanied by thought blocking (TB) phenomena. The entropy that quantifies the complexity of the spontaneous coupling has been used to describe the observed transitions. According to our findings, the high synchrony-derived entropy (SE) defines a metastable state, where formations of cortical areas are able to coordinate transiently under the demands of stimulus-oriented processes or other internal cognitive associations. It was also found that the disruption of the sensitive balance to the side of oversynergy (overconnectedness) rather than the side of independence (coincidental coupling) is relevant with functional fixations under the specific symptom of schizophrenia. An introduced measure relative to the persistence of coupling indicated that the overcoupled brain areas exhibit a kind of "stiffness" in processing incoherent phasic components. Our consideration enhances the understanding of the role the metastability plays in the interpretation of deeply subjective phenomena, such as AVHs and TBs that affect the normal information routing in the brain.

1. Introduction

The oscillatory activity of the brain reflects the collective action or the functional convergence of neuronal subunits that are interacted in a larger set. The coherent activity is considered to serve either the local or the large-scale neuronal communication. The strength and duration of this neuronal coordination is modulated by various cognitive demands. The origin of these demands can be either stimulus-specific conveying information about their cause or internally induced from processes that reflect contents of perceptions, thoughts, imagination, and various mental states. This coordinative mechanism may allow different perceptual features of an object, different aspects of a moving scene, separate remembered parts of a significant experience, and even different ideas that arise in a conversation to be bound together into a more associative-defined entity [1–3]. Coordination dynamics imply the availability and capacity of the brain cites to collectively act under the demands of stimulus-oriented processes or other internal cognitive associations. Under this consideration, metastability is defined as a state where individual parts of the brain preserve their tendencies to function autonomously and at the same time to exhibit coordinated activity [4–8]. In this state, coherent and incoherent neuronal activities occur in a critical region between segregation and integration, respectively, a condition that exhibits similarities with the thermodynamic phase transitions observed in an excited system [3, 9]. In general, if these transitions (metastable state) are involved in the continuous flow of mental processes and contribute in the formation of new information, they should be detected under conscious states, reflecting a dynamical view of the coupling behaviour. Furthermore, irregularities of these transitions may interpret the abnormal brain functioning observed in nosological entities such as schizophrenia [10–17].

Considering the above, the present study is aimed at investigating probable disruption of metastability associated with the disruption of the mental processes occurred during the rare symptom of thought blocking in schizophrenia or in other words the consistency of phenomenal and electrophysiological findings. Thought blocking (TB) is a disorder of thought, usually induced by underlying psychotic processes. The phenomenon is characterized by regular interruptions in the stream of thought. Bleuler [18] described that "the phenomenon is developed rapidly and occurred in transitory episodes of varying duration, with blocking not only the stream of thought but also the entire psyche, involving the processes of attention, perception, memory, speech, and motility." In the psychiatric bibliography, TB symptoms constitute core symptoms of schizophrenia and are attributed to the form and not to the content of the thought process [19]. These symptoms are rare and should be differentiated from the spontaneous distraction in the flow of thought occurring in normal individuals [20]. In our experience [21], phase synchrony analyses during dense and persisting auditory verbal hallucination (AVH) states that led to TBs have shown prolonged periods of strong coupling among the left temporal area and the remaining central and frontal cortical areas. The observed common mode of synchrony fluctuation lasted from 0.5 to 2 seconds, and it had been detected in a time window of 4 seconds referring to the denotation of the subjective experience of the symptom. The observation was found to engage, mostly, at the left temporal area and the remaining central and frontal brain areas. In this work [21], the methodological procedure was focused on the immediate vicinity of the symptom (symptom capture approach) and not on long-lasting resting-state EEG samples, which is the case of the present analysis.

In the present study, we examined the profile of the resting-state spontaneous coupling of EEG samples obtained from (a) normal healthy subjects, (b) a set of surrogates (see Methods section), (c) subjects suffering from persisted auditory verbal hallucinations and TBs (TB patients), and (d) a set of non-TB patients. The synchrony-derived entropy has been applied to quantify the complexity that governs the distribution of the average phase coherence (APC) values obtained from long-length resting-state EEG. As a rule, the APC computation, for all the included in the study samples, has been performed in segments of variable length, by giving us the ability to investigate the dependence between the APC values and the length of a given time window. The introduced approach allowed us to evaluate the persistence of coupling by means of the "rate of coupling loss," a parameter relevant to the temporal characteristics of the phase locking. From our findings, there are indications that AVH and TB symptoms are disturbances in the connectivity level that concern unregulated excessive coordination. This functional overintegration was found to be relevant to functional fixations that led to the inhibition of processing noticed in the neurophenomenological level. The observation is similar with a disruption in the temporal structure to the side of overconnectedness. In the same line of evidence, disruption of the coordination mechanism, to the side of independence, may contribute in the disorganization syndrome in schizophrenia [4, 17, 22]. Both disturbances may be considered as irregularities of a fragile equilibrium between the segregated and collective functioning that envelope the metastable regime.

2. Methods

The TB patient group consisted of data based on recordings from twelve patients (5 males, 7 females, mean age: 32 ± 5, duration of illness: 13 ± 4 years, mean PANSS score: 78 ± 3), with drug-resistant spontaneous AVHs and with prominent experience of TBs during the recording periods. The non-TB patient group included recordings from twelve schizophrenic patients (8 men, 4 women, mean age: 33 ± 7; duration of illness: 12 ± 7 years; mean PANSS score: 65 ± 7) who, at the time of enrollment, did not exhibit AVH and TB symptoms. All subjects were seated in a light and sound-attenuated, double skin Faraday cage. Electrodes (Fp1, Fp2, F7, F3, Fz, F4, F8, FT7, FC3, FCz, FC4, FT8, T7, C3, Cz, C4, T8, TP7, CP3, CPz, CP4, TP8, P7, P3, Pz, P4, P8, O1, Oz, O2, and earlobes as mean electrical reference) were configured on the scalp, using a standard cap. Recordings of the horizontal-plane eye-movement potentials were made by two electrodes fixed 1 cm bilateral to the outer canthus of each eye. The skin resistance of each electrode was kept below 10 kΩ for the entire recording session, and the sampling rate was set to 500 samples per second. The recruitment of patients, the criteria for their inclusion in the present study, and the EEG data pretreatment have been previously described in detail [10, 21]. Additionally, EEG samples from twelve healthy volunteers (7 males and 5 females with mean age of 30 ± 5 years) have been included in the group of normals (labelled normals). As a rule, three recordings with 4 min duration for each corresponding participated group case have been segmented in a considerable number of epochs, covering the entire resting-state recording. A series of test intervals ranging from 400 to 2000 ms have also been considered in our analysis, while the standard segmentation width for the computation of APC was kept at 1000 ms for the entire study. Due to the robustness against the influence of noise, APC (see (3)) could be considered as a stable measure for phase synchronization in biological time series such as the EEG [23]. The following (1) and (2) are the analytic representations of two time series $x(t)$ and $y(t)$ following the Hilbert transformation:

$$z_x(t) = x(t) + j\tilde{x}(t) = a_x(t)e^{j\phi_x(t)}, \quad (1)$$

$$z_y(t) = y(t) + j\tilde{y}(t) = a_y(t)e^{j\phi_y(t)}, \quad (2)$$

where $j\tilde{x}(t)$ and $j\tilde{y}(t)$ are the imaginary parts of the complex variables $z_x(t)$ and $z_y(t)$, respectively, and a_x and a_y and $\phi_x(t)$ and $\phi_y(t)$ are the instantaneous amplitude and phase, respectively [24]. The measure R (see (3)) expresses the average phase coherence of a couple of N point segments, with 1 and 0 to be the limits of a strong and a weak coupling, respectively [24].

$$R = \left| \frac{1}{N} \sum_{k=1}^{N-1} e^{j(\phi_x(n) - \phi_y(n))} \right|. \quad (3)$$

An equal number of surrogate data sets have been also analyzed in the same manner as the original EEG data. The applied method was based on the rank-shuffled surrogate, a procedure that affects the temporal structure by generating artificial data sets by randomly shuffling the rank of the original signals [25]. We have also examined the efficacy of the followed procedure in the evaluation of phase synchrony data following the study of Sun et al. [26]. Finally, the distributions of the APC values, obtained from the different groups, have been subjected to entropy computations, introducing this way, a descriptor of the APC complexity, the synchrony-derived entropy (SE) based on Shannon's entropy [27].

$$SE = \frac{\sum_{k=1}^{n} s_k \log s_k}{\log (n)}, \quad (4)$$

where n is the number of synchrony bins and s the synchrony values counted in each bin. SE constitutes a measure of information relative to the mode of coupling and could detect the preference of the connectivity for a given period. The high entropy values reflect flatness of the APC distribution denoting irregularity, instability, and lack of preference in the mode of coupling, while the low values are associated with prolonged phase locking.

The SE values that concern the TB patient group data were calculated from the resting-state EEG segments during prolonged periods (even several minutes) where dense hallucinatory states and TBs dominate. Always, the patients were instructed, immediately after the recovery from the thought blocking state, to annotate the past experience using an optical switch. This symptom capture approach was found more efficient in capturing isolated or sparse symptoms by considering the SE values found in association with the annotation [21]. After a detailed description of the experimental protocol, all subjects gave written informed consent and the University Mental Health Research Institute ethics committee approval was obtained. The experimental procedure was conducted in accordance with the Declaration of Helsinki [28].

3. Results

In the present study, we investigate the continuous flow of patterns that the interconnected brain areas generate reflecting the instantaneous mode of connectivity. Four representative cases were chosen: a normal subject, a surrogate data set, a patient under dense AVHs who additionally exhibited TBs, and a non-TB patient, respectively. Figure 1(a) represents the spontaneous variability of APC values corresponded to a 40 sec EEG segment obtained from a representative healthy subject. The phase coupling has been computed within the alpha EEG spectral region, among the left temporal, and the remaining brain sites. The attached map to the right indicates the spatial distribution of the observed coupling schemes, and it is compatible with the spatial characteristics of resting-state coupling under closed eye condition. The observation is congruent with the transient and nonstationary processes that characterize the normal brain functioning, and it was found to be common in all analyzed normal data sets. Accordingly, the estimated entropy (blue line appeared in Figure 1(e)) indicated a relatively flat distribution (SE = 0.81), denoting that the examined system does not exhibit any specific preference in the mode of coupling.

Similarly, the spontaneous coupling obtained from a representative surrogate data set shows a morphological complexity analogous to a system, that is, its active units exhibit coincidental coupling (Figure 2(b)). The corresponding map indicated the lack of any spatial preference in the distribution of the coupling values. On the other hand, the distribution of synchrony values indicated a relative flatness (black line appeared in Figure 1(e)); analogously, the entropy value was found even higher (SE = 0.92) than in the normal subject.

The complexity of coupling is seen different from the other analyzed cases in the instance of the excessive and broadly distributed oscillatory states recorded from a representative patient under a dense hallucinatory state that led to thought blocking. Figure 1(c) illustrates that several brain sites vary their resting-state coupling in a common mode with explicit preference to the high integration. As it is shown, the strong coupling was found lasted several seconds, while release of locking appeared intermittently. The distribution of APC values exhibited a peak relative to the prolonged temporal and spatial locking (red line appeared in Figure 1(e)). Accordingly, the estimated entropy during the majority of the persistent coupling instances was found within the range of 0.50 to 0.65 indicated, thus, a system having tendency to a relative stability. The attached map shows the spatial preference of the high coupling occurrences. It has to be noticed that in the majority of patient data, the coupling variability exhibited morphological similarities with the previously described representative case. The APC values appeared in Figure 1(d) concern the spontaneous variability of a non-TB patient. The formation did not show instances of persisting overcoupling, while the estimated entropy (green line appeared in Figure 1(e)) indicated a relatively flat distribution (SE = 0.85), denoting that the examined system does not exhibit any specific preference in the mode of coupling.

The dependence between the length of the analysis window (400 to 2000 ms) and the measured coupling, revealed different coupling behaviour among the four groups studied. The differences of the APC values for the standard interval (1000 ms) denoted by the blue box was found to be statistically significant (ANOVA $F(3, 44) = 84.11$, $p < 0.001$) (Figure 2(a)). Specifically, the difference between the non-TB patients and TB patients was found to be statistically significant (ANOVA $F(1, 22) = 34.4$, $p < 0.001$). The fitted lines define the "rate of synchrony loss" a parameter relevant to the amount of phasic components that could influence the balance between coherence-incoherence as a function of the

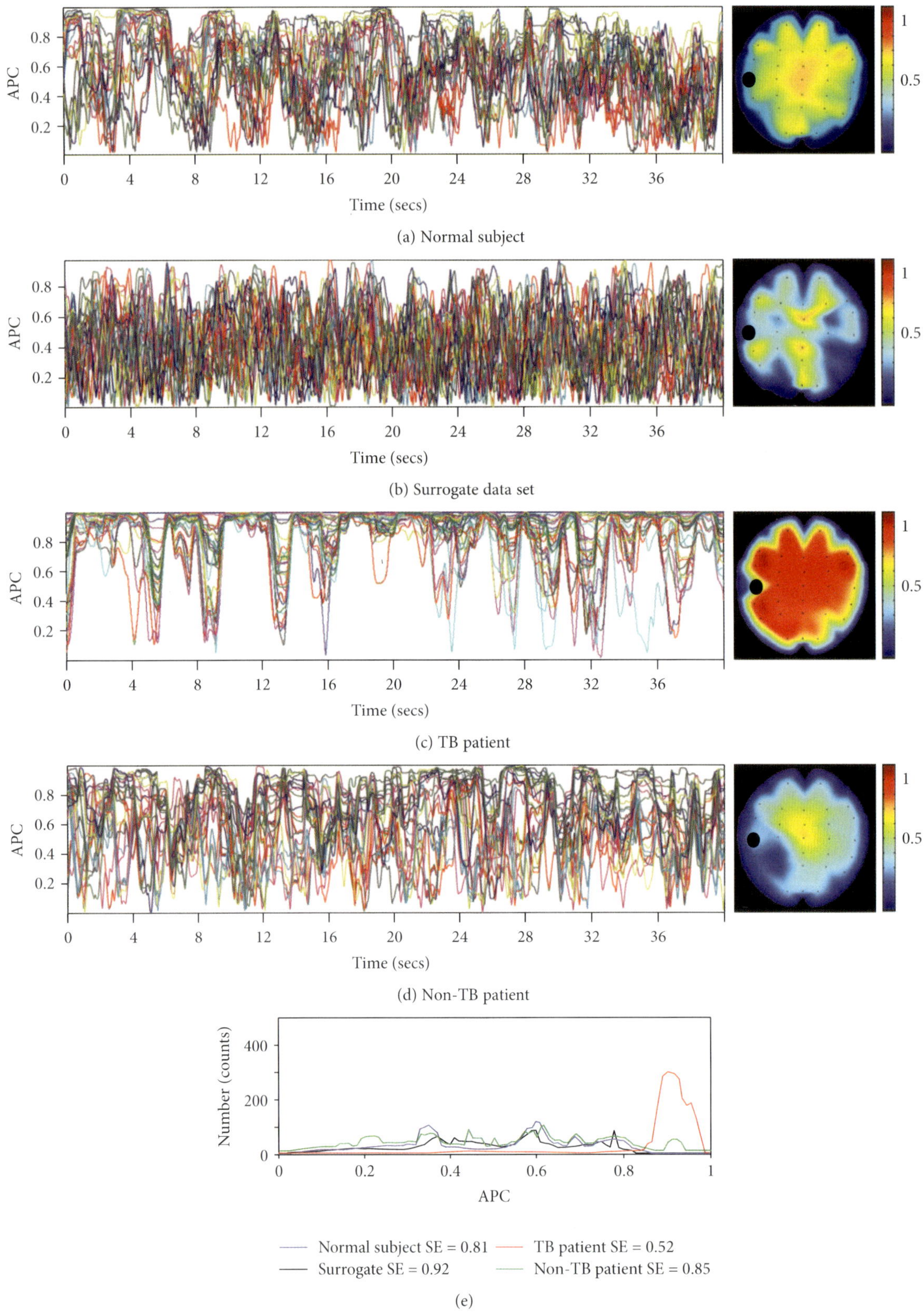

Figure 1: Representative resting-state APC values corresponding to a normal subject (a), a surrogate data set (b), a non-TB patient (c), and to a TB patient under persistent AVHs that led to TBs (d), respectively. Each line of plots represents the coupling between the left temporal region and the remaining brain sites during a representative 40 sec window. The spatial distribution of the coupling mode is shown for each case with an attached map to the right. The distributions of the APC values, measured for each case, are shown in (e). Synchrony-derived entropy values estimated for each of the four distributions are given under the graph, respectively.

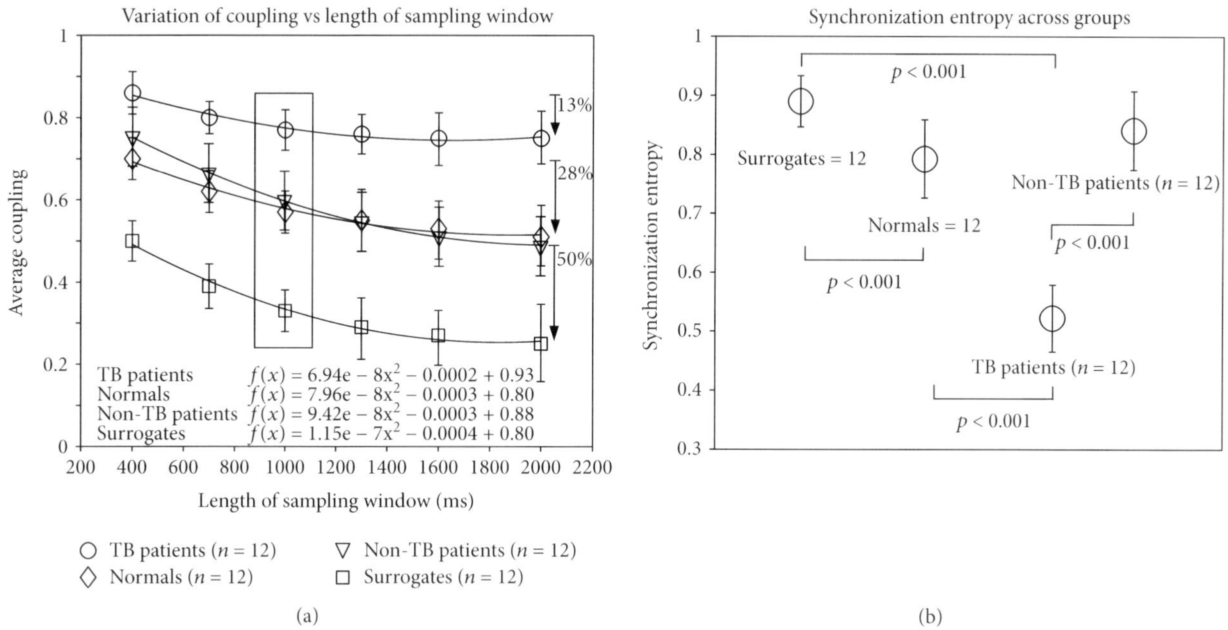

FIGURE 2: Average APC ± SD values versus length of the analysis window for TB patients, non-TB patients, normals, and surrogate group, respectively. (a) The fit models represent the rate of loss as a function of the length of the analysis window. The downward arrows indicate the "loss of coupling" as percentage of the initial values for each group, respectively. The blue frame includes the standard interval (1000 ms) values, where the differences among the four groups were found statistically significant. In (b), the average synchronization entropy values (SE ± SD) across the four groups are shown. Pairwise comparison of entropy values using the Mann–Whitney rank-sum test shows significant differences ($p < 0.001$) in the group pairs: normals-TB patients, normals-surrogates, surrogates-TB patients, and TB patients-non-TB patients.

length of the analysis window. The fast decay of the fitted lines indicates fast release of the coupling and vice versa. The group of surrogates exhibits the lower persistence since phase coherence is clearly symptomatic. The mean values of normals maintained a clear distance from the surrogates with the rate of loss found relatively lower. The non-TB patients indicated a fitted line relatively identical to that of normals. The TB patient data exhibited increased mean values of coupling well separated from the other groups, while the values observed in the long lengths indicated saturation of synchrony loss which is equivalent to prolonged coupling. More specifically, the difference between the non-TB patients and TB patients was found to be statistically significant (ANOVA $F(1, 22) = 34.4$, $p < 0.001$). This finding allowed us to associate the abnormal coupling (fixation) with the disruption of the mental flow, observed explicitly in the group of TB patients.

Additionally, pairwise comparison of synchronization entropy values across the four groups using the Mann–Whitney rank-sum test showed significant differences ($p < 0.001$) observed between arranged group pairs: normal-TB patients, normal-surrogates, surrogates-TB patients, and TB patients-non-TB patients, respectively (Figure 2(b)).

4. Discussion

Various complex systems, both natural and synthetic, exhibiting coherent and incoherent phenomena, have been computationally modeled using arrangements of weakly coupled oscillators [29, 30]. Simulation studies revealed a number of specific coupling behaviours and critical states that could influence the analysis strategies and consequently the understanding of brain functioning. The metastable chimera state based on the activity of community-organized oscillators has shown to generate a large repertoire of transient (metastable) states, where collective action and segregation coexist [31]. The abovementioned findings, although are in need of further theoretical understanding, exhibit similarities with those observed in the neurophenomenal level. In the brain level, functional segregation and integration are considered to be organizational aspects that reflect the collective and the independent activity of the neuronal components, respectively. These aspects also define the broader regions of irregularity and regularity, respectively [1, 4, 5, 7]. The normal brain functioning implies that the participating units retain their intrinsic mode of functioning (individuality and specificity), while at the same time these units participate collectively in transient schemes under various cognitive demands [17]. In this sense, a less defined and, thus, a more adaptive neuronal functioning could enhance the creation of new information. On the other hand, prolonged periods of excessive coherence (excessive synergy) in complex dynamical systems could be characterized as pathological. In the ground of a completely different neurophysiological-neuroanatomical mechanism, the severe oscillatory states occurred in the case of epileptic seizures were found to be associated with periods of impaired consciousness [13, 32].

The current work tries to reveal the involvement of the temporal organization, during a distinguished symptom of schizophrenia that led to interruptions of the thought. More precisely, we attempted to interpret the intermitted brain functioning in the phenomenal level, through specific irregularities of the metastable balance observed in the resting-state activity. TB symptoms are considered to be abnormalities of the flow of thought, and they could be conceived possibly as interruptions in the continuous information processing, due to the repetitive intrusions of hallucinations experienced by the subjects [21]. This point of view is in agreement to the theoretical consideration of Chapman [33] who stated that "the thought blocks are relevant with overload condition in the information processing." The fact that the oscillatory mechanisms are affected during these symptoms of schizophrenia [10] led us to investigate the mode that excessive collective action is reflected the resting-state spontaneous coupling.

Several measures have been proposed to characterize quantitatively the interplay between the complementary tendencies of independent and collective actions. Tononi et al. [34] defined a statistical measure for the amount of "structure" within a system's dynamics, as expression of its "complexity" with its value being high for systems with subsets of large mutual statistical dependencies. In a later study by Tononi and Edelman [35], in the theoretical level, different parts of such systems can engage in separate activity and yet remain interdependent. An analysis, by Seth et al. [36], concerning the strengths and limitations of three quantitative measures of dynamical complexity in the neural systems underlying consciousness, neural complexity, information integration, and causal density, has shown that none of these measures alone could capture the multidimensional complexity of a working neuronal system. However, any approach that quantifies complex organizational aspects, such as segregation and integration, with a single descriptor, could be considered simplistic, and criticism is needed for the interpretation of the findings. As discussed by Kelso and Tognoli [1], the empirical characterization of a system's behaviour, in terms of transitory states, encounters some difficulties. It is crucial, before any attempt to find signatures of a metastable state, to identify from the continuous stream of brain activity (flow of mental processes) some segments corresponding to specific neurophenomenological regimes. Thus, in our study, the phenomenal disruption has been associated with a pathological connectedness. The synchronization entropy findings provide a statistical description of brain connectivity by measuring the average amount of information in a probability distribution. In our study, this descriptor was found to be sensitive enough in detecting changes in the temporal structure of brain functioning. The continuous fluctuation of coupling values, as denoted by the high SE values, reflects the widespread oscillations across the distributed cortical areas and suggests the nonstationary nature of the brain. This could be an interim state where both segregation and integration coexist by serving the availability of the neuronal assemblies to participate in the production of mental information. In the case of thought blocks (TB patients), the excessive production of information as defined by the notably low entropy values was found to restrain significantly the normal flow of mental contents. Although a common nosological background exists, the non-TB patients did not exhibit active symptoms (AVHs, TBs), neither the previously described erroneous mode of coupling. Referring to the disrupted connectivity, the disorder of the metastable sensitive balance between large-scale integration and independent processing in the cortex, in favor of independent processing, has been suggested to be involved in the disorganization syndrome in schizophrenia [11]. Schizophrenia is a multifaced disorder including delusional, hallucinatory, and formal thought disorders. These symptoms seem to be based on the background of disturbed connectivity which allows the manifestation of erroneous and autonomous symptoms that leads to phenomenal abnormalities in the stream of consciousness [37].

The domination of the frontotemporal excessive coupling (see Figure 1(c)), during the experience of TB symptoms, was found to restrain the spontaneous synchrony variability, impeding the continuous information processing. The prolonged phase locking implies that the coordinated cortical sites emerge and relay within frontotemporal areas uniformly unchanged informational contents. Map appeared in Figure 1(c) illustrates persistent coupling, possibly caused by failure of the feedback regulatory mechanism to manage the excessive coupling and in extend to the organization of the rhythmical activity. In this view, the understudied system became more stable, incapable to produce information, and consequently slothful. The low entropy findings indicated lower complexity. This assumption is in agreement with a shift from the metastable regime, characterized by transient patterns of synchrony, to episodes of prolonged stability, characterized by stationary coupling. In general, a synchronization index reflects the ratio between the coherent and incoherent contents of two activities assessed in a given time window. Based on the transitory nature of brain coupling, it is assumed that high spontaneous synchrony should be principally measured, in short time windows. Along this line of thinking, the introduced analysis regarding the persistence of coupling, allowed us to classify the different coupling preferences of the four groups. More specifically, the persistent cortical connectedness, under the specific symptoms of TB patients, indicated that the overcoupled brain areas exhibited a kind of "stiffness" in processing incoherent phasic components. This state is associated with the fixation of the functional specialization due to overintegration. The fact that the coupling profile of the non-TB patients was found to be clearly separated from that of TB patients supports further the existence of a common ground between the abnormal coupling and the findings at the phenomenal level. According to our findings, synchrony-derived entropy effectively describe the disruption occurred in a critical equilibrium between the segregated and collective functioning under abnormal coupling states. This consideration may contribute in the understanding of the role that metastability plays in the interpretation of deeply subjective phenomena related with the diminished processing of information in the brain level.

Acknowledgments

The authors are grateful to Dr. Nikolaos Melis for his valuable comments and discussions.

References

[1] J. A. S. Kelso and E. Tognoli, "Toward a complementary neuroscience: metastable coordination dynamics of the brain," in *Neurodynamics of Cognition and Consciousness*, L. I. Perlovsky and R. Kozma, Eds., pp. 39–59, Springer-Verlag, Berlin, Heidelberg, 2007.

[2] A. A. Fingelkurts, A. A. Fingelkurts, and C. F. H. Neves, "Natural world physical, brain operational, and mind phenomenal space-time," *Physics of Life Reviews*, vol. 7, no. 2, pp. 195–249, 2010.

[3] A. A. Fingelkurts, A. A. Fingelkurts, and C. F. H. Neves, "Consciousness as a phenomenon in the operational architectonics of brain organization: criticality and self-organization considerations," *Chaos, Solitons & Fractals*, vol. 55, pp. 13–31, 2013.

[4] S. L. Bressler and J. A. S. Kelso, "Cortical coordination dynamics and cognition," *Trends in Cognitive Sciences*, vol. 5, no. 1, pp. 26–36, 2001.

[5] A. A. Fingelkurts and A. A. Fingelkurts, "Making complexity simpler: multivariability and metastability in the brain," *The International Journal of Neuroscience*, vol. 114, no. 7, pp. 843–862, 2004.

[6] J. A. S. Kelso, "Behavioral and neural pattern generation: the concept of neurobehavioral dynamical systems," in *Cardiorespiratory and Motor Coordination*, H. P. Koepchen and T. Huopaniemi, Eds., pp. 224–238, Springer-Verlag, Berlin, 1991.

[7] A. A. Fingelkurts and A. A. Fingelkurts, "Information flow in the brain: ordered sequences of metastable states," *Information*, vol. 8, no. 1, p. 22, 2017.

[8] J. A. S. Kelso, *Dynamic Patterns: The Self-Organization of Brain and Behavior*, MIT Press, Cambridge, 1995, (Chapter 2 and 3).

[9] Y. Kuramoto, *Chemical Oscillations, Waves, and Turbulence*, Springer-Verlag, Berlin, 1984.

[10] E. Angelopoulos, E. Koutsoukos, A. Maillis, G. N. Papadimitriou, and C. Stefanis, "Cortical interactions during the experience of auditory verbal hallucinations," *The Journal of Neuropsychiatry and Clinical Neurosciences*, vol. 23, no. 3, pp. 287–293, 2011.

[11] S. L. Bressler, "Cortical coordination dynamics and the disorganization syndrome in schizophrenia," *Neuropsychopharmacology*, vol. 28, no. S1, pp. S35–S39, 2003.

[12] K. J. Friston, "The disconnection hypothesis," *Schizophrenia Research*, vol. 30, no. 2, pp. 115–125, 1998.

[13] E. Koutsoukos, A. Maillis, C. Papageorgiou, S. Gatzonis, C. Stefanis, and E. Angelopoulos, "The persistent and broadly distributed EEG synchronization might inhibit the normal processing capability of the human brain," *Neuroscience Letters*, vol. 609, pp. 137–141, 2015.

[14] W. A. Phillips and S. M. Silverstein, "Convergence of biological and psychological perspectives on cognitive coordination in schizophrenia," *The Behavioral and Brain Sciences*, vol. 26, no. 1, pp. 65–82, 2003.

[15] P. J. Uhlhaas, C. Haenschel, D. Nikolic, and W. Singer, "The role of oscillations and synchrony in cortical networks and their putative relevance for the pathophysiology of schizophrenia," *Schizophrenia Bulletin*, vol. 34, no. 5, pp. 927–943, 2008.

[16] N. D. Wolf, F. Sambataro, N. Vasic et al., "Dysconnectivity of multiple resting-state networks in patients with schizophrenia who have persistent auditory verbal hallucinations," *Journal of Psychiatry & Neuroscience*, vol. 36, no. 6, pp. 366–374, 2011.

[17] A. A. Fingelkurts and A. A. Fingelkurts, "Alpha rhythm operational architectonics in the continuum of normal and pathological brain states: current state of research," *International Journal of Psychophysiology*, vol. 76, no. 2, pp. 93–106, 2010.

[18] E. Bleuler, *Dementia Praecox or the Group of Schizophrenias*, International Universities Press, New York, NY, USA, 1950.

[19] P. J. McKenna, *Schizophrenia and Related Syndromes*, Oxford University Press, Oxford, 1994.

[20] N. C. Andreasen, "Thought, language, and communication disorders: diagnostic significance," *Archives of General Psychiatry*, vol. 36, no. 12, pp. 1325–1330, 1979.

[21] E. Angelopoulos, E. Koutsoukos, A. Maillis, G. N. Papadimitriou, and C. Stefanis, "Brain functional connectivity during the experience of thought blocks in schizophrenic patients with persistent auditory verbal hallucinations: an EEG study," *Schizophrenia Research*, vol. 153, no. 1-3, pp. 109–112, 2014.

[22] M. J. Cuesta and V. Peralta, "Integrating psychopathological dimensions in functional psychoses: a hierarchical approach," *Schizophrenia Research*, vol. 52, no. 3, pp. 215–229, 2001.

[23] F. Mormann, K. Lehnertz, P. David, and C. E. Elger, "Mean phase coherence as a measure for phase synchronization and its application to the EEG of epilepsy patients," *Physica D: Nonlinear Phenomena*, vol. 144, no. 3-4, pp. 358–369, 2000.

[24] M. G. Rosenblum and J. Kurths, "Analysing synchronization phenomena from bivariate data by means of the Hilbert transform," in *Nonlinear Analysis of Physiological Data*, H. Kantz, J. Kurths, and G. Mayer-Kress, Eds., pp. 91–99, Springer-Verlag, 1998.

[25] J. Theiler, S. Eubank, A. Longtin, B. Galdrikian, and J. Doyne Farmer, "Testing for nonlinearity in time series: the method of surrogate data," *Physica D: Nonlinear Phenomena*, vol. 58, no. 1–4, pp. 77–94, 1992.

[26] J. Sun, X. Hong, and S. Tong, "Phase synchronization analysis of EEG signals: an evaluation based on surrogate tests," *IEEE Transactions on Biomedical Engineering*, vol. 59, no. 8, pp. 2254–2263, 2012.

[27] C. E. Shannon, "A mathematical theory of communication," *Bell System Technical Journal*, vol. 27, no. 3, pp. 379–423, 1948.

[28] World Medical Association, "WMA Declaration of Helsinki: ethical principles for medical research involving human subjects," in *Proceedings of the 64thWMA General Assembly*, Fortaleza, 2013Available at. http://www.wma.net/en/30publications/10policies/b3/index.html.

[29] A. Pikovsky, M. Rosenblum, and J. Kurths, *Synchronization: A Universal Concept in Nonlinear Sciences*, Cambridge University Press, Cambridge, 2001.

[30] Y. Kuramoto and D. Battogtokh, "Coexistence of coherence and incoherence in nonlocally coupled phase oscillators," *Nonlinear Phenomena and Complex Systems*, vol. 5, pp. 380–385, 2002.

[31] M. Shanahan, "Metastable chimera states in community-structured oscillator networks," *Chaos*, vol. 20, no. 1, pp. 013108–0131085, 2010.

[32] M. Arthuis, L. Valton, J. Régis et al., "Impaired consciousness during temporal lobe seizures is related to increased long-distance cortical-subcortical synchronization," *Brain*, vol. 132, no. 8, pp. 2091–2101, 2009.

4

Exploring the Neuroplastic Effects of Biofeedback Training on Smokers

Niki Pandria,[1,2] Alkinoos Athanasiou,[1] Nikos Terzopoulos,[1] Evangelos Paraskevopoulos,[1,2] Maria Karagianni,[1] Charis Styliadis,[1] Chrysoula Kourtidou-Papadeli,[3] Athanasia Pataka,[4] Evgenia Lymperaki,[5] and Panagiotis D. Bamidis[1]

[1]*Lab of Medical Physics, School of Medicine, Faculty of Health Sciences, Aristotle University of Thessaloniki (AUTH), 54124 Thessaloniki, Greece*
[2]*Northern Greece Neurofeedback Center, Thessaloniki, Greece*
[3]*Aeromedical Center of Thessaloniki, Thessaloniki, Greece*
[4]*Pulmonary Department, Oncology Unit, "G. Papanikolaou" General Hospital, Aristotle University of Thessaloniki, Thessaloniki, Greece*
[5]*Department of Medical Laboratories, Alexander Technological Educational Institute of Thessaloniki, Sindos, Greece*

Correspondence should be addressed to Niki Pandria; npandria@auth.gr

Academic Editor: Luigi Trojano

Smoking and stress cooccur in different stages of a nicotine addiction cycle, affecting brain function and showing additive impact on different physiological responses. Resting-state functional connectivity has shown potential in identifying these alterations. Nicotine addiction has been associated with detrimental effects on functional integrity of the central nervous system, including the organization of resting-state networks. Prolonged stress may result in enhanced activation of the default mode network (DMN). Considering that biofeedback has shown promise in alleviating physiological manifestations of stress, we aimed to explore the possible neuroplastic effects of biofeedback training on smokers. Clinical, behavioral, and neurophysiological (resting-state EEG) data were collected from twenty-seven subjects before and after five sessions of skin temperature training. DMN functional cortical connectivity was investigated. While clinical status remained unaltered, the degree of nicotine dependence and psychiatric symptoms were significantly improved. Significant changes in DMN organization and network properties were not observed, except for a significant increase of information flow from the right ventrolateral prefrontal cortex and right temporal pole cortex towards other DMN components. Biofeedback aiming at stress alleviation in smokers could play a protective role against maladaptive plasticity of connectivity. Multiple sessions, individualized interventions and more suitable methods to promote brain plasticity, such as neurofeedback training, should be considered.

1. Introduction

Resting-state brain activity involves the recruitment and activation of a number of subcomponents of the brain, such as the visual (VN), salience (SN), ventral and dorsal attention (VAN and DAN), sensorimotor (SMN), frontoparietal control (FPCN), and cinguloopercular control networks (COCN) [1, 2]. Among those networks that have been identified, the default mode network (DMN) has drawn attention as a state of organized baseline brain function [3]. It has been suggested to be involved in self-awareness and self-referential thought processes and episodic memory [4]. The exact definition of DMN nodes shows some variation between studies. Nonetheless, a number of important DMN nodes can be safely identified with the posterior cingulate cortex (PCC), precuneus (PCU), medial and lateral prefrontal cortices (mPFC, dlPFC, and vlPFC), inferior parietal cortex (IPC), and areas of the temporal lobe, including the lateral temporal cortex (LTC), the temporal pole (TPC), and middle temporal lobe (mTL) [3–5].

A chronic smoking habit has been associated with negative functional and structural effects on the central nervous system. These effects include decreased neurocognitive capacity, as well as the atrophy of grey and white matter of the brain in frontal, prefrontal, cingulate, temporal, and frontoparietal sites, among others [6]. Functional brain connectivity has also been shown to be affected in smoking, characterized by a disorganization of efficiency-related resting-state network topological properties. Heavy smokers showed lower global efficiency of both whole-brain network and DMN, as well as increased clustering and greater path lengths [7]. Moreover, these changes were associated with the severity and duration of smoking-habit abuse. Resting-state connectivity of prefrontal areas, involved in the facilitation of drug response- and reward-related mechanisms, has been shown to be enhanced in smokers and such findings have been suggested as biomarkers of addiction [8]. In general, DMN connectivity appears to show some impairment and decrease in smokers [4, 5, 9] but other functional brain networks, especially those involved in executive functions and cognition, are also affected by the addiction [9, 10].

Moreover, stress that is present in different stages of the nicotine addiction cycle seems [11, 12] to affect the organization of DMN [13, 14]. In a recent study by Soares et al. [13], prolonged stress was found to lead to greater activation of resting-state networks including the DMN, DAN, VAN, SM, and VN networks. Focusing on DMN, they found that stress resulted in the augmented activation of DMN, mainly in the inferior parietal cortex, medial prefrontal cortex, and medial orbitofrontal, precuneus, and posterior cingulate cortex. Increased activation of anterior DMN components could suggest an increase in self-subjective thoughts and a dynamic interplay between regions associated with emotional processing and cognitive functions. Moreover, the enhanced activation of inferolateral parietal lobes, along with the precuneus, could be linked to episodic memory retrieval and longer emotional stimuli processing. Similar findings of DMN activation were shown in another recent study investigating the role of social stress in resting-state networks, using the cyberball task [14]. Although the salience network (SN) and executive control network (ECN) remained stable, following a cyberball task DMN increased its connectivity with hubs of SN, high-order visual areas, and sensorimotor areas shifting the brain towards a more vigilant and attentive state.

Although smokers commonly report that smoking constitutes a technique to relieve negative emotions and cope with stressful conditions, it seems that stress is an aggravating factor that is present in every stage of the nicotine addiction cycle, forming "Nesbitt's paradox" [12, 15–18]. Modulating Flay's stage model of smoking [19], stress seems to be apparent at the preparatory stage of smoking, as individuals characterized by higher stress levels seem to be at high risk of adopting a smoking habit [20]. Furthermore, acute chronic stressors [21], perceived stress [22, 23], childhood adverse experiences [24], and negative life events [23, 25] have been found to increase the risk for smoking uptake and therefore for smoking initiation and experimentation. Smoking status was found to vary with diverse stress indices [26–29], and stressful conditions were found to lead to an increase of smoking urge [30], amount [31, 32], and intensity [33–35]. Moreover, a causal link between stress and smoking seems to be well-established during the maintenance phase [12]. Increased stress was also observed when comparing stress levels at different time conditions, resulting in relapse (prior to quitting and 1 month, 3 months, and 6 months of abstinence). However, stress levels were differentiated depending on the outcome of abstinence. In more detail, smokers who remained abstinent experienced a steady decrease in stress over time, while those who failed to quit smoking or were abstinent for only a brief period were consistently characterized by relatively high stress levels [36]. Moreover, the association between stress and relapse was shown to be robust, as 35% to 100% of smokers reported that lapses occurred while experiencing stress-related situations or negative affective states [37–40] and those who relapsed due to stress progressed very quickly to another lapse episode [41].

Considering that smoking and stress are shown to have additive impact on different physiological responses such as heart rate, blood pressure, and cortisol output [30, 42–44], they could also affect DMN connectivity and/or DMN network properties in a combined way. In this framework, our research protocol was introduced in order to objectively measure the impact of neuromodulation in DMN connectivity. Biofeedback (BF) has been established as a promising intervention for anxiety or stress-related conditions [45]. It allows the subjects to voluntarily influence their sympathetic activity providing real-time feedback of a physiologic measure such as skin temperature, heart rate, or electrodermal activity (EDA) [46, 47]. Recently, Critchley et al. [47] explored the mechanisms of sympathetic tone modulation using EDA training. They revealed a specific activation in the right anterior cingulate/ventromedial prefrontal cortex, left anterior cingulate, and left cerebellar vermis on intentional relaxation through BF training. Another reliable marker of stress lies with skin temperature [48], which seems to be affected by smoking along with vascular resistance in fingers, volumetric blood flow through tissues, and arterial perfusion [49–51]. Thus, skin temperature BF training could be beneficial for smokers to deal with stress.

To the best of our knowledge, this the first study that aims to investigate the possible impact of BF on DMN of active smokers through mediating stress. Furthermore, effects of BF training on smoking status were also explored using clinical data and behavioral evaluation.

2. Materials and Methods

2.1. Participants. We recruited twenty-seven smokers (male : female, 9 : 18) with a mean age of 50.52 years (range: 24–75, standard deviation (SD): 12.364). The participants were recruited in the context of the SmokeFreeBrain project [52] following the inclusion and exclusion criteria of the neurofeedback clinical study protocol (https://clinicaltrials.gov/ct2/show/NCT02991781). All subjects signed an informed

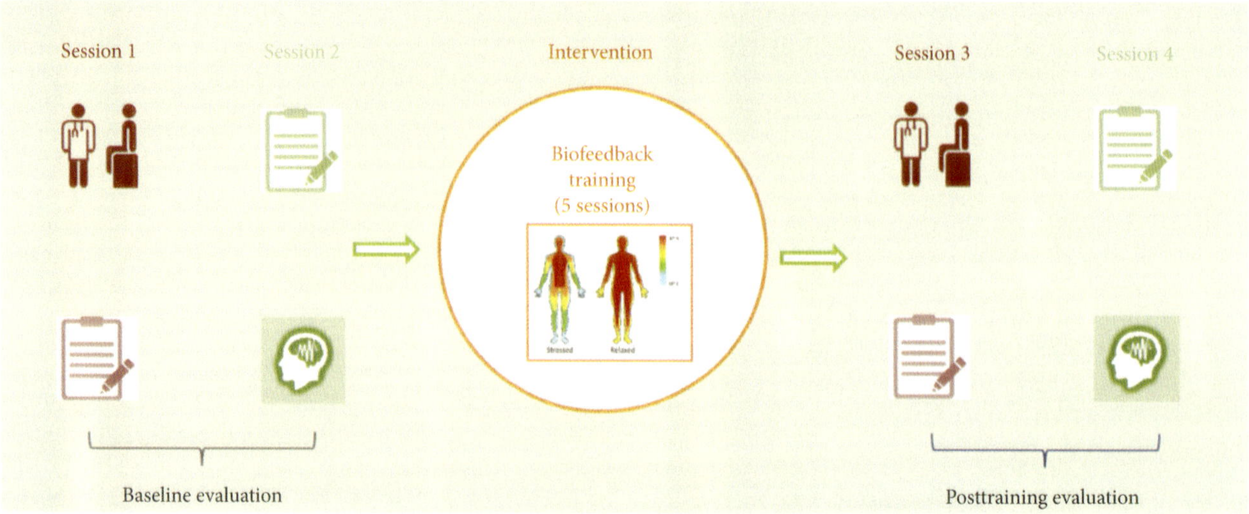

Figure 1: The different phases of the experimental protocol included two preintervention and two postintervention sessions with the participants, undergoing clinical, behavioral, and electrophysiological evaluation. The intervention phase included five biofeedback training sessions.

consent form, prior to their inclusion, in compliance with the Code of Ethics of the World Medical Association (Declaration of Helsinki). Inclusion criteria were the following: (1) active smokers (more than ten cigarettes per day), (2a) either being unemployed for at least three months and between eighteen to thirty-five years old, or (2b) being diagnosed with asthma or chronic obstructive pulmonary disease (COPD) with an age greater than thirty years old. Exclusion criteria included diagnosis of neurological, mental or psychiatric illness and drug-resistant epilepsy. Three (3) out of 27 participants were young and unemployed adults, sixteen (16) out of 27 were asthma patients, and eight (8) out of 27 were COPD patients. The study (design, methodology, and experimental protocol) was approved by the Bioethics Committee of the Medical School of the Aristotle University of Thessaloniki.

2.2. Experimental Design. Each participant went through a detailed clinical examination, which is a prerequisite for the SmokeFreeBrain (SFB) project (http://smokefreebrain.eu/). Specifically, each participant, after checking for eligibility criteria, underwent a baseline clinical evaluation (session 1, Figure 1) prior to which eligibility criteria were tested. Session 1 took place either at the private practice of a collaborator physician or at the Respiratory Failure Unit of "G. Papanikolaou" General Hospital. If a participant was eligible, demographic, medical, and behavioral data were collected. Demographics included age, years of education, gender, body mass index (BMI), number of cigarettes per day, and cigarette dependence in months.

Clinical evaluation included pulmonary function tests such as spirometry with parameters of forced expiratory flow in 1 second (FEV1), forced vital capacity (FVC), expiratory ratio (%FEV1/FVC), forced expiratory flow at the middle half of the FVC (FEF25–75%), and measurement of exhaled carbon monoxide levels (CO), as well as a blood sampling for the evaluation of total oxidative stress/total oxidative capacity (TOS/TOC), and vitamin E. In the current study, we just analyzed TOS/TOC scores both before and after the intervention.

Behavioral assessment was performed by administrating a battery of behavioral tests and questionnaires validated or adapted for the Greek population. These were the following: Fagerström Test for Nicotine Dependence [53], Motivation [54], The Contemplation Ladder [55], Minnesota Nicotine Withdrawal Scale [56], Beck Depression Inventory [57], State-Trait Anxiety Inventory [58], General Health Test [59], Rosenberg Self-Esteem Scale [60], and World Health Organization Quality of Life Instrument—Brief [61]. In addition, the COPD patients completed the COPD Assessment Test score [62] and the COPD and Asthma Sleep Impact Scale [63], while asthma patients answered the Asthma Control Test [64].

In session 2 (Figure 1), a baseline neuropsychological evaluation was performed administrating the Stroop Test [65], Trail-Making Test A and B [66], and Digit Span Test [67], along with an electrophysiological assessment through electroencephalographic recordings (EEG) in different conditions. EEG recordings were performed with a Nihon Kohden 128-channel EEG recording system and an active electrode cap (actiCAP 128Ch, Brain Products) according to the high-resolution EEG 10-5 international electrode system [68]. Recordings took place inside the electromagnetically shielded and sound-attenuated room of the Medical Physics Laboratory, before and after the biofeedback training. They were performed at a sampling rate of 1000 Hz, while electrode impedances of the brain signal, ground electrode, and references were kept lower than 10 kΩ. EEG was recorded during four different conditions, including eyes open (EO) (5 minutes), eyes fixated in a smoking-related image (EF) (1 minute), eyes closed (EC) (5 minutes), and a multifeature auditory mismatch negativity measurement according to the guidelines of Näätänen et al. [69] (15 min in duration). In the current manuscript, eyes-closed data were analyzed following the suggestions by Raichle et al.

[3], where resting-state is defined as a task-free state in which the individuals rest quietly awake with eyes closed.

The intervention phase (Figure 1) consisted of five 30-minute sessions of skin temperature training. Each training session included, at the start, an introduction to stress-coping techniques of 15-minute length and a one-minute baseline peripheral temperature recording. These were followed by 30 minutes of skin temperature training as suggested by Peniston and Kulkosky [70]. Participants sat comfortably on a reclined chair across a computer monitor resting their nondominant hand on the lap or a pillow. A sensitive thermistor was placed in the middle fingertip of their nondominant hand. The training goal at each session was to achieve temperature enhancement while receiving an audiovisual feedback. When the temperature exceeded an autoadjusted threshold, a puzzle was being formed accompanied by a pleasant auditory stimulus as described in [71]. In the posttraining phase (sessions 3 and 4), the followed procedures were identical to the baseline. Additionally, in the posttraining clinical evaluation, urine samples were collected to assess cotinine levels in our participants apart from the procedures already described for the baseline screening.

In later phases of the intervention, as part of the SmokeFreeBrain project, multiple sessions of alpha-theta neurofeedback training are introduced, but this is not discussed in the current study.

2.3. Total Oxidative Capacity/Total Oxidative Stress (TOC/TOS). After blood draw, blood samples were centrifuged for 10 min at 2000*g* and 4°C, and serum samples (1 ml), divided in two or three microcentrifuge tubes, were stored at −80°C. The average time lapse between sample collection and freezing was 90 minutes. Determination of the peroxides was performed by the reaction of a peroxidase with peroxides in the sample followed by the conversion of tetramethyl benzidine to a colored product. After the addition of a stop solution, the samples were measured at 450 nm in a microliter plate reader. The quantification was performed by the delivered calibrator.

2.4. Data Preprocessing and Resting-State Connectivity. The Brain Electrical Source Analysis software (BESA research, version 6.0, Megis Software, Heidelberg, Germany) was used for the preprocessing of the EEG data in EC condition. Data were visually inspected to detect bad channels. Bad channels detected along with ground and reference electrodes (AFz and FCz, resp.) were interpolated via an interpolation algorithm of the BESA software. A high-pass filter with a cutoff frequency at 1 Hz was chosen to remove low-frequency signals along with a low-pass filter with a cutoff frequency at 30 Hz removing high-frequency signals. Furthermore, a notch filter was used at 50 Hz in order to eliminate the industrial noise. Independent component analysis (ICA) decomposition was performed in the current screen of the EEG data (60 seconds) using the principal component analysis (PCA) technique. In more detail, the method underlying the ICA analysis is the extended ICA algorithm [72]. The dimensionality of data was reduced by PCA before ICA by ignoring all PCA components that explain less than 1% of the variance. Linear drifts, heart modulation, muscle contamination, artifacts induced by the participant's movements, and high-frequency noise were characterized as artifactual sources and removed. After reconstructing the whole dataset excluding noisy ICA components, data were visually inspected.

Ten random epochs of equal length (4 seconds) were extracted using ten random triggers and exporting an interval of 4000 ms around the triggers (−2000 ms to +2000 ms). An equal number of epochs (epochs = 10) was exported for both baseline and posttraining EEG recordings (EC).

Afterwards, the lead field matrix was obtained by the eConnectome toolbox relating 2054 scalp triangles to 7850 cortical dipoles [73, 74]. The lead field matrix is provided by means of a three-layer BEM model based on the Colin27 MNI brain [75]. The dipoles were restricted to the gray matter with perpendicular orientations towards the local cortical surface. Minimum norm estimate (MNE) was performed to solve the inverse problem by minimizing the source space energy given that the source dipoles' power is constrained by the cortex physiology [76]. Tikhonov regularization was applied through the Regularization Toolbox [77] to find the MNE solution. Additionally, we created eighteen custom-defined ROIs representing important nodes of the default mode network (DMN) at the surface of the cortex cortical model, in order to proceed to the computation of connectivity (Figure 2). The ROI time series signal was computed by averaging the signal of all included cortical current dipoles. ROI time series were computed for each node at each of the ten 4-second epochs for each subject.

The functional cortical connectivity between the 18 custom-defined nodes of DMN was evaluated by means of the directed transfer function (DTF) metric [78] with significance testing using surrogate data. DTF is a Granger causality measure [79] that uses the multivariate autoregressive model (MVAR) and describes the information flow between the node j and the node i at frequency f, producing weighted directed graphs. The order of the MVAR model was set to ten, based on SBC and FPE criteria as computed by the eConnectome software. For our analysis, DTF networks were computed at the frequency band of alpha rhythm at 8–12 Hz as alpha rhythm is the dominant brain rhythm at idling rest [80, 81]. DTF was computed between ROI time series of the network nodes at each of the ten 4-second epochs for each subject, producing 27*10*2 adjacency matrices (for the pre- and posttime conditions). The DTF adjacency matrices, corresponding to resting-state connectivity networks, were then compared between pre- and posttime conditions, in order to identify significantly altered connections. For this, we tested by false discovery rate (FDR) with 5000 permutations, using the NBS toolbox [82]. Following the aforementioned analysis design, we further explored possible differences in resting-state networks depending on gender.

2.5. Network Analysis. Network analysis was performed using the Brain Connectivity Toolbox (BCT) [83] for alpha band networks. The topological properties of the connectivity adjacency matrices were calculated using graph network analysis at each epoch for each subject. The topological

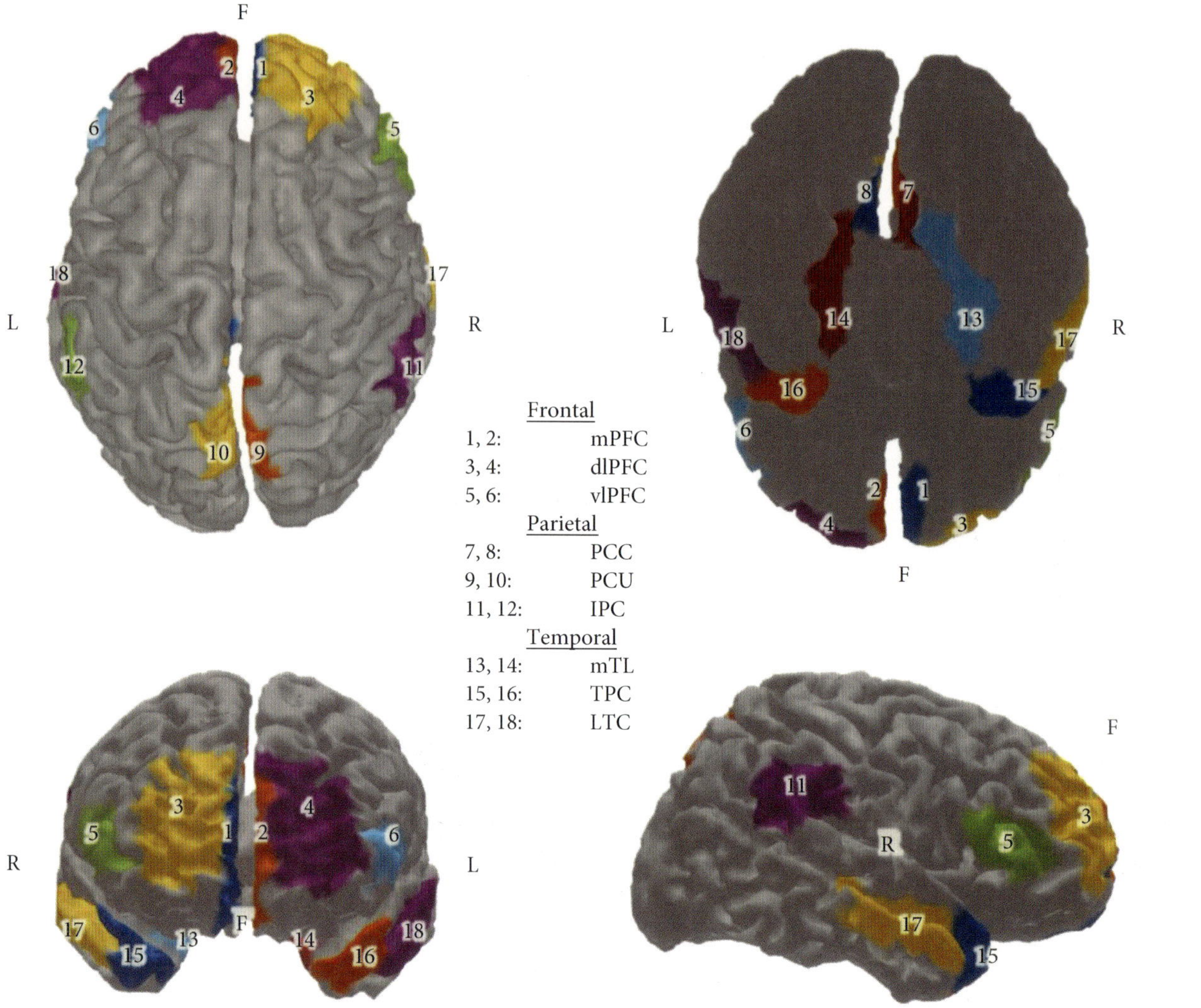

Figure 2: Defined regions of interest (ROIs) of the default mode network (DMN) on the Colin27 brain model. 1 and 2: medial prefrontal cortex (mPFC), 3 and 4: dorsolateral prefrontal cortex (dlPFC), 5 and 6: ventrolateral prefrontal cortex (vlPFC), 7 and 8: posterior cingulate cortex (PCC), 9 and 10: precuneus (PCU), 11 and 12: inferior parietal cortex (IPC), 13 and 14: medial temporal lobe (mTL), 15 and 16: temporal pole cortex (TPC), and 17 and 18: lateral temporal cortex (LTC). Even numbers correspond to the left hemisphere and odd numbers to the right hemisphere.

properties were then averaged across epochs for each subject, producing two average values of each property (detailed below) for the resting-state network of each subject, one at the pre- and one at the posttime condition. Characteristic path length (CPL), mean clustering coefficient (CC), and density (D), as well as the small-world (SW) measures were computed [84, 85]. Moreover, the in- and out-strengths values for each of the 18 nodes of the network were also calculated.

Characteristic path length (CPL) is the average shortest distance between node i and all other nodes, and it is considered as measure of integration [86, 87]. Mean clustering coefficient (CC), a measure of segregation, indicates the graph nodes' tendency to be organized in triangles [88, 89]. Density (D) is the number of actual connections among network nodes divided by the maximum possible connections. Small-world (SW) networks (small-world scalar is defined in [90, 91]) are characterized by a short path length that is indicative of communication efficiency along with a high clustering coefficient which represents a high suborganization [92, 93]. In our study, the comparison of CPL and CC in the SW metric was made against 10,000 random networks with the same number of connections and density to connectivity networks. The in-strength metric for each node (IS) was defined as the sum of the weights of all incoming connections to that node. The out-strength metric for each node (OS) was calculated by adding the weights of outgoing connections from that node [83, 85].

2.6. Statistical Analysis. All statistical analyses were performed using the IBM SPSS (version 23) and the level at which the null hypothesis is rejected was set as 5 out of 100 ($a = 0.05$).

2.6.1. Demographic Data. Demographic data were tested for normality assumption by visual inspection of histograms, normal Q-Q plots, and boxplots, checking skewness and kurtosis parameters [94–96], and using formal normality tests (Shapiro-Wilk test and Kolmogorov-Smirnov test) [97, 98] in order to calculate the appropriate measures of centrality and variation. As the variables age, education years, BMI index, and smoking dependence in months were approximately normally distributed, mean and standard deviation were calculated while median and interquartile range were calculated for the number of daily cigarettes. Moreover, we investigated gender differences in demographic data. Normality assumption was tested for demographics between male and female participants. Depending on the normality assumption, either t-test for independent samples or the Mann–Whitney U test was performed.

2.6.2. Clinical Data. Total oxidative stress/total oxidative capacity (TOS/TOC) was analyzed at the two time conditions in the twenty-two participants out of twenty-seven as the rest of the samples were not available. Differences in oxidative stress were initially explored using paired t-test, as they were continuous variables and approximately normally distributed. Exhaled CO levels were also compared both before and after biofeedback training using paired t-test. Additionally, we explored gender differences in clinical data. Using repeated measures analysis of variance, with gender as a covariate factor, could be an analysis of choice, but this was not followed because normality assumption was not met in every cell of the analysis. Thus, within-group changes in TOS and CO levels, respectively, were explored using the Wilcoxon Signed Ranks test or paired t-test after grouping by gender. Between-group differences of clinical data at the two time points were compared between male and female cohorts using the Mann–Whitney U test or independent samples t-test.

2.6.3. Behavioral Data. Total scores collected by neuropsychological tests and questionnaires such as the Fagerström Test, Minnesota Nicotine Withdrawal Scale, Beck Depression Inventory II (BDI II), State-Trait Anxiety Inventory I (STAI I) and II (STAI II), General Health Test, Rosenberg Self-Esteem Scale, and Motivation test were analyzed in this study. More precisely, score differences both before and after biofeedback training were calculated for each test or questionnaire. Score differences were tested for normality assumption using the aforementioned methodology (Section 2.6.1). Depending on normality assumption, different analyses were planned (paired t-tests or Wilcoxon Signed Ranks tests). However, total scores of Fagerström Test at the two time points were also converted into ordinal variables using the following formula: (a) scores from 0 to 3 were coded as low dependent, (b) scores from 4 to 6 were coded as medium dependent, and (c) scores from 7 to 10 were coded as high dependent [53]. In this case, differences between different levels of dependence at the two time points were investigated performing the McNemar-Bowker Test. In the case where differences between different levels of dependence reached statistical significance (p values < 0.05), McNemar tests were performed by two. In this case, p values were corrected for multiple comparisons using Bonferroni correction.

Gender differences were further explored in behavioral data. As data did not fit in the assumptions of repeated-measures ANOVA with a covariate, an alternative design was preferred. Score differences in neuropsychological tests and questionnaires were calculated and then tested for normality assumption between male and female participants. Depending on the normality assumption of score differences, within-group comparisons were performed using either paired t-test or the Wilcoxon Signed Ranks test after grouping data by gender. Independent samples t-test or the Mann–Whitney U tests were run for between-group comparisons.

2.6.4. Network Properties. Network properties such as CPL, mean CC, D, and SW, as well as IS and OS were calculated for each participant at the two time points. Differences (posttraining values − pretraining values) were computed for each property at the two time conditions and then tested for normality assumption. Different analyses were performed, either paired t-tests or the Wilcoxon Signed Ranks tests, at each network property depending on normality assumption. Possible within- and between-group differences depending on gender were explored using the same methodology as the one used in clinical and behavioral data.

3. Results

3.1. Demographic Data. The participants (male : female, 9 : 18) had a mean age of 50.52 years (range: 24–75, standard deviation (SD): 12.364), 15.04 mean education years (range: 3–27; SD: 4.743), and a mean BMI index of 26.31 (SD: 4.899). The median number of cigarettes smoked per day was 20 (range: 12.50–60.00 (cigarettes); IQR: 20.0–40.0) and mean smoking dependence was 358.50 months (range: 48–650 (months), SD: 152.95). Comparisons of demographics between male and female participants did not reveal any significant differences (education: $U = 44.00$; $p = 0.059$; BMI: $t = 1.356$; df $= 25$; $p = 0.187$; number of cigarettes per day: $U = 59.00$; $p = 0.241$; smoking dependence in months: $t = 1.477$; df $= 25$; $p = 0.152$) apart from age ($U = 40.00$; $p = 0.035$). More precisely, male participants were older than female participants (age—male: 58.00 (46.50, 70.00); female: 49.50 (41.00, 55.50)).

3.2. Clinical Data. Total oxidative stress seems to be nonsignificantly reduced after five sessions of BF training compared to the pretraining phase (TOS pretraining: 281.395; TOS posttraining: 222.506; $t = 1.014$; df $= 21$; $p = 0.322$). However, 13 out of 22 participants (59.09%) showed a TOS decrease at the posttraining phase evaluation. Exhaled CO levels were unaffected by the intervention as a nonsignificant increase was observed (exhaled CO levels pretraining (mean): 16.11; exhaled CO levels posttraining (mean): 16.89; $t = -0.496$; df $= 26$; $p = 0.624$). Although, the smoking status of the group does not seem to be significantly affected, 5 out of 27 participants (18.52%) showed exhaled CO levels lower than 8 ppm. A CO cutoff value of 8 ppm has been proposed to be able to discriminate smokers from nonsmokers [99, 100]. Exploring within-group changes and gender differences in TOS and

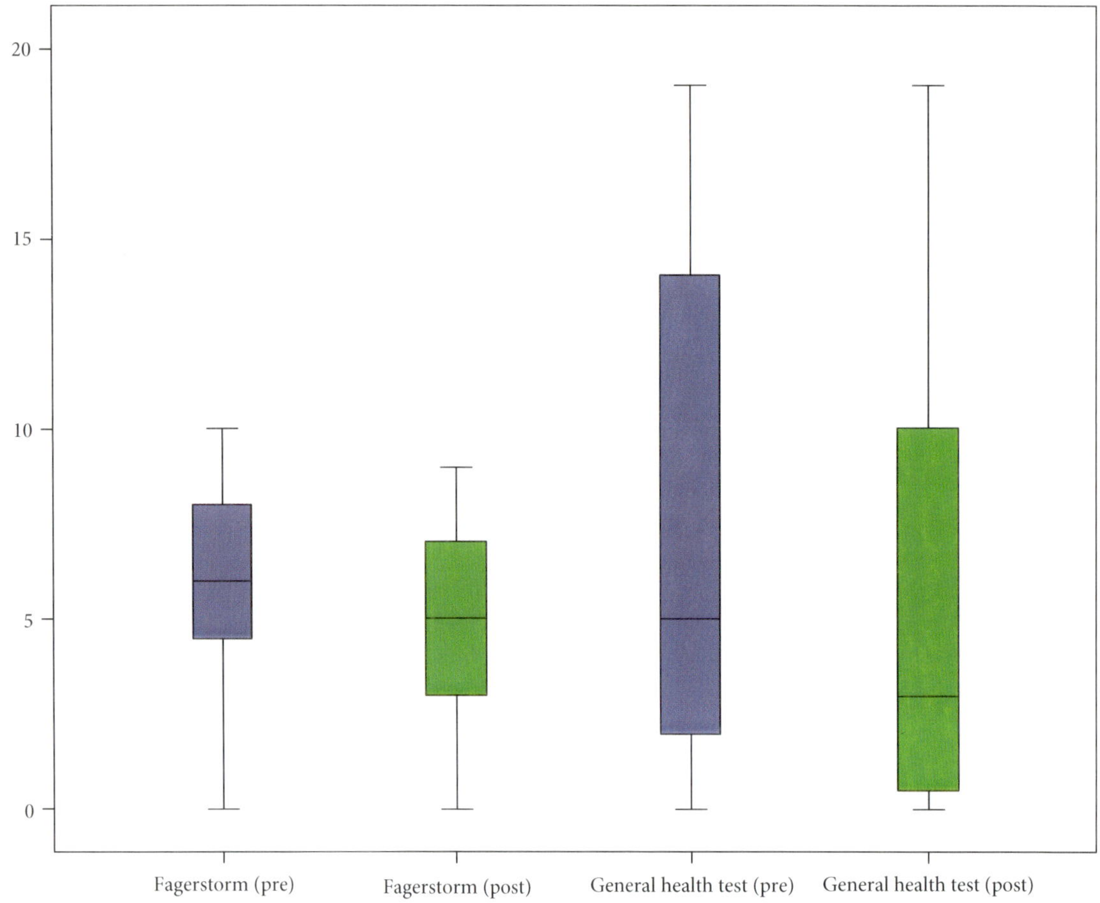

FIGURE 3: Boxplots of scores in Fagerström and General Health Tests at the two time points (pretraining, posttraining).

TABLE 1: A contingency table of participants regarding their nicotine dependence category at pretraining and posttraining phases.

Nicotine dependence in participants (pretraining)	Nicotine dependence in participants (posttraining)			Total
	Low-nicotine dependent	Moderate-nicotine dependent	High-nicotine dependent	
Low-nicotine dependent	5	0	0	5
Moderate-nicotine dependent	4	6	1	11
High-nicotine dependent	0	4	7	11
Total	9	10	8	27

exhaled CO levels, respectively, we did not find significant results (within-group CO: female: $W = -1.403$; $p = 0.161$; male: $W = -0.491$; $p = 0.623$; TOS: female: $t = -0.145$; df = 13; $p = 0.887$; male: $t = -1.261$; df = 7; $p = 0.248$; between-group TOS: $t = 1.143$; df = 20; $p = 0.267$; exhaled CO levels: $U = 71.00$; $p = 0.606$).

3.3. Behavioral Data. Analyzing behavioral data at the two time points, significant findings were observed in the Fagerström Test ($W = -2.404$; $p = 0.016$) and in the General Health Test ($W = -2.003$; $p = 0.045$). More precisely, scores in both tests were found to be decreased at the posttraining phase (Fagerström pretraining (median): 6.0; Fagerström posttraining (median): 5.0; General Health Test pretraining (median): 5.0; and General Health Test posttraining (median): 3.0) (Figure 3).

When Fagerström scores at the two time points were recoded into ordinal data according to the test guidelines, differences nearly reached significance ($\chi^2 = 5.80$; df = 3; $p = 0.055$; see below Table 1). Performing post hoc tests, no significant results between different levels of nicotine dependence were found (all p values > 0.05, Bonferroni corrected). As displayed in Figure 4, the number of participants with low-nicotine dependence increased (from 5 to 9 participants) whereas the number of participants with moderate- and high-nicotine dependence decreased (from 11 to 10 and from 11 to 8 participants, resp.).

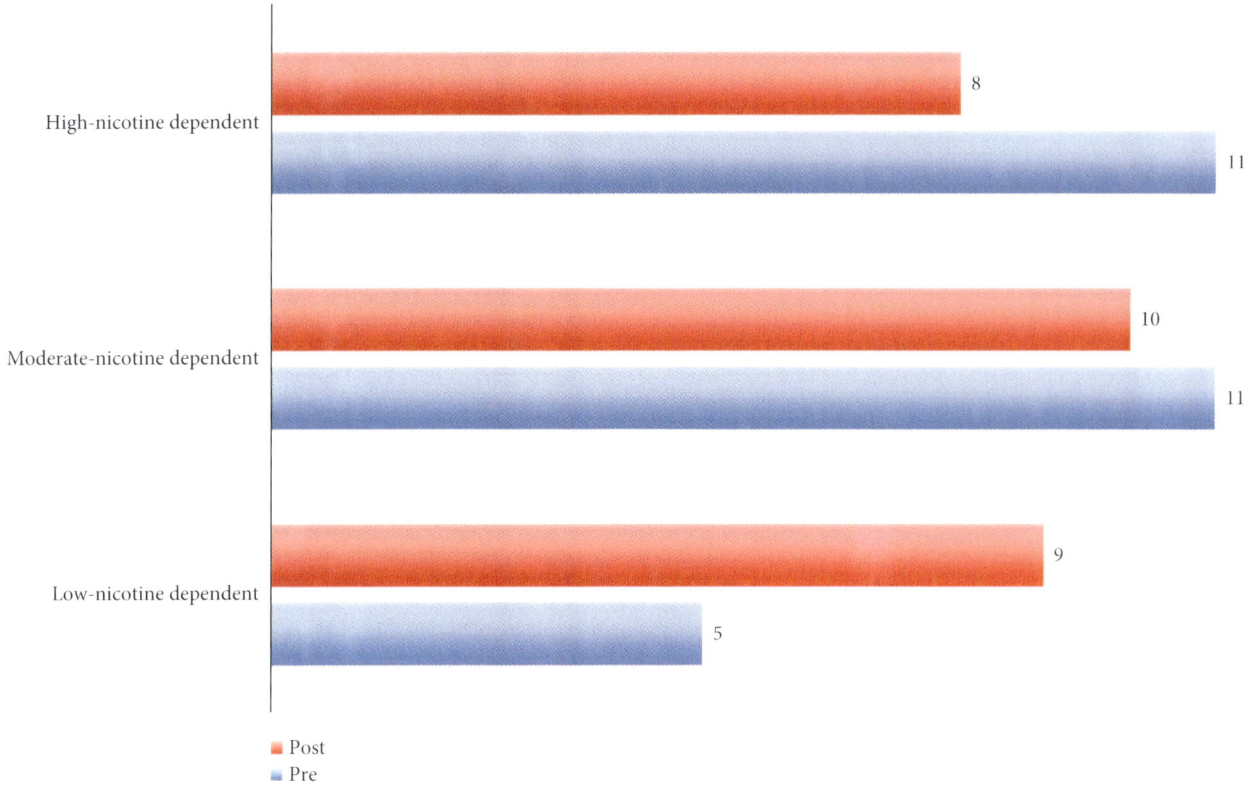

FIGURE 4: Number of participants in different nicotine dependence levels at the two time points of training.

In more detail, subjects who were characterized as low-nicotine dependent preserved their level of dependence whereas four moderate dependent participants turned to low-nicotine dependence level. Six participants remained at the moderate dependence level, as were initially characterized, while only one increased the level of dependence to high-nicotine dependence. Furthermore, four highly nicotine-dependent participants moved to the level of moderate dependence while at the same time seven preserved their level of nicotine dependence (Table 1).

Additionally, participants scored lower in the General Health Test which is considered as an overall screening tool for detecting psychiatric disorders [101] ($W = -2.003$; $p = 0.045$; General Health Test pretraining (median): 5.0; General Health Test posttraining (median): 3.0; see Figure 3).

Furthermore, participants seem to nonsignificantly decrease their withdrawal symptoms along with depressive and anxiety symptomatology as scores at Minnesota Nicotine Withdrawal Scale, BDI II, STAI I, and STAI II were observed to be decreased when comparing the two time conditions (Minnesota Nicotine Withdrawal Scale pretraining (mean): 28.185; Minnesota Nicotine Withdrawal Scale posttraining (mean): 24.815; BDI II pretraining (median): 16.0; BDI II posttraining (median): 14.0; STAI I pretraining (median): 40.50; STAI I posttraining (median): 38.50; STAI II pretraining (median): 50.0; and STAI II posttraining (median): 46.0). Subjective self-esteem was found to be slightly increased (Rosenberg pretraining (median): 20.0; Rosenberg posttraining (median): 20.136) after five sessions of skin temperature training while motivation scores were reduced (Motivation pretraining (mean): 32.444; Motivation posttraining (mean): 30.889). However, changes observed in the aforementioned tests when comparing the participants' scores at the two time conditions did not reach statistical significance (BDI II: $W = -0.243$; $p = 0.808$; STAI I: $W = -0.241$; $p = 0.809$; STAI II: $W = -1.590$; $p = 0.112$; Rosenberg: $W = -0.607$; $p = 0.544$; Motivation: $t = 1.129$; $df = 26$, $p = 0.269$). Additionally, planned comparisons in behavioral data between male and female participants did not result in significant gender differences (Minnesota Nicotine Withdrawal Scale: $U = 69.00$; $p = 0.536$; Fagerström Nicotine Dependence: $U = 44.00$; $p = 0.051$; BDI: $t = 0.704$; $df = 23$; $p = 0.488$; STAI I: $t = 0.764$; $df = 24$; $p = 0.452$; STAI II: $U = 58.00$, $p = 0.426$; General Health Test: $U = 63.50$; $p = 0.360$; Rosenberg: $U = 66.50$; $p = 0.450$; Motivation: $t = 1.654$; $df = 9.975$; $p = 0.129$). Female smokers did not show significant changes in any behavioral aspect tested (all p values > 0.05) while male smokers showed a significantly reduced degree of nicotine dependence (before training: 6.00, (5.50, 8.50); after training: 5.00, (3.00, 6.50); $W = -2.254$; $p = 0.024$) and scores at the General Health Test (before training: 7.00, (1.00, 15.50); after training: 3.00, (0.00, 10.00); $W = -2.154$; $p = 0.031$).

3.4. Resting-State Functional Connectivity Networks. The comparison of resting-state functional connectivity networks ($27^{*}10^{*}2$, where 27 is the number of participants, 10 is the number of epochs per subject, and 2 is the time conditions (pretraining, posttraining)) using the aforementioned NBS methodology (false discovery rate) did not produce any

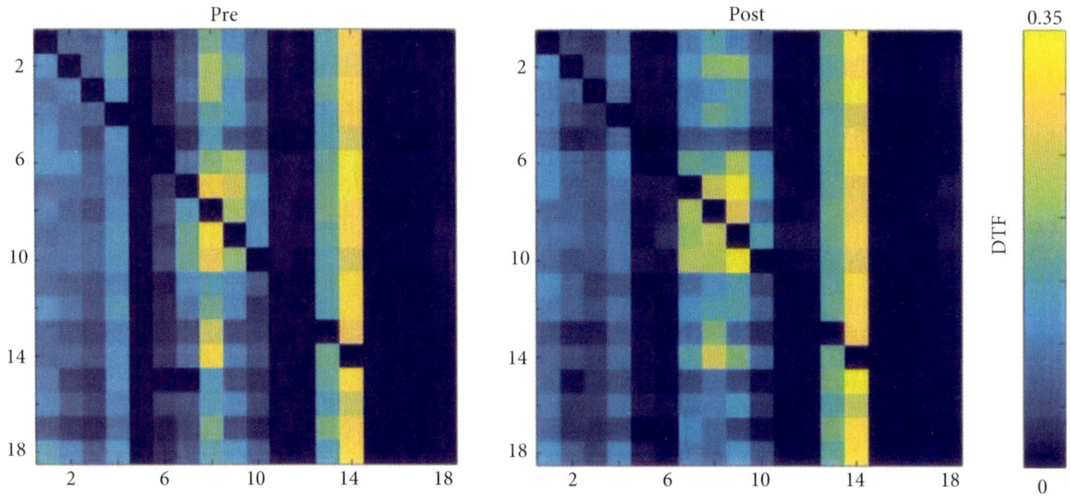

Figure 5: Adjacency matrices (average of all subjects across all epochs) of the resting-state network at prebiofeedback and postbiofeedback time conditions. Adjacency rows and columns correspond to the ROI labels defined in Figure 2.

significant results. Moreover, comparisons of resting-state functional connectivity networks depending on gender did not result in any significant changes. For visualization purposes, the resting-state functional connectivity networks were averaged by time condition (across all epochs and all subjects for pre- and posttime conditions). The grand averages for each time condition were depicted both as adjacency matrices (Figure 5) and as connectivity maps (Figure 6) using the BrainNet Viewer toolbox [102]. The mTL nodes bilaterally were identified as the most important hubs of information transfer, driving connections to almost every other node of the network at both time conditions (Figure 6). Connections originating from the left mTL, which were also above 50% of max information transfer, were also observed to be denser and presented greater information transfer than those from the right mTL. No node was disconnected from the resting-state network. Also, a cluster of nodes driving connections among themselves and to frontal area nodes was also identified involving the PCC and PCU nodes bilaterally and especially at the left hemisphere. These findings were relatively constant at both time conditions. With regards to total outgoing connection strengths (outflow) by network node, visualization was made using the eConnectome graphical tool (Figure 7). The nodes that contributed the most outgoing information flow to the resting-state network were the left and right mTL, left PCC, right PCU, left dlPFC, and right mPFC (Figure 7), both at pre and posttime conditions.

3.5. Network Properties. Exploring network properties (CC, CPL, D, and SW) at the two time conditions, we observed a slight increase in the network's density (D pretraining (mean): 0.432; D posttraining (mean): 0.444) whereas minimal decreases were found in other network properties such as mean CC (mean CC pretraining (mean): 0.068; mean CC posttraining (mean): 0.064), CPL (CPL pretraining (mean): 3.950; CPL posttraining (mean): 3.834) and SW (SW pretraining (median): 1.176; SW posttraining (median): 1.160). However, differences in the network's properties at the two time conditions did not reach statistical significance (mean CC: $t = 0.786$; df = 26; $p = 0.439$; CPL: $t = 0.889$; df = 26; $p = 0.382$; D: $t = -0.776$; df = 26; $p = 0.445$, SW: $W = -0.048$; $p = 0.962$). Similar findings were revealed when comparing network property changes at the two time points between male and female smokers (CPL: $t = 0.595$; df = 25; $p = 0.557$; CC: $t = -0.987$; df = 25; $p = 0.333$; D: $t = 0.435$; df = 25; $p = 0.667$; SW: $U = 69.00$; $p = 0.537$). Additionally, within-group comparisons did not reveal any significant change in network properties at both male and female participants (CPL—female: $t = -0.362$; df = 17; $p = 0.722$; male: $t = -1.063$; df = 8; $p = 0.319$; CC—female: $t = -1.084$; df = 17; $p = 0.293$; male: $t = 0.512$; df = 8; $p = 0.622$; D—female: $t = 0.830$; df = 17; $p = 0.418$; male: $t = 0.098$; df = 8; $p = 0.924$; SW—female: $W = -0.370$; $p = 0.711$; male: $W = -0.415$; $p = 0.678$).

The outflow of two nodes, as measured by out-strength, right vlPFC (Figure 8), and right TPC (Figure 9) was marginally significantly higher in the posttraining resting-state networks (right vlPFC pretraining (median): 0.0202; right vlPFC posttraining (median): 0.0728; right vlPFC: $W = -1.844$, $p = 0.065$; right TPC pretraining (median): 0.0242; right TPC posttraining (median): 0.0434; right TPC: $W = -1.890$, $p = 0.059$). Both nodes contributed connections to every other network node and to each other. Neither node was among the top contributors to network outflows in either time condition.

By exploring gender differences in inflow and outflow change, respectively, significant differences between male and female participants were found only in the outflow of the left mPFC ($t = -2.551$; df = 24.594; $p = 0.017$) and left PCU ($t = -2.780$; df = 24.982; $p = 0.010$). In more detail, networks of male smokers showed a greater change of outflow of these two nodes from pre- to posttraining compared to the female smokers (outflow change in left mPFC (mean (SD))—male smokers: 0.32 (0.24); female smokers: −0.07 (0.56); outflow change in left PCU (mean (SD))—male smokers: 0.32 (0.26); female smokers: −0.10 (0.54)).

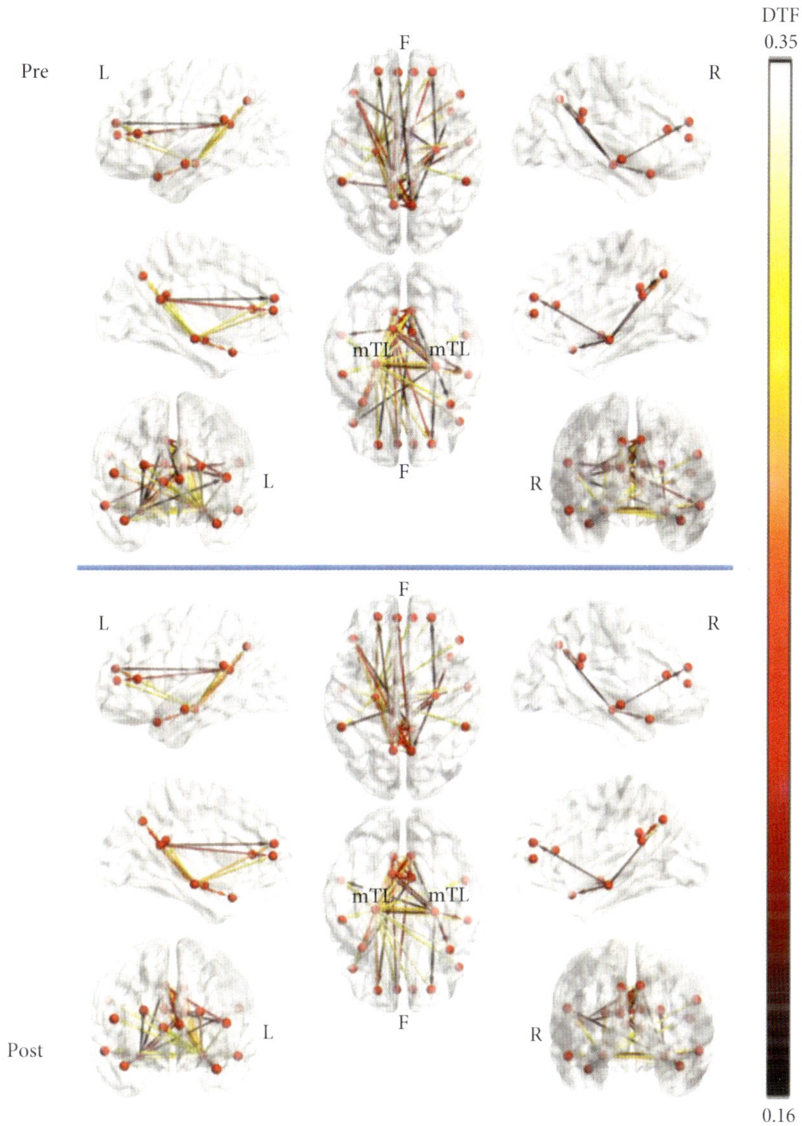

Figure 6: Connectivity maps of the resting-state network at pre- and posttime conditions (averaged for all subjects, across all epochs), only depicting connections above 50% of the max information flow. No statistically significant differences were computed for the whole network connectivity by NBS-FDR. The network is mainly driven at both conditions by the bilateral mTL nodes that both reach almost every network node and each other.

Within-group comparisons at the two time conditions revealed a significant increase in female participants' network inflow of right TPC ($W = -2.199$; $p = 0.028$; before training: 0.018 (0.005, 0.037); after training: 0.054 (0.017, 0.105)). In addition, a significant increase in male participants' network outflow out of the left mPFC ($t = 4.088$; $\mathrm{df} = 8$; $p = 0.003$; before training: 1.07 (0.24); after training: 1.39 (0.43)) and left PCU ($t = 3.785$; $\mathrm{df} = 8$; $p = 0.005$; before training: 1.28 (0.37); after training: 1.60 (0.39)) was also revealed.

4. Discussion

The main aim of the current study is to assess the impact of skin temperature biofeedback on cortical connectivity during resting state in a group of active smokers. Both stress and smoking induce changes in the connectivity between the main hubs of the resting-state networks of the cortex [103]. Hence, the goal of the present study was to investigate whether a biofeedback intervention that aims to alleviate the stress induced during a smoking-cessation attempt might play a protective role, affecting the reorganization of the resting-state cortical networks. A schematic representation of the research area explored is displayed in Figure 10. To this aim, we used a multimodal approach investigating clinical, behavioral, and neurophysiological (EEG) indices before and after the application of 5 sessions of skin temperature biofeedback. Stress seems to be involved at every stage of the nicotine dependence cycle, as we have already mentioned, from preparation to initiation of smoking up to episodes of relapse (Figure 10(b)). Individuals characterized by higher stress levels can be considered at high risk of adopting a smoking habit [20]. Various stress characteristics

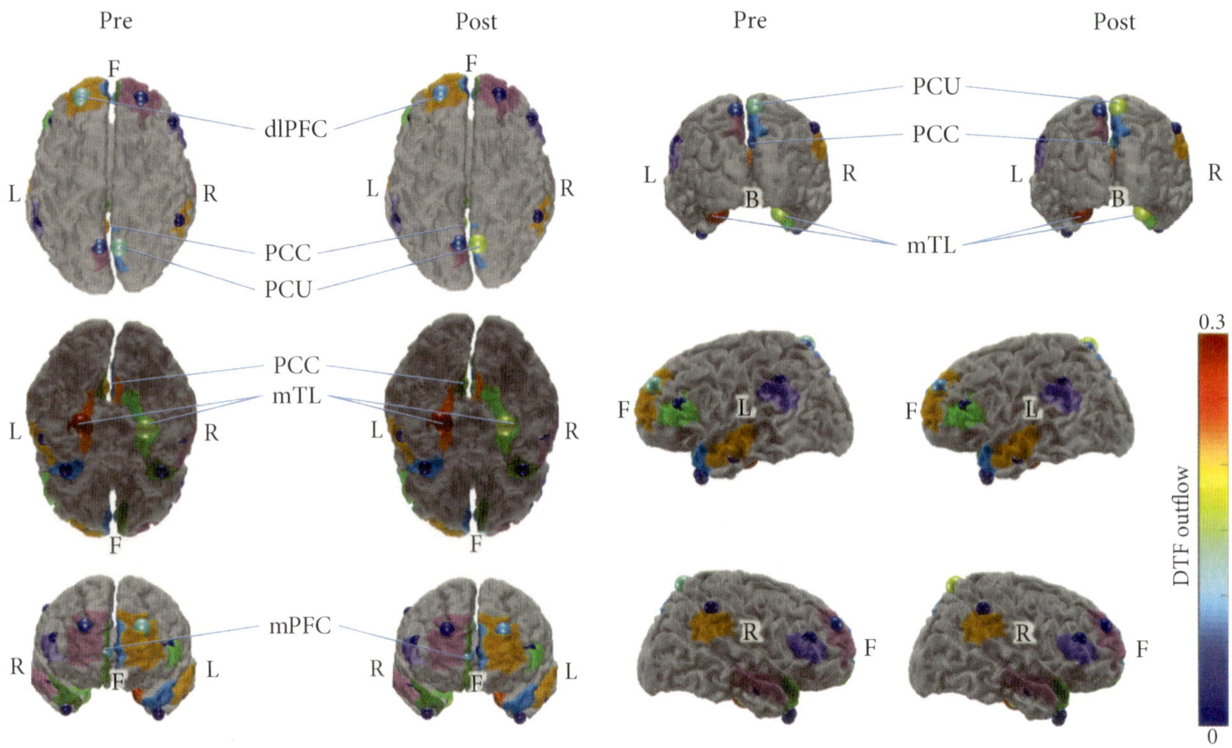

FIGURE 7: DTF outflows (out-strength) of each node of the resting-state network at pre- and posttime conditions, averaged for all subjects, across all epochs. Most significant contributions to outflow were observed for the following nodes: bilateral mTL (especially left), left PCC, right PCU, left dlPFC, and right mPFC.

and indices have been associated with different stages of the cycle [21–29, 31–35]. Although a causal link between stress and smoking appears well established, it has not been clarified whether and how intervening to alleviate stress can also meaningfully impact the behavioral aspects of a smoking habit. If such an effect can be identified, the mechanisms could be explored along the lines of covarying effects on different levels of brain function, the organization of resting-state self-referential networks, such as the DMN, being an obvious target. In this case, a protective role of biofeedback on the organization of cortical networks and stress reduction could present a meaningful connection that needs to be further investigated.

Regarding the physiological mechanisms of smoking-induced stress, multiple compounds of cigarette smoke, many of them being prooxidant and oxidant, are capable of increasing free radicals and enhancing oxidative stress in the organism [104, 105]. Free radicals are responsible for oxidative damage on multiple cellular tissues' constituents such as membrane protein lipids and DNA [106]. Additionally, the imbalance between the increased production of free radicals and decreased capacity of antioxidants leads to complicated pathological responses including an inflammatory immune response [107]. Results indicated that the total oxidative stress showed a nonsignificant decrease in the post-, compared to the preintervention measurement, implying that at a clinical level, 5 sessions of skin temperature biofeedback did not cause a significant decrease of stress-related clinical indices. Nonetheless, 13 out of 22 participants achieved a TOS decrease. Similarly, exhaled CO levels did not show significant change, indicating that the participants' smoking status [100, 108] was preserved. Although many factors could affect the exhaled CO levels, smoking constitutes the most likely cause [108]. Multiple studies have explored the optimal cutoff to discriminate smokers to nonsmokers, suggesting CO cutoffs of 6 ppm [108, 109], 8 ppm [99, 100], or 10 ppm [110, 111]. Even if our results did not suggest a significant change in the smoking status of the group, 5 participants to the total group of 27 showed exhaled CO levels lower than 8 ppm.

The behavioral data show an inconsistent result: while depressive and anxiety symptomatology was not significantly reduced, significant results were reached regarding the degree of nicotine dependence and the psychiatric symptomatology of the subjects, both of which appeared improved. Cortical functional connectivity between the 18 custom-defined nodes of DMN was evaluated by means of the DTF [78]. Importantly, the cortical network analysis revealed that biofeedback intervention did not cause a complete reorganization of the functional connectivity of the 18 nodes of DMN. Nonetheless, the analysis of the network properties of the resting-state network before and after the intervention revealed that there was a significant difference in the outflow of two nodes: the right vlPFC and the right TPC that both showed significantly greater out-strength in the postintervention resting-state networks compared to the preintervention measurement. This variation of results may be interpreted as an indication that biofeedback interventions,

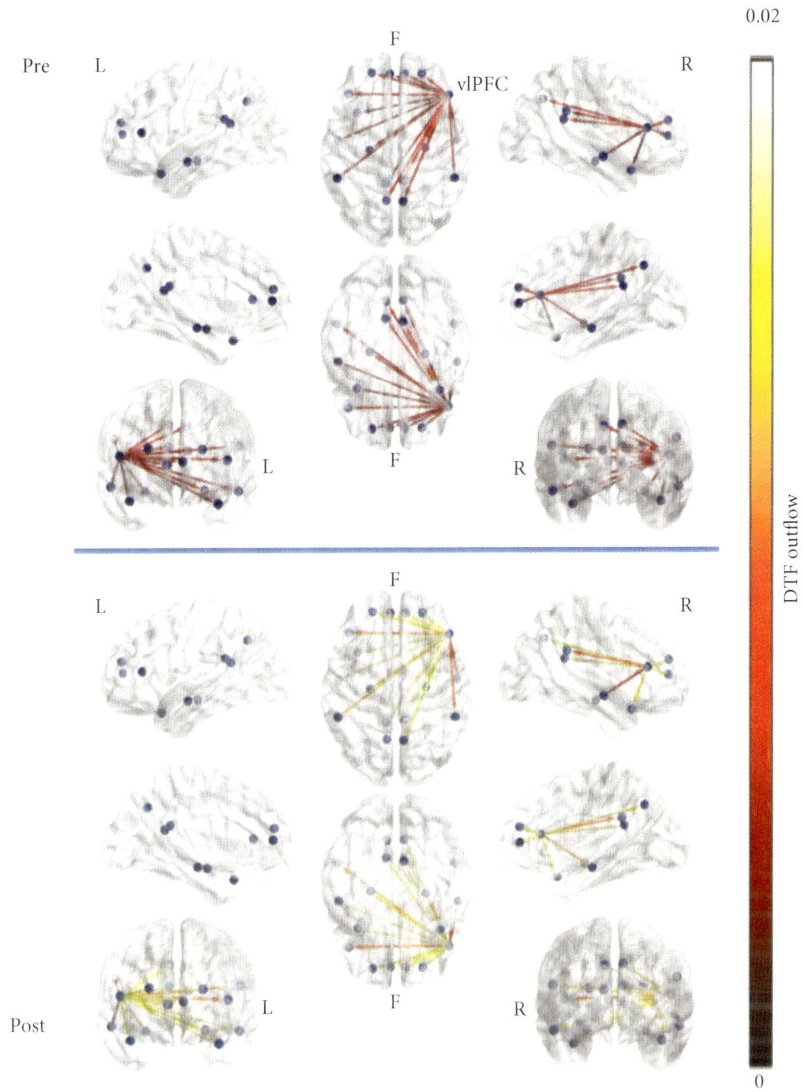

FIGURE 8: DTF outflow (outgoing weighted connections) of the right ventrolateral prefrontal cortex (vlPFC) node of the resting-state network at pre- and posttime conditions, averaged for all subjects, across all epochs. The node outflow was marginally significantly higher after biofeedback.

aiming at reducing stress in active smokers, could play a protective role against the addiction-related dysfunction of the resting-state functional connectivity [112]. Nonetheless, limitations of the intervention as applied in the current study may have reduced the corresponding effect size, hence limiting the effectiveness of the intervention.

The exploration of the properties of the pre- and postintervention networks revealed that the out-strength of the right vlPFC showed a significant increase in the postintervention compared to the preintervention measurement. vlPFC is a cortical region which is correlated to response inhibition and shows great involvement in addictive behaviors [113], while it is hypothesized to account for the declined cognition associated with addiction [114]. It shows anatomical connectivity with subcortical structures, such as the striatum and putamen [115] and temporal areas [116], supporting its role in emotional and working memory circuits. Based on the fact that vlPFC is strongly involved in working memory [117], its increased connectivity with the resting-state network could show a heightened attention involvement during the resting state [103] which may be related to smoking abstinence, as previous research shows [114]. Abnormal connectivity between medial PFC and lateral PFC in smokers has also been found in a previous resting-state fMRI study [118], highlighting the role of this region in nicotine addiction. A prominent theory regarding vlPFC is that it acts as a "circuit breaker" of ongoing cognitive processes when motivationally salient stimuli appear [119]. Its connections to the major nodes of the DMN imply a stronger coupling of large-scale resting networks, including the salience, default, and executive control networks in nicotine addiction. This finding is also in line with previous research in the field [112]. Importantly, the increase of its outgoing functional connectivity to the prominent DMN nodes indicates a positive reorganization of the network, minimizing negative affective states as well as deficits in cognitive abilities related with nicotine

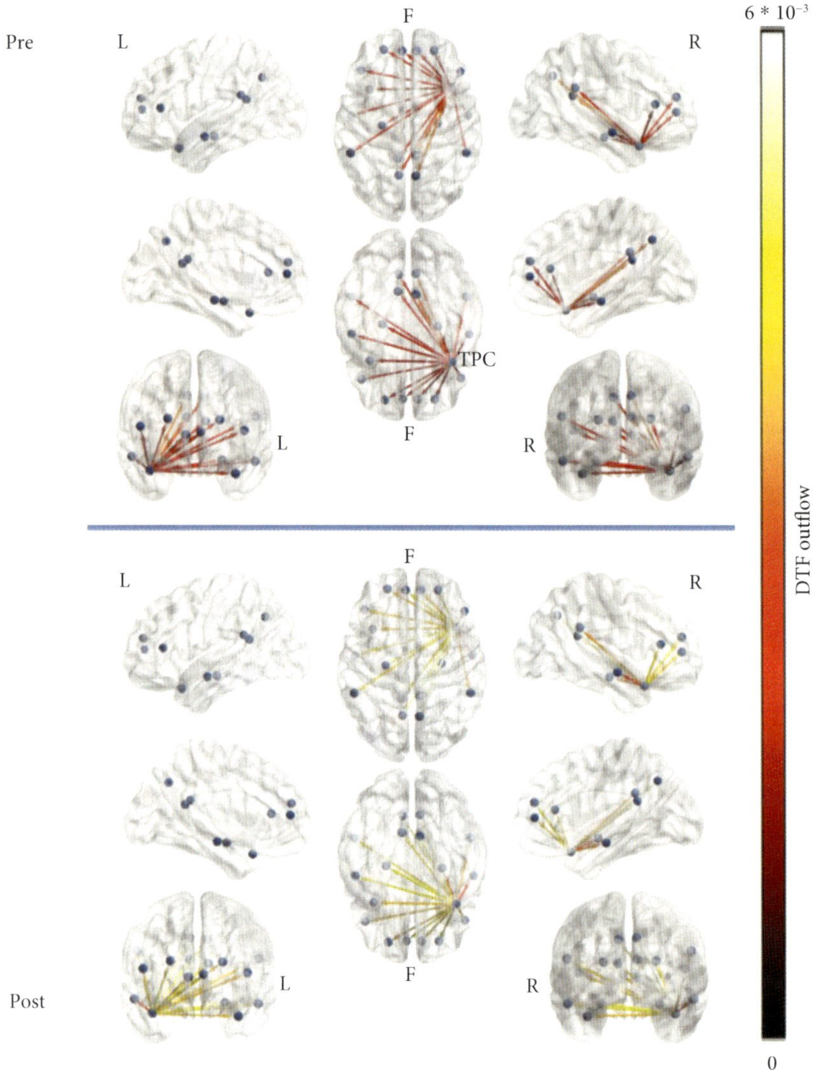

FIGURE 9: DTF outflow (outgoing weighted connections) of the right temporal pole cortex (TPC) node of the resting-state network at pre- and posttime conditions, averaged for all subjects, across all epochs. The node outflow was marginally significantly higher after biofeedback.

addiction. This is an interpretation which may be supported by the recent three-network model of addiction proposed by Sutherland et al. [120]. The fact that the increase of out-strength of this region compared to the rest of the network does not cause reorganization of the overall network, as shown in the corresponding analysis, is probably due to the fact that this node was not among the top contributors to the network outflows in either time condition.

Similarly to the network properties of vlPFC, the TPC also reveals a significant increase in its out-strength connectivity to the rest of the DMN nodes in the post- compared to the preintervention measurement. This region has been implicated in autobiographical memory in normal subjects [121]; it participates in various high-order cognitive functions including emotional processing [122], and it is highly associated with the DMN. A recent fMRI study also associates this region with nicotine dependence severity [123], while the reduced functional connectivity of this region is associated with emotional dysfunction [124]. Hence, the increase of TPC functional connectivity outflow could be indicative that the biofeedback intervention may have contributed to a protective reorganization in the DMN. A possible mechanism can be explored along the enhancement of network components that are related to positive emotional and autobiographical processing. The TPC has been associated with the integration of information from diverse modalities and has been shown to strengthen its coupling to the areas it modulates through emotional music [125]. Our BF paradigm incorporates pleasant relaxing audio and video, that is played on when the subject succeeds in the temperature increase task, suggesting a possible mechanism for the observed enhancement of TPC connectivity. Furthermore, female participants also significantly increased inflow to this area, something that could be explored along the lines of gender differences, since females have been shown to be more responsive to emotional stimuli [126]. In accordance to the vlPFC results, the significant out-strength or in-strength increases of TPC did not reorganize the overall DMN. This

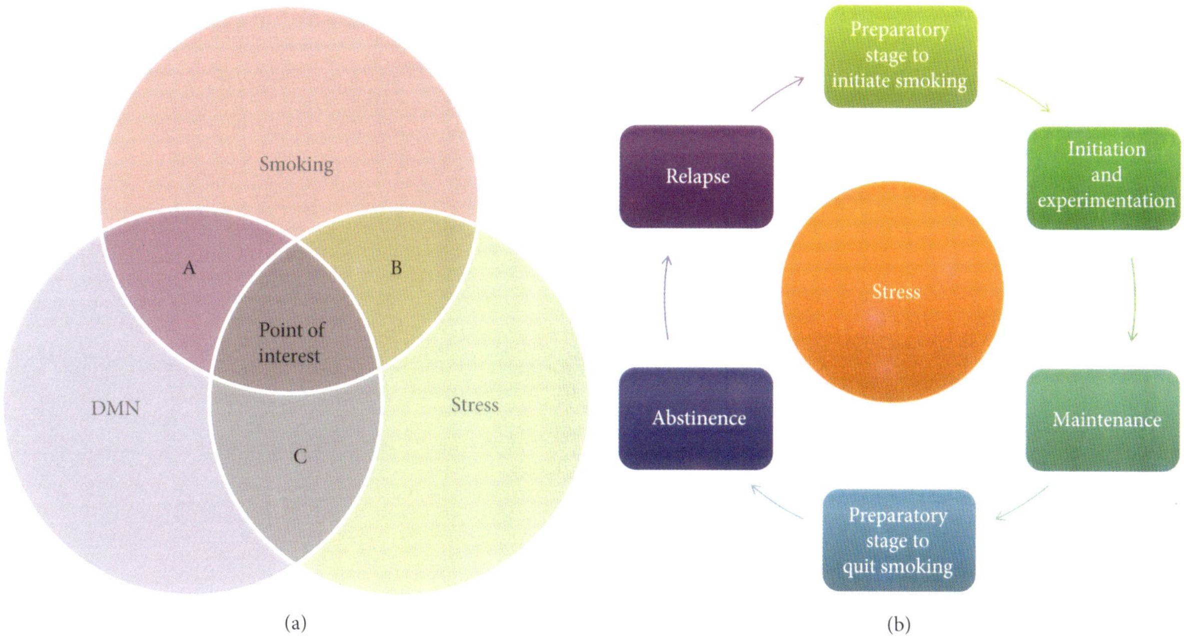

FIGURE 10: A schematic representation of research areas explored (a) and of the relation of nicotine addiction cycle to stress (b). The nicotine addiction cycle seems to involve stress at every stage from preparation to initiation of smoking up to relapse.

may be grounded to the fact that TPC was not a strong contributor in the outflow of the overall DMN. Nonetheless, the increase of its out-flow is significant, supporting the interpretation of protective neuroplastic resting-state connectivity changes induced by the biofeedback intervention.

Significant increases were also indeed found in male participants' network outflow out of the left mPFC and left PCU after BF training, both being core nodes of the DMN. Although these nodes presented in general higher outflow than right vlPFC and right TPC, they still did not count among the top outflow contributors of the network either before or after training and, thus, they also did not cause overall network reorganization. It has been proposed that mPFC is involved in learning associations of multimodal information and corresponding emotional responses [127], while PCU is involved in episodic memory retrieval and emotional stimuli processing. In the meantime, as already mentioned, a number of studies have reported neurocognitive dysfunction in stress and smoking, associated with addiction, award-related mechanisms, and emotional association, as portrayed in enhanced connectivity of prefrontal areas and the precuneus [6–14]. BF training, through its own award-related mechanism, could be activating the affected areas in a similar way, thus suggesting an improvement of the person's capability to learn a positive neurocognitive response, previously affected by addiction and stress. It is unclear whether this response can be explained in terms of gender differences; its sustainability in time remains to be investigated as well.

As we already discussed, despite some promising indications, a number of limitations should be identified. A limited number of sessions were only performed in the current study limiting the possible effectiveness of the intervention. However, the number of training sessions was chosen close to that suggested by Peniston and Kulkosky [70]. Also, the sessions were more than those used in Hartwell et al. [128]. To the best of our knowledge, guidelines for optimal skin temperature training intensity in adult smokers have not been established yet. Additionally, planned comparisons depending on gender revealed a significant difference in age between male and female smokers included in this study. Male smokers were older than female smokers as most of them were COPD patients. As repeated-measures analysis of variance with covariates could not be performed due to deviations from analysis assumptions, the age effect could not be controlled, consisting a limitation of our analysis. Moreover when considering the effect of neuromodulation, it can be argued that neurofeedback is a more direct and more appropriate method to promote plasticity of functional connectivity networks and should be incorporated into an intervention designed to take advantage of an existing causal link of stress and smoking with regards to brain connectivity. This is also the case with the SmokeFreeBrain project, where multiple sessions of neurofeedback are also introduced in later phases of the intervention. In our future work, we aim to longitudinally investigate the effects of both methods in the resting-state networks of smokers. Along that line, approaches tailored to individual needs could also be considered. Finally, a more detailed approach to resting-state network connectivity could explore the effects of neuromodulation, as an intervention for stress and smoking, on resting-state network interdependencies, among the DMN and the networks tasked with salience, attention, and executive functions.

5. Conclusions

The clinical status of active smokers was not significantly modified after five sessions of biofeedback training. The behavioral data showed mixed results; while depressive and anxiety symptomatology were not significantly reduced, significant improvement was observed in the degree of nicotine dependence and the psychiatric symptomatology of the subjects. The cortical network analysis revealed that this type of short-term biofeedback training did not lead to a complete reorganization of the functional connectivity of the DMN nodes. However, marginally significant differences in the information outflow of two nodes, the right vlPFC and the right TPC, towards the other DMN nodes were indeed found. These information outflow enhancements from both nodes to the prominent DMN nodes may indicate a positive reorganization of the network, minimizing negative affective states. However, these increases in information outflow were not sufficient to reorganize the overall DMN connectivity as the nodes implicated were not among the top contributors in the outflow of the overall DMN. Our results could be interpreted as an indication that short-term biofeedback training, focusing on stress alleviation in active smokers, may play a protective role against the addiction-related dysfunction of resting-state functional connectivity, thereby preparing the grounds for extended neurofeedback training.

Ethical Approval

This study was conducted in accordance with the Declaration of Helsinki (1964) and its following amendments. Approval was obtained by the Bioethics Committee of the Medical School of the Aristotle University of Thessaloniki.

Acknowledgments

The study was conducted in the framework of the SmokeFreeBrain project funded by the European Union's Horizon 2020 research and innovation program under the agreement stipulated under Grant no. 681120.

References

[1] K. Christoff, Z. C. Irving, K. C. R. Fox, R. N. Spreng, and J. R. Andrews-Hanna, "Mind-wandering as spontaneous thought: a dynamic framework," *Nature Reviews Neuroscience*, vol. 17, no. 11, pp. 718–731, 2016.

[2] E. DuPre and R. N. Spreng, "Structural covariance networks across the life span, from 6 to 94 years of age," *Network Neuroscience*, vol. 1, no. 3, pp. 302–323, 2017.

[3] M. E. Raichle, A. M. MacLeod, A. Z. Snyder, W. J. Powers, D. A. Gusnard, and G. L. Shulman, "A default mode of brain function," *Proceedings of the National Academy of Sciences of the United States of America*, vol. 98, no. 2, pp. 676–682, 2001.

[4] J. Tanabe, E. Nyberg, L. F. Martin et al., "Nicotine effects on default mode network during resting state," *Psychopharmacology*, vol. 216, no. 2, pp. 287–295, 2011.

[5] R. R. Wetherill, Z. Fang, K. Jagannathan, A. R. Childress, H. Rao, and T. R. Franklin, "Cannabis, cigarettes, and their co-occurring use: disentangling differences in default mode network functional connectivity," *Drug and Alcohol Dependence*, vol. 153, pp. 116–123, 2015.

[6] G. E. Swan and C. N. Lessov-Schlaggar, "The effects of tobacco smoke and nicotine on cognition and the brain," *Neuropsychology Review*, vol. 17, no. 3, pp. 259–273, 2007.

[7] F. Lin, G. Wu, L. Zhu, and H. Lei, "Altered brain functional networks in heavy smokers," *Addiction Biology*, vol. 20, no. 4, pp. 809–819, 2015.

[8] A. C. Janes, L. D. Nickerson, B. d B. Frederick, and M. J. Kaufman, "Prefrontal and limbic resting state brain network functional connectivity differs between nicotine-dependent smokers and non-smoking controls," *Drug and Alcohol Dependence*, vol. 125, no. 3, pp. 252–259, 2012.

[9] B. J. Weiland, A. Sabbineni, V. D. Calhoun, R. C. Welsh, and K. E. Hutchison, "Reduced executive and default network functional connectivity in cigarette smokers," *Human Brain Mapping*, vol. 36, no. 3, pp. 872–882, 2015.

[10] L. E. Hong, H. Gu, Y. Yang et al., "Association of nicotine addiction and nicotine's actions with separate cingulate cortex functional circuits," *Archives of General Psychiatry*, vol. 66, no. 4, pp. 431–441, 2009.

[11] G. Tsourtos, P. R. Ward, and R. Muller, "Smoking and stress: the double-edged sword of living in a disadvantaged area," *Australasian Medical Journal*, vol. 1, no. 1, pp. 1–17, 2008.

[12] J. D. Kassel, L. R. Stroud, and C. A. Paronis, "Smoking, stress, and negative affect: correlation, causation, and context across stages of smoking," *Psychological Bulletin*, vol. 129, no. 2, pp. 270–304, 2003.

[13] J. M. Soares, A. Sampaio, L. M. Ferreira et al., "Stress impact on resting state brain networks," *PLoS One*, vol. 8, no. 6, article e66500, 2013.

[14] B. Clemens, L. Wagels, M. Bauchmüller, R. Bergs, U. Habel, and N. Kohn, "Alerted default mode: functional connectivity changes in the aftermath of social stress," *Scientific Reports*, vol. 7, article 40180, 2017.

[15] O. F. Pomerleau and C. S. Pomerleau, "Research on stress and smoking: progress and problems," *British Journal of Addiction*, vol. 86, no. 5, pp. 599–603, 1991.

[16] D. Choi, S. Ota, and S. Watanuki, "Does cigarette smoking relieve stress? Evidence from the event-related potential (ERP)," *International Journal of Psychophysiology*, vol. 98, no. 3, pp. 470–476, 2015.

[17] D. G. Gilbert, "Paradoxical tranquilizing and emotion-reducing effects of nicotine," *Psychological Bulletin*, vol. 86, no. 4, pp. 643–661, 1979.

[18] A. C. Parrott, "Nesbitt's Paradox resolved? Stress and arousal modulation during cigarette smoking," *Addiction*, vol. 93, no. 1, pp. 27–39, 1998.

[19] B. R. Flay, "Youth tobacco use: risks, patterns, and control," in *Nicotine addiction: Principles and Management*, C. T. Orleans and J. D. Slade, Eds., pp. 365–384, Oxford University Press, New York, NY, USA, 1993.

[20] D. Patton, G. E. Barnes, and R. P. Murray, "Personality characteristics of smokers and ex-smokers," *Personality and Individual Differences*, vol. 15, no. 6, pp. 653–664, 1993.

[21] J. J. Koval, L. L. Pederson, C. A. Mills, G. A. McGrady, and S. C. Carvajal, "Models of the relationship of stress, depression, and other psychosocial factors to smoking behavior: a

comparison of a cohort of students in grades 6 and 8," *Preventive Medicine*, vol. 30, no. 6, pp. 463–477, 2000.

[22] S. Dugan, B. Lloyd, and K. Lucas, "Stress and coping as determinants of adolescent smoking behavior 1," *Journal of Applied Social Psychology*, vol. 29, no. 4, pp. 870–886, 1999.

[23] L. Siqueira, M. Diab, C. Bodian, and L. Rolnitzky, "Adolescents becoming smokers: the roles of stress and coping methods," *The Journal of Adolescent Health*, vol. 27, no. 6, pp. 399–408, 2000.

[24] R. F. Anda, J. B. Croft, V. J. Felitti et al., "Adverse childhood experiences and smoking during adolescence and adulthood," *JAMA*, vol. 282, no. 17, pp. 1652–1658, 1999.

[25] J. J. Koval and L. L. Pederson, "Stress-coping and other psychosocial risk factors: a model for smoking in grade 6 students," *Addictive Behaviors*, vol. 24, no. 2, pp. 207–218, 1999.

[26] T. L. Conway, R. R. Vickers Jr, H. W. Ward, and R. H. Rahe, "Occupational stress and variation in cigarette, coffee, and alcohol consumption," *Journal of Health and Social Behavior*, vol. 22, no. 2, pp. 155–165, 1981.

[27] W. L. Hellerstedt and R. W. Jeffery, "The association of job strain and health behaviours in men and women," *International Journal of Epidemiology*, vol. 26, no. 3, pp. 575–583, 1997.

[28] J. Ogden and T. Mtandabari, "Examination stress and changes in mood and health related behaviours," *Psychology & Health*, vol. 12, no. 2, pp. 289–299, 1997.

[29] A. Steptoe, J. Wardle, T. M. Pollard, L. Canaan, and G. J. Davies, "Stress, social support and health-related behavior: a study of smoking, alcohol consumption and physical exercise," *Journal of Psychosomatic Research*, vol. 41, no. 2, pp. 171–180, 1996.

[30] K. A. Perkins, J. E. Grobe, C. Fonte, and M. Breus, ""Paradoxical" effects of smoking on subjective stress versus cardiovascular arousal in males and females," *Pharmacology, Biochemistry, and Behavior*, vol. 42, no. 2, pp. 301–311, 1992.

[31] L. H. Epstein and F. L. Collins Jr, "The measurement of situational influences of smoking," *Addictive Behaviors*, vol. 2, no. 1, pp. 47–53, 1977.

[32] J. E. Rose, S. Ananda, and M. E. Jarvik, "Cigarette smoking during anxiety-provoking and monotonous tasks," *Addictive Behaviors*, vol. 8, no. 4, pp. 353–359, 1983.

[33] D. R. Cherek, "Effects of acute exposure to increased levels of background industrial noise on cigarette smoking behavior," *International Archives of Occupational and Environmental Health*, vol. 56, no. 1, pp. 23–30, 1985.

[34] G. L. Mangan and J. F. Golding, *The Psychopharmacology of Smoking*, Cambridge University Press, New York, 1984.

[35] C. S. Pomerleau and O. F. Pomerleau, "The effects of a psychological stressor on cigarette smoking and subsequent behavioral and physiological responses," *Psychophysiology*, vol. 24, no. 3, pp. 278–285, 1987.

[36] S. Cohen and E. Lichtenstein, "Perceived stress, quitting smoking, and smoking relapse," *Health Psychology*, vol. 9, no. 4, pp. 466–478, 1990.

[37] T. H. Brandon, S. T. Tiffany, K. M. Obremski, and T. B. Baker, "Postcessation cigarette use: the process of relapse," *Addictive Behaviors*, vol. 15, no. 2, pp. 105–114, 1990.

[38] R. Borland, "Slip-ups and relapse in attempts to quit smoking," *Addictive Behaviors*, vol. 15, no. 3, pp. 235–245, 1990.

[39] K. M. Cummings, C. R. Jaén, and G. Giovino, "Circumstances surrounding relapse in a group of recent exsmokers," *Preventive Medicine*, vol. 14, no. 2, pp. 195–202, 1985.

[40] S. Shiffman, "Relapse following smoking cessation: a situational analysis," *Journal of Consulting and Clinical Psychology*, vol. 50, no. 1, pp. 71–86, 1982.

[41] S. Shiffman, M. Hickcox, J. A. Paty, M. Gnys, J. D. Kassel, and T. J. Richards, "Progression from a smoking lapse to relapse: prediction from abstinence violation effects, nicotine dependence, and lapse characteristics," *Journal of Consulting and Clinical Psychology*, vol. 64, no. 5, pp. 993–1002, 1996.

[42] M. C. Davis and K. A. Matthews, "Cigarette smoking and oral contraceptive use influence women's lipid, lipoprotein, and cardiovascular responses during stress," *Health Psychology*, vol. 9, no. 6, pp. 717–736, 1990.

[43] J. M. MacDougall, L. Musante, S. Castillo, and M. C. Acevedo, "Smoking, caffeine, and stress: effects on blood pressure and heart rate in male and female college students," *Health Psychology*, vol. 7, no. 5, pp. 461–478, 1988.

[44] O. F. Pomerleau and C. S. Pomerleau, "Cortisol response to a psychological stressor and/or nicotine," *Pharmacology, Biochemistry, and Behavior*, vol. 36, no. 1, pp. 211–213, 1990.

[45] K. S. Calderon and W. W. Thompson, "Biofeedback relaxation training: a rediscovered mind-body tool in public health," *American Journal of Health Studies*, vol. 19, no. 4, pp. 185–194, 2004.

[46] J. N. Demos, *Getting Started with Neurofeedback*, W.W. Norton & Co., 2005.

[47] H. D. Critchley, R. N. Melmed, E. Featherstone, C. J. Mathias, and R. J. Dolan, "Brain activity during biofeedback relaxation: a functional neuroimaging investigation," *Brain*, vol. 124, no. 5, pp. 1003–1012, 2001.

[48] P. Karthikeyan, M. Murugappan, and S. Yaacob, "Descriptive analysis of skin temperature variability of sympathetic nervous system activity in stress," *Journal of Physical Therapy Science*, vol. 24, no. 12, pp. 1341–1344, 2012.

[49] R. Morecraft, W. F. Blair, T. D. Brown, and R. H. Gable, "Acute effects of smoking on digital artery blood flow in humans," *The Journal of Hand Surgery*, vol. 19, no. 1, pp. 1–7, 1994.

[50] L. N. A. van Adrichem, S. E. R. Hovius, R. van Strik, and J. C. van der Meulen, "Acute effects of cigarette smoking on microcirculation of the thumb," *British Journal of Plastic Surgery*, vol. 45, no. 1, pp. 9–11, 1992.

[51] R. M. Gilbert and M. A. Pope, "Early effects of quitting smoking," *Psychopharmacology*, vol. 78, no. 2, pp. 121–127, 1982.

[52] P. D. Bamidis, E. Paraskevopoulos, E. Konstantinidis, D. Spachos, and A. Billis, "Multimodal e-Health services for smoking cessation and public health: the SmokeFreeBrain project approach," *Studies in Health Technology and Informatics*, vol. 245, pp. 5–9, 2017.

[53] T. F. Heatherton, L. T. Kozlowski, R. C. Frecker, and K. O. Fagerstrom, "The Fagerström test for nicotine dependence: a revision of the Fagerström tolerance questionnaire," *Addiction*, vol. 86, no. 9, pp. 1119–1127, 1991.

[54] S. J. Curry, L. Grothaus, and C. McBride, "Reasons for quitting: intrinsic and extrinsic motivation for smoking cessation in a population-based sample of smokers," *Addictive Behaviors*, vol. 22, no. 6, pp. 727–739, 1997.

[55] L. Biener and D. B. Abrams, "The contemplation ladder: validation of a measure of readiness to consider smoking cessation," *Health Psychology*, vol. 10, no. 5, pp. 360–365, 1991.

[56] J. R. Hughes and D. Hatsukami, "Signs and symptoms of tobacco withdrawal," *Archives of General Psychiatry*, vol. 43, no. 3, pp. 289–294, 1986.

[57] A. T. Beck, C. H. Ward, M. Mendelson, J. Mock, and J. Erbaugh, "An inventory for measuring depression," *Archives of General Psychiatry*, vol. 4, no. 6, p. 561, 1961.

[58] C. D. Spielberger, R. L. Gorsuch, R. Lushene, P. R. Vagg, and G. A. Jacobs, *Manual for the State-Trait Anxiety Inventory*, Consulting Psychologists Press, Palo Alto, CA, USA, 1983.

[59] D. P. Goldberg and V. F. Hillier, "A scaled version of the General Health Questionnaire," *Psychological Medicine*, vol. 9, no. 1, p. 139, 1979.

[60] M. Rosenberg, *Society and the adolescent self-image*, Princeton University Press, Princeton, NJ, USA, 1965.

[61] The Whoqol Group, "The World Health Organization quality of life assessment (WHOQOL): development and general psychometric properties," *Social Science & Medicine*, vol. 46, no. 12, pp. 1569–1585, 1998.

[62] R. F. Pokrzywinski, D. M. Meads, S. P. McKenna, G. A. Glendenning, and D. A. Revicki, "Development and psychometric assessment of the COPD and Asthma Sleep Impact Scale (CASIS)," *Health and Quality of Life Outcomes*, vol. 7, no. 1, p. 98, 2009.

[63] P. W. Jones, G. Harding, P. Berry, I. Wiklund, W.-H. Chen, and N. Kline Leidy, "Development and first validation of the COPD Assessment Test," *The European Respiratory Journal*, vol. 34, no. 3, pp. 648–654, 2009.

[64] E. P. Grammatopoulou, N. Stavrou, P. Myrianthefs et al., "Validity and reliability evidence of the Asthma Control Test—ACT in Greece," *Journal of Asthma*, vol. 48, no. 1, pp. 57–64, 2011.

[65] J. R. Stroop, "Studies of interference in serial verbal reactions," *Psychological Monographs*, vol. 18, no. 6, pp. 643–662, 1935.

[66] T. N. Tombaugh, "Trail Making Test A and B: normative data stratified by age and education," *Archives of Clinical Neuropsychology*, vol. 19, no. 2, pp. 203–214, 2004.

[67] D. Wechsler, *WAIS-R Manual: Wechsler Adult Intelligence Scale-revised*, Psychological Corporation, 1981.

[68] R. Oostenveld and P. Praamstra, "The five percent electrode system for high-resolution EEG and ERP measurements," *Clinical Neurophysiology*, vol. 112, no. 4, pp. 713–719, 2001.

[69] R. Näätänen, S. Pakarinen, T. Rinne, and R. Takegata, "The mismatch negativity (MMN): towards the optimal paradigm," *Clinical Neurophysiology*, vol. 115, no. 1, pp. 140–144, 2004.

[70] E. G. Peniston and P. J. Kulkosky, "Alpha-theta brainwave training and beta-endorphin levels in alcoholics," *Alcoholism, Clinical and Experimental Research*, vol. 13, no. 2, pp. 271–279, 1989.

[71] P. Niki, K. Maria, F. Christos, and B. Panagiotis, "Exploring the efficacy of biofeedback training in smoking addiction: a SFB pilot study," *Frontiers in Human Neuroscience*, vol. 10, 2016.

[72] T. W. Lee, M. Girolami, and T. J. Sejnowski, "Independent component analysis using an extended infomax algorithm for mixed subgaussian and supergaussian sources," *Neural Computation*, vol. 11, no. 2, pp. 417–441, 1999.

[73] F. Babiloni, F. Cincotti, C. Babiloni et al., "Estimation of the cortical functional connectivity with the multimodal integration of high-resolution EEG and fMRI data by directed transfer function," *NeuroImage*, vol. 24, no. 1, pp. 118–131, 2005.

[74] B. He, Y. Dai, L. Astolfi, F. Babiloni, H. Yuan, and L. Yang, "eConnectome: a MATLAB toolbox for mapping and imaging of brain functional connectivity," *Journal of Neuroscience Methods*, vol. 195, no. 2, pp. 261–269, 2011.

[75] A. C. Evans, D. L. Collins, S. R. Mills, E. D. Brown, R. L. Kelly, and T. M. Peters, "3D statistical neuroanatomical models from 305 MRI volumes," in *1993 IEEE Conference Record Nuclear Science Symposium and Medical Imaging Conference*, vol. 3, pp. 1813–1817, San Francisco, CA, USA, October-November 1993.

[76] H. Becker, L. Albera, P. Comon, R. Gribonval, F. Wendling, and I. Merlet, "Brain-source imaging: from sparse to tensor models," *IEEE Signal Processing Magazine*, vol. 32, no. 6, pp. 100–112, 2015.

[77] P. C. Hansen, "Regularization tools version 4.0 for Matlab 7.3," *Numerical Algorithms*, vol. 46, no. 2, pp. 189–194, 2007.

[78] C. Wilke, Lei Ding, and Bin He, "Estimation of time-varying connectivity patterns through the use of an adaptive directed transfer function," *IEEE Transactions on Biomedical Engineering*, vol. 55, no. 11, pp. 2557–2564, 2008.

[79] C. W. J. Granger, "Investigating causal relations by econometric models and cross-spectral methods," *Econometrica*, vol. 37, no. 3, p. 424, 1969.

[80] D. M. Groppe, S. Bickel, C. J. Keller et al., "Dominant frequencies of resting human brain activity as measured by the electrocorticogram," *NeuroImage*, vol. 79, pp. 223–233, 2013.

[81] P. Capotosto, C. Babiloni, G. L. Romani, and M. Corbetta, "Resting-state modulation of alpha rhythms by interference with angular gyrus activity," *Journal of Cognitive Neuroscience*, vol. 26, no. 1, pp. 107–119, 2014.

[82] A. Zalesky, A. Fornito, and E. T. Bullmore, "Network-based statistic: identifying differences in brain networks," *NeuroImage*, vol. 53, no. 4, pp. 1197–1207, 2010.

[83] M. Rubinov and O. Sporns, "Complex network measures of brain connectivity: uses and interpretations," *NeuroImage*, vol. 52, no. 3, pp. 1059–1069, 2010.

[84] A. Athanasiou, M. A. Klados, C. Styliadis, N. Foroglou, K. Polyzoidis, and P. D. Bamidis, "Investigating the role of alpha and beta rhythms in functional motor networks," *Neuroscience*, vol. 378, pp. 54–70, 2018.

[85] A. Athanasiou, N. Terzopoulos, N. Pandria et al., "Functional brain connectivity during multiple motor imagery tasks in spinal cord injury," *Neural Plasticity*, vol. 2018, Article ID 9354207, 20 pages, 2018.

[86] O. Sporns and R. Kötter, "Motifs in brain networks," *PLoS Biology*, vol. 2, no. 11, p. e369, 2004.

[87] O. Sporns, "Graph theory methods for the analysis of neural connectivity patterns," in *Neuroscience Databases*, pp. 171–185, Springer US, Boston, MA, 2003.

[88] G. Fagiolo, "Clustering in complex directed networks," *Physical Review E*, vol. 76, no. 2, article 026107, 2007.

[89] J.-P. Onnela, J. Saramäki, J. Kertész, and K. Kaski, "Intensity and coherence of motifs in weighted complex networks," *Physical Review E*, vol. 71, no. 6, article 065103, 2005.

[90] N. Pandria, L. Kovatsi, A. B. Vivas, and P. D. Bamidis, "Resting-state abnormalities in heroin-dependent individuals," *Neuroscience*, vol. 378, pp. 113–145, 2018.

[91] J. Liu, J. Liang, W. Qin et al., "Dysfunctional connectivity patterns in chronic heroin users: an fMRI study," *Neuroscience Letters*, vol. 460, no. 1, pp. 72–77, 2009.

[92] D. J. Watts and S. H. Strogatz, "Collective dynamics of "small-world" networks," *Nature*, vol. 393, no. 6684, pp. 440–442, 1998.

[93] O. Sporns and J. D. Zwi, "The small world of the cerebral cortex," *Neuroinformatics*, vol. 2, no. 2, pp. 145–162, 2004.

[94] D. P. Doane and L. E. Seward, "Measuring skewness: a forgotten statistic?," *Journal of Statistics Education*, vol. 19, no. 2, 2011.

[95] D. Cramer, "Fundamental statistics for social research," in *Step-by-Step Calculations and Computer Techniques Using SPSS for Windows*, Routledge, London and New York, 1998.

[96] D. Cramer and D. Howitt, *The SAGE Dictionary of Statistics*, SAGE Publications, 2004.

[97] N. M. Razali and Y. B. Wah, "Power comparisons of Shapiro-Wilk, Kolmogorov-Smirnov, Lilliefors and Anderson-Darling tests," *Journal of Statistical Modeling and Analytics*, vol. 2, no. 1, pp. 21–33, 2011.

[98] S. S. Shapiro and M. B. Wilk, "An analysis of variance test for normality (complete samples)," *Biometrika*, vol. 52, no. 3-4, pp. 591–611, 1965.

[99] N. J. Wald, M. Idle, J. Boreham, and A. Bailey, "Carbon monoxide in breath in relation to smoking and carboxyhaemoglobin levels," *Thorax*, vol. 36, no. 5, pp. 366–369, 1981.

[100] M. J. Jarvis, H. Tunstall-Pedoe, C. Feyerabend, C. Vesey, and Y. Saloojee, "Comparison of tests used to distinguish smokers from nonsmokers," *American Journal of Public Health*, vol. 77, no. 11, pp. 1435–1438, 1987.

[101] S. A. Willmott, J. A. P. Boardman, C. A. Henshaw, and P. W. Jones, "Understanding general health questionnaire (GHQ-28) score and its threshold," *Social Psychiatry and Psychiatric Epidemiology*, vol. 39, no. 8, pp. 613–617, 2004.

[102] M. Xia, J. Wang, and Y. He, "BrainNet Viewer: a network visualization tool for human brain connectomics," *PLoS One*, vol. 8, no. 7, article e68910, 2013.

[103] A. C. Janes, S. Farmer, A. L. Peechatka, B. . B. Frederick, and S. E. Lukas, "Insula-dorsal anterior cingulate cortex coupling is associated with enhanced brain reactivity to smoking cues," *Neuropsychopharmacology*, vol. 40, no. 7, pp. 1561–1568, 2015.

[104] J. L. Smith and R. E. Hodges, "Serum levels of vitamin C in relation to dietary and supplemental intake of vitamin C in smokers and nonsmokers," *Annals of the New York Academy of Sciences*, vol. 498, pp. 144–152, 1987.

[105] E. M. Park, Y. M. Park, and Y. S. Gwak, "Oxidative damage in tissues of rats exposed to cigarette smoke," *Free Radical Biology & Medicine*, vol. 25, no. 1, pp. 79–86, 1998.

[106] B. Halliwell, "Oxidants and human disease: some new concepts," *The FASEB Journal*, vol. 1, no. 5, pp. 358–364, 1987.

[107] F. Ozguner, A. Koyu, and G. Cesur, "Active smoking causes oxidative stress and decreases blood melatonin levels," *Toxicology and Industrial Health*, vol. 21, no. 10, pp. 21–26, 2005.

[108] E. T. Middleton and A. H. Morice, "Breath carbon monoxide as an indication of smoking habit," *Chest*, vol. 117, no. 3, pp. 758–763, 2000.

[109] J. Hung, C.-H. Lin, J.-D. Wang, and C.-C. Chan, "Exhaled carbon monoxide level as an indicator of cigarette consumption in a workplace cessation program in Taiwan," *Journal of the Formosan Medical Association*, vol. 105, no. 3, pp. 210–3, 2006.

[110] P. Tønnesen, J. Nørregaard, K. Mikkelsen, S. Jørgensen, and F. Nilsson, "A double-blind trial of a nicotine inhaler for smoking cessation," *JAMA*, vol. 269, no. 10, pp. 1268–1271, 1993.

[111] D. E. Jorenby, S. S. Smith, M. C. Fiore et al., "Varying nicotine patch dose and type of smoking cessation counseling," *JAMA*, vol. 274, no. 17, pp. 1347–1352, 1995.

[112] J. R. Fedota and E. A. Stein, "Resting-state functional connectivity and nicotine addiction: prospects for biomarker development," *Annals of the New York Academy of Sciences*, vol. 1349, no. 1, pp. 64–82, 2015.

[113] S. Morein-Zamir and T. W. Robbins, "Fronto-striatal circuits in response-inhibition: relevance to addiction," *Brain Research*, vol. 1628, Part A, pp. 117–129, 2015.

[114] M. M. Sweitzer, C. F. Geier, M. A. Addicott et al., "Smoking abstinence-induced changes in resting state functional connectivity with ventral striatum predict lapse during a quit attempt," *Neuropsychopharmacology*, vol. 41, no. 10, pp. 2521–2529, 2016.

[115] Y.-J. Chen, Y. C. Lo, Y. C. Hsu et al., "Automatic whole brain tract-based analysis using predefined tracts in a diffusion spectrum imaging template and an accurate registration strategy," *Human Brain Mapping*, vol. 36, no. 9, pp. 3441–3458, 2015.

[116] E. Takahashi, K. Ohki, and D.-S. Kim, "Diffusion tensor studies dissociated two fronto-temporal pathways in the human memory system," *NeuroImage*, vol. 34, no. 2, pp. 827–838, 2007.

[117] X. Fang, Y. Zhang, Y. Zhou et al., "Resting-state coupling between core regions within the central-executive and salience networks contributes to working memory performance," *Frontiers in Behavioral Neuroscience*, vol. 10, p. 27, 2016.

[118] X. Zhang, B. J. Salmeron, T. J. Ross et al., "Anatomical differences and network characteristics underlying smoking cue reactivity," *NeuroImage*, vol. 54, no. 1, pp. 131–141, 2011.

[119] M. Corbetta and G. L. Shulman, "Control of goal-directed and stimulus-driven attention in the brain," *Nature Reviews Neuroscience*, vol. 3, no. 3, pp. 201–215, 2002.

[120] M. T. Sutherland, M. J. McHugh, V. Pariyadath, and E. A. Stein, "Resting state functional connectivity in addiction: lessons learned and a road ahead," *NeuroImage*, vol. 62, no. 4, pp. 2281–2295, 2012.

[121] R. L. Buckner, S. E. Petersen, J. G. Ojemann, F. M. Miezin, L. R. Squire, and M. E. Raichle, "Functional anatomical studies of explicit and implicit memory retrieval tasks," *The Journal of Neuroscience*, vol. 15, no. 1, pp. 12–29, 1995.

[122] L. Fan, J. Wang, Y. Zhang, W. Han, C. Yu, and T. Jiang, "Connectivity-based parcellation of the human temporal pole using diffusion tensor imaging," *Cerebral Cortex*, vol. 24, no. 12, pp. 3365–3378, 2014.

[123] E. D. Claus, S. K. Blaine, F. M. Filbey, A. R. Mayer, and K. E. Hutchison, "Association between nicotine dependence severity, BOLD response to smoking cues and functional connectivity," *Neuropsychopharmacology*, vol. 38, no. 12, pp. 2363–2372, 2013.

[124] J. D. Bremner, M. Narayan, L. H. Staib, S. M. Southwick, T. McGlashan, and D. S. Charney, "Neural correlates of memories of childhood sexual abuse in women with and without posttraumatic stress disorder," *American Journal of Psychiatry*, vol. 156, no. 11, pp. 1787–1795, 1999.

[125] C. Pehrs, J. Zaki, L. H. Schlochtermeier, A. M. Jacobs, L. Kuchinke, and S. Koelsch, "The temporal pole top-down modulates the ventral visual stream during social cognition," *Cerebral Cortex*, vol. 27, no. 1, pp. 777–792, 2017.

[126] C. Lithari, C. A. Frantzidis, C. Papadelis et al., "Are females more responsive to emotional stimuli? A neurophysiological study across arousal and valence dimensions," *Brain Topography*, vol. 23, no. 1, pp. 27–40, 2010.

[127] D. R. Euston, A. J. Gruber, and B. L. McNaughton, "The role of medial prefrontal cortex in memory and decision making," *Neuron*, vol. 76, no. 6, pp. 1057–1070, 2012.

[128] K. J. Hartwell, J. J. Prisciandaro, J. Borckardt, X. Li, M. S. George, and K. T. Brady, "Real-time fMRI in the treatment of nicotine dependence: a conceptual review and pilot studies," *Psychology of Addictive Behaviors*, vol. 27, no. 2, pp. 501–509, 2013.

5

Hand Dexterity Impairment in Patients with Cervical Myelopathy: A New Quantitative Assessment using a Natural Prehension Movement

Masao Omori,[1] **Satoshi Shibuya**,[2] **Tsuyoshi Nakajima**,[2] **Takashi Endoh**,[3] **Shinya Suzuki**,[4] **Shun Irie**,[2] **Ryohei Ariyasu**,[2] **Satoshi Unenaka**,[5] **Hideto Sano**,[1] **Kazutaka Igarashi**,[1] **Shoichi Ichimura**,[1] and **Yukari Ohki**[2]

[1]*Department of Orthopaedic Surgery, Kyorin University School of Medicine, 6-20-2 Shinkawa, Mitaka, Tokyo 181-8611, Japan*
[2]*Department of Integrative Physiology, Kyorin University School of Medicine, 6-20-2 Shinkawa, Mitaka, Tokyo 181-8611, Japan*
[3]*Faculty of Human Development and Education, Uekusa Gakuen University, 1639-3 Ogura-cho, Wakaba-ku, Chiba 264-0007, Japan*
[4]*Department of Physical Therapy, School of Rehabilitation, Health Sciences University of Hokkaido, 1757 Kanazawa, Tobetsucho, Ishikari-gun, Hokkaido 061-0293, Japan*
[5]*Department of Sports Education, School of Lifelong Sport, Hokusho University, 23 Bunkyodai, Ebetsu, Hokkaido 069-0833, Japan*

Correspondence should be addressed to Masao Omori; omori_masao@hotmail.co.jp

Academic Editor: Norbert Kovács

Cervical myelopathy (CM) caused by spinal cord compression can lead to reduced hand dexterity. However, except for the 10 sec grip-and-release test, there is no objective assessment system for hand dexterity in patients with CM. Therefore, we evaluated the hand dexterity impairment of patients with CM objectively by asking them to perform a natural prehension movement. Twenty-three patients with CM and 30 age-matched controls were asked to reach for and grasp a small object with their right thumb and index finger and to subsequently lift and hold it. To examine the effects of tactile afferents from the fingers, objects with surface materials of differing textures (silk, suede, and sandpaper) were used. All patients also underwent the Japanese Orthopedic Association (JOA) test. Preoperative patients showed significantly greater grip aperture during reach-to-grasp movements and weaker grip force than controls only while attempting to lift the most slippery object (silk). Patients, immediately after surgery, ($n = 15$) tended to show improvements in the JOA score and in reaction time and movement time with respect to reaching movements. Multiple regression analysis demonstrated that some parameters of the prehension task could successfully predict subjective evaluations of dexterous hand movements based on JOA scores. These results suggest that quantitative assessments using prehension movements could be useful to objectively evaluate hand dexterity impairment in patients with CM.

1. Introduction

Cervical myelopathy (CM) is a condition caused by spinal cord compression associated with disc herniation, cervical spondylosis, and congenital stenosis [1]. CM generally causes sensory disturbances of the upper and lower extremities (e.g., numbness or pain), reduced hand dexterity, gait disturbance, and urinary dysfunction. In severe cases, surgical treatment is applied to relieve compression of the spinal cord (i.e., decompressive surgery). Hence, appropriate functional outcome measures are necessary to determine the disease severity, progression of the disorder, and effectiveness of surgical treatment.

Several subjective scales have been developed to assess clinical deficits in CM patients: the European Myelopathy Score [2], Nurick Score [3], Cooper Myelopathy Score [4], and the Japanese Orthopedic Association (JOA) score [5]. The JOA score has been widely used in Japan, and high degrees of inter- and intraobserver reliability have been confirmed [6]. Upper and lower extremity impairments caused by CM have also been evaluated objectively using several scales. For example, with respect to the lower extremity, the 30 m walking test [7], 10 sec step test [8], and triangle step test [9] have been developed. As a scale for the upper extremity, the 10 sec grip-and-release test is frequently used in Japan to evaluate hand function in myelopathy patients [10]. Recently, our group also proposed functional assessment of the proximal arm muscle in CM patients using target-reaching movements [11]. However, movements in the 10 sec grip-and-release test are quite different from the daily actions performed with the upper extremity. In fact, patients with CM have difficulty in manipulating relatively small objects (e.g., buttons or tableware) with their fingers during activities of daily living (i.e., reduced hand dexterity), in which fine motor control of the fingers via various sensory feedback mechanisms is necessary. Therefore, we assume that a natural prehension movement could be useful as an objective measure for characterizing hand dexterity impairments. To verify this hypothesis, we first compared preoperative patients and age-matched control subjects using a newly developed prehension task, which involved asking patients to reach and pick up objects of various surface textures [12]. We aimed to determine if this prehension task is suitable for assessing hand dexterity in patients with CM.

2. Materials and Methods

2.1. Participants. Twenty-three patients diagnosed with cervical spondylosis myelopathy (15 men and eight women; 65.0 ± 14.8 years old, mean ± SD) and 30 age-matched controls (12 men and 18 women; 63.4 ± 17.2 years old) participated in this study. A chi-squared test with Yates' correction confirmed that participant type (i.e., patients and controls) and gender were independent of each other ($\chi^2_1 = 2.38$, $p > 0.12$). Mean symptom duration was 18.0 ± 23.5 months. Neurological segment diagnosis indicated impairments of the C3 level ($n = 1$), C4 level ($n = 1$), C5 level ($n = 8$), C6 level ($n = 8$), and C7 level ($n = 5$). Magnetic resonance imaging was used in all patients both pre- and postoperatively. Signal changes were detected in all but six patients on T2-weighted imaging but in only seven patients on T1-weighted imaging. All participants were right-handed and had normal or corrected-to-normal vision. All were unaware of the purpose of the experiment. This study was approved by the institutional human review committee at the Kyorin University School of Medicine (approval number 498), and all participants provided written informed consent in accordance with the Helsinki Declaration. Fifteen of the 23 patients (65%) who participated in the preoperative experiment underwent decompression surgery using expansive open-door laminoplasty ($n = 13$) or anterior spinal fusion ($n = 2$). Immediately after surgery (14.6 ± 6.5 days), they underwent the assessment a second time.

2.2. JOA Score. As a conventional clinical scale based on patient symptoms, the JOA score for CM was applied to all participants (Table 1). Although the JOA score originally included the functions of the lower extremity and bladder, only the scores regarding the upper extremity were used for

Table 1: Japanese Orthopedic Association score for cervical compressive myelopathy.

Dysfunction score
A. Motor function
I. Fingers
0 = unable to feed oneself with any tableware, including chopsticks, a spoon, or fork, and/or unable to fasten buttons of any size
1 = can manage to feed oneself with a spoon and/or a fork but not with chopsticks
2 = either chopstick feeding or writing is possible but not practical, and/or large buttons can be fastened
3 = either chopstick feeding or writing is clumsy but practical, and/or cuff buttons can be fastened
4 = normal
II. Shoulder and elbow (evaluated by MMT score of the deltoid or biceps muscles, whichever is weaker)
−2 = MMT ≤ 2
−1 = MMT 3
−0.5 = MMT 4
0 = MMT 5
III. Lower extremity
0 = unable to stand up and walk by any means
0.5 = able to stand up but unable to walk
1 = unable to walk without a cane or other support on a level
1.5 = able to walk without a support but with a clumsy gait
2 = walks independently on a level but needs support on stairs
2.5 = walks independently when going upstairs but needs support when going downstairs
3 = capable of fast walking but clumsily
4 = normal
B. Sensory function
I. Upper extremity
0 = complete loss of touch and pain sensation
0.5 = 50% or below of normal sensation and/or severe pain or numbness
1 = over 60% of normal sensation and/or moderate pain or numbness
1.5 = subjective numbness of a slight degree without any objective sensory deficit
2 = normal
II. Lower extremity (same as I)
III. Trunk (same as I)
C. Bladder function
0 = urinary retention and/or incontinence
1 = sense of retention and/or dribbling and/or thin stream and/or incomplete continence
2 = urinary retardation and/or pollakiuria
3 = normal

MMT: manual muscle testing.

two domains in the present study: motor function of the fingers (AI in Table 1: range 0–4) and sensory function of the upper extremity (BI in Table 1: range 0–2). Accordingly, the total score of motor and sensory functions ranged from 0–6 (AI + BI).

2.3. Apparatus and Procedures. Participants were seated in front of a wooden desk, on which a cubical object (4 cm per side, 70 g weight) was positioned in the participant's midsagittal plane, 43 cm from the front edge of the desktop (Figure 1(a)). A detachable surface material selected from silk, suede, or sandpaper was attached on two sides, which faced each other and were contacted by the participant's thumb and index finger (thick lines in Figure 1(b)). The object had an integrated force measurement system (see below), which could measure the perpendicular force exerted to each side by the thumb or index finger (i.e., grip force; arrows in Figure 1(b)). To detect movement initiation, an electrostatic touch sensor (2 × 2 cm) was positioned 13 cm to the participant's right side. The center-to-center distance between the object and the touch sensor was 36 cm. A blackboard stood immediately behind the object, on which a marker was attached 10 cm from the desktop as a height target when lifting the object.

All participants completed three conditions with different surface materials, the order of which was fixed to prevent slips: sandpaper, suede, and then silk (i.e., from the least slippery material to the most slippery). Each condition was composed of 10 successive trials. Before each trial, participants were instructed to position their right hand on the touch sensor and put tips of their right thumb and index finger together ("Start" in Figure 1(c)). After delivery of a first auditory stimulus (a pure tone at 500 Hz) as the "go" signal, participants reached for and grasped the object with their right thumb and index finger as soon and accurately as possible ("Reach and Grasp" in Figure 1(c)). Subsequently, they lifted the object to the target marker on the blackboard and held it there until a second tone was provided approximately 3 s after the initiation of holding ("Lift" in Figure 1(c)). After the second tone, the participant was allowed to put the object on the desktop again and return their right hand to the starting position. The participants took a rest of 3 min between conditions, during which the experimenter altered the surface material. In total, the experiment took about 20–30 min to complete.

2.4. Data Acquisition and Dependent Variables. Using an electromagnetic motion tracking system (The MotionMonitor; Innovative Sports Training, Inc., Chicago, IL, USA), the following three positions of the right hand were sampled three-dimensionally at 100 Hz: tips of the thumb, index finger, and wrist (i.e., styloid process of the radius). Grip force signals from the thumb and index finger were measured by two channels of strain gauges (KFG-2N-120-C1-11L1M2R, Kyowa Co., Tokyo, Japan) at 100 Hz that were mounted on the surfaces of two sides of the object. The grip forces from the two channels were averaged. Movement initiation was detected by the touch sensor.

Using the SC/ZOOM system (Physiology Section; IMB, University of Umea, Sweden), we extracted the following seven parameters from the raw data; (1) reaction time (RT): time from the auditory "go" signal to movement initiation; (2) movement time (MT): time from movement initiation to the time at which either the thumb or index finger contacted the object first (i.e., touch object); (3) maximum grip aperture (MGA): maximum distance between the thumb and index finger during the reach-to-grasp movement; (4) time of maximum grip aperture (ToMGA): time from movement initiation to the time at which the MGA occurred; (5) position of MGA (PoMGA): the distance between the object and the location where the MGA occurred; (6) normalized movement distance (NMD): the wrist trajectory distance from the start position to the touch object divided by the direct distance; and (7) grip force: mean grip force from 3.0–3.5 sec after touching the object. This period corresponded to a late holding phase, during which stable grip forces could be recorded in all participants.

For statistical analysis, we excluded the first three of 10 trials in each condition because unstable grip forces were sometimes observed. Parameters 1–6 were averaged across the seven remaining trials and three conditions in each participant. Grip force (7) was computed in each condition. Statistical analyses were performed using STATISTICA version 10.0 (StatSoft Inc., Tulsa, OK, USA), and a p value of <0.05 indicated statistical significance.

3. Results

3.1. Kinematics of Reach-to-Grasp Movements: Patients versus Controls. All patients in the current study could complete the reach-to-grasp movement using all three materials. Figure 2 represents the trajectories of the thumb (red), index finger (blue), and wrist (gray) during movements in one healthy control (Figure 2(a)) and two patients (Figures 2(b) and 2(c)). Qualitatively, each digit in the healthy control tended to move straight toward the target object, with the distance between the two fingertips (i.e., grip aperture) increasing from the initial position. Additionally, the healthy control showed lower intertrial variability in their movements. In contrast, the patients tended to show curved trajectories and higher variability in their movements. Additionally, the timing and size of grip aperture differed greatly among the patients. For example, some patients (Figure 2(b)) exhibited excessive grip aperture relative to object size, although the aperture started from the same initial position as in healthy controls. On the other hand, some other patients also (Figure 2(c)) tended to spread their fingers from the middle of the reaching phase, which makes PoMGA closer to the object.

Quantitative analysis found some significant differences between the control and patients, especially with respect to grip aperture (Figure 3). The average MGA was significantly greater in the patients (11.4 ± 2.5 cm, mean ± SD) than healthy controls (9.7 ± 1.4 cm) ($t_{32} = 3.0$, $p < 0.01$; Welch's two-sample t-test; Figure 3(a)). Although no difference was detected between the patients and healthy controls with respect to MT ($p > 0.3$), the patients took more time to reach

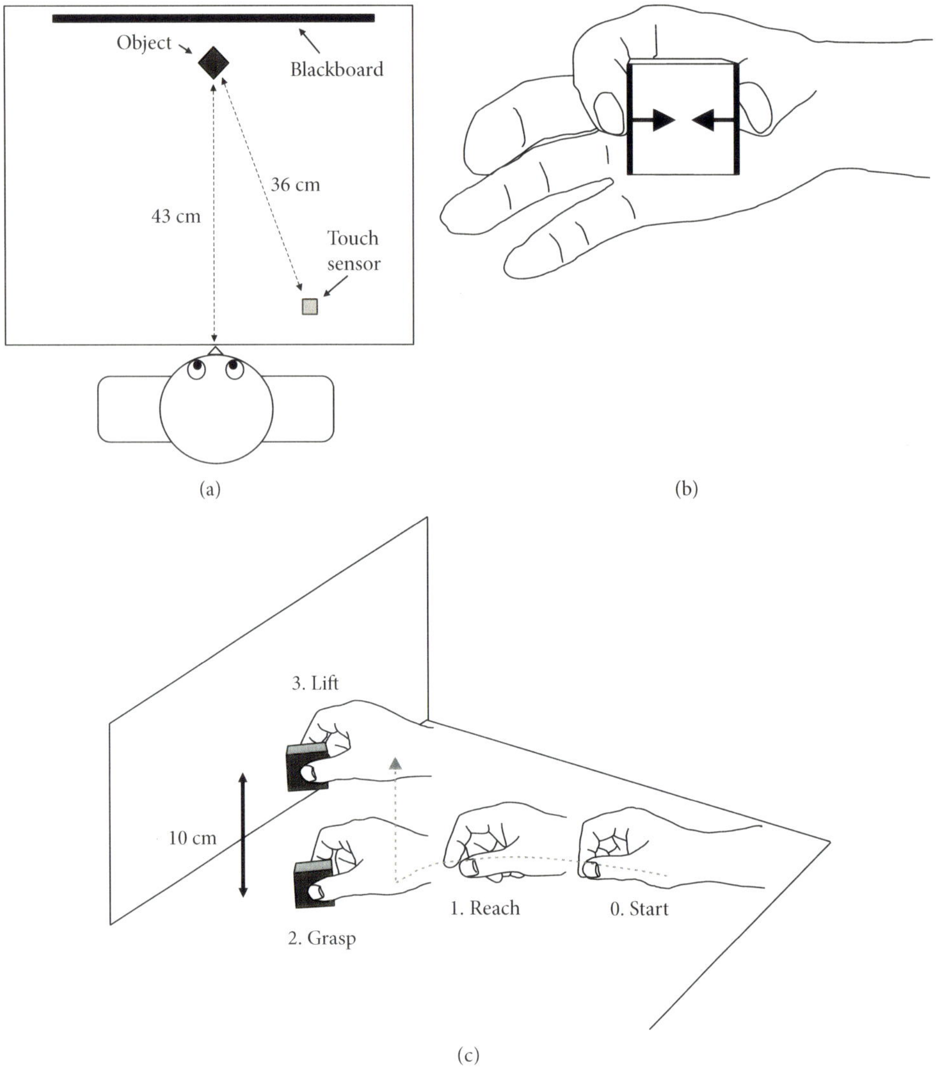

FIGURE 1: Experimental setup and prehension task. (a) Top view of the experimental setup. (b) Grip force during holding the object. The object had a force measurement system, which could measure perpendicular force to each side exerted to each side by the thumb or index finger. (c) Prehension task included three movement components: (1) reaching, (2) grasping, and (3) lifting.

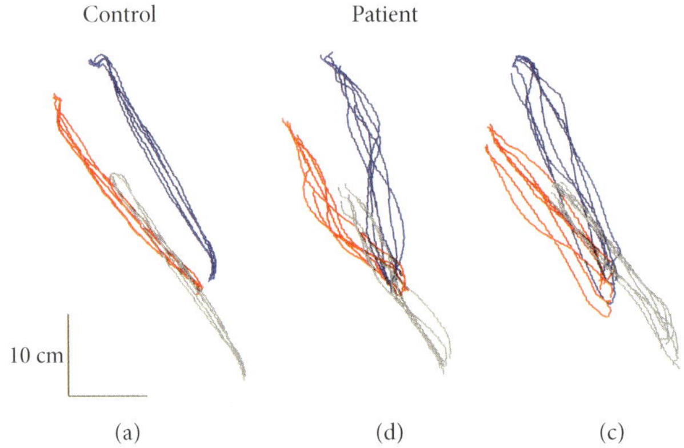

FIGURE 2: Representative examples of superimposed 2D trajectories during reach-to-grasp movements in one control subjects (a) and two patients (b–c). Red, blue, and gray lines indicate trajectories of the thumb and index finger and wrist, respectively.

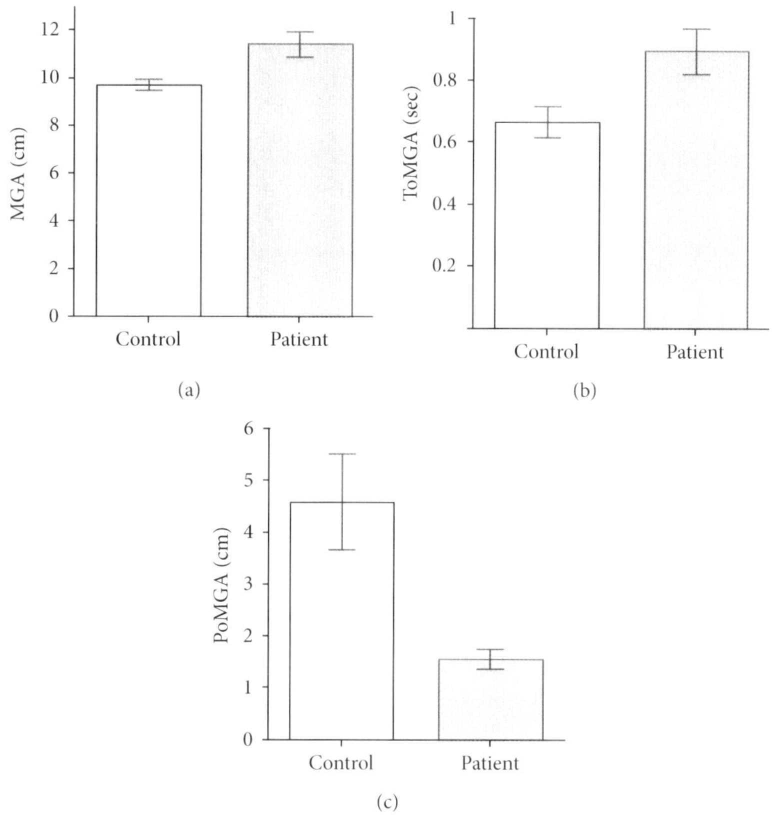

FIGURE 3: Averaged data of the control (white bars) and preoperative patients (gray bars) with regard to maximum grip aperture. (a) Maximum grip aperture (MGA). Maximum value of distance between the thumb and index finger during reach-to-grasp movements. (b) Time of maximum grip aperture (ToMGA). Time from movement initiation to time at which the MGA occurred. (c) Position of maximum grip aperture (PoMGA). The position at which the MGA occurred relative to the object.

the MGA (ToMGA; 0.89 ± 0.35 s versus 0.67 ± 0.28 s; patients versus controls) ($t_{42} = 2.6$, $p < 0.05$; Figure 3(b)) and consequently the location at which the MGA occurred was closer to the object (PoMGA: 1.6 ± 1.0 versus 4.6 ± 5.1 cm) ($W = 128.0$, $p < 0.01$; Wilcoxon rank-sum test; Figure 3(c)). Additionally, the NMD of patients (1.1 ± 0.1) was significantly shorter than that of controls (1.2 $+0.2$) ($t_{41} = 3.2$, $p < 0.01$; Table 2). With respect to RT, there were no significant differences between patients and controls ($p > 0.5$).

3.2. Grip Forces: Patients versus Controls. Figures 4(a) and 4(b) represent the grip force profiles of three conditions in one control and one patient, respectively. The grip forces of the control increased steeply and were modulated by surface materials. The greatest force was obtained when the most slippery material was used (i.e., silk; dashed line), whereas the least force was used when the nonslip material was picked up (i.e., sandpaper; solid line). In contrast, the patient's grip force increased moderately, and material-dependent force modulations were not observed. Statistical analysis for all participants using two-way analysis of variance (ANOVA) with repeated measures in one factor (subject [2: patient and control] × material [3: silk, suede, and sandpaper]) demonstrated that the main effect of material ($F_{2,\ 102} = 20.9$, $p < 0.01$) and the interaction between the two ($F_{2,\ 102} = 3.1$, $p < 0.05$) were significant. According to post hoc multiple comparisons (Fisher's least significant difference), greater grip forces were produced under the silk condition than the sandpaper and suede conditions in controls ($p < 0.01$) and patients ($p < 0.05$) (Figures 4(c) and 4(d)). However, in comparisons between the controls and patients, only the grip force in the silk condition showed a nearly significant difference (controls versus patients: 6.4 ± 4.3 versus 4.8 ± 1.9 N; $p = 0.07$). Otherwise, there were no differences between the two groups ($p > 0.3$).

3.3. Postoperative Changes. Immediately after surgery, 15 of 23 patients who underwent surgery repeated the same prehension task. Hence, we compared the data between the pre- and postoperative states. In the reach-to-grasp movement, RT (pre versus post; 0.52 ± 0.25 versus 0.46 ± 0.22 s: $t_{14} = 2.05$, $p = 0.06$, paired t-test) and MT (1.15 ± 0.55 versus 0.94 ± 0.32 s: $t_{14} = 1.81$, $p = 0.09$) tended to decrease after surgery (Table 2), although these differences did not reach statistical significance ($p = 0.05$). For the remaining parameters (i.e., MGA, ToMGA, PoMGA, and NMD), no significant differences were detected ($p > 0.2$). With respect to grip force, two-way ANOVA (period [2: pre- and postoperation] × material [3: silk, suede, and sandpaper]) showed that the main effect of period ($p > 0.2$) and the interaction between the two ($p > 0.8$) were not significant. However, the main effect

Table 2: Summarized data from prehension movement analysis and JOA score.

Parameter	Control	Patient	
		Preop	Postop
Number male/female	30 12/18	23 15/8	15 12/3
Age	63.4 ± 17.2	65.0 ± 14.8	63.9 ± 15.8
Reach-to-grasp movement			
Reaction time [RT] (sec)	0.53 ± 0.19	0.50 ± 0.24	0.46 ± 0.22 (0.52 ± 0.25)
Movement time [MT] (sec)	1.01 ± 0.37	1.12 ± 0.43	0.94 ± 0.32 (1.15 ± 0.55)
Maximum grip aperture [MGA] (cm)	9.71 ± 1.35	11.4 ± 2.46**	11.7 ± 2.62 (11.5 ± 2.53)
Time of maximum grip aperture [ToMGA] (ms)	0.67 ± 0.28	0.89 ± 0.35*	0.78 ± 0.33 (0.91 ± 0.44)
Position of maximum grip aperture [PoMGA] (cm)	4.58 ± 5.09	1.55 ± 0.96§§	1.27 ± 0.67 (1.43 ± 0.70)
Normalized movement distance [NMD]	1.22 ± 0.18	1.11 ± 0.07**	1.08 ± 0.05 (1.10 ± 0.08)
Grip force (N)			
Sandpaper	4.18 ± 3.56	3.88 ± 2.08	3.88 ± 2.08
Suede	4.68 ± 3.81	3.86 ± 1.68	3.73 ± 1.84 (4.24 ± 1.82)
Silk	6.39 ± 4.27	4.79 ± 1.94	4.34 ± 2.84 (5.06 ± 2.14)
JOA score			
Motor function of fingers	—	1.91 ± 1.12	2.40 ± 1.12 (2.13 ± 1.25)
Sensory function of the upper extremity	—	1.11 ± 0.50	1.37 ± 0.52 (1.10 ± 0.47)
Total (motor + sensory)	—	3.02 ± 1.31	3.77 ± 1.28† (3.23 ± 1.55)

Values are expressed as mean ± SD. JOA test was not performed for normal controls (–). Values in parentheses indicate preoperative values of 15 patients.*Statistically significant difference from control ($p < 0.05$, Welch two sample t-test). ** Statistically significant difference from control ($p < 0.01$, Welch two sample t-test). §§Statistically significant difference from control ($p < .01$, Wilcoxon rank-sum test). †Statistically significant different from preoperation ($p < .05$, paired sample t-test).

of material was statistically significant ($F_{2,\ 28} = 8.4$, $p < 0.01$). Post hoc analysis using Tukey's honest significant difference test found that grip force in the silk condition (4.7 ± 2.5 N) was significantly greater than that in the sandpaper condition (3.3 ± 1.7 N; $p < 0.01$).

3.4. JOA Scores for the Upper Extremity. The JOA score for the upper extremity showed that the preoperative patients had obvious damage in two domains: motor (1.9 ± 1.1, normal = 4: $t_{22} = 8.9$, $p < 0.01$, one sample t-test) and sensory (1.1 ± 0.5, normal = 2: $t_{22} = 8.6$, $p < 0.01$) scores (Table 2). The total score of motor and sensory domains was 3.0 ± 1.3 (normal = 6; $t_{22} = 10.9$, $p < 0.01$). For the patients who underwent surgery ($n = 15$), we examined whether postoperative recovery could be observed using a paired t-test or Wilcoxon signed-rank test. As a result, significant improvements after surgery were identified with respect to total score (pre- versus postoperative: 3.2 ± 1.6 versus 3.8 ± 1.3; $t_{14} = 2.78$, $p < 0.05$). A similar tendency was also observed for sensory function ($t_{14} = 1.95$, $p = 0.07$) but not for motor function ($p > 0.1$; Wilcoxon signed-rank test).

3.5. Regression and Correlation Analyses. To verify the clinical validity of the quantitative assessment system for hand dexterity impairment applied in this study, we performed regression analyses between parameters obtained from the test and the JOA score. Here, we used the combined data ($n = 38$) of the pre- and postoperative patients. Table 3 shows the correlation coefficients between motor and sensory scores of the JOA scale and the parameters of the task. The motor and sensory scores of the JOA scale did not correlate significantly.

Some parameters correlated with JOA scores. For example, the motor score significantly correlated with MT ($r = -0.63$; $p < 0.01$) and RT ($r = -0.47$; $p < 0.01$). Although the motor score evaluates dexterous finger movements (Table 1), it did not correlate with grip forces irrespective of the surface material of the object. In contrast, the sensory score correlated significantly with a different parameter: grip force of the suede condition ($r = -0.33$; $p < 0.05$). Interestingly, the correlation coefficient showed a negative value; patients with good sensory function exerted weaker grip force in the condition.

We further examined whether parameters obtained from the current task (explanatory variables) could explain the motor score assessed from the JOA score (object variable) using multiple regression analysis and selected explanatory variables to yield an appropriate regression model using the forward-stepwise method. As a result, a significant regression model was found ($F_{5,\ 30} = 8.09$, $p < 0.01$, adjusted $r^2 = 0.50$). Figure 5 shows a scatter plot between the motor scores predicted from the model (abscissa) and the observed scores (ordinate). The significant predictors were MT ($\beta = -0.91$, $p < 0.01$), ToMGA ($\beta = 0.47$, $p < 0.05$), and grip forces in the suede ($\beta = -0.55$, $p < 0.05$) and silk conditions ($\beta = 0.48$, $p < 0.05$).

Similar analyses were performed for sensory and total scores. The sensory score could not be explained by the current variables ($F_{2,\ 33} = 2.67$, $p = 0.08$, adjusted $r^2 = 0.09$). The total JOA score showed an intermediate value

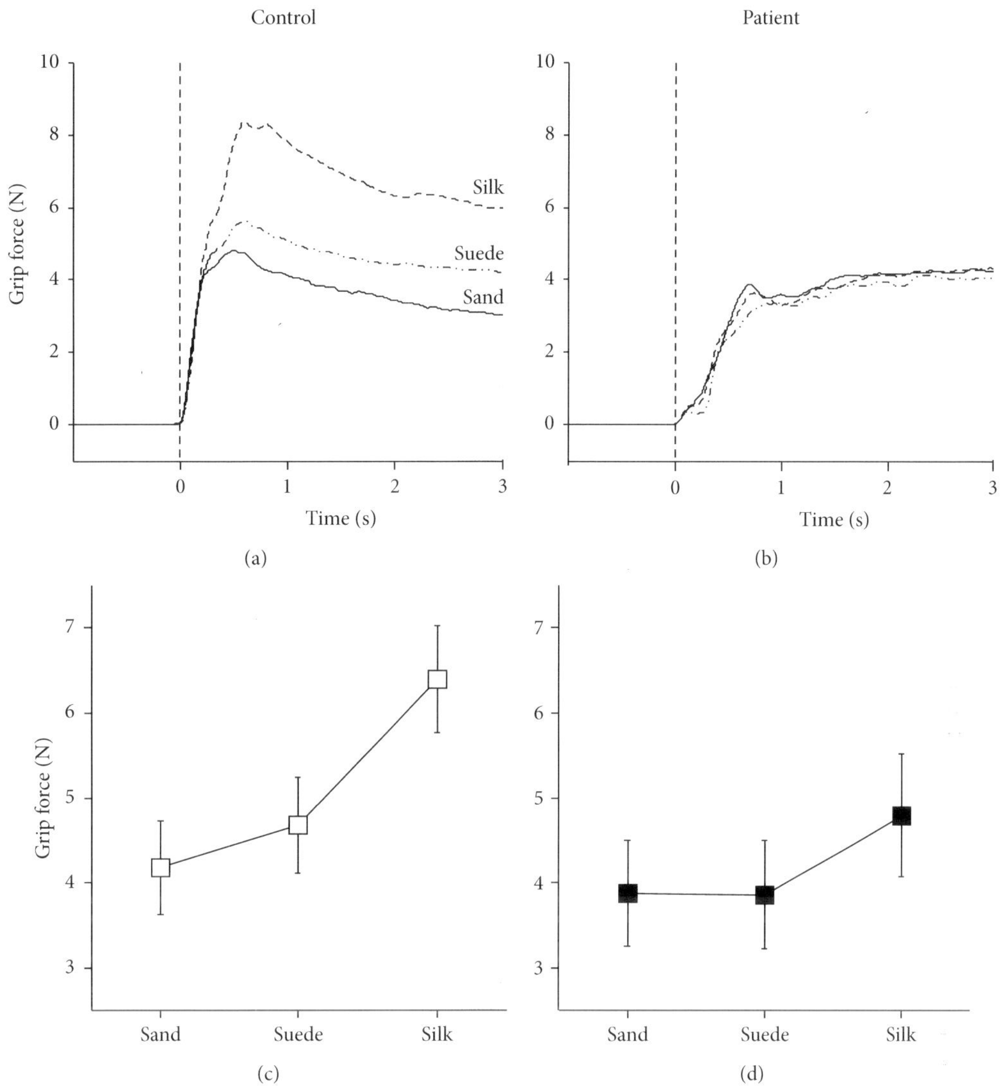

FIGURE 4: Grip force. Representative example of mean grip force profiles of one control subject (a) and one patient (b). A sold line, long dashed double-dotted line, and dashed line indicate sandpaper, suede, and silk conditions, respectively. The zero of x-axis (dotted vertical line) represents the starting time of lifting movement. Averaged grip forces of three conditions in the controls (c) and patients (d). Error bars denote ± 1.0SE.

between motor and sensory scores ($F_{5,\ 30} = 4.57$, $p < 0.01$, adjusted $r^2 = 0.34$). Significant predictors for the latter were MT ($\beta = -0.71$, $p < 0.05$) and grip force in the suede condition ($\beta = -0.58$, $p < 0.05$).

4. Discussion

In this study, we used a natural prehension movement task to quantitatively examined hand dexterity impairment in patients with CM. Previously, this task has been used in studies of monkeys to verify dexterous finger movement ability after damage to the neuronal system [13, 14]. For this reason, we believed that it would be useful for assessing hand dexterity in patients with CM and aimed to test this hypothesis.

In the present study, preoperative patients had decreased performance compared to controls, mainly with respect to grip aperture control and grip force modulation. Immediately after surgery, the patients showed improvements in JOA score and shortening of RT and MT compared to controls. Multiple regression analysis demonstrated that several parameters from the prehension task could explain the dysfunctions of finger movements in daily life according to the JOA score. These results suggest that analysis of this natural prehension task shows promise for objectively evaluating the current severity of CM with respect to hand dexterity impairments.

Traditionally, the reach-to-grasp movement is thought to consist of two components: transport or reaching (i.e., the hand is moved toward the object) and grasping (i.e., hands or fingers are preshaped in anticipation of contact with the object) [15]. Previous studies in healthy humans have reported that the MGA occurs at approximately 60–70% of the reaching duration [16, 17], suggesting a tight coupling between the two components. The current results in age-

TABLE 3: Correlation coefficients between all parameters using combined data from pre-and postoperative patients ($n = 38$).

Parameter	2	3	4	5	6	7	8	9	10	11
1. JOA (motor)	.31	−.47**	−.63**	−.28	−.06	−.21	−.32	−.11	−.15	.09
2. JOA (sensory)		.05	−.03	−.11	−.05	.16	−.15	−.26	−.33*	−.24
3. RT			.59**	.42**	.27	.01	.48**	.02	−.12	−.27
4. MT				.71**	−.06	.20	.41*	.02	.07	−.06
5. MGA					.13	.05	.41*	−.02	−.12	−.14
6. ToMGA						−.08	.33	.10	.10	−.06
7. PoMGA							.27	.10	.03	−.04
8. NMD								.27	.18	.17
9. Grip force (sand)									.68**	.44**
10. Grip force (suede)										.80**
11. Grip force (silk)										

*$p < 0.05$, **$p < 0.01$. JOA: Japanese Orthopedic Association score; RT: reaction time; MT: movement time; MGA: maximum grip aperture; ToMGA: time of maximum grip aperture; PoMGA: position of maximum grip aperture; NMD: normalized movement distance.

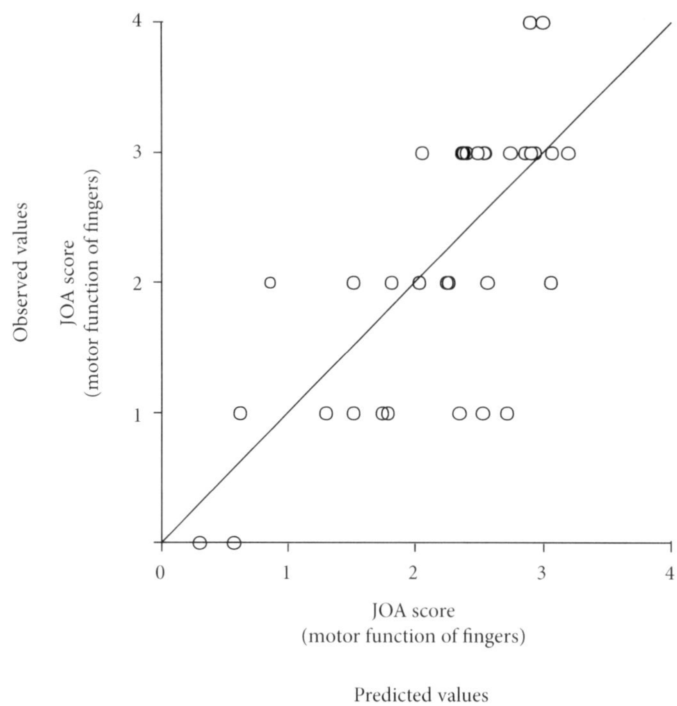

FIGURE 5: A scatter plot regarding the JOA score (motor function of fingers: normal = 4) between predicted values according to a multiple regression analysis (abscissa) and the observed values (ordinate). A diagonal line means an exact match between the two values.

matched controls were consistent with this principle (66%, 0.67 s/1.01 s, ToMGA/MT). However, in the patients, the MGA occurred much later (80%, 0.90 s/1.12 s) and immediately before contact with the object (i.e., PoMGA). Moreover, the patients showed evidence of excessive MGA compared to the controls. We assume that changes in grip aperture control were caused by pyramidal tract damage in the spinal cord [13]. However, these changes may also reflect decreased somatosensory information associated with CM (sensory score of JOA: 1.11 ± 0.45; normal = 2). Gentilucci et al. [18] examined the role of tactile information from the hand during reach-to-grasp movements by providing local anesthesia to the participants' fingertips. The results showed that blocking tactile afferents mainly influenced the kinematics of the finger-opening phase: the duration of this phase was extended and MGA increased. The results in patients in this study are consistent with these findings and might provide evidence for the importance of somatosensory inputs from the hand in grip aperture control.

When picking up a small object up using the index finger and thumb, people can modulate their grip force adequately based on the friction between the skin of the finger and the object (i.e., the more slippery the object, the greater the grip force) [12]. However, the force modulation ability of CM patients was decreased in this study. In particular, patients were unable to exert higher grip force when attempting to pick up the most slippery object (i.e., silk) when compared to controls. There are at least two reasons for impaired grip force modulation in these patients. One is that the patients' finger muscle strength was decreased due to CM so that the patients could not produce a strong grip force despite being able to complete the task. It is known that patients with CM show lower scores (<20 times) on the 10 sec grip-and-release test [10], which is correlated with gripping power to some extent [19]. Hence, in this study, we infer that patients' maximum grip forces would be weakened. The other reason is that patients' failure to adapt to different surficial materials (i.e., frictions) was caused by sensory dysfunction in the hand, as mentioned above. A human study involving the administration of local anesthesia to the index finger and thumb demonstrated that the adaptation to friction between the skin and the object was strongly dependent on cutaneous afferent input [12].

In this study, in contrast to the silk condition, the grip forces under the suede and sandpaper conditions in patients were not different from those of controls. Because the patients could exert stronger forces in the sandpaper condition, the forces of these two conditions could be less influenced by muscle strength. Indeed, the forces correlated moderately with the sensory JOA score. If patients have a good sensory function, they use weaker grip forces for the materials, as observed in healthy controls [12].

Postoperatively, JOA score was significantly improved, although it was still far from the normal value. In the prehension task, postoperative changes were confirmed only in the reaching component (i.e., shortening of the RT and MT) but not in the grasping and lifting components. The difference between the reaching and grasping (or lifting) components could be partially explained by direct and indirect motor pathways from the motor cortex to spinal motoneurons during control of the upper extremity. Animal studies in cats and monkeys have demonstrated that reaching movements are less influenced than finger manipulations after spinal pyramidotomy (i.e., surgical severance of the direct pathway [i.e., pyramidal tract] by creating a partial lesion of the lateral funiculus) at the C5 level [13, 14]. This effect would be caused by an indirect pathway (i.e., interneuronal systems), including propriospinal neurons at the C3–C4 level, which mediate corticomotoneuronal inputs to the proximal arm muscles predominantly [20]. The existence of the C3–C4 propriospinal neuron system in humans has also been suggested from electrophysiological findings [21, 22]. Accordingly, the current results might reflect different time courses of recovery processes between the direct and indirect pathways after surgery. Similar dissociation in movement impairments and their recovery was also observed in patients with CM [11]. To corroborate this hypothesis, we need to perform further follow-up investigations of postoperative changes using this prehension task.

While the grasping and lifting components are unable to detect clear recovery immediately after surgery, our multiple regression analysis showed that the parameters in the prehension task could explain the current motor dysfunction of fingers in activities of daily living (e.g., fastening buttons) according to the JOA score (motor score) (adjusted $r^2 = 0.50$; $p < 0.01$). The selected explanatory variables included all movement components (reaching [MT], grasping [ToMGA], and lifting [grip forces of the suede and silk conditions]). At first sight, it is unusual that the reaching component (MT) is included in the variables because the reaching and grasping components are independent [15]. However, in a study of monkeys involving pyramidotomy, it was shown that the animal could pinch food pellets with the index finger and thumb after a recovery period [13, 14]. The authors suggested that this recovery could be induced by interneuronal systems, which mediate corticomotoneuronal inputs to the proximal arm muscles in the normal condition [20]. Thus, it is possible that the interneuronal systems could contribute to the recovery of dexterous hand movements even in patients with CM. The contribution of interneuronal systems was also suggested in a previous study with CM patients [11]. Otherwise, the ToMGA and grip forces of the suede and silk conditions indicate the functioning of the pyramidal tract, sensory functions, and muscle strength of the hand muscles. Thus, dexterous hand movements are supported by different neuronal systems.

There are several limitations to this study should be discussed. First, the CM patients in the current study could complete the task. Thus, the current method cannot be applied to patients with severe impairments. Second, we did not follow the recovery of patients over a long-term period. To evaluate recovery in the long term, future studies will be needed. Third, we fixed the order of the surface materials to make the task easier for patients. Finally, we analyzed data from patients with compression at different spinal levels. In the future, we need to collect detailed data to the clarify effects of compression level on the findings of the present study.

5. Conclusions

The results of this study suggest that prehension movement analysis could be efficient and valid for the objective evaluation of current impairment of hand dexterity in patients with CM.

Authors' Contributions

Masao Omori and Satoshi Shibuya contributed equally to this work.

Acknowledgments

The authors would like to thank Mrs. C. Okada for her help with data analysis. Table 1 is reproduced from K. Igarashi et al. [11], [under the Creative Commons Attribution License/public domain]. This work was supported by the Japan Society for the Promotion of Science (KAKENHI), Grant nos. 23500617 and 26120002 to Yukari Ohki.

References

[1] T. A. Mattei, C. R. Goulart, J. B. Milano, L. P. F. Dutra, and D. R. Fasset, "Cervical spondylotic myelopathy: pathophysiology, diagnosis, and surgical techniques," *ISRN Neurology*, vol. 2011, Article ID 463729, 5 pages, 2011.

[2] J. Herdmann, M. Linzbach, M. Krzan, J. Dvorák, and W. J. Bock, "The European Myelopathy Score," in *Advances in Neurosurgery*, B. L. Bauer, M. Brock, and M. Klinger, Eds., Springer, Berlin, 1994.

[3] S. Nurick, "The pathogenesis of the spinal cord disorder associated with cervical spondylosis," *Brain*, vol. 95, no. 1, pp. 87–100, 1972.

[4] B. W. Chiles III, M. A. Leonard, H. F. Choudhri, and P. R. Cooper, "Cervical spondylotic myelopathy: patterns of neurological deficit and recovery after anterior cervical decompression," *Neurosurgery*, vol. 44, no. 4, pp. 762–769, 1999.

[5] K. Hirabayashi, K. Watanabe, K. Wakano, N. Suzuki, K. Satomi, and Y. Ishii, "Expansive open-door laminoplasty for cervical spinal stenotic myelopathy," *Spine*, vol. 8, no. 7, pp. 693–699, 1983.

[6] K. Yonenobu, K. Abumi, K. Nagata, E. Taketomi, and K. Ueyama, "Interobserver and intraobserver reliability of the Japanese Orthopaedic Association scoring system for evaluation of cervical compression myelopathy," *Spine*, vol. 26, no. 17, pp. 1890–1894, 2001.

[7] A. Singh and H. A. Crockard, "Quantitative assessment of cervical spondylotic my elopathy by a simple walking test," *The Lancet*, vol. 354, no. 9176, pp. 370–373, 1999.

[8] Y. Yukawa, F. Kato, K. Ito et al., "Ten second step test as a new quantifiable parameter of cervical myelopathy," *Spine*, vol. 34, no. 1, pp. 82–86, 2009.

[9] H. Mihara, S. Kondo, A. Murata, K. Ishida, T. Niimura, and M. Hachiya, "A new performance test for cervical myelopathy: the triangle step test," *Spine*, vol. 35, no. 1, pp. 32–35, 2010.

[10] K. Ono, S. Ebara, T. Fuji, K. Yonenobu, K. Fujiwara, and K. Yamashita, "Myelopathy hand. New clinical signs of cervical cord damage," *The Journal of Bone & Joint Surgery*, vol. 69-B, no. 2, pp. 215–219, 1987.

[11] K. Igarashi, S. Shibuya, H. Sano, M. Takahashi, K. Satomi, and Y. Ohki, "Functional assessment of proximal arm muscles by target-reaching movements in patients with cervical myelopathy," *The Spine Journal*, vol. 11, no. 4, pp. 270–280, 2011.

[12] R. S. Johansson and G. Westling, "Roles of glabrous skin receptors and sensorimotor memory in automatic control of precision grip when lifting rougher or more slippery objects," *Experimental Brain Research*, vol. 56, no. 3, pp. 550–564, 1984.

[13] S. Sasaki, T. Isa, L. G. Pettersson et al., "Dexterous finger movements in primate without monosynaptic corticomotoneuronal excitation," *Journal of Neurophysiology*, vol. 92, no. 5, pp. 3142–3147, 2004.

[14] Y. Nishimura, H. Onoe, Y. Morichika, S. Perfiliev, H. Tsukada, and T. Isa, "Time-dependent central compensatory mechanisms of finger dexterity after spinal cord injury," *Science*, vol. 318, no. 5853, pp. 1150–1155, 2007.

[15] M. Jeannerod, "The timing of natural prehension movements," *Journal of Motor Behavior*, vol. 16, no. 3, pp. 235–254, 1984.

[16] S. Chieffi and M. Gentilucci, "Coordination between the transport and the grasp components during prehension movements," *Experimental Brain Research*, vol. 94, no. 3, pp. 471–477, 1993.

[17] M. Santello and J. F. Soechting, "Gradual molding of the hand to object contours," *Journal of Neurophysiology*, vol. 79, no. 3, pp. 1307–1320, 1998.

[18] M. Gentilucci, I. Toni, E. Daprati, and M. Gangitano, "Tactile input of the hand and the control of reaching to grasp movements," *Experimental Brain Research*, vol. 114, no. 1, pp. 130–137, 1997.

[19] Y. Yukawa, H. Nakashima, K. Ito, M. Machino, S. Kanbara, and F. Kato, "Quantifiable tests for cervical myelopathy; 10-s grip and release test and 10-s step test: standard values and aging variation from 1230 healthy volunteers," *Journal of Orthopaedic Science*, vol. 18, no. 4, pp. 509–513, 2013.

[20] B. Alstermark and S. Sasaki, "Integration in descending motor pathways controlling the forelimb in the cat. 15. Comparison of the projection from excitatory C3-C4 propriospinal neurones to different species of forelimb motoneurones," *Experimental Brain Research*, vol. 63, no. 3, pp. 543–556, 1986.

[21] E. Pierrot-Deseilligny, "Propriospinal transmission of part of the corticospinal excitation in humans," *Muscle & Nerve*, vol. 26, no. 2, pp. 155–172, 2002.

[22] T. Nakajima, T. Tazoe, M. Sakamoto et al., "Reassessment of non-monosynaptic excitation from the motor cortex to motoneurons in single motor units of the human biceps brachii," *Frontiers in Human Neuroscience*, vol. 11, no. 19, 2017.

6

Cognitive-Enhancing Effect of a Hydroethanolic Extract of *Crinum macowanii* against Memory Impairment Induced by Aluminum Chloride in BALB/c Mice

Mohammed S. Jilani,[1] Dexter Tagwireyi,[1] Louis L. Gadaga,[1] Charles C. Maponga,[2] and Cosmas Mutsimhu[1]

[1]*Drug and Toxicology Information Service (DaTIS), School of Pharmacy and Department of Clinical Pharmacology, College of Health Sciences, University of Zimbabwe, P.O. Box A 178, Avondale, Harare, Zimbabwe*
[2]*School of Pharmacy, University of Zimbabwe, P.O. Box MP167, Mount Pleasant, Harare, Zimbabwe*

Correspondence should be addressed to Mohammed S. Jilani; saaqibj@gmail.com

Academic Editor: Antonio Orlacchio

Crinum macowanii is a bulbous plant indigenous to many parts of Southern Africa. Extracts of *C. macowanii* have gained interest since the discovery of various alkaloids, few of which possess acetylcholinesterase inhibitory activity. The present study was performed to evaluate the effect of a crude hydroethanolic extract of *C. macowanii* against aluminum chloride-induced memory impairment in mice using the Morris water maze and the novel object recognition task. *C. macowanii* (10, 20, and 40 mg/kg p.o) was administered daily for five weeks, while donepezil (3 mg/kg p.o) was used as the positive control. *C. macowanii* at a dosage of 40 mg/kg showed a significantly lower escape latency than the negative control ($P < 0.0001$) and was found to be comparable to donepezil 3 mg/kg in the Morris water maze test. *C. macowanii* at 40 mg/kg exhibited a significantly higher discrimination index than aluminum chloride-treated mice in the novel object recognition task. The results may support the usefulness of *C. macowanii* in the management of dementia and related illnesses.

1. Introduction

Alzheimer's disease (AD) is a chronic neurodegenerative disease characterized by cognitive dysfunction, psychiatric, and behavioral disturbances [1]. Hallmark pathological characteristics of AD include the deposition of amyloid-β (Aβ) plaques and neurofibrillary tangles in the brain accompanied by synaptic dysfunction [2]. This is the amyloid hypothesis, which postulates that amyloid deposits in the brain are the main cause of AD [3], while the Tau hypothesis suggests that abnormalities in the hyperphosphorylated tau protein are the cause of AD [4]. Early-onset familial Alzheimer's disease is an uncommon form of AD caused by a mutation in one of at least three genes: PSEN1, APP gene, and PSEN2 [5]. Oxidative stress also appears to be a major cause of AD-related pathologies caused by oxidative reactive species [5]. AD is incurable, and presently, there is no treatment that can retard the progression of the disease [6]. The cholinergic hypothesis concludes that the loss of cholinergic function results in memory loss and disruption of cognitive function [7, 8].

Current treatment of AD revolves around the increase in cholinergic transmission between the synaptic cleft by the use of acetylcholinesterase inhibitors (AChEi). These drugs include galantamine, rivastigmine, and donepezil [9]. These medications do not slow the progression of the disease; however, they do provide a modest but consistent improvement in functional and cognitive ability [10]. Since rivastigmine and galantamine are both related to natural products [11], there may still be a benefit in investigating more naturally occurring compounds in order to discover other and perhaps more effective AChEi.

The Amaryllidaceae family contains 1310 species which are widely distributed, and *Crinum* is an important genus of this family [12]. Over the years, alkaloids have been identified as the main active constituents of interest in *Crinum* species. These include lycorine-, crinine-, belladine-, galanthamine-, lycorinine-, and tazettine-type alkaloids [12–14].

Crinum macowanii (CM), a member of the *Crinum* genus, is known as *umduze* or *dururu* in the southern African languages of isiNdebele and Shona, respectively, and has a variety of medicinal uses [15]. Various alkaloids which have been isolated from CM include lycorine, 1-O-acetyllycorine, crinine, powelline, crinamine, crinamidine, 3-O-acetylhamayne, 1-epideacetylbowdensine, and cherylline [16]. Some of these alkaloids such as lycorine have been reported to possess acetylcholinesterase (AChE) inhibitory activity [17] and hence could be of benefit in treating dementia. In fact, a recent study reported that a crude hydroethanolic extract of CM had nootropic-like activity in a scopolamine-induced amnesia BALB/c mouse model [18]. However, while the scopolamine AD mouse model used in the aforementioned study [18] is commonly used for assessing nootropic-like activity in rodents, it only assesses cognitive enhancement resulting from the increase in the neurotransmitter—acetylcholine. Yet evidence in the literature suggests that AD is primarily caused by neurodegeneration. Thus, it is possible that the results seen in the study could not be replicated in a model which exhibits neurodegeneration. There is, therefore, a need to validate the results seen by Mugwagwa and colleagues [18] in a model that may be closer to AD. Hence, in this study, we have investigated the possible nootropic effects of CM using the aluminum chloride-induced dementia mouse model. This model not only causes learning memory impairment and cognitive decline in mice but also results in neurodegeneration [19–21].

In order to investigate these effects, the Morris water maze (MWM) and novel object recognition (NOR) test protocols were used. In addition to the behavioral tests, we also investigated the AChE inhibitory and free radical scavenging activity.

2. Materials and Methods

2.1. Plant Collection. Fresh bulbs of *C. macowanii* were collected in November 2014 at the University of Zimbabwe (UZ) grounds, Harare coordinates 17°47′14.5″S 31°03′06.4″ E. The plant sample was authenticated by a taxonomist from the Botanical Gardens and National Herbarium in Harare. A total number of 24 bulbs were collected for this study.

2.2. Preparation of Crude Extract. The crude extract was prepared as described by Mugwagwa et al. [18]. Briefly, fresh bulbs of *C. macowanii* were washed with water and peeled. They were dried under a shade for a period of 3 weeks. To ensure complete drying, the scales were further oven-dried at 55 degrees Celsius. The dried scales were reduced to fine powder using a Thomas Scientific Mill Model 4 (Thomas-Wiley Laboratory, USA) with a sieve size of 1 mm. A total of 1.1 kg of dried powder was obtained. The powder was then macerated in aqueous ethanol (70% *v*/*v*, up to 8 L) (1 : 10 *w*/*v*). To ensure the extraction of alkaloids, the maceration was continued for 72 hours with occasional shaking at room temperature. The mixture was then filtered to remove the bulky material using a mutton cloth. The finer material was filtered out by the process of vacuum filtration using Merck number 454 filter paper. This solution was concentrated using a Heidolph instrument, which was the Rotavapor 4000 (Heidolph, Germany). The resultant paste was freeze-dried using Heto Lab Equipment, Heto Freeze Dryer 3 (Heto-Holten A/S, Denmark), for 48 hours to obtain 102 g of the powdered crude extract. This powder was stored in a cool dark place in a desiccator.

2.3. Animals. Male BALB/c mice (22-37 g) were purchased from the animal house at the University of Zimbabwe. The mice were housed at the animal holding room in the Clinical Pharmacology Department of the University of Zimbabwe and were allowed to acclimatize for a period of one week. A natural hour light/dark cycle at room temperature was maintained, while a standard pellet diet was made freely accessible. Tap water was provided *ad libitum*. Authorization to use laboratory animals for the research project was granted by the Joint Research and Ethical Committee (JREC approval number: JREC/121/15).

2.4. Drugs and Reagents. Donepezil hydrochloride (DONZ) (Actavis Limited, India) and crude extract of *C. macowanii* were used. Aluminum chloride (ALCL) was obtained from the School of Pharmacy, University of Zimbabwe. Normal saline was used as the vehicle for both the CM and the DONZ. Acetylcholinesterase enzyme assay kit was purchased from Sigma Aldrich, South Africa. DPPH (2,2-Diphenyl-1-(2,4,6-trinitrophenyl)hydrazyl) and ascorbic acid were obtained from the Biochemistry Department, University of Zimbabwe. The study was partly funded by the researcher and the School of Pharmacy, University of Zimbabwe.

2.5. Grouping and Treatment Schedule. Mice were randomly put into six different groups. Tails of each mouse were marked with a nontoxic marker.

The mice were divided into 6 groups with 6 mice in each group. The experimental design was conducted as described by Mugwagwa et al. [18] and Linardaki et al. [22]. The experimental design was as follows:

Group 1: CM 10 mg/kg/day, p.o. + ALCL 50 mg/kg/day p.o. for 5 weeks
Group 2: CM 20 mg/kg/day, p.o. + ALCL 50 mg/kg/day p.o. for 5 weeks
Group 3: CM 40 mg/kg/day, p.o. + ALCL 50 mg/kg/day p.o. for 5 weeks
Group 4: DONZ 3 mg/kg/day, p.o. + ALCL 50 mg/kg/day p.o. for 5 weeks (positive control)
Group 5: water p.o. (vehicle control); for 5 weeks
Group 6: ALCL 50 mg/kg/day p.o. (negative control) 5 weeks

ALCL was given 30 minutes before DONZ and CM extract to avoid possible interactions between aluminum and other substances.

After 5 weeks, the mice were subjected to the MWM and the NOR test. Following the behavioral tests, the acetylcholinesterase enzyme test and the DPPH free radical scavenging test were performed. In addition, FT-IR and LC-MS fingerprinting analysis of the same extract were also conducted.

2.6. Behavioral Tests

2.6.1. Morris Water Maze Test (MWM). The water maze used was a large metallic circular pool painted black on the inside (110 cm diameter and 40 cm in height). Water (20 ± 1°C) was filled to a depth of 30 cm. The water maze area was divided into four equal quadrants, and a colorless escape circular platform (10 cm in diameter and 25 cm in height) was located in the south-west quadrant. The experiment was monitored using a camera which was positioned directly above the pool. The MWM task was performed as described by Bromley-Brits et al. [23]. Briefly, the experiment was conducted over a period of 6 days. Each mouse was gripped at the base of the tail and gently placed in the water, and time was noted for the mouse to find the platform (escape latency). Mice were given 4 trials per day. On day 1, the platform was made visible by the water being 1 cm below the platform. On days 2–5, the platform was submerged below the water. Day 6 was the probe trial in which the platform was completely removed, and the amount of time spent by the mouse in the target quadrant (south-west) was noted. Each animal was allowed 90 seconds to locate the platform. If an animal failed to locate the platform within this period, it was gently guided to the platform. The animal was left on the platform for 5 s upon locating it. The mouse was then dried with a towel and placed back in the cage.

2.6.2. Novel Object Recognition (NOR) Task. The NOR task was conducted as described by Mugwagwa et al. [18] to assess short-term and long-term memory. The apparatus consisted of an open rectangular box made of plastic with the following dimensions: 43 cm × 31 cm × 16 cm. The experiment was monitored by a camera placed directly above the arena. The test consisted broadly of 2 phases: a sample and test phase. During the sample phase, 2 identical objects (white, square container) were placed equidistant from each other. The mouse was placed in the arena for 5 minutes and then placed back in the cage. The process was repeated for all the animals. The apparatus was cleaned with ethanol between each trial interval so as to remove any olfactory clues which could have been left behind during previous trials. The position of the identical and novel objects was interchanged from left to right in order to prevent bias for a particular location. The same procedure was conducted for the test phase; however, one object was replaced by a novel object (green plastic toy bus). After 5 days, the same procedure was repeated except that the test phase was conducted 24 hrs after the sample phase. The time taken to explore an object was noted.

Object exploration was defined as the mouse licking, sniffing, touching the objects with the paws, or if its head was oriented towards the object within a distance of 2 cm.

The following parameters were measured: time (in seconds) spent exploring familiar object (T_f), time (in seconds) spent exploring the novel object (T_n), and total time (in seconds) spent exploring both objects ($T_f + T_n$). The percentage of discrimination index (DI%) was determined using the following equation:

$$\mathrm{DI}(\%) = \left(\frac{T_n}{T_n + T_f}\right) \times 100, \quad (1)$$

where DI = discrimination index, T_n = time (in seconds) spent exploring the novel object, and T_f = time (in seconds) spent exploring the familiar object.

2.7. Biochemical Tests

2.7.1. Acetylcholinesterase Enzyme Activity Test. Three mice from each study group were sacrificed, and their brains were isolated. The acetylcholinesterase enzyme (AChE) activity test was performed using the AChE enzyme kit from Sigma Aldrich, which measures the AChE activity of the brain homogenate. The assay is based on the Ellman method in which thiocholine, produced by AChE, reacts with 5,5¢-dithiobis (2-nitrobenzoic acid) to form a colorimetric (412 nm) product, which is proportional to the AChE activity present. The isolated brain samples were homogenized with 0.1 M phosphate buffer, pH 7.5, followed by centrifugation at 14,000 rpm. The supernatant was used for the assay. The following equation was used to calculate the ACHE activity:

$$\text{AChE activity(units/L)} = \frac{A_{2\,\text{min}} - A_{10\,\text{min}}}{A_{\text{calib}} - A_{\text{blank}}} \times n \times 200, \quad (2)$$

where 200 = equivalent activity (units/L) of the calibrator when assayed—read at 2 minutes and 10 minutes, n = dilution factor, $A_{2\text{min}}$ = absorbance of the calibrator at 2 minutes, $A_{10\text{min}}$ = absorbance of the calibrator at 10 minutes, $A_{\text{calibrator}}$ = absorbance of the calibrator at 10 minutes, and A_{blank} = absorbance of the blank at 10 minutes.

2.7.2. DPPH Radical Scavenging Assay. The free radical scavenging effect of CM was examined using the method employed by Doreddula et al. [24]. Briefly, one mL of 0.2 mM DPPH solution in methanol was mixed with the 1 mL extracts of 3.2, 6.3, 12.5, 25, 50, 100, 200, and 400 μg/mL concentrations, respectively. Absorbance was measured at 517 nm after incubation of the mixture in the dark for 20 min. The free radical scavenging activity of CM was determined by comparing its absorbance with that of a blank solution. Ascorbic acid was used as a reference standard.

The ability to scavenge the DPPH radical was calculated using the following equation:

$$\text{DPPH radical scavenging activity}(\%) = \frac{A_b - A_s}{A_b} \times 100, \quad (3)$$

where A_b = absorbance of the blank and A_s = absorbance of the sample.

2.8. Fingerprinting of the Extract of Crinum macowanii. Phytochemical fingerprinting of the extract used in this study was done using LC-MS and FT-IR analysis. In addition, rudimentary qualitative phytochemical screening was conducted to identify possible secondary metabolites in the extract.

2.8.1. LC-MS Analysis. LC-MS analysis was carried out using an Agilent HPLC 1260 System, and an Agilent Q-TOF 6530 mass spectrometer was used as the detector for fingerprinting the extract. 1 mg of free dried sample extract was dissolved in 1 mL of methanol : water (50 : 50) by volume. The resulting mixture was transferred into a 5 mL syringe and filtered through a 0.22 μm acrosdisc syringe filter into an HPLC vial for LC-MS/MS analysis. Gradient elution with composition as follows: solvent A: (water with 0.1% formic acid), solvent B: acetonitrile with 0.1% formic acid, and injection volume: 5 μL. Column temperature was maintained at 40°C and with a total run time of 27 minutes. The LC-Q-TOF-MS data was analyzed using Agilent Technologies Mass Hunter Software Version B.07.03 (509).

2.8.2. FT-IR Analysis. A Fourier-transform infrared (FT-IR) spectrophotometer was used to identify the characteristic functional groups in the extract as a further fingerprint. A portion of the freeze-dried sample was placed on the FT-IR plate with a spatula, and the spectrum was read after background subtraction using the Perkin Elmer Analyst software version 10.5.2.

2.8.3. Phytochemical Screening. Rudimentary phytochemical screening was performed as described by Yadav et al. 2014 [25]. Phytochemical tests were performed for tannins, flavonoids, alkaloids, steroids, glycosides, and saponins.

(a) Alkaloids: test for alkaloids. The crude extract was mixed with 2 mL of 1% HCl and heated gently. Mayer's and Wagner's reagents were then added to the mixture. The turbidity of the resulting precipitate was taken as evidence for the presence of alkaloids

(b) Steroids: test for steroid. The crude extract was mixed with 2 mL of chloroform and concentrated sulfuric acid was added sidewise. A red color produced in the lower chloroform layer indicated the presence of steroids

(c) Glycosides: test for glycosides Liebermann's test. The crude extract was mixed with each of 2 mL of chloroform and 2 mL of acetic acid. The mixture was cooled in ice. Carefully concentrated sulfuric acid was added. A color change from violet to blue to green indicated the presence of a steroidal nucleus, i.e., glycone portion of a glycoside

(d) Saponins: test for saponins. The crude extract was mixed with 5 mL of distilled water in a test tube, and it was shaken vigorously. The formation of stable foam was taken as an indication for the presence of saponins

(e) Flavonoids: alkaline reagent test. The crude extract was mixed with 2 mL of 2% solution of NaOH. An intense yellow color was formed which turned colorless on the addition of a few drops of diluted acid which indicated the presence of flavonoids

3. Data Analysis

All the results were expressed as mean ± SEM. Data for the MWM test were analyzed by analysis of variance (ANOVA) followed by Tukey's post hoc test in GraphPad Instat package version 7.03. Data analysis for the NOR task was evaluated using one-way analysis of variance (ANOVA) followed by Dunnett's Multiple Comparison tests in GraphPad Prism (version 7.03).

Two-way repeated measures (mixed model) ANOVA followed by Bonferroni posttests were used to compare the two objects in the object recognition task in GraphPad Prism (version 7.03). Data for the biochemical tests were analyzed using two-way analysis of variance (ANOVA) followed by post hoc multiple comparisons using Bonferroni tests. $P < 0.05$ was considered significant.

4. Results

4.1. Morris Water Maze. The effect of *Crinum macowanii* at three doses (10, 20, and 40 mg/kg) on aluminum chloride-induced memory impairment was investigated. The MWM behavioral test was utilized to assess the escape latencies (EL) and time spent in the target quadrant (TSTQ) expressed in seconds.

Results for the EL for all groups are shown in Figure 1(a). There were significant differences in the EL amongst the groups during the course of 5 days ($f = 37.43$, $P < 0.0001$). There was also a significant difference in the EL between mice in the CM 40 mg/kg group and Aluminum chloride (ALCL) group ($P < 0.0001$) with a mean EL of 26.77 ± 1.67 s and 56.43 ± 2.84 s, respectively. A significant difference was also noted between the DONZ 3 mg/kg group and ALCL group ($P < 0.0001$). No significant difference in EL was seen between CM group at 40 mg/kg and DONZ 3 mg/kg group ($P < 0.9070$). The EL for the ALCL group (mean of 56.43 ± 2.84 s) was significantly higher than the vehicle control group (water, mean of 40.53 ± 2.3 s). The DONZ 3 mg/kg group demonstrated the lowest EL (23.54 ± 1.64 s) followed by the CM at 40 mg/kg group (26.77 ± 1.67 s). Comparing the three dosage groups of CM, the CM at 40 mg/kg group showed the lowest EL followed by the CM at 20 and 10 mg/kg groups.

On day 6, the probe trial was performed wherein the time each mouse spent in the target quadrant (TSTQ) was noted. Results are shown in Figure 1(b). The ALCL group spent the least amount of time in the target quadrant (4.5 ± 1.2 s), while the highest was seen with the DONZ 3 mg/kg group (28.83 ± 2.13 s). No significant difference was seen in the time spent in the target quadrant between DONZ 3 mg/kg and CM 40 mg/kg ($P = 0.9358$). The CM 40 mg/kg treated group showed significantly more time spent in the target quadrant than the ALCL-treated group ($P < 0.0001$).

4.2. Novel Object Recognition Test. The NOR test assessed short-term and long-term memory function. It consisted of a sample and test phase. The discrimination index (DI) was calculated for each trial of the test phase to assess the preference for the novel object.

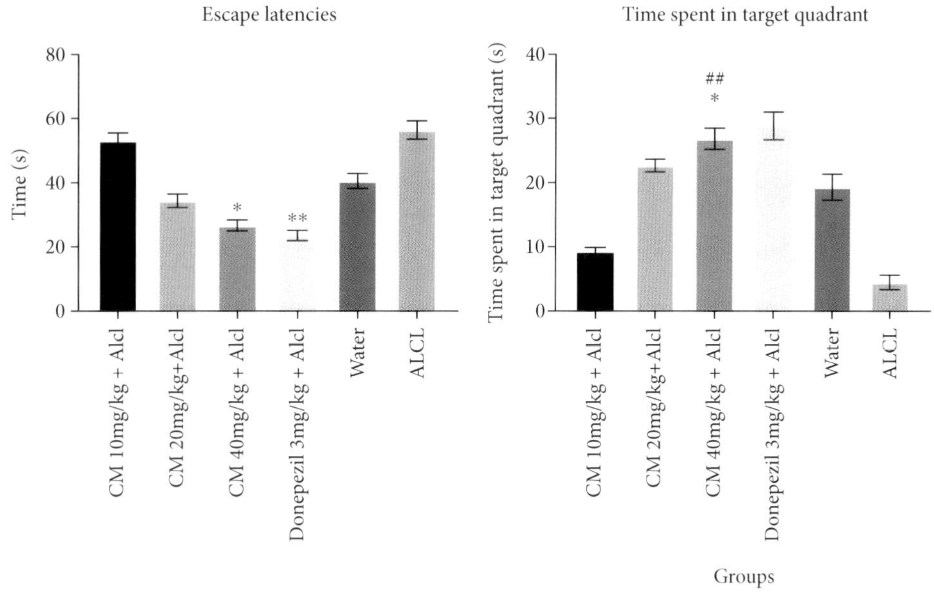

(a) (b)

FIGURE 1: (a) Escape latencies (s) for all groups from day 1 to day 5. Effect of *Crinum macowanii* (10, 20, and 40 mg/kg) on Morris water maze task. *versus ALCL, $P < 0.0001$, **versus ALCL, $P < 0.0001$. One-way analysis of variance followed by Tukey's post hoc test. (b) Time (s) spent in the target quadrant. * versus donepezil, $P = 0.9538$, ## versus ALCL-treated group, $P < 0.0001$.

The DI for the short-term phase is shown in Figure 2(c). During the short-term phase, there was no significant difference in the DI amongst the groups except between the CM 40 mg/kg and ALCL groups ($P < 0.0316$). The DI for the CM 40 mg/kg group (%DI = 58.97 ± 1.05) was higher than the DONZ 3 mg/kg group (% DI = 53.62 ± 2.1) during the short-term memory task, although this was not significant ($P = 0.4509$). During the short-term memory test, the DI was above 50% for all groups except for the ALCL-treated group (% DI = 49.1 ± 3.55). The same was observed for the long-term memory test (% DI = 46.58 ± 3.76).

During the long-term memory test shown in Figure 2(f) the DONZ 3 mg/kg treated group showed a significantly higher DI than the ALCL group ($P < 0.0071$).

During the sample phase of the short-term memory test, there was no significant difference in the time spent exploring each identical object ($P > 0.05$). In the test phase of the short-term memory test, CM 40 mg/kg treated mice spent significantly more time exploring the novel object than the familiar object ($P = 0.0180$).

During the sample phase of the long-term memory test, there was no significant difference in the time spent exploring each identical object ($P > 0.05$). The CM 10, 20, and 40 mg/kg, DONZ 3 mg/kg, and the control (water) treated mice spent more time exploring the novel object; however, this difference was not significant. In both test phases for short and long-term memory, the ALCL-treated mice showed more time exploring the familiar object than the novel object. This again was not statistically significant.

4.3. Acetylcholinesterase Enzyme Activity Test. The results for the AChE test are shown in Figure 3. The CM-treated group at 40 mg/kg exhibited significantly decreased acetylcholinesterase enzyme (AChE) activity as compared to the ALCL-treated group ($P < 0.0001$) and the control group ($P = 0.0013$). The donepezil-treated group showed the lowest AChE activity (1421 ± 23.75UL) followed by the CM 40 mg/kg treated group (2549 ± 28.65UL). The donepezil-treated group was seen to have a significantly lower AChE activity than the ALCL-treated group ($P < 0.0001$).

4.4. DPPH Radical Scavenging Assay. DPPH radical scavenging activity is shown in Figure 4. A dose-dependent increase in free radical scavenging activity was seen with an increased dose of CM; however, the DPPH free radical scavenging activity of ascorbic acid was significantly higher ($P < 0.0001$) than that of CM at all concentrations.

4.5. Results for Fingerprinting

4.5.1. LC-MS Analysis. The results for LC-MS chemical fingerprint are presented in Figure 5. The extract used in this study showed a number of prominent links. As this was meant to only be a fingerprint, no attempt was made at trying to identify the compounds associated with the respective retention times and mass to charge ratios.

4.5.2. FT-IR Analysis. The FT-IR fingerprint of the compound suggested the presence of various functional groups, which included alkyl, ketone, aldehyde, carboxylic acids, esters, and amide groups. This is presented in Figure 6.

4.5.3. Phytochemical Screening. Rudimentary phytochemical screening of the crude hydroethanolic extract of CM suggested the presence of alkaloids, steroids, glycosides, saponins, and flavonoids.

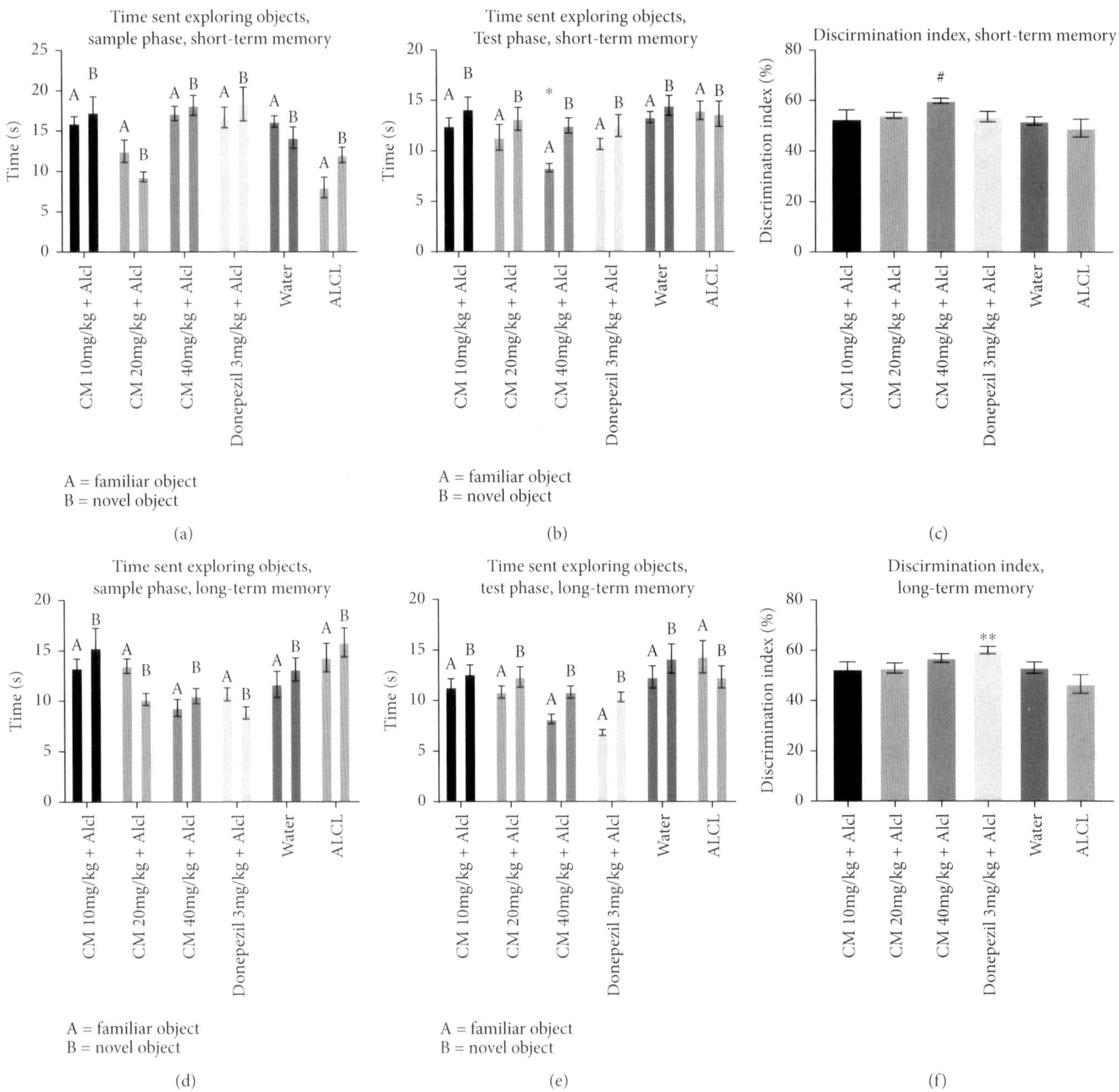

FIGURE 2: (a) Novel object recognition test, short-term memory, and sample phase. (b) Novel object recognition test, test phase, and short-term memory. (c) Novel object recognition test, discrimination index for short-term memory. Effect of *Crinum macowanii* (CM) (10, 20, and 40 mg/kg) on the short-term memory object recognition task: (a) exploration times in the sample phase, (b) exploration times in the test phase, and (c) discrimination index. $^{*}P = 0.0180$ novel object versus familiar object, $^{\#}P = 0.0358$ versus ALCL. ((a) and (b)) Two-way repeated measures (mixed model) ANOVA followed by Bonferroni posttests. (c) One-way analysis of variance followed by Dunnett's Multiple Comparison tests. (d) Novel object recognition test, sample phase, and long-term memory. (e) Novel object recognition test, test phase, and long-term memory. (f) Novel object recognition test, discrimination index, and long-term memory. Effect of *Crinum macowanii* (CM) (10, 20, and 40 mg/kg) on the long-term memory object recognition task: (d) exploration times in the sample phase, (e) exploration times in the test phase, and (f) discrimination index. ($^{**}P = 0.0071$ versus ALCL). ((d) and (e)) Two-way repeated measures (mixed model) ANOVA followed by Bonferroni posttests. (f) One-way analysis of variance followed by Dunnett's Multiple Comparison tests.

5. Discussion

The current study investigated the effect of a hydroethanolic extract of *Crinum macowanii* bulbs in the aluminum mouse model for Alzheimer's disease using the novel object recognition task and the Morris water maze test for assessing memory function.

Memory function in animal models is generally assessed using various behavioral tasks. We have employed the Morris water maze and novel object recognition task. The MWM

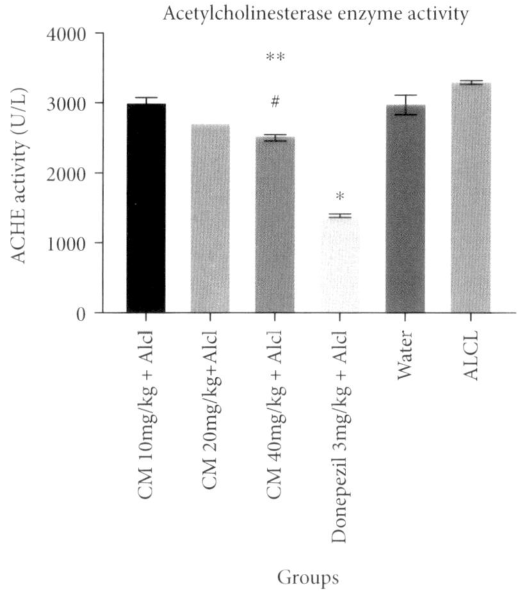

FIGURE 3: Acetylcholinesterase enzyme activity assay. Effect of *C. macowanii* on AChE activity in the brain homogenate of mice. Values are mean ± SEM. Data was analyzed by two-way ANOVA followed by Bonferroni multiple comparisons test. $^{*}P < 0.0001$ versus the control group; $^{\#}P = 0.0013$ versus the control group; $^{**}P < 0.001$ versus the ALCL-treated group.

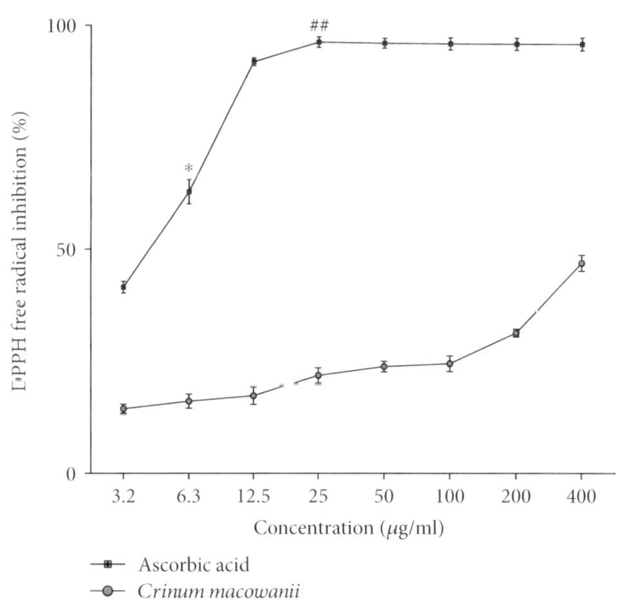

FIGURE 4: DPPH free radical scavenging activity of a crude extract of *Crinum macowanii*. DPPH radical scavenging activity of *Crinum macowanii* and ascorbic acid. The data are the representative of three independent experiments. Values are mean ± SEM. The data were analyzed by two-way ANOVA followed by Bonferroni multiple comparisons test. CM versus AA, $^{*}P < 0.0001$; CM versus AA, $^{\#\#}P < 0.0001$.

test is one of the main behavioral tests used to assess memory function, has the ability to differentiate between spatial and nonspatial memory deficits [26], and can also evaluate learning and relearning [27]. A previous study which evaluated the antiamnesic activity of CM suggested that the extract of CM may be used in the treatment of AD [18]. The study, however, did not utilize the MWM. Moreover, the animal model employed in this current study is known to mimic AD more closely than the scopolamine mouse model.

β-amyloid protein *($A\beta P$)* is a peptide resulting from the cleavage of the amyloid precursor protein. This is the basis of the amyloid cascade hypothesis which suggests that the accumulation of $A\beta P$ results in the pathogenesis of AD [28, 29]. It has been demonstrated that the polymerization of $A\beta P$ is enhanced by aluminum [30]. Orally administered aluminum was seen to increase the amount of $A\beta P$ in mice [31]. This suggests that the aluminum mouse model is a relevant animal model for AD. The fact that aluminum has a role to play in the amyloid hypothesis and is an abundant metal which can be commonly ingested by humans makes the aluminum mouse model a relevant model for studying the pathogenesis of AD. In this study, the ALCL-treated mice showed the highest EL and the least time spent in target quadrant, which implied memory impairment due to aluminum.

In the MWM test, a decreased EL during 5 days of trials and an increase in time spent in the target quadrant on the 6th day indicated improved memory function. CM at a dosage of 40 mg/kg showed a significant memory-enhancing effect as compared to the negative control (ALCL) and the vehicle control (water). The CM 40 mg/kg group was also seen to possess similar memory-enhancing effects as the positive control group—DONZ, which is one of the currently approved medications for treating AD. The DONZ 3 mg/kg group showed the lowest EL, although not significantly different than the CM 40 mg/kg group. This suggests that CM at 40 mg/kg was comparable to DONZ 3 mg/kg in improving memory function. The significantly shorter EL of the CM 40 mg/kg treated group as compared to the control group suggests that the *C. macowanii* extract improved memory function in the MWM test against aluminum chloride-induced memory impairment. A dose-dependent decrease in EL was seen in all treatment groups of CM with an increase in dose of the extract.

The probe trial on day 6th was performed by removing the platform from the maze. The time spent in the target quadrant by each mouse was noted and a longer amount of time spent in the target quadrant indicated improved memory function. Similar results were observed during the probe trial, wherein the DONZ group spent the longest time in the target quadrant, but no significant difference was seen in time spent in the target quadrant between the DONZ 3 mg/kg and the CM 40 mg/kg groups. CM 40 mg/kg treated mice spent significantly more time in the target quadrant than the ALCL group. The results of the EL and time spent in the target quadrant indicate that CM extract attenuated aluminum-induced spatial memory impairment.

The novel object recognition test was used to assess short- and long-term memory. The present study evaluated the use of *C. macowanii* extract for its memory enhancing effect against aluminum chloride-induced memory impairment in mice.

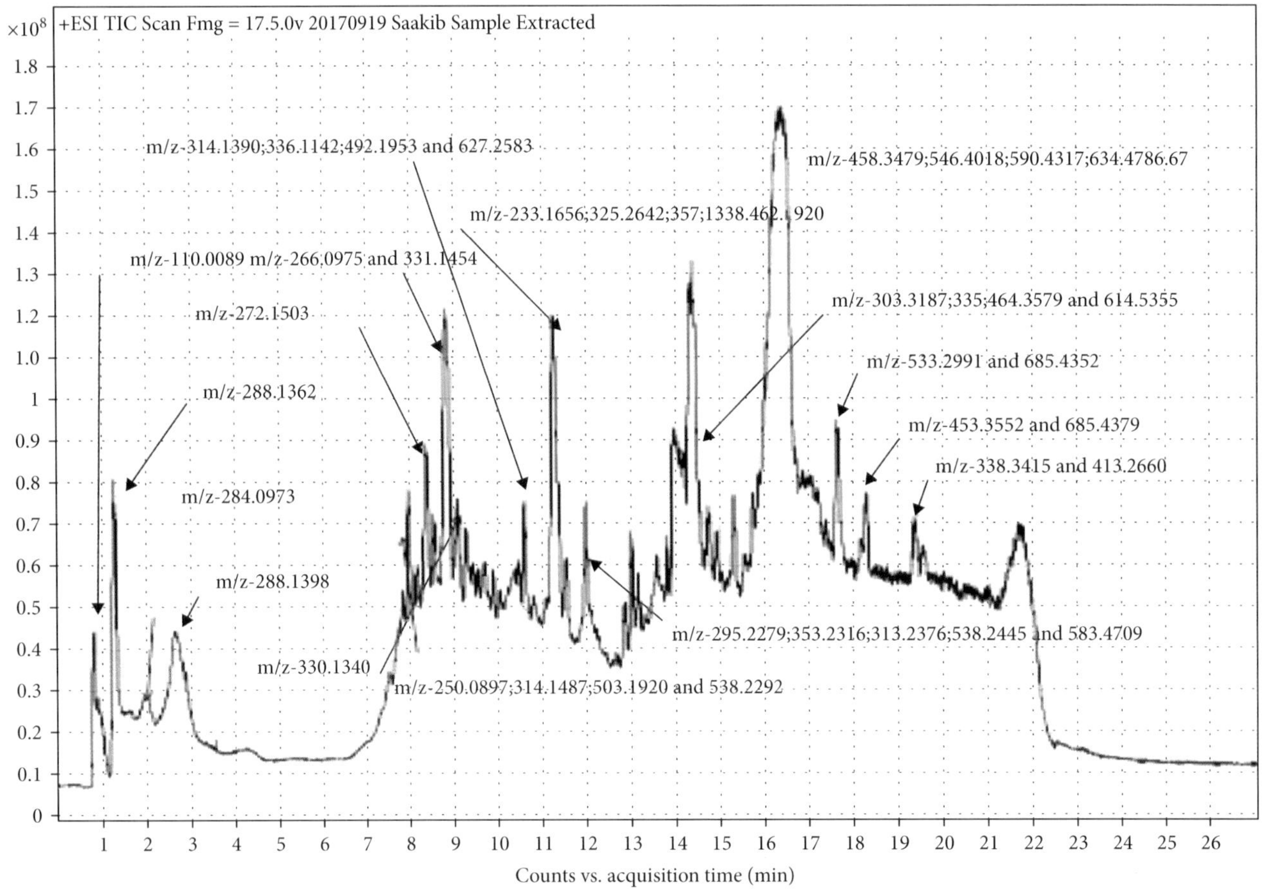

FIGURE 5: The LC-MS fingerprint of a crude hydroethanolic extract of *C. macowanii*. The LC-MS fingerprint of a crude hydroethanolic extract of *C. macowanii* with prominent peaks.

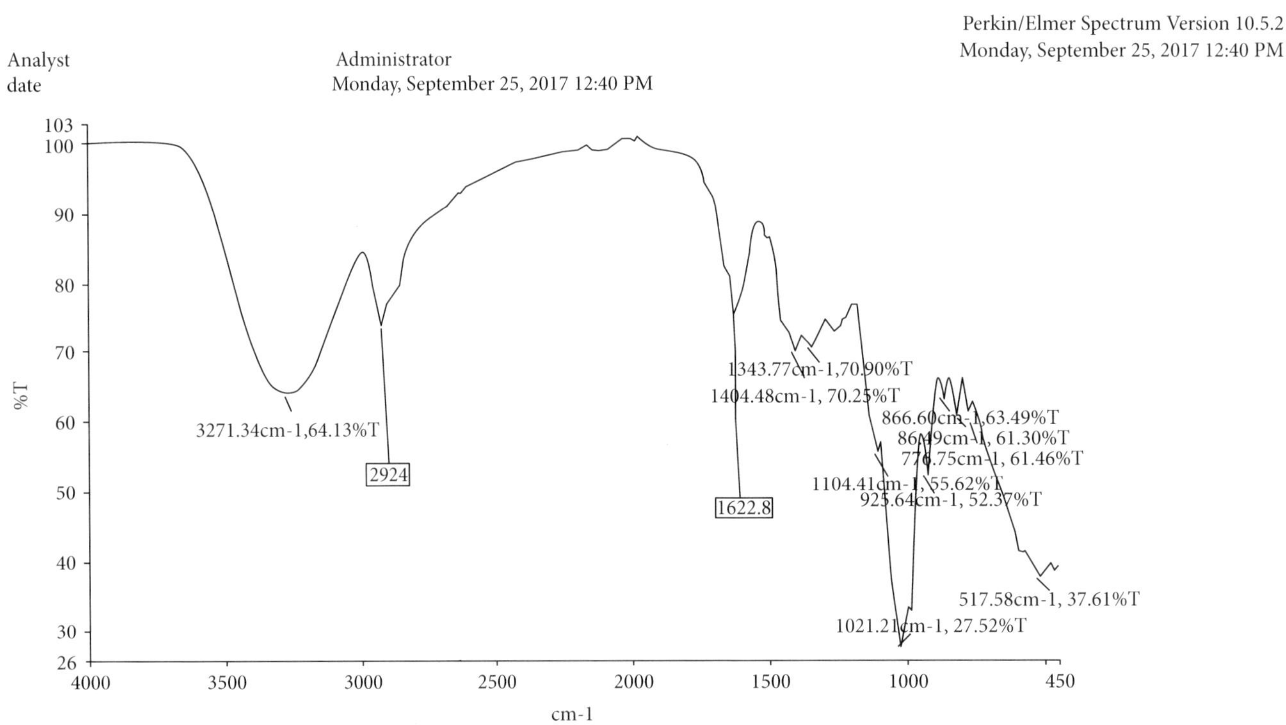

FIGURE 6: FT-IR spectrum of a hydroethanolic extract of *Crinum macowanii* showing the most prominent peaks.

Although there was no significant difference in time spent exploring each identical object in the sample phase for short-term memory, significant differences were seen in the test phase.

CM 40 mg/kg treated mice spent significantly more time exploring the novel object than the familiar object ($P = 0.0180$) for the short-term memory task. This was also confirmed by the percentage of discrimination indices which showed a significant difference as compared to the negative control—ALCL. The increase in DI and exploration time of the novel object in mice treated with *C. macowanii* at 40 mg/kg suggested short-term memory enhancing activity. During the long-term memory task for the test phase, no group showed any significant preference for exploring the novel object. Hence, it may be said that none of the doses of *C. macowanii* can be helpful for improving long-term memory against aluminum-induced memory impairment.

Mugwagwa et al. [18] have demonstrated that CM failed to attenuate memory deficits caused by scopolamine in the short-term memory task of NOR. However, CM at high doses showed long-term memory enhancing activity. In contrast, this study has shown that CM was more effective in improving short-term memory rather than long-term memory in the NOR task. The reason for the difference is unclear but may be due to the different mouse models used in each study.

Various studies have reported the presence of alkaloids in CM, while acetylcholinesterase inhibitory activity has also been reported in some [17]. We know that AD is a result of neurodegeneration which results in a decrease in cholinergic transmission in the brain [32]. An effective treatment strategy to improve AChE function is to inhibit the enzyme-acetylcholinesterase which is responsible for the breakdown of acetylcholine, thereby increasing the amount of acetylcholine. CM is an ideal candidate since we have established that the extract does inhibit AChE. The AChE activity test was performed to assess the enzyme inhibitory activity of CM. A higher enzyme activity indicates an inverse relation with the amount of acetylcholine present in the brain. The AChE assay exhibited a dose-dependent decrease in AChE activity in the CM-treated groups. Isolated samples obtained from the brains of the CM-treated groups showed a significantly lower AChE activity than the ALCL-treated group and the control group. The outcome of this study shows that CM has an inhibitory effect on the enzyme—AChE. The AChE activity is likely due to the presence of alkaloids such as lycorine [17].

The DPPH free radical scavenging assay was performed to assess the antioxidant activity of the crude extract of CM. Although a dose-dependent increase of free radical scavenging activity was seen with an increased dose of CM, the activity was significantly less than that of ascorbic acid.

Phytochemical screening chemical tests for the hydroethanolic extract of CM showed the presence of glycosides, alkaloids, saponins, steroids, and flavonoids. The presence of flavonoids may play a neuroprotective role in AD.

The pathogenesis of AD is a complex process resulting from many factors such as ingestion of toxic metals, e.g., aluminum, the decrease in cholinergic transmission, the presence of amyloid protein, and/or neurodegeneration caused by free radicals. These AD-like pathologies may potentially be treated by CM since this study has shown CM to possess AChE inhibitory activity and antioxidant activity. Furthermore, CM has shown to attenuate ALCL-induced memory deficits in the MWM and NOR tasks.

6. Conclusion

The hydroethanolic crude extract of *C. macowanii* at a dose of 40 mg/kg showed short-term memory enhancing activity in the NOR task. The same was not demonstrated in the long-term memory task. *C. macowanii* at high doses demonstrated a memory-enhancing effect in the Morris water maze test which was seen to be comparable to that of donepezil. Hence, it may be concluded that *C. macowanii* at high doses ameliorates aluminum chloride-induced memory deficits in mice in the Morris water maze and novel object recognition test and may be of potential benefit in treating AD and related disorders.

Abbreviations

AChE: Acetylcholinesterase
AChEi: Acetylcholinesterase inhibitor
Aβ: Amyloid beta
AD: Alzheimer's disease
ALCL: Aluminum chloride
CM: *Crinum macowanii*
DONZ: Donepezil
DI: Discrimination index
EL: Escape latency
FT-IR: Fourier-transform infrared spectroscopy
LC-MS: Liquid chromatography–mass spectrometry
MWM: Morris water maze
NOR: Novel object recognition.

Acknowledgments

The authors are thankful to the School of Pharmacy, Department of Biochemistry and the Department of Clinical Pharmacology, University of Zimbabwe for the usage of the laboratory facilities. The plant was authenticated by Mr. Chapano from the Botanical Gardens and National Herbarium.

References

[1] A. Burns and S. Iliffe, "Alzheimer's disease," *BMJ*, vol. 338, p. b158, 2009.

[2] J. Sevigny, P. Chiao, T. Bussière et al., "The antibody aducanumab reduces Aβ plaques in Alzheimer's disease," *Nature*, vol. 537, no. 7618, pp. 50–56, 2016.

[3] J. Hardy and D. Allsop, "Amyloid deposition as the central event in the aetiology of Alzheimer's disease," *Trends in Pharmacological Sciences*, vol. 12, no. 10, pp. 383–388, 1991.

[4] A. Mudher and S. Lovestone, "Alzheimer's disease-do tauists and baptists finally shake hands?," *Trends in Neurosciences*, vol. 25, no. 1, pp. 22–26, 2002.

[5] L. Bertram and R. E. Tanzi, "Thirty years of Alzheimer's disease genetics: the implications of systematic meta-analyses," *Nature Reviews Neuroscience*, vol. 9, no. 10, pp. 768–778, 2008.

[6] J. Folch, D. Petrov, M. Ettcheto et al., "Current research therapeutic strategies for Alzheimer's disease treatment," *Neural Plasticity*, vol. 2016, Article ID 8501693, 15 pages, 2016.

[7] R. Bartus, R. Dean, B. Beer, and A. Lippa, "The cholinergic hypothesis of geriatric memory dysfunction," *Science*, vol. 217, no. 4558, pp. 408–414, 1982.

[8] J. L. Cummings and C. Back, "The cholinergic hypothesis of neuropsychiatric symptoms in Alzheimer's disease," *The American Journal of Geriatric Psychiatry*, vol. 6, no. 2, Supplement 1, pp. S64–S78, 1998.

[9] M. Farlow, "A clinical overview of cholinesterase inhibitors in Alzheimer's disease," *International Psychogeriatrics*, vol. 14, Supplement 1, pp. 93–126, 2002.

[10] N. Herrmann, S. A. Chau, I. Kircanski, and K. L. Lanctôt, "Current and emerging drug treatment options for Alzheimer's disease," *Drugs*, vol. 71, no. 15, pp. 2031–2065, 2011.

[11] A. P. Murray, M. B. Faraoni, M. J. Castro, N. P. Alza, and V. Cavallaro, "Natural AChE inhibitors from plants and their contribution to Alzheimer's disease therapy," *Current Neuropharmacology*, vol. 11, no. 4, pp. 388–413, 2013.

[12] J. Refaat, M. S. Kamel, M. A. Ramadan, and A. A. Ali, "Crinum and an endless source of bioactive principles: a review. Part 1-Crinum alkaloids: lycorine-type alkaloids," *International Journal of Pharmaceutical Sciences and Research*, vol. 3, no. 7, pp. 1883–1890, 2012.

[13] J. Refaat, M. S. Kamel, M. A. Ramadan, and A. A. Ali, "Crinum and an endless source of bioactive principles: a review, part II. Crinum alkaloids: crinine-type alkaloids," *International Journal of Pharmaceutical Sciences and Research*, vol. 3, no. 9, p. 3091, 2012.

[14] J. Refaat, M. S. Kamel, M. A. Ramadan, and A. A. Ali, "Crinum, III, an endless source of bioactive principles: a review. Part 1*crinum alkaloids*: belladine-, galanthamine-, lycorenine-, tazettine-type alkaloids and other minor types," *International Journal of Pharmaceutical Sciences and Research*, vol. 3, no. 10, p. 3630, 2012.

[15] A. Maroyi, "A review of ethnoboatany, therapeutic value, phytochemistry and pharmacology of Crinum macowanii Baker: a highly traded bulbous plant in Southern Africa," *Journal of Ethnopharmacology*, vol. 194, pp. 595–608, 2016.

[16] E. E. Elgorashi, S. E. Drewes, and J. Van Staden, "Organ-to-organ and seasonal variation in alkaloids from Crinum macowanii," *Fitoterapia*, vol. 73, no. 6, pp. 490–495, 2002.

[17] E. E. Elgorashi, G. I. Stafford, and J. van Staden, "Acetylcholinesterase enzyme inhibitory effects of Amaryllidaceae alkaloids," *Planta Medica*, vol. 70, no. 3, pp. 260–262, 2004.

[18] A. T. Mugwagwa, L. L. Gadaga, W. Pote, and D. Tagwireyi, "Antiamnesic effects of a hydroethanolic extract of *Crinum macowanii* on scopolamine-induced memory impairment in mice," *Journal of Neurodegenerative Diseases*, vol. 2015, Article ID 242505, 9 pages, 2015.

[19] G. M. Berlyne, J. Ben Ari, E. Knopf, R. Yagil, G. Weinberger, and G. M. Danovitch, "Aluminium toxicity in rats," *Lancet*, vol. 299, no. 7750, pp. 564–568, 1972.

[20] J. R. McDermott, A. I. Smith, K. Iqbal, and H. M. Wisniewski, "Brain aluminum in aging and Alzheimer disease," *Neurology*, vol. 29, no. 6, pp. 809–814, 1979.

[21] F. Ashall and A. M. Goate, "Role of the β-amyloid precursor protein in Alzheimer's disease," *Trends in Biochemical Sciences*, vol. 19, no. 1, pp. 42–46, 1994.

[22] Z. I. Linardaki, M. G. Orkoula, A. G. Kokkosis, F. N. Lamari, and M. Margarity, "Investigation of the neuroprotective action of saffron (*Crocus sativus* L.) in aluminum-exposed adult mice through behavioral and neurobiochemical assessment," *Food and Chemical Toxicology*, vol. 52, pp. 163–170, 2013.

[23] K. Bromley-Brits, Y. Deng, and W. Song, "Morris water maze test for learning and memory deficits in Alzheimer's disease model mice," *Journal of Visualized Experiments*, no. 53, 2011.

[24] S. K. Doreddula, S. R. Bonam, D. P. Gaddam, B. S. R. Desu, N. Ramarao, and V. Pandy, "Phytochemical analysis, antioxidant, antistress, and nootropic activities of aqueous and methanolic seed extracts of ladies finger (*Abelmoschus esculentus* L.) in mice," *The Scientific World Journal*, vol. 2014, Article ID 519848, 14 pages, 2014.

[25] M. Yadav, S. Chatterji, S. K. Gupta, and G. Watal, "Preliminary phytochemical screening of six medicinal plants used in traditional medicine," *International Journal of Pharmacy and Pharmaceutical Sciences*, vol. 6, no. 5, pp. 539–542, 2014.

[26] R. D'Hooge and P. P. De Deyn, "Applications of the Morris water maze in the study of learning and memory," *Brain Research Reviews*, vol. 36, no. 1, pp. 60–90, 2001.

[27] A. V. Terry Jr and J. J. Buccafusco, "Spatial navigation (water maze) tasks," in *Methods of Behavior Analysis in Neuroscience*, pp. 169–182, CRC Press, 2009.

[28] J. Hardy and D. J. Selkoe, "The amyloid hypothesis of Alzheimer's disease: progress and problems on the road to therapeutics," *Science*, vol. 297, no. 5580, pp. 353–356, 2002.

[29] O. Wirths, G. Multhaup, and T. A. Bayer, "A modified β-amyloid hypothesis: intraneuronal accumulation of the β-amyloid peptide - the first step of a fatal cascade," *Journal of Neurochemistry*, vol. 91, no. 3, pp. 513–520, 2004.

[30] M. Kawahara and M. Kato-Negishi, "Link between aluminum and the pathogenesis of Alzheimer's disease: the integration of the aluminum and amyloid cascade hypotheses," *International Journal of Alzheimer's Disease*, vol. 2011, Article ID 276393, 17 pages, 2011.

[31] D. Praticò, K. uryu, S. Sung, S. Tang, J. Q. Trojanowski, and V. M. Y. Lee, "Aluminum modulates brain amyloidosis through oxidative stress in APP transgenic mice," *The FASEB Journal*, vol. 16, no. 9, pp. 1138–1140, 2002.

[32] D. Schuster, M. Spetea, M. Music et al., "Morphinans and isoquinolines: acetylcholinesterase inhibition, pharmacophore modeling, and interaction with opioid receptors," *Bioorganic & Medicinal Chemistry*, vol. 18, no. 14, pp. 5071–5080, 2010.

7

Face-to-Face or Telematic Cognitive Stimulation in Patients with Multiple Sclerosis and Cognitive Impairment: Why Not Both?

C. Guijarro-Castro,[1] Y. Aladro-Benito,[2] A. Sánchez-Musulim,[3] A. Belen-Caminero,[4] I. Pérez Molina,[5] I. Gómez-Moreno,[1] L. Gómez-Romero,[1] J. Millán-Pascual,[6] M. J. Laredo,[2] and M. Cerezo-García[2]

[1]*Sección de Neurología, Hospital Virgen de la Luz, Cuenca, Spain*
[2]*Sección de Neurología, Hospital Universitario de Getafe de Madrid, Madrid, Spain*
[3]*Hospital Santa Bárbara de Puertollano, Ciudad Real, Spain*
[4]*Sección de Neurología, Hospital Ntra. Sra. de Sonsoles de Ávila, Ávila, Spain*
[5]*Hospital Universitario Virgen de la Salud de Toledo, Toledo, Spain*
[6]*Sección de Neurología, Hospital La Mancha Centro de Alcazar de San Juan, Ciudad Real, Spain*

Correspondence should be addressed to C. Guijarro-Castro; cristina.guijarro@sen.es

Academic Editor: Lambros Messinis

Introduction. Cognitive impairment (CI) affects 40–65% of patients with multiple sclerosis (MS). Few studies address telematic cognitive stimulation (TCS) in MS. The objective of this study is to evaluate the efficacy and impact of telestimulation or distance cognitive stimulation (TCS), with and without the support of face-to-face cognitive stimulation (FCS) in cognitive impairment in MS. *Methods.* Multicentre, prospective, randomised, controlled study. We will include 98 MS patients with EDSS ≤ 6, symbol digit modality test (SDMT) $\leq$ Pc 25, and Multiple Sclerosis Neuropsychological Screening Questionnaire (MSNQ) > 26 points. Patients will be randomised into 3 groups, a TCS group, a mixed TCS/FCS group, and a control group. CS is performed 3 days a week for 3 months. Processing speed, memory, attention, and executive functions will be rehabilitated. FCS will include ecological exercises and strategies. EDSS and a cognitive evaluation (SDMT, CTMT, PASAT, and TAVEC), MSNQ, psychological impact scales (MSIS), and depression (BDI) will be carried out, baseline, postrehabilitation, and also 6 and 12 months later, to evaluate the effect of CS in the longer term. *Conclusion.* This study could help to establish the usefulness of TCS or, in its absence, TCS with face-to-face help for CI in MS. The interest lies in the clear benefits of remote rehabilitation in the daily life of patients.

1. Introduction

Multiple sclerosis (MS), a chronic demyelinating disease, is characterised by a heterogeneous set of symptoms that can lead to severe disability and have an impact on accessibility to medical services, functional capacity of the patient, and health-related quality of life (HRQOL) [1].

Cognitive impairment (CI) affects 40–65% of patients and mainly involves information processing speed (IPS), attention, executive functions, and memory. It becomes more frequent as the disease evolves, but may appear in early stages and be independent of physical disability. IC correlates mainly with cerebral atrophy estimated by magnetic resonance (MR) volumetric techniques [2–4]. In MS, deficits in concentration, attention, working memory, IPS, and executive functions, predominantly in problem solving and abstract reasoning [5], are more frequently observed. Deficits vary from series to series in relation to, among other factors, the neuropsychological batteries used and the type of patient studied. Two neuropsychological batteries have been widely accepted for the study of CI in MS, the Rao Brief Battery (BRB-N) [6], and the MACFIMS (Minimal Assessment of

Cognitive Function in Multiple Sclerosis) [7]. Both have the inconvenience of administration time, 30 and 90 minutes, respectively, and require qualified personnel. The Symbol Digit Modalities Test (SDMT) (about 2 minutes for execution) has been proposed as a screening test because of its high sensitivity and specificity to discriminate patients with and without CI. It is a good tool in longitudinal studies because of its reproducibility [8]. Recently, the BICAMS (Brief International Cognitive Assessment of Multiple Sclerosis) has been proposed as a new screening battery. This has been validated in 28 countries and supported by different neurological associations. It takes 15 minutes, can be performed by nonspecialised staff, and includes the California Verbal Learning Test-II (CVLT-II), the Brief Visuospatial Memory Test-Revised, and the SDMT [9].

There is no pharmacological treatment for CI in MS [10]. There is a sufficient consensus on the protective role of intellectual enrichment in the development of CI in dementia and aging. In MS, the work is with lower numbers but the results are similar: level of education and the intellectual enrichment maintained by leisure activities such as reading, among others, diminish the deleterious effect of the lesional load and atrophy in cognition [11, 12]. There are few studies that analyse the effect of cognitive rehabilitation on MS's cognitive dysfunction [13]. Recent analyses by Cochrane [14, 15] show that intensive training, specifically in memory, seems to have a clear benefit. Fifteen phase III studies with a total of 989 participants are included, but the risk of bias is low in only 7 of these and heterogeneity is important. The results are more contradictory with attention; there is little work with rehabilitation programmes aimed at treating IPS and executive functions [8, 9, 14, 15]. Functional MRI studies have shown that this CS activates the prefrontal and cingulate cortexes [16].

1.1. Justification and Hypotheses. No comparative studies comparing telematic (TCS) and face-to-face stimulation (FCS) with neuropsychologists are currently known. Telestimulation would offer clear advantages for the patient, given its lower interruption in their daily activities, work, social life, and so forth. With the design of this randomised and controlled pilot study, we want to compare individualised training by TCS with face-to-face support, with individualised training only by TCS.

1.2. Objectives of the Study

1.2.1. Main Goal. The main goal is to evaluate the efficacy and impact of TCS with and without FCS support on CI.

1.2.2. Secondary Objectives

(1) Evaluate the degree of patient satisfaction with the TCS programme.

(2) Evaluate adherence to treatment with the TCS programmes.

(3) Evaluate if the changes obtained with the rehabilitation treatment are maintained at 6 and 12 months of the CS.

2. Material and Methods

This is an experimental, prospective, randomised, controlled, minimally interventional, and multicentre study.

The study is being carried out in the following hospitals, with the approval of the Research Ethics Committee of each centre: Hospital Virgen de la Luz (Cuenca), Hospital Universitario Virgen de la Salud (Toledo), Hospital Santa Bárbara (Ciudad Real), Hospital Virgen de Sonsoles (Ávila), Hospital Valdepeñas (Ciudad Real), and Hospital Universitario de Getafe (Madrid).

Patients with MS according to the McDonald Criteria, 2010 (1917) from multiple sclerosis consultations ranging from 18–65 years old, EDSS (Expanded Disability Status Scale, 1983) ≤ 6, with a score of >26 in the Multiple Sclerosis Neuropsychological Screening Questionnaire (MSNQ) [17] and/or $\leq$Pc 25 in the SDMT [18], have signed informed consent.

Exclusion criteria are severe cognitive impairment (defined by the Mini-Mental State Examination (MMSE) scores ≤ 26) [19], being free of attacks and/or treatment with corticosteroids 30 days before the first cognitive assessment, presence of other CNS disease, history of vascular or traumatic brain damage, and psychiatric disorder or psychotropic substance abuse that may interfere with the test performance.

The patients included will be randomised into 3 groups: (1) TCS group, patients will receive only telematic intervention for 3 days each week; (2) mixed TCS/FCS group, patients will receive telematic intervention for 2 days more FCS for one day each week; and (3) control group. The face-to-face rehabilitation will be performed with 2 neuropsychologists in groups of five patients. As in the design of another recent clinical trial on cognitive rehabilitation, our control group will be assigned to the waiting list, providing the opportunity to participate in the cognitive rehabilitation programme once the study has been completed [20].

2.1. Neurological and Neuropsychological Evaluation. Patients from all three groups will undergo a neuropsychological evaluation that includes the domains of IPS, attention, memory, and executive functions, before starting CS (baseline visit), at the end of 12 weeks of treatment (visit 2) and at 6 and 12 months.

The neurological and neuropsychological evaluation is detailed as follows:

(1) Disability: EDSS, baseline, and after training

(2) Neuropsychological testing

 (i) Processing speed: SDMT [18], Comprehensive Trail Making Test (CTMT) CTMT 1 [21]

 (ii) Attention: CTMT 2 y 3 [20]

 (iii) Executive functions: PASAT 3 (Paced Auditory Serial Addition Test) [22], CTMT 4 and 5, verbal fluency (phonological and semantic)

(iv) Memory: Spain-Complutense Verbal Learning Test (TAVEC) (Spanish version of the California Verbal Learning Test) [23]

(3) Self-administered questionnaires

(i) Risk for neuropsychological impairment and self-perceived cognitive quality of life: MSNQ [17]

(ii) Fatigue: Fatigue Severity Scale (FSS) and Fatigue Impact Scale (FIS) [24]

(iii) Physical and psychosocial impact of MS: Multiple Sclerosis Impact Scale (MSIS-29) [25]

(iv) Depression: Beck Depression Inventory (BDI) [26]

(v) Satisfaction measure: satisfaction questionnaire

2.1.1. Cognitive Stimulation Programme

(1) Cognitive Telestimulation Programme. A state-of-the-art cognitive stimulation application will be installed on the latest generation devices (computers, tablets, and smartphones). This platform is based on a web resource and mobile applications and uses games, validated [27, 28] and selected by expert neuropsychologists. This computer programme has been validated in fibromyalgia, healthy students and children with attention deficit hyperactivity disorder [27, 28]. It has different training settings ("full brain," "athletes," "students," "drivers," "executives," "over 60," and "children") and allows users to obtain a profile of the advances obtained by cognitive stimulation. In addition, they are sent reminder messages to perform assigned tasks. They have 62 games classified according to the predominant cognitive domain, "perception and speed," "memory," "attention," and "executive functions."

At each training session, patients will perform 4 sets (one from each cognitive domain), with an estimated time of 15 minutes for all four games.

(2) Cognitive Stimulation Face-to-Face in Cognitive Strategies. It will be based on exercises and teach strategies with ecological exercises based on principles of optimisation, compensation, and restoration, to improve cognition (one session), attention (2 sessions), memory (2 sessions), and executive functions (one session on inhibition and another on problem solving). There will be 3 more sessions for presentation and adherence to the programme, feedback on the CS software, and evaluation of the programme.

2.2. Statistical Analysis. We have calculated the sample size with an online platform (http://Fisterra.com). The sample size estimate is based on an analysis of the MSIS. Starting from a population of 450 patients with MS, a sample size of 98 patients with CI and MS representative of MSIS has been calculated.

The SPSS.22.0 program will be used for statistical analysis.

The primary outcome was a cognitive performance measured by improvement in SDMT, PASAT, CTMT and TAVEC, and self-perceived psychosocial impact (MSNQ, MSIS-29).

Continuous variables will be expressed as mean and standard deviation or median and 25th and 75th percentiles and categorical variables as percentages. The normal distribution of the data will be verified by the Kolmogorov–Smirnov test. To compare baseline demographic, clinical, and neuropsychological variables between groups, one-way ANOVA or Kruskal-Wallis will be used for quantitative variables and Chi-square or Fisher's exact test for categorical variables.

The effect of CS on cognitive performance was measured in each group (named "intragroup") comparing cognitive scores before and after treatment using an ANCOVA (analysis of covariance) adjusted by depression level or Friedman test for independent samples. To compare outcomes in cognitive scores between groups, an ANCOVA adjusted by sex, age, education level, baseline cognitive scores, and depression level will be used. The same procedure will be employed to analyse the effect of CS on MSIS and MSNQ as daily life impact measures.

Patients will be stratified in 2 groups: cognitive improvement and no changes/impairment in order to evaluate if age, sex, EDSS, educational level, baseline cognitive status, and FCS support (independent variables) have a capacity of predicting the cognitive improvement (dependent variable) through a logistic regression model. Cognitive improvement is defined as a gain > 1.5 S.D. in the score in at least 2 cognitive tests.

This study has been awarded a grant for research in the XIII Call for Research Grants of 2016 from the Mutua Madrileña Foundation.

3. Discussion

Telemedicine (TM) is the exchange of medical information between two different physical locations. The goals of TM are to provide services that cannot be managed face-to-face and improve the efficiency of existing ones. The use of TM to clinically monitor MS patients has been shown to improve Health-related quality of life (HRQOL), reducing the cost of associated medical services [29]. A randomised clinical trial has shown that cognitive behavioural therapy was an effective treatment for fatigue in MS, using an internet-based version programme consisting of eight interactive sessions with clinical psychologists [30]; although studies with a greater number of patients are needed.

A recent Spanish study demonstrated the usefulness of TM to assess gait disability in MS patients, especially in the most disabled. The gait distance evaluation included a video of self-performed neurological examination and specific multimedia questionnaires, together with the measurements of a triaxial accelerometer [31].

Several studies about impact of cognitive rehabilitation in MS, although with methodology limitations [32], show some improvements in attention, IPS, executive functions, and working memory [33, 34]. They have few patients and are not comparable and thus do not confirm the effectiveness reported. Cochrane has performed a systematic review on TCS in MS patients, including studies using telecommunication technology in their environment [35]. They included nine randomised clinical trials ($N = 531$ participants, 469 patients included) investigating a variety of TCS interventions in adults with MS. These interventions were complex, with more than one rehabilitation component, and included physical activity and management of behavioural and educational symptoms. The methodological quality was considered low. They conclude that there is "low-level" evidence for TCS interventions in reducing short-term disability and fatigue, functional activities, fatigue, pain, insomnia, and long-term psychological symptoms. The data was limited on the evaluation of the process (the satisfaction of the participants and the therapists), and no cost analysis was performed [35]. Despite the paucity of data and the low level of evidence, partly explained by methodological problems, such interventions could be an alternative method of functional and cognitive rehabilitation in MS patients, although more robust trials are needed to prove clinical effectiveness and the cost of these interventions [35, 36].

Several authors have reported that adaptation to these computer programmes is good. Amato et al. observed a benefit only in sustained attention tasks in a randomised trial conducted on 88 patients, using training with specific computerized training and nonspecific training for one hour twice a week. Regardless of the training received, the patients' perception was positive [37]. The same results in adaptation to the programme have recently been published with an application for mobile devices with memory exercises [38].

The main dilemma in this issue is that there are no programmes, computer programme or on-site, that have demonstrated superiority; then, there is no recommendation in this regard. Even more, we do not know what is the therapeutic window for cognitive rehabilitation. The efficacy of CS in neurodegenerative diseases, as MS, today is subject of controversy; maybe, it only allows a better adaptation to cognitive dysfunction.

Nevertheless, a recent Cochrane review of 2016 finds that the benefit of cognitive rehabilitation is clear in MS patients with cognitive impairment, at least in memory [39]. MS is a progressive disease, and CS can, through the neuronal plasticity of a young brain, meet both expectations: functional improvement and cognitive improvement. Other authors believe that CS does not improve cognitive performance but reduces perceived deficit in MS patients [36, 40]. Like other authors [41], we think that both goals can be achieved, as in stroke and brain damage.

This project aims to evaluate whether this type of intervention may be an alternative method in the treatment of patients with MS and cognitive impairment, given the need for more studies that prove the clinical effectiveness and cost of these interventions [30].

4. Conclusion

The design of our study aims to answer the question of the validity of TCS in MS patients with CI, since it has not been shown to have the same ability to maintain cortical functions as is attributed to FCS. The interest lies in the clear benefits of remote rehabilitation for patients' daily lives.

In our opinion, a feasible, cost-effective alternative that could respond to this need would be the combination of both forms of training; since in our experience, patients with CI require supervision and training in the cognitive therapy to be applied, whether face-to-face or remote.

We considered that this study could help to establish the usefulness of TCS; or in its absence, TCS with FCS helps in MS patients with CI.

Authors' Contributions

C Guijarro-Castro, Y Aladro-Benito, M Cerezo-García, and M. J. Laredo did the conceptualization. All the authors did the resource and data curation. Y Aladro-Benito and M Cerezo-García did the formal analysis. All the authors did the investigation. C Guijarro-Castro, Y Aladro-Benito, and M Cerezo-García did the writing and preparing of the original draft. All the authors did the writing, review, and editing. All authors read and approved the final manuscript.

Acknowledgments

The authors thank Mutua Madrileña Foundation and Hospital Nacional de Parapléjicos Foundation for their support.

References

[1] C. Guijarro-Castro, S. Moreno-García, F. Bermejo-Pareja, and J. Benito-León, "Calidad de vida relacionada con la salud en Esclerosis Múltiple," *Revista Española de Esclerosis Múltiple*, vol. 13, pp. 17–23, 2010.

[2] N. D. Chiaravalloti and J. DeLuca, "Cognitive impairment in multiple sclerosis," *The Lancet Neurology*, vol. 7, no. 12, pp. 1139–1151, 2008.

[3] G. C. DeLuca, R. L. Yates, H. Beale, and S. A. Morrow, "Cognitive impairment in multiple sclerosis: clinical, radiologic and pathologic insights," *Brain Pathology*, vol. 25, no. 1, pp. 79–98, 2015.

[4] C. Guijarro-Castro, M. Muñoz-Pasadas, and A. Martínez-Alvárez, "El Symbol Digit Modality Test no discrimina pacientes de Síndrome Radiológico Aislado de controles sanos," in *Comunicación en la LVXIII Reunión Anual de la SEN*, Valencia, 2015.

[5] B. A. Parmenter, B. Weinstock-Guttman, N. Garg, F. Munschauer, and R. HB Benedict, "Screening for cognitive impairment in multiple sclerosis using the symbol digit modalities test," *Multiple Sclerosis*, vol. 13, pp. 152–157, 2007.

[6] S. M. Rao, *A Manual for the Brief, Repeatable Battery of Neuropsychological Tests in Multiple Sclerosis*, National Multiple Sclerosis Society, New York, 1990.

[7] R. H. B. Benedict, D. Cookfair, R. Gavett et al., "Validity of the minimal assessment of cognitive function in multiple sclerosis (MACFIMS)," *Journal of the International Neuropsychological Society*, vol. 12, no. 4, pp. 549–558, 2006.

[8] M. P. Amato, E. Portaccio, B. Goretti et al., "Relevance of cognitive deterioration in early relapsing-remitting MS: a 3-year follow-up study," *Multiple Sclerosis Journal*, vol. 16, no. 12, pp. 1474–1482, 2010.

[9] D. W. Langdon, M. P. Amato, J. Boringa et al., "Recommendations for a brief international cognitive assessment for multiple sclerosis (BICAMS)," *Multiple Sclerosis Journal*, vol. 18, pp. 891–898, 2012.

[10] M. P. Amato, D. Langdon, X. Montalban et al., "Treatment of cognitive impairment in multiple sclerosis: position paper," *Journal of Neurology*, vol. 260, no. 6, pp. 1452–1468, 2013.

[11] R. H. Benedict, S. A. Morrow, B. Weinstock Guttman, D. Cookfair, and D. J. Schretlen, "Cognitive reserve moderates decline in information processing speed in multiple sclerosis patients," *Journal of the International Neuropsychological Society*, vol. 16, no. 05, pp. 829–835, 2010.

[12] J. F. Sumowski, M. A. Rocca, V. M. Leavitt et al., "Brain reserve and cognitive reserve protect against cognitive decline over 4.5 years in MS," *Neurology*, vol. 82, no. 20, pp. 1776–1783, 2014.

[13] E. M. Rosti-Otajärvi and P. I. Hämäläinen, "Neuropsychological rehabilitation for multiple sclerosis," *Cochrane Database of Systematic Reviews*, vol. 2, 2014.

[14] R. das Nair, H. Ferguson, D. L. Stark, and N. B. Lincoln, "Memory rehabilitation for people with multiple sclerosis," *Cochrane Database of Systematic Reviews*, vol. 3, 2012.

[15] R. das Nair, K. J. Martin, and N. B. Lincoln, "Memory rehabilitation for people with multiple sclerosis," *Cochrane Database of Systematic Reviews*, vol. 3, 2016.

[16] L. Parisi, M. A. Rocca, P. Valsasina, L. Panicari, F. Mattioli, and M. Filippi, "Cognitive rehabilitation correlates with the functional connectivity of the anterior cingulate cortex in patients with multiple sclerosis," *Brain Imaging and Behavior*, vol. 8, no. 3, pp. 387–393, 2014.

[17] R. H. Benedict, F. Munschauer, R. Linn et al., "Screening for multiple sclerosis cognitive impairment using a self-administered 15-item questionnaire," *Multiple Sclerosis Journal*, vol. 9, no. 1, pp. 95–101, 2003.

[18] J. C. Arango-Lasprilla, D. Rivera, G. Rodríguez et al., "Symbol digit modalities test: normative data for the Latin American Spanish speaking adult population," *NeuroRehabilitation*, vol. 37, no. 4, pp. 625–638, 2015.

[19] M. F. Folstein, S. E. Folstein, and P. R. McHugh, ""Mini-mental state". A practical method for grading the cognitive state of patients for the clinician," *Journal of Psychiatric Research*, vol. 12, no. 3, pp. 189–198, 1975.

[20] O. Rilo, J. Peña, N. Ojeda et al., "Integrative group-based cognitive rehabilitation efficacy in multiple sclerosis: a randomized clinical trial," *Disability and Rehabilitation*, vol. 40, no. 2, pp. 208–216, 2018.

[21] T. N. Tombaugh, "Trail making test A and B: normative data stratified by age and education," *Archives of Clinical Neuropsychology*, vol. 19, no. 2, pp. 203–214, 2004.

[22] D. M. A. Gronwall, "Paced auditory serial-addition task: a measure of recovery from concussion," *Perceptual and Motor Skills*, vol. 44, no. 2, pp. 367–373, 1977.

[23] M. J. Benedet and M. A. Alejandre, *TAVEC: test de aprendizaje verbal España-Complutense: manual*, TEA Ediciones, Madrid, 1998.

[24] L. B. Krupp, N. G. LaRocca, J. Muir-Nash, and A. D. Steinberg, "The fatigue severity scale. Application to patients with multiple sclerosis and systemic lupus erythematosus," *Archives of Neurology*, vol. 46, no. 10, pp. 1121–1123, 1989.

[25] J. Hobart, D. Lamping, R. Fitzpatrick, A. Riazi, and A. Thompson, "The multiple sclerosis impact scale (MSIS-29): a new patient-based outcome measure," *Brain*, vol. 124, no. 5, pp. 962–973, 2001.

[26] A. T. Beck, C. H. Ward, M. Mendelson, J. Mock, and J. Erbaugh, "An inventory for measuring depression," *Archives of General Psychiatry*, vol. 4, no. 6, pp. 561–571, 1961.

[27] M. Fernández-Sanchez, J. Sánchez, J. M. Diago, and J. M. Bescos, "Neuropsychological rehabilitation in fibromialgia patients. Effects of an online cognitive training program," in *Conference on Recent Advances in Neurorrehabilitation (ICRAN2013)*, Valencia, 2013.

[28] P. Fernández-Sanchez Barjola, J. Sánchez, J. M. Diago, and J. M. Bescos, "Evaluación de los efectos de un programa de brainfitness online sobre el rendimiento académico y neuropsicológico de un grupo de estudiantes universitarios," in *IN:X Congreso Andaluz de Neuropsicología: Rehabilitación Neuropsicológica en la Infancia y la Adolescencia*, Cádiz, 2013.

[29] N. Sola-Valls, Y. Blanco, M. Sepúlveda, E. Martinez-Hernandez, and A. Saiz, "Telemedicine for monitoring MS activity and progression," *Current Treatment Options in Neurology*, vol. 17, no. 11, p. 47, 2015.

[30] R. Moss-Morris, P. McCrone, L. Yardley, K. van Kessel, G. Wills, and L. Dennison, "A pilot randomised controlled trial of an internet-based cognitive behavioural therapy self-management programme (MS Invigor8) for multiple sclerosis fatigue," *Behaviour Research and Therapy*, vol. 50, no. 6, pp. 415–421, 2012.

[31] N. Sola-Valls, Y. Blanco, M. Sepúlveda et al., "Walking function in clinical monitoring of multiple sclerosis by telemedicine," *Journal of Neurology*, vol. 262, no. 7, pp. 1706–1713, 2015.

[32] A. M. Plohmann, L. Kappos, W. Ammann et al., "Computer assisted retraining of attentional impairments in patients with multiple sclerosis," *Journal of Neurology, Neurosurgery, & Psychiatry*, vol. 64, no. 4, pp. 455–462, 1998.

[33] A. Vogt, L. Kappos, P. Calabrese et al., "Working memory training in patients with multiple sclerosis - comparison of two different training schedules," *Restorative Neurology and Neuroscience*, vol. 27, no. 3, pp. 225–235, 2009.

[34] F. Mattioli, C. Stampatori, D. Zanotti, G. Parrinello, and R. Capra, "Efficacy and specificity of intensive cognitive rehabilitation of attention and executive functions in multiple sclerosis," *Journal of the Neurological Sciences*, vol. 288, no. 1-2, pp. 101–105, 2010.

[35] F. Khan, B. Amatya, J. Kesselring, and M. Galea, "Telerehabilitation for persons with multiple sclerosis," *Cochrane Database of Systematic Reviews*, vol. 9, no. 4, 2015.

[36] N. B. Lincoln, R. das Nair, L. Bradshaw et al., "Cognitive rehabilitation for attention and memory in people with multiple sclerosis: study protocol for a randomised controlled trial (CRAMMS)," *Trials*, vol. 16, no. 1, p. 556, 2015.

[37] M. Amato, B. Goretti, R. Viterbo et al., "Computer-assisted rehabilitation of attention in patients with multiple sclerosis: results of a randomized, double-blind trial," *Multiple Sclerosis Journal*, vol. 20, no. 1, pp. 91–98, 2014.

[38] A. Tacchino, L. Pedullà, L. Bonzano et al., "A new App for at-home cognitive training: description and pilot testing on patients with multiple sclerosis," *JMIR mHealth and uHealth*, vol. 3, no. 3, 2015.

[39] R. das Nair, K. Martin, and N. B. Lincoln, "Memory rehabilitation for people with multiple sclerosis," *Cochrane Database of Systematic Reviews*, no. 3, 2016.

[40] A. Mäntynen, E. Rosti-Otajärvi, K. Koivisto, A. Lilja, H. Huhtala, and P. Hämäläinen, "Neuropsychological rehabilitation does not improve cognitive performance but reduces perceived cognitive deficits in patients with multiple sclerosis: a randomised, controlled, multi-centre trial," *Multiple Sclerosis Journal*, vol. 20, no. 1, pp. 99–107, 2014.

[41] A. Cerasa, F. Tomaiuolo, and A. Quattrone, "Which is the goal of cognitive rehabilitation in multiple sclerosis: the improvement of cognitive performance or the perception of cognitive deficits?," *Multiple Sclerosis Journal*, vol. 20, no. 1, pp. 124-125, 2014.

8

Neuroprotective Effect of DAHP via Antiapoptosis in Cerebral Ischemia

Yanhua Qin,[1] Weiming Hu,[2] Yang Yang,[3] Zhiying Hu,[4] Weiyun Li,[3] and Marong Fang[3]

[1]*Department of Psychiatry, Sir Run Run Shaw Hospital, Zhejiang University School of Medicine, Hangzhou, China*
[2]*Department of Psychiatry, The Third Hospital of Quzhou, Quzhou, China*
[3]*Institute of Neuroscience, Zhejiang University School of Medicine, Hangzhou, China*
[4]*Department of Obstetrics and Gynecology, Hangzhou Red Cross Hospital, Hangzhou, China*

Correspondence should be addressed to Marong Fang; fangmaro@zju.edu.cn

Academic Editor: Tauheed Ishrat

Aberrant production of nitric oxide following inducible nitric oxide synthase (iNOS) expression has been implicated in cell death and contributes to ischemic brain injury. Tetrahydrobiopterin (BH4) is an essential cofactor of NOS activity. Herein, we evaluated antiapoptotic and anti-inflammatory effects of diamino-6-hydroxypyrimidine (DAHP), a guanosine 5′-triphosphate cyclohydrolase 1 (GTPCH1) inhibitor on focal cerebral ischemia-reperfusion injury by middle cerebral artery occlusion and reperfusion (MCAO) and investigated the underlying mechanism. Sprague-Dawley rats were divided into five groups. Experimental groups were subjected to 1.5 h transient MCAO. T2-weighted imaging was performed to evaluate brain edema lesions in the stroke rats. Infarct volume was estimated by 2,3,5-triphenyltetrazolium chloride (TTC) staining after 24 h reperfusion. Western blotting and immunohistochemistry were performed to detect iNOS, caspase-3, Bcl-2, COX-2, and TNF-α protein expressions. Apoptosis was determined by TUNEL staining. T2 hyperintensity changes were observed in primary ischemic region. DAHP pretreatment significantly suppressed iNOS overexpression, caspase-3, and TNF-α. There was also attenuation of neuronal apoptosis with decrement in proteins Bcl-2 and COX-2 expressions. On the basis of our results, we hypothesize DAHP to have a neuroprotective function against focal cerebral ischemia and might attenuate brain injury by decreasing reactive oxygen species (ROS) production, subsequently inhibiting apoptosis.

1. Introduction

Localized reduction of brain blood flow can result in cerebral ischemia, and prolonged ischemia causes brain infarction, which in turn could result in death [1]. There are two kinds of stroke—ischemic strokes, which are caused by blood clots, and hemorrhagic strokes. Statistics pertaining to demise of individuals following ischemic cardiovascular stroke in 2008 was 7.3 million, with 6.2 million individuals dying from stroke or other cerebrovascular disease in 2008. Stroke or cerebrovascular diseases account for about 4.9% (about 450000 people) of total deaths in low-income countries, thus making it the sixth most common cause of death [2]. Similarly, in 2011, stroke or cerebrovascular diseases accounted for 12.8% (4.91 million people) and 8.9% (790000 people) of total deaths in middle-income and developed countries, respectively, thus making it the second common cause of death in these countries [3].

Thrombolytic therapy, which is deliquescing of blood clot, has been reported to be the optimum therapy for ischemic stroke. Effectiveness of this therapy lies in it being executed within the first 6 hours (the golden hours) following onset of stroke symptoms. Nevertheless, many patients miss the golden hours and are treated with antiplatelet aggregation drugs such as aspirin. Antiplatelet aggregations drugs have the tendency of decreasing risk of reattack; however, they neither allay nor reverse damage caused by stroke [4].

Multitudinous researches have been done on inflammatory response and apoptosis caused by strokes in humans. Several different cytokines are implicated in inflammatory process. These cytokines once stimulated could either upregulate or downregulate substrates, resulting in excessive production of ROS such as hydroxyl radicals (OH^-), superoxide anions ($O_2^{(-)}$), and hydrogen peroxide (H_2O_2) as well as reactive nitrogen species (RNS) such as nitric oxide (NO) and peroxynitrite ($OONO^-$) [5]. Aberrant production of ROS and RNS further results in cell and tissue injury. Some of the cytokines implicated in inflammation include caspase-3 (C3), inducible nitric oxide syntheses (iNOS), and tumor necrosis factor α (TNF-α) [6].

Production of RNS has been associated with nitric oxide syntheses (NOS). Both endothelial NOS (eNOS) and neuronal NOS (nNOS) are expressed constitutively whereas iNOS expression is induced by proinflammatory cytokines such as TNF-α. Increased NOS activity has been reported to be accompanied by GTPCH 1 activation and tetrahydrobiopterin (BH4) formation [7]. BH4 is a requisite for NOS to produce nitric oxide (NO); thus, decreased BH4 curtails production of NO and oxidative stress [8]. BH4 is susceptible to oxidation by ROS, and inflammatory cytokines can increase BH4 synthesis. However, inflammation can also oxidate BH4 due to increasing production of ROS, which in turn forms dihydrobiopterin (BH2) and ultimately biopterin (B) [9]. BH4 synthesis mainly occurs from substrate GTP via a de novo pathway comprised of three steps, with GTP cyclohydrolase 1 (GTPCH 1) being the rate-limiting enzyme under normal conditions. Inhibition of BH4 synthesis via diamino-6-hydroxypyrimidine (DAHP; 0.5 g/kg IP) [10], the inhibitor of GTPCH 1, was reported to abate production of BH4 levels, iNOS activity, and $ONOO^-$ levels as well as cerebral infraction [8]. Though hampering of endogenous brain BH4 rate-limiting enzyme GTPCH 1 with DAHP reduces cerebral infarction via iNOS activity inhibition, its neuronal protective mechanism remains elusive. In view of this, our study was aimed at elucidating the mechanistic neuronal protection by DAHP, subsequently providing a theoretical basis in the development of clinical drugs for ischemia stroke treatment.

2. Materials and Method

2.1. Animal Preparation. All animal procedures and protocols were performed in accordance with the Guide for the Care and Use of Laboratory Animals (NIH publication, 85-23, revised 1996) and were reviewed and approved by the Ethics Committee for the Use of Experimental Animals in Zhejiang University. All male adult Sprague-Dawley (SD) rats (Zhejiang University Laboratory Animal Breeding and Research Center, Hangzhou, China) were housed at a constant temperature (25°C) and humidity (50–60%) under a regular 12 h light/dark schedule, with free access to food and water before and after ischemic induction. Seventy-five adult male Sprague-Dawley rats (weighing 250–300 g) were randomly assigned to 5 groups: normal control ($n = 15$), sham group ($n = 15$), middle cerebral artery occlusion (MCAO, $n = 15$), MCAO with DAHP treatment (0.5 g/kg IP, dissolved in 0.5 ml dimethyl sulfoxide (DMSO)) 12 hours before ischemia ($n = 15$), and MCAO with vehicle (0.5 ml DMSO IP) 12 hours before ischemia ($n = 15$). Both DMSO and DAHP were purchased from Sigma-Aldrich Co., USA.

2.2. Induction of Cerebral Ischemic Reperfusion Injury. Methods of cerebral ischemic reperfusion injury were from previous research [11]. Rats were anesthetized with chloral hydrate (400 mg/kg) intraperitoneally. Under anesthesia, right common carotid arteries (CCA), external carotid artery (ECA), and internal carotid artery (ICA) were exposed via a ventral midline incision of the neck. After carefully isolating CCA and separating from the adjacent vagus nerve, CCA and ECA were ligatured with two surgical wires. An incision was made distal to the CCA ligation. Then, a piece of 26/0 monofilament nylon suture with its tip slightly rounded by heat was inserted through the right CCA incision and advanced a distance of 18 mm from the carotid bifurcation toward the origin of right middle cerebral artery, thus occluding blood flow to cortex and striatum. After 150 minutes, reperfusion was accomplished by careful withdrawal of nylon suture; CCA was ligatured distal to the incision, with muscular tissue and skin sewed up. Finally, animals were put into their respective cages. MRI was employed to ascertain successfulness of model. 24 hours after surgery, rats were anesthetized again, and brains were rapidly removed for TTC stain, TUNEL assay, and immunohistochemistry.

2.3. MRI Scanning. Rat brains were scanned in a 1.5-Tesla (T) MRI animal scanner (MAGNETOM Trio with TIM system, Siemens, Erlangen, Germany) with the MRI parameters setting at TE = 92 ms, TR = 3620 ms, FOV = $8 \times 8\ cm^2$, M = 256×256, NA = 2, thickness = 2 mm, and gap = 0 mm.

2.4. TTC for Infarct Volume Assessment. Each brain was cut at 2 mm intervals from the frontal pole using a rat brain matrix. Sections were stained with 2% 2,3,5-triphenyltetrazolium chloride (TTC, Sigma-Aldrich Co., USA) at 37°C for 10 minutes, fixed in 4% paraformaldehyde overnight, and photographed.

2.5. Apoptosis Assay. Terminal deoxynucleotidyl transferase-mediated UTP end labeling (TUNEL) assay was conducted by using a TUNEL detection kit following the manufacturer's instruction (Roche, Mannheim, Germany). Extent of TUNEL was normalized to total nuclear content using 4′,6-diamidino-2-phenylindole (DAPI) staining. Sections were treated with 5 μg/ml proteinase K for 2 minutes at room temperature and rewashed with PBS. Then, sections were treated with a TUNEL reaction mixture at 37°C for 1 hour. DAPI (Sigma-Aldrich Co., USA) was diluted in PBS. For DAPI staining, a 500x stock solution was diluted to 10x PBS; 100 μl of this 10x DAPI solution was then added into each section to achieve a final DAPI loading solution of 10 μM. 10 minutes after, unincorporated DAPI solution was removed and 500 μl of fresh PBS was added to sections. TUNEL-stained sections stained with DAPI were visualized with a confocal laser scanning inverted microscope (Meta Zeiss LSM 510). Positive cells were counted in 5 random fields per section at 200x magnification.

2.6. Immunohistochemistry. 24 hours following reperfusion, animals were deeply anesthetized with 4% chloral hydrate and then perfused transcardially with 500 ml of 0.9% saline, followed by 4% paraformaldehyde in 0.01 M PBS. Brains were removed, postfixed in a 4% paraformaldehyde solution, and transferred to a 30% sucrose solution prior to processing for immunostaining. Brains were then frozen and sectioned coronally. Sections were incubated for 15 minutes with 3% hydrogen peroxide in methanol to block endogenous peroxidases and then blocked for 1 hour with 0.3% Triton X-100/ 10% normal goat serum in 0.01 M PBS. Then, sections were incubated with primary antibody anti-iNOS, TNF-α, COX-2, caspase-3, and Bcl-2 (rabbit, 1 : 200, Thermo Fisher Scientific, Waltham, MA) overnight at 4°C. After a thorough washing in PBS, sections were incubated with HRP-conjugated goat anti-rabbit IgG (1 : 200; Santa Cruz Biotechnology, CA) for 1 hour and then visualized with 3,3′-diaminobenzidine (DAB, Sigma-Aldrich Co., USA). Positive cells in each section were counted at 200x magnification.

2.7. Western Blot Analysis. Total protein was extracted from right brain tissues of each group. Protein concentration of extract was determined by Bio-Rad DC protein assay. Equal amounts of tissue extracts containing 30 μg of total protein were boiled for 5 minutes. Denatured proteins were separated by SDS-PAGE and transferred to polyvinylidene difluoride (PVDF) membrane in a Bio-Rad Trans-Blot apparatus. Membranes were blocked with TBST containing 5% nonfat milk for 2 hours at room temperature and then incubated with primary rabbit polyclonal anti-COX-2 (1 : 300), anti-Bcl-2 (1 : 500), anti-iNOS (1 : 300), and anti-caspase-3 (1 : 300) on a platform shaker overnight at 4°C. Equivalent loading of protein across all test lanes was confirmed by subsequent β-actin immunoblots (anti-β-actin 1 : 200; Biomeda) after incubation with horseradish peroxidase-conjugated goat anti-rabbit antibody (1 : 3000; Jackson ImmunoResearch Laboratories, USA) for 1 hour at room temperature and ECL detection.

2.8. Statistical Analysis. Data are presented as mean ± stand ard error of mean (SEM). One-way analysis of variance (ANOVA) was used to determine statistical significance with SPSS 16.0 program. Comparison among groups was performed by ANOVA followed by LSD-Fisher post hoc test. A P value of <0.05 was considered statistically significant. All statistical analysis and graphs were performed or generated with GraphPad Prism Version 4.0 (GraphPad Prism Software Inc., CA).

3. Results and Discussion

3.1. MRI Assessment of MCAO Model. MRI is considered to be the most sensitive tool in evaluation of brain edema lesions in stroke victims. After 24 hours of surgery, T2-weighted imaging was performed in stroke rats and T2 hyperintensity changes were observed in primary ischemic region. Representative image is shown in Figure 1. Infarct lesion was observed 24 hours after reperfusion in our MCAO model.

3.2. DAHP Curtails Infarct Volume. In evaluating DAHP neuroprotectiveness, infarct volume was measured at 24 hours following reperfusion. Brains of rats were stained with 2% TTC to obtain infarct volume. Unstained areas (negative TTC stains) that appeared white were defined as infarct regions whereas normal regions appeared red (Figure 2(a)). Infarct volume (mm^3) was calculated as 2 mm (thickness of the slice) × sum of the infarction area (mm^2) in all slices using computerized planimetry (PC-based image tool software). As evidenced in Figure 2(b), infarct volume of the DAHP group was significantly decreased in comparison to the MCAO group ($^*P < 0.05$, versus DAHP-treated group). No cerebral infarction was observed in the sham group. Infarct volume suggests DAHP plays a neuroprotective role in brain infarction.

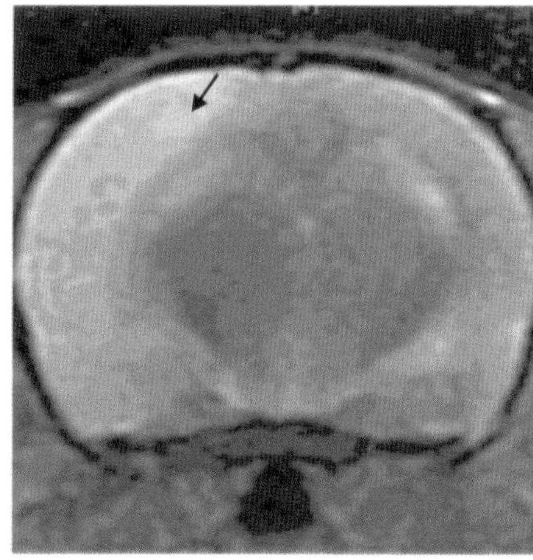

Figure 1: Infarct region performed T2 hyperintensity changes. T2-weighted magnetic resonance image revealed an abnormally increased T2 signal in the primary ischemic region (arrow).

3.3. DAHP Mitigates Neuronal Apoptosis. TUNEL-positive cell represents apoptotic cell. As illustrated in Figure 3(a), at 24 hours following reperfusion, number of apoptotic cells in penumbral area and infarct zone was observed. TUNEL method can identify DNA fragmentation of apoptotic cells. As depicted in Figure 3(b), in comparison to sham rats, number of TUNEL-positive cells was significantly increased in both MCAO and DMSO groups ($^{\#}P < 0.05$, versus sham group). In the DAHP treated group, number of TUNEL-positive cells was significantly decreased relative to both MCAO and DMSO groups ($^*P < 0.05$, versus DAHP-treated group). These results suggest DAHP could effectively obviate apoptotic cells following onset of stroke.

3.4. Immunohistochemistry. Inflammatory cytokine expression in an MCAO rat model was detected via immunohistochemistry analysis in penumbral and stroke area at 24 hours after reperfusion. Positive staining cells were brown in color (Figure 4). Bcl-2, TNF-α, caspase-3, cyclooxygenase-2 (COX-2), and iNOS expressions in rat cortex were delineated, and the integral optical density (IOD) was measured with Image-Pro Plus 6.0 software. In comparison to MCAO group, DAHP suppressed the expressions of apoptotic cytokines, caspase-3, TNF-α, and iNOS ($^*P <$ 0.05 versus DAHP-treated group); however, expressions of antiapoptotic cytokines, Bcl-2, and COX-2 were stimulated

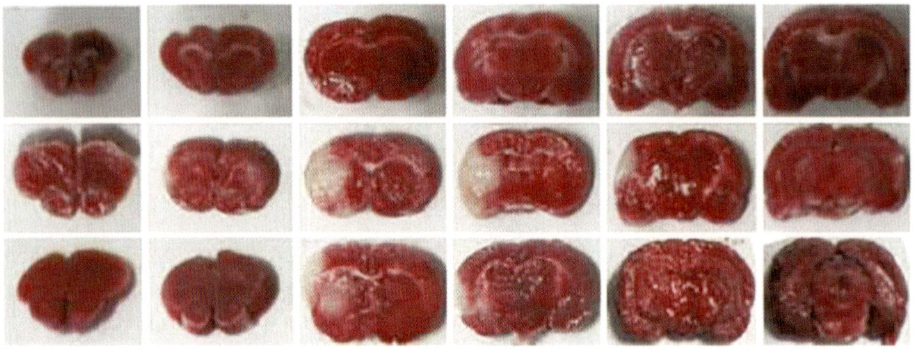

(a)

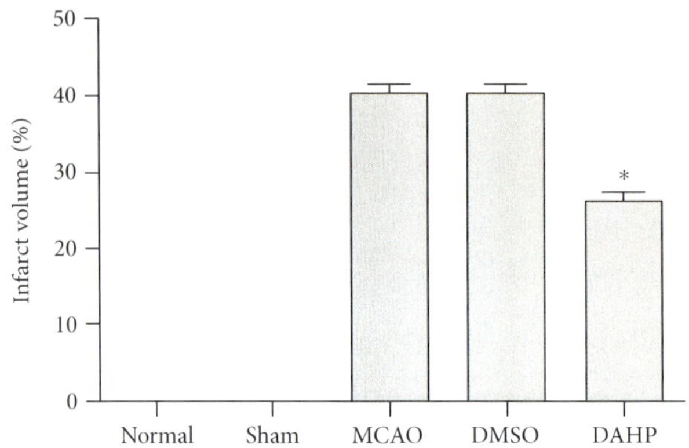

(b)

FIGURE 2: (a) Unstained areas (negative TTC stains) were defined as infarct regions, while normal regions appeared red. (b) Bar graph represents the infarct volume from TTC staining in various groups (mean ± SEM, $n = 6$, $^*P < 0.05$ versus the DAHP-treated group). Infarct volume markedly decreased in the DAHP-treated group, compared with the MCAO group ($n = 6$, $^*P < 0.05$ versus the DAHP-treated group).

($^*P < 0.05$ versus the DAHP-treated group) (Figure 5). Cytokine expressions between MCAO and DMSO groups were not statistically different ($P > 0.05$).

3.5. Western Blotting. Western blotting was used to quantify cytokine protein expression in MCAO rat models. In comparison to MCAO group, expressions of apoptotic cytokines, caspase-3, TNF-α, and iNOS were suppressed by DAHP ($^*P < 0.05$ and $^{**}P < 0.05$ versus DAHP-treated group) (Figures 6(a), 6(c), and 6(d)). However, antiapoptotic cytokine expressions of Bcl-2 and COX-2 were stimulated ($^*P < 0.05$ versus the DAHP-treated group) (Figures 6(b) and 6(e)). Cytokine expressions between MCAO and DMSO groups were not statistically different.

3.6. Discussion. We evidence neuroprotectiveness of DAHP in an MCAO rat model and report our findings following Western blot and immunohistochemical analyses as well as TUNEL staining.

Stroke is a global health problem and the leading cause of adult disability in the United States. Thrombolytic therapy is currently the most effective treatment. However, there is a concomitant increased risk of bleeding coupled with irreversibility of damage caused. In view of this, exploration of alternative therapeutics for ischemia stroke in clinical setting is paramount. In our study, we occluded blood flow to the brain and subsequently cut off immediate oxygen supply to neurons. In our study, we occluded blood flow to the brain and subsequently cut off immediate oxygen supply to neurons, leading to death of cells (Figure 2(a)).

In this study, iNOS expression was suppressed via DAHP which is possibly due to inhibition of GTPCH 1 activity to decrease BH4 synthesis. This was in contrast with previous studies that reported iNOS protein level to be not downregulated but with a reduced activity [8]. Accumulated toxic products, ROS and RNS, can tip the balance between life and death [12]. RNS and ROS can break DNA and induce lipid peroxidation, protein nitrosylation of cell membrane and organelle damage of cell and tissue. Thus, downregulated iNOS by DAHP resulted in less RNS and ROS, which in turn decreased neuronal injury [13].

Apoptotic cell death pathways implicated in brain injury following cerebral ischemia have been elucidated [10]. Apoptosis is a form of cell death and is composed of two pathways—intrinsic pathway (mitochondrial pathway) and extrinsic pathway. Furthermore, the central role of apoptosis is ascribed to its elimination of dying cells so as to maintain normal development [14]. Excessive apoptosis, however, is presented in some pathological conditions such as stroke intracerebral hemorrhage, cancer, autoimmune disorders, and heart disease [15, 16]. Various reactive oxygen and nitrogen species (ROS/RNS) regulate apoptosis.

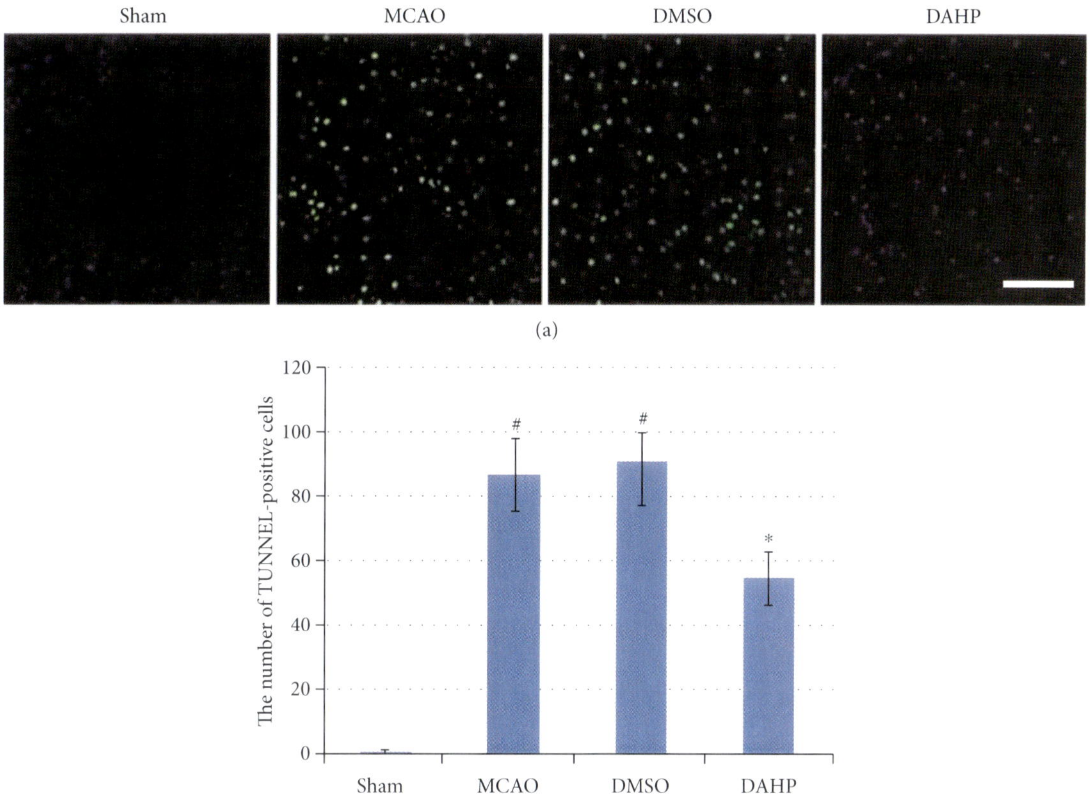

Figure 3: (a) Representative feature of TUNEL-positive cells in the ischemia area. (b) Bar graph reflected the TUNEL-positive staining score in each group (mean ± SEM, $n = 6$, $^{*}P < 0.05$ versus the DAHP-treated group). Ischemic reperfusion caused much neuron apoptosis; this can be demonstrated by the MCAO group ($^{\#}P < 0.05$ versus the sham group) with reduced neuron apoptosis compared with the MCAO group ($n = 6$, $^{*}P < 0.05$), and DMSO failed to attenuate apoptosis.

ROS and RNS have been demonstrated to have both pro- and antiapoptotic roles depending on a variety of factors such as type of cells involved, redox state of cell, as well as flux and dose of NO. Also, RNS and ROS can trigger inflammation via disparate cytokines such as TNF-α and caspase-3. As a proinflammatory cytokine, TNF-α has been reported to activate apoptosis through either intrinsic or extrinsic pathway via activation of caspase-3 by caspase-8 ([17]). Caspase-3 is a member of caspase family, which are essential initiators and executioners in apoptosis; caspase-3 acts as an executioner [18]. Caspase-3 has been reported to be overexpressed in myocardial infarction [19]. We found caspase-3 to be excessively expressed in infarct lesions of MCAO group. In essence, apoptosis plays an essential role in stroke pathology, while DAHP treatment markedly decreased caspase-3 protein in our study; thus, DAHP neuroprotective effects might arise following suppression of proapoptotic factors. Besides, members of Bcl-2 family, the major regulators of mitochondrial apoptotic pathway, are associated with pro- and antiapoptosis [20]. Antiapoptotic effect of Bcl-2 protein has been reported to be so because of Bcl-2 possessing four BH domains [5]. Additionally, Bcl-2 can suppress the level of free radicals or regulate cellular antioxidants to impede apoptosis [21]. Decreased infarct volume and upregulated Bcl-2 in our DAHP group implies DAHP proffered protection to neurons from death, possibly via antiapoptosis.

COX-2's role in cerebral infarction is presently ambiguous. COX-2 activation protects cardiomyocytes against oxidative stress [22]. Inhibition of COX-2 exacerbates inflammation and hippocampal neuronal death induced by seizures [23]. Hippocampal neuronal cells are attenuated in COX-2-deficient mouse death following transient forebrain ischemia [23, 24]. COX-2 is a major mediator implicated in inflammation and ischemic stroke [25]. In our study, COX-2 expression was upregulated more in DAHP group than in MCAO and DMSO groups. Thus, we hypothesize COX-2 might play a protective role in brain injury. We believe that following occlusion of blood flow to the brain, protective effect of COX-2 was set in motion against neuronal death, and with the assistance of DAHP, its expression and protective effect was enhanced, subsequently culminating in curtailed inflammation and RNS.

4. Conclusions

In summation, DAHP attenuates brain injury in a rat model through iNOS signaling pathway as well as apoptosis.

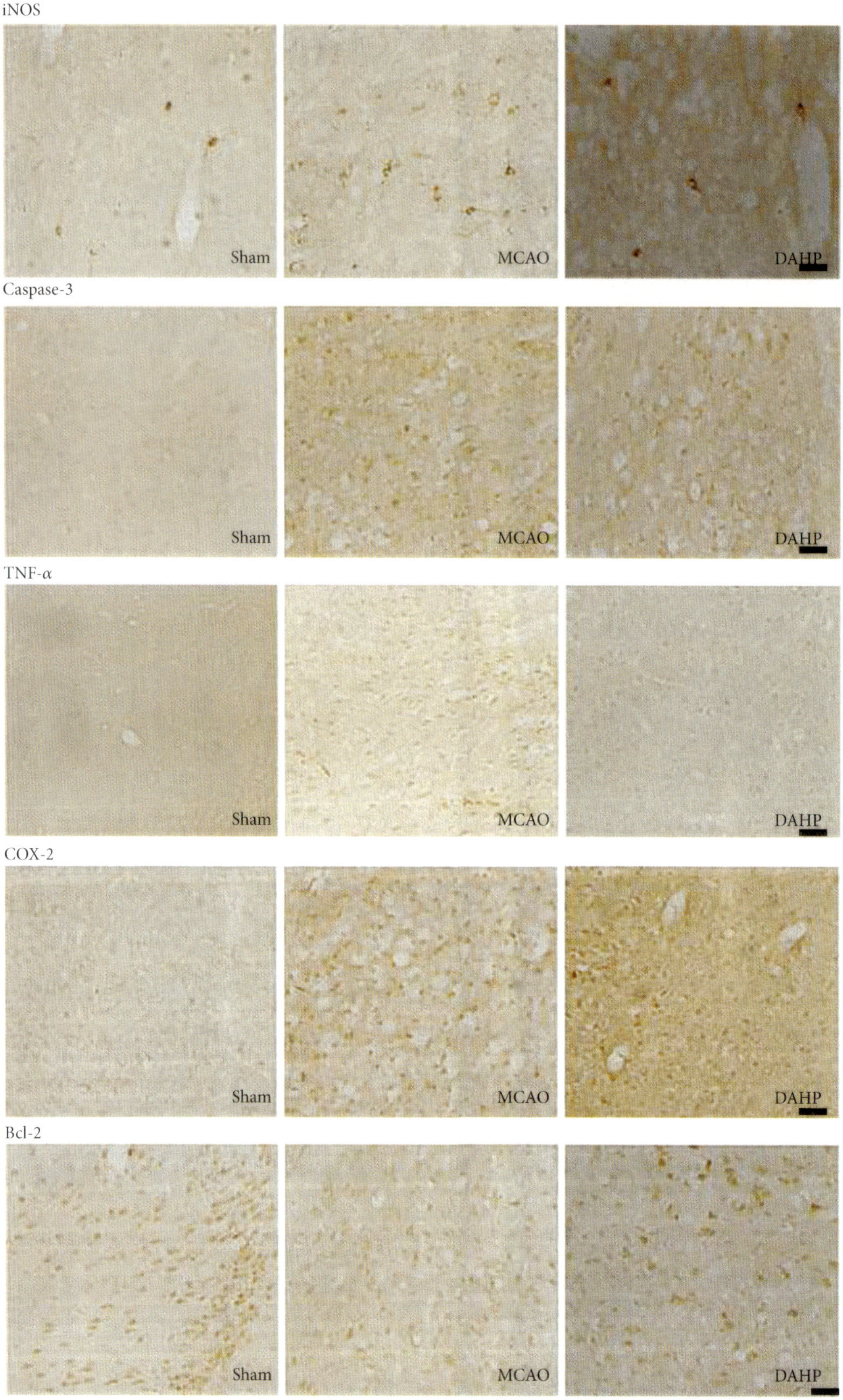

FIGURE 4: Immunohistochemistry staining shown in penumbral and stroke areas at 24 h after reperfusion. DAHP downregulated the expression levels of caspase-3, TNF-α, and iNOS, but upregulated the levels of Bcl-2 and COX-2, when compared with the MCAO group.

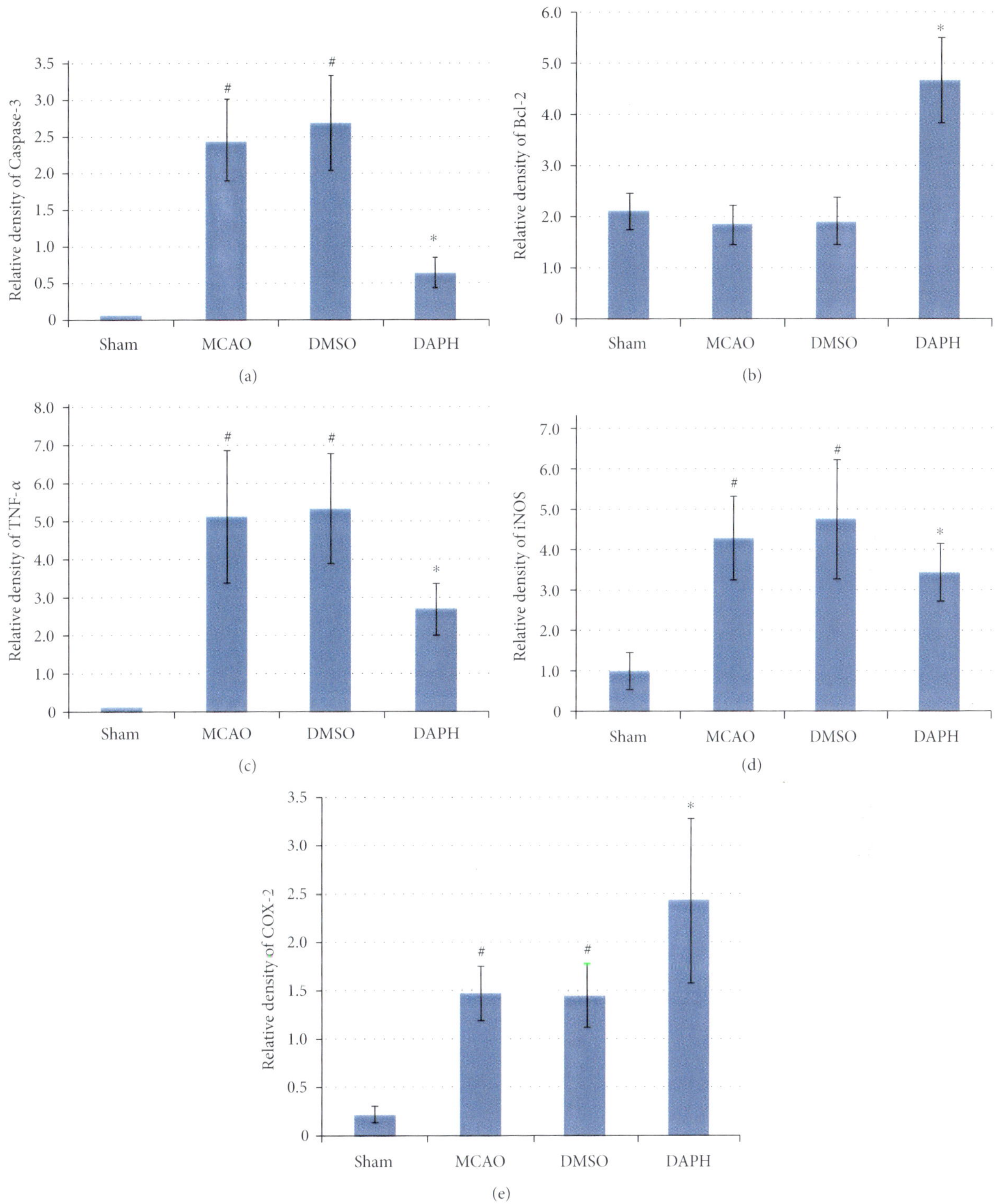

FIGURE 5: Expression levels for some inflammation cytokines in the rat cortex in penumbral and stroke areas were quantified by IOD with Image Pro Plus 6.0 software. (a) DAHP downregulated the caspase-3 expression ($^{*}P < 0.05$, versus the DAHP-treated group). Ischemic reperfusion induced a substantial caspase-3 expression ($^{\#}P < 0.05$, versus the sham group), which was significantly attenuated by DAHP but not vehicle treatment and MCAO groups ($n = 4$, $^{*}P < 0.05$, versus the DAHP-treated group). (b) DAHP increased Bcl-2 expression. The total Bcl-2 expression was significantly increased 24 h after ischemic reperfusion in the DAHP group ($n = 4$, $^{*}P < 0.05$, versus the DAHP-treated group), relative to MCAO or vehicle treatment. (c) DAHP reduced TNF-α expression. Ischemic reperfusion induced a substantial increase in TNF-α expression ($^{\#}P < 0.05$, versus the sham group), which reduced in the DAHP-treated group ($n = 3$, $^{*}P < 0.05$, versus the DAHP-treated group). (d) DAHP attenuated iNOS expression. Ischemic reperfusion induced a substantial increase in iNOS expression ($^{\#}P < 0.05$, versus the sham group), which was significantly attenuated by DAHP ($n = 4$, $^{*}P < 0.05$, versus the DAHP-treated group). (e) DAHP induced COX-2 expression; DAHP increased COX-2 expression ($n = 4$, $^{*}P < 0.05$, versus the DAHP-treated group).

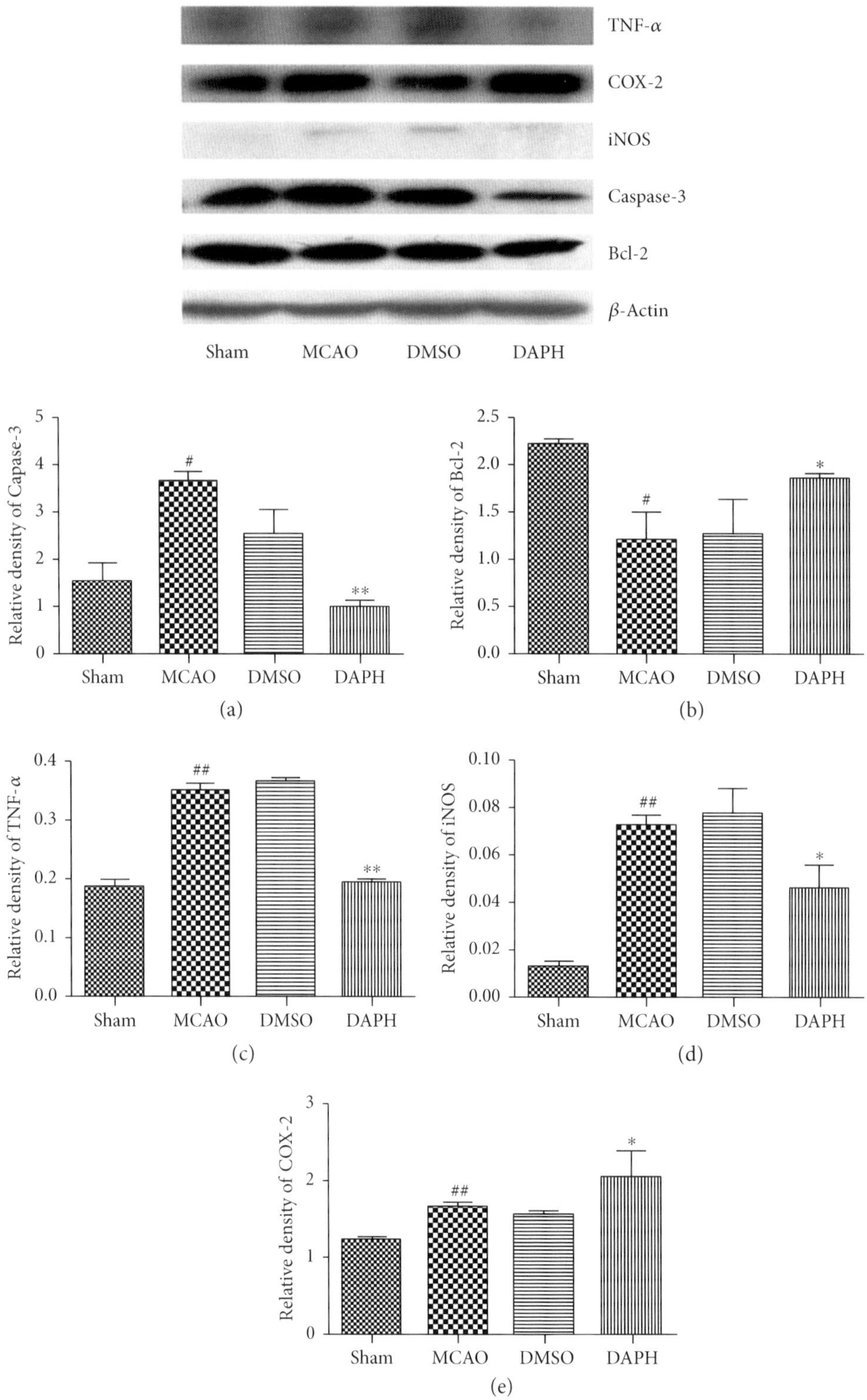

FIGURE 6: Protein expression levels for inflammation cytokines in the rat cortex in penumbral and stroke areas were quantified by Western blotting. (a, c, d) DAHP downregulated caspase-3, TNF-α, and iNOS protein expression. Ischemic reperfusion induced a substantial caspase-3, TNF-α, and iNOS expression in the vehicle treatment and MCAO groups ($^{\#}P < 0.05$, versus the sham group), which was significantly attenuated by DAHP ($^{*}P < 0.05$ and $^{**}P < 0.05$, versus the DAHP-treated group). (b) DAHP increased Bcl-2 expression ($^{*}P < 0.05$, versus the DAHP-treated group). Total Bcl-2 expression was significantly increased 24 h after ischemic reperfusion in the DAHP group, relative to MCAO or vehicle treatment. (e) DAHP induced COX-2 protein expression. Ischemic reperfusion induced COX-2 expression in the MCAO- and DMSO-treated groups, but COX-2 expression was more upregulated in the DAHP group than in the MCAO and DMSO groups ($^{*}P < 0.05$, versus the DAHP-treated group). $^{\#\#}P < 0.05$, versus the sham group (c–e).

Authors' Contributions

Marong Fang designed the experiments; Yanhua Qin drafted the manuscript; Yanhua Qin, Zhiying Hu, Yang Yang, and Weiyun Li performed the experiments; and Marong Fang analyzed the data and revised the manuscript. All authors read and approved the final manuscript.

Acknowledgments

The authors wish to acknowledge the contributions of Drs. Henry Davies, Benson O.A. Botchway, and Xiaoxue Du as well as Ms. Yuting Jiang in the revision of the manuscript as well as providing technical skills. This work was supported by the National Natural Science Foundation of China (no. 81671138).

References

[1] J. Galea and D. Brough, "The role of inflammation and interleukin-1 in acute cerebrovascular disease," *Journal of Inflammation Research*, vol. 6, pp. 121–128, 2013.

[2] W. J. van der Spuy and E. Pretorius, "Interrelation between inflammation, thrombosis, and neuroprotection in cerebral ischemia," *Reviews in the Neurosciences*, vol. 23, no. 3, pp. 269–278, 2012.

[3] M. B. Yilmaz, M. Tonge, H. Emmez, F. Kaymaz, and M. Kaymaz, "Neuroprotective effects of quetiapine on neuronal apoptosis following experimental transient focal cerebral ischemia in rats," *Journal of Korean Neurosurgical Association*, vol. 54, no. 1, pp. 1–7, 2013.

[4] X. Zhan, B. P. Ander, G. Jickling et al., "Brief focal cerebral ischemia that simulates transient ischemic attacks in humans regulates gene expression in rat peripheral blood," *Journal of Cerebral Blood Flow & Metabolism*, vol. 30, no. 1, pp. 110–118, 2010.

[5] G. Condorelli, R. Roncarati, J. Ross et al., "Heart-targeted overexpression of *caspase3* in mice increases infarct size and depresses cardiac function," *Proceedings of the National Academy of Sciences of the United States of America*, vol. 98, no. 17, pp. 9977–9982, 2001.

[6] C. D. Munhoz, B. García-Bueno, J. L. M. Madrigal, L. B. Lepsch, C. Scavone, and J. C. Leza, "Stress-induced neuroinflammation: mechanisms and new pharmacological targets," *Brazilian Journal of Medical and Biological Research*, vol. 41, no. 12, pp. 1037–1046, 2008.

[7] V. H. Oidor-Chan, E. Hong, F. Pérez-Severiano et al., "Fenofibrate plus metformin produces cardioprotection in a type 2 diabetes and acute myocardial infarction model," *PPAR Research*, vol. 2016, Article ID 8237264, 14 pages, 2016.

[8] G. A. Kidd, H. Hong, A. Majid, D. I. Kaufman, and A. F. Chen, "Inhibition of brain GTP cyclohydrolase I and tetrahydrobiopterin attenuates cerebral infarction via reducing inducible NO synthase and peroxynitrite in ischemic stroke," *Stroke*, vol. 36, no. 12, pp. 2705–2711, 2005.

[9] K. Noguchi, N. Hamadate, T. Matsuzaki et al., "Improvement of impaired endothelial function by tetrahydrobiopterin in stroke-prone spontaneously hypertensive rats," *European Journal of Pharmacology*, vol. 631, no. 1-3, pp. 28–35, 2010.

[10] Y. Yang, K. Gao, Z. Hu et al., "Autophagy upregulation and apoptosis downregulation in DAHP and triptolide treated cerebral ischemia," *Mediators of Inflammation*, vol. 2015, Article ID 120198, 12 pages, 2015.

[11] S. Bai, Z. Hu, Y. Yang et al., "Anti-inflammatory and neuroprotective effects of triptolide via the NF-κB signaling pathway in a rat MCAO model," *The Anatomical Record*, vol. 299, no. 2, pp. 256–266, 2016.

[12] A. Gangwar, S. Paul, Y. Ahmad, and K. Bhargava, "Competing trends of ROS and RNS-mediated protein modifications during hypoxia as an alternate mechanism of NO benefits," *Biochimie*, vol. 148, pp. 127–138, 2018.

[13] A. Lopez, J. A. Lorente, J. Steingrub et al., "Multiple-center, randomized, placebo-controlled, double-blind study of the nitric oxide synthase inhibitor 546C88: effect on survival in patients with septic shock," *Critical Care Medicine*, vol. 32, no. 1, pp. 21–30, 2004.

[14] B. Montico, A. Nigro, V. Casolaro, and J. Dal Col, "Immunogenic apoptosis as a novel tool for anticancer vaccine development," *International Journal of Molecular Sciences*, vol. 19, no. 2, 2018.

[15] H. Prentice, P. M. Gharibani, Z. Ma et al., "Neuroprotective functions through inhibition of ER stress by taurine or taurine combination treatments in a rat stroke model," *Advances in Experimental Medicine and Biology*, vol. 975, pp. 193–205, 2017.

[16] J. Zhou, X. An, J. Dong et al., "IL-17 induces cellular stress microenvironment of melanocytes to promote autophagic cell apoptosis in vitiligo," *The FASEB Journal*, 2018.

[17] B. J. van Raam and G. S. Salvesen, "Proliferative versus apoptotic functions of caspase-8: hetero or homo: the caspase-8 dimer controls cell fate," *Biochimica et Biophysica Acta (BBA) - Proteins and Proteomics*, vol. 1824, no. 1, pp. 113–122, 2012.

[18] C. Laulier and B. S. Lopez, "The secret life of Bcl-2: apoptosis-independent inhibition of DNA repair by Bcl 2 family members," *Mutation Research/Reviews in Mutation Research*, vol. 751, no. 2, pp. 247–257, 2012.

[19] L. Galluzzi, O. Kepp, C. Trojel-Hansen, and G. Kroemer, "Mitochondrial control of cellular life, stress, and death," *Circulation Research*, vol. 111, no. 9, pp. 1198–1207, 2012.

[20] W. Li, Y. Yang, Z. Hu, S. Ling, and M. Fang, "Neuroprotective effects of DAHP and triptolide in focal cerebral ischemia via apoptosis inhibition and PI3K/Akt/mTOR pathway activation," *Frontiers in Neuroanatomy*, vol. 9, p. 48, 2015.

[21] I. Kim, W. Xu, and J. C. Reed, "Cell death and endoplasmic reticulum stress: disease relevance and therapeutic opportunities," *Nature Reviews Drug Discovery*, vol. 7, no. 12, pp. 1013–1030, 2008.

[22] N. P. Dowd, M. Scully, S. R. Adderley, A. J. Cunningham, and D. J. Fitzgerald, "Inhibition of cyclooxygenase-2 aggravates doxorubicin-mediated cardiac injury in vivo," *The Journal of Clinical Investigation*, vol. 108, no. 4, pp. 585–590, 2001.

[23] D. S. Lee, B. Li, N. K. Im, Y. C. Kim, and G. S. Jeong, "4,2′,5′-Trihydroxy-4′-methoxychalcone from *Dalbergia odorifera* exhibits anti-inflammatory properties by inducing heme oxygenase-1 in murine macrophages," *International Immunopharmacology*, vol. 16, no. 1, pp. 114–121, 2013.

9

Effects of *Ficus umbellata* (Moraceae) Aqueous Extract and 7-Methoxycoumarin on Scopolamine-Induced Spatial Memory Impairment in Ovariectomized Wistar Rats

Stéphane Zingue,[1,2] Harquin Simplice Foyet,[3] Sefirin Djiogue,[2] Yannick Ezo'o Ezo'o,[1] Hervé Hervé Ngatanko Abaïssou,[2] Pafroumi Fachagbo,[1] and Dieudonné Njamen[2,3]

[1]*Department of Life and Earth Sciences, Higher Teachers' Training College, University of Maroua, P.O. Box 55, Maroua, Cameroon*
[2]*Department of Animal Biology and Physiology, Faculty of Science, University of Yaoundé 1, P.O. Box 812, Yaoundé, Cameroon*
[3]*Department of Biological Sciences, Faculty of Science, University of Maroua, P.O. Box: 814, Maroua, Cameroon*

Correspondence should be addressed to Stéphane Zingue; stephanezingue@gmail.com and Dieudonné Njamen; dnjamen@gmail.com

Academic Editor: Jesus Pastor

The present work was undertaken to evaluate the ability of *F. umbellata* aqueous extract and its major component 7-methoxycoumarin (MC) to improve scopolamine-induced spatial memory impairment in ovariectomized Wistar rats. For this to be done, 10 sham-operated and 30 postmenopausal-like rats were randomly distributed in eight groups ($n = 5$) and treated with distilled water (2 mL/250 g), estradiol valerate (1 mg/kg BW), piracetam (1.5 mg/kg BW), *F. umbellata* aqueous extract (50 and 200 mg/kg BW), or MC (1 mg/kg BW) for 21 consecutive days. Before and after the memory impairment with scopolamine (2 mg/kg BW), animals underwent behavioral evaluations on Y- and radial mazes. As results, age and ovariectomy did not induce significant changes in the reference memory errors. While age decreased working memory errors, ovariectomy increased it. The MC as well as *F. umbellata* extract significantly increased ($p < 0.01$) the percentage of spontaneous alternation and decreased ($p < 0.001$) working and spatial reference memory errors and anxiety parameters (rearing and grooming) in ovariectomized rats. MC significantly reduced ($p < 0.05$) the MDA level, but resulted in an increase in GSH level in brain homogenates. These results suggest that MC is endowed with neuroprotective effects and could account for the neuroprotective effects of *F. umbellata* in rats.

1. Introduction

Estrogens are steroidal hormones mainly produced by ovaries, which greatly fluctuate during women's lifespan and decline with menopause [1]. Numerous studies indicate that estrogens have neuroprotective effects either by direct activation of estrogen receptors (ERs), which are located in the brain, or by activation of receptors of other neuroprotective factors [1]. Studies in female rodents have shown that a decrease in plasmatic estrogen levels following ovariectomy enhances brain damage under neurodegenerative conditions [2, 3] and increases amyloid-β oligomers in a mouse model of Alzheimer's disease (AD) [4]. AD is the most frequent form of dementia and is an age-related neurodegenerative disease characterized by a loss or decline in memory and severe cognitive as well as behavioral impairments [5]. According to the World Alzheimer Report [6], 46.8 million people worldwide have dementia, out of which 60 to 70% are AD patients. To date, the pathophysiology of AD remains unclear, but it is considered that the β-amyloid and tau protein aggregation, reduced acetylcholine (ACh), and glutamatergic deficit are principal agents of the pathogenesis of AD [7]. However, age, genetic predisposition, stress, emotions, and the sudden drop in estrogen levels after menopause are nowadays recognized as risk factors that may contribute to AD symptoms [8, 9].

Hormone replacement therapy (HRT) has been used for many years to treat symptoms of menopause, including hot flushes and depression. Prospective studies have shown that it enhances cognitive skills in postmenopausal women [10]. Nevertheless, a long-term use of HRT is associated with adverse effects such as increased risks of endometrial and breast cancers, stroke, and pulmonary thromboembolism [11–13]. Hence, many women resort to natural health remedies as alternative therapies to treat menopausal symptoms [14]. Plant preparations and plant-derived compounds (phytoestrogens) are being considered as natural alternative to hormone replacement therapy.

Ficus umbellata (Moraceae) is a tropical tree commonly called "Mewed" in "Guiziga." Its back is used in indigenous medicine for the treatment of menopause-related physiological disorders [15]. Just like *F. sur*, *F. platyphylla*, *F. ovata*, *F. ingens*, and *F. glumosa*, it is used to treat some nervous system disorders such as dementia, neuralgia, and epilepsy [15, 16]. Previous studies revealed the transactivation of ERα in a reporter gene assay induces significant estrogen-like effects on estrogen target organs (uterus, vagina, and mammary gland) in rats when treated with *F. umbellata* aqueous and methanol extracts. These extracts also brought about a significant decrease in the frequency of occurrence of hot flushes in experimental rats. The major component of these extracts after isolation and characterization was found to be 7-methoxycoumarin (MC) [17]. Additionally, MC exhibited estrogen-like and tissue-selective effects in vitro on cell-based assay and in vivo on Wistar rats [18]. In the present study, the neuroprotective potential of MC as well as *F. umbellata* aqueous extract was evaluated using scopolamine-induced spatial memory impairment in ovariectomized Wistar rats. The investigation focused on number of entries, the percentage of spontaneous alternation, and working and spatial reference memory errors. Since scopolamine-induced memory deficits are accompanied with oxidative damage, oxidative stress biomarkers (MDA and GSH levels) were also assessed.

2. Materials and Methods

2.1. Chemicals. Estradiol valerate (Progynova® 2 mg) was purchased from Delpharm (Lille, France). UPLC-grade solvents methanol, acetonitrile (ACN), methyl tert-butyl ether (MTBE), water, scopolamine, piracetam, and formic acid (FA) were purchased from Sigma-Aldrich (Saint-Quentin-Fallavier, France). Penicillin (xtapen®) was provided by CSPC Zhongnuo Pharmaceutical (Shijiazhuang City, China). Diclofenac (Dicloecnu®) was provided by ECNU Pharmaceutical (Yanzhou City, China).

2.2. Plant Material and Preparation of F. umbellata Extracts. Stem bark of *F. umbellata* was harvested in Yaounde (centre region, Cameroon) in September 2013. This botanical sample was authenticated by Mister Victor Nana, botanist at the National Herbarium of Cameroon (HNC) by comparison to the specimens deposited under the voucher number 99/HNC. After shade drying and grinding, 2000 g of powder was macerated in water at room temperature (5 L of solvent × 3, 48 h per extraction). The combined solutions were filtered with Whatman paper number 4 and evaporated using an oven with ventilation (40°C, during 48 h) to yield 229.8 g of aqueous crude extract. Alternatively, 2700 g of the powder was macerated in 95% methanol at room temperature (5 L of solvent × 3, 48 h per extraction). The combined solutions were evaporated under reduced pressure (337 mbar at 40°C) using a rotary evaporator to yield 162 g of a methanol crude extract (MeOH).

2.3. Isolation of 7-Methoxycoumarin (MC). UPLC chromatograms of *F. umbellata* aqueous as methanol extracts showed that MC is their major compound (Supplementary Data 1). After a bioguided fractionation of *F. umbellata* methanol extract, MC was isolated [17]. Figure 1 shows a summary of the physicochemical properties of MC.

2.4. Animals. Healthy young female Wistar rats aged four weeks, weighing (~ 150 g), were used in this study. These rats were purchased from the breeding facility of the Animal Physiology Laboratory of the University of Yaounde I (Cameroon). Animals were housed in clean polyacrylic cages in a light-controlled room (approx. 12 h light/dark), and temperature was maintained around 25°C. A soy-free rat chow diet was provided to the animals with water ad libitum. The composition of animal diet was as follows: corn (36.7%), bone flour (14.5%), wheat (36.6%), fish flour (4.8%), crushed palm kernel (7.3%), sodium chloride (0.3%), and vitamin complex (Olivitazol® 0.01%). Housing of animals and all experiments were conducted in accordance with the principles and procedures of the European Union legislation on the use of animals for scientific purposes (Directive 2010/63/EU) adopted by the Cameroon Institutional National Ethic Committee, Ministry of Scientific Research and Technology Innovation (reg. number FWA-IRD 0001954).

2.5. Study Design. At the beginning of the experiment, 5 rats aged 2.5 months underwent behavioral evaluations on Y- and radial mazes in order to record basic data (BD). Afterwards, ketamine (50 mg/kg BW; ip) and diazepam (10 mg/kg BW; ip) anesthesia were used. 30 rats were bilaterally ovariectomized using the dorsal approach, and 10 others were sham-operated. Animals were allowed for (84) days for the setup of menopausal-like conditions [19–21], followed by the random distribution of animals (now aged 5.5 months) into eight groups ($n = 5$). Groups I (SHAM 1) and II (SHAM 2) were sham-operated rats and received distilled water. Groups III to VIII were ovariectomized rats treated as follows: Group III received distilled water and served as negative control (OVX). Group IV served as positive control 1 and received estradiol valerate (1 mg/kg BW). Group V served as positive control 2 and received piracetam, a nootropic drug that exhibits cognition-enhancing properties [22] at a dose of 1.5 mg/kg BW. Groups VI and VII received the *F. umbellata* aqueous extract at the doses of 50 and 200 mg/kg, respectively. Group VIII received the MC at the dose of 1 mg/kg. Distilled water was used as a vehicle for the dissolution of substances which were administered orally using a feeding tube (2 mL/250 g) for three weeks (a single dose per day).

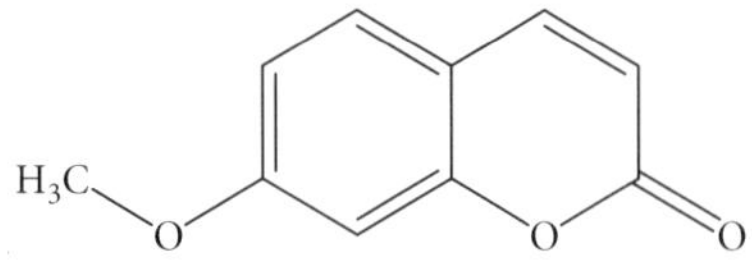

FIGURE 1: 7-Methoxycoumarin (molecular weight = 176.1 M; molecular formula = $C_{10}H_8O_3$) [17].

Piracetam and MC were given intraperitoneally (0.3 mL/250 g). However, parallel injections/gavages of vehicle were given so that all rats had the same administration experiences. Behavioral testing was achieved between the 12th and 21st days of treatment. On the last day of treatment, scopolamine (2 mg/kg) was administered as a single dose 30 min after drug administration through intraperitoneal (ip) injection route to all the groups except group I (SHAM 1). Exceptionally this day, behavioral testing was done before and after scopolamine injection. A right hemisphere of each animal's brain was homogenized to give 20% (*w*/*v*) homogenate in an ice-cold sodium buffer (0.1 M, pH 7.3). The homogenate was centrifuged at 3000 ×g for 15 min at 4°C. The supernatant was stored at −20°C for the determination of some oxidative stress biomarkers.

2.6. Behavioral Testing

2.6.1. Y-Maze Test. Short-term memory was assessed by spontaneous alternation behavior in the Y-maze task as previously reported by Foyet et al. [23]. Briefly, the maze consisted of three arms (35 cm long, 25 cm high, and 10 cm wide) and an equilateral triangular central area. Each rat was placed in a randomized order at the end of one arm and allowed to move freely through the maze for 8 min. An arm entry was counted when the hind paws of the rat were completely within the arm. Spontaneous alternation behavior was defined as three consecutive entries in three different arms (i.e., A, B, C or B, C, A, etc.). The percentage alternation score (PAS) was calculated by the following formula: PAS = [total alternation number/(total number of entries − 2)] × 100. Furthermore, the total number of arm entries was used as a measure of general activity of the animals. The maze was wiped clean with 70% ethanol between each animal to minimize odor cues [23, 24].

Anxiety negatively influences learning activity and new information storage; some anxiety parameters such as frequency of rearing and grooming [25] were therefore recorded during the Y-maze test.

2.6.2. Radial Arm Maze. In this study, the radial arm maize was used to assess working memory and reference memory as previously reported by Hritcu et al. [26]. This apparatus was a wooden platform raised 50 cm above the floor, consisting of 8 arms (48 cm long × 12 cm wide). All the arms numbered 1–8 extended radially from a central area (32 cm in diameter). A food cup containing a single 50 mg food pellet was placed at the end of each arm. Visual cues were placed around the maze and maintained in their positions throughout the testing period. In order to maintain at 85% of their free feeding weight, the animals were kept on restricted diet over a week prior to the performance of the maze task with free access to water ad libitum. Before the trial training for recording sequences of alternation in the radial maze arms, three rats were placed in the central platform of the radial maze and allowed to explore freely and consume the food distributed on the central platform and arms. The food was progressively restricted to the arms and the food cups. During the trial training, a rat is placed on the central platform and allowed to explore until all the 5 baits had been consumed or until 5 minutes has elapsed. During the eight-day tests, each animal is placed individually on the central platform of the radial maze facing an arm for the assessment of reference memory and working memory. Five arms (numbers 1, 2, 4, 5, and 7) out of 8 were baited throughout the training days. The number of reference memory errors (entering an arm that was not baited) and working memory errors (entering an arm containing food, but previously entered) was measured. An arm entry was counted when all the four limbs of the animal were within the arm. 70% ethanol was used to clean the maze after the passage of each rat in order to reduce residual odors [26, 27].

2.7. Histological Analysis. The histomorphology of the brain was performed from 5 μm sections of paraffin-embedded tissues following hematoxylin-eosin staining. Brains were photographed at 40x magnification using the complete Zeiss equipment consisting of a microscope Axioskop 40 connected to a computer where the image was transferred, and analyzed with the MRGrab1.0 and AxioVision 3.1 software, all provided by Zeiss (Hallbergmoos, Germany).

2.8. Biochemical Analysis

2.8.1. Total Content of Reduced Glutathione GSH. To measure the reduced glutathione (GSH) level, the brain homogenate in sodium buffer (0.1 M, pH 7.3) was taken. The procedure was followed as previously described by Shamnas et al. [28]. Briefly, the homogenate was mixed with an equal volume of trichloroacetic acid (TBA, 20%) containing 1 mM EDTA to precipitate the proteins. The mixture was allowed to stand for 5 minutes prior to centrifugation. The supernatant (200 μL) was then transferred to a new set of test tubes to which was each added 1.8 mL of Ellman's reagent (5,5′-dithiobis-2-nitrobenzoic acid) (0.1 mM) prepared in 0.3 M phosphate buffer with 1% sodium citrate solution. Then, the content in all the test tubes was made up to the volume of 2 mL with distilled water. After the completion of the total reaction, the solutions were measured at 412 nm against a blank. Absorbance values were then compared with a standard curve generated from GSH.

2.8.2. Determination of MDA Level. Malondialdehyde (MDA), which is a measure of lipid peroxidation, was spectrophotometrically measured using the thiobarbituric acid assay as reported by Padurariu et al. [29]. Briefly, 200 μL of brain homogenate was added and mixed with 1 mL of 50% trichloroacetic acid in 0.1 M HCl and 1 mL of 26 mM thiobarbituric acid. After vortex mixing, samples were maintained at 95°C for 20 minutes. Furthermore, samples were centrifuged at 800 ×g for 10 minutes and supernatants were read at 532 nm. A calibration curve was constructed using MDA as standard, and the results were expressed as mM/mg protein.

2.9. Statistical Analysis. Results were presented as means ± s tandard error of the mean (SEM). All formula and functions were calculated with Microsoft Excel software. Data analysis was performed with GraphPad Prism 5.0 software. The normal distribution of data was assessed by Shapiro-Wilk test, and the distribution was found normal ($p = 0.5$). Further, the one-way ANOVA test was followed by the Newman-Keuls post hoc test; a stepwise multiple comparison procedure was used to identify sample means that are significantly different from each other. Differences were considered significant at a probability level of 5% ($p < 0.05$).

3. Results

3.1. Effect of Age and Ovariectomy on Short-Term and Long-Term Memories. As observed in Figure 2, age has no effect on number of entries (Figure 2(a)) in the Y-maze. Indeed, no significant change was noted in normal rats aged 5.5 months (SHAM 1) as compared to the basic data (BD) recorded in youngest animal (2.5 months). Figure 2(b) shows that the percentage of spontaneous alternation behavior significantly ($p < 0.001$) increased with age. Furthermore, ovariectomy significantly ($p < 0.001$) increased the number of entries (Figure 2(a)) but significantly ($p < 0.05$) reduced the percentage of spontaneous alternation as compared to the age-matched normal animal (SHAM 1).

Age and ovariectomy did not induce significant changes in the reference memory errors (Figure 2(d)), while normal rats aged 5.5 months made less working memory errors than the youngest ones did (2.5 months), although significant ($p < 0.01$) only on day 1 of the experiment (Figure 2(c)). The ovariectomized rats made more working memory errors as compared to the age-matched normal rats (Figure 2(c)). Interestingly, the ovariectomized rats took a significantly ($p < 0.001$) lower time to collect baits as compared to the normal group (Figure 2(e)). It is worth noting that working memory error and reference memory error as well as the time taken to collect all baits decreased continuously throughout the experiment in all groups.

3.2. Effect of Age and Ovariectomy on Anxiety Parameters. The number of rearing and grooming significantly ($p < 0.001$) decreased in normal rats aged 5.5 months as compared to youngest rats (2.5 months) (Figure 3). Ovariectomy significantly ($p < 0.001$) increased these parameters as compared to aged-matched normal rats (SHAM 1).

3.3. Effects of 7-Methoxycoumarin and F. umbellata Extract on Short-Term Memory. Before memory impairment with scopolamine, ovariectomized rats (OVX) had a significantly higher ($p < 0.001$) number of entries into the arms of the Y-maze than normal rats (SHAM 2). *F. umbellata* aqueous extract treatment at both doses (50 and 200 mg/kg) significantly ($p < 0.001$) reduced this parameter just like piracetam (1.5 mg/kg) as compared to the OVX group (Figure 4(a)). Thirty minutes after injection of scopolamine, the number of entries significantly ($p < 0.001$) increased in normal rats treated with scopolamine (SHAM 2 + SCOP) as compared to the age-matched normal group, which did not receive scopolamine (SHAM 1). No significant change was observed between all animals to which scopolamine was administered (Figure 4(b)).

Figure 4(c) shows a nonsignificant decrease in the percentage of spontaneous alternations behavior with ovariectomy before the administration of scopolamine. There was a nonsignificant increase in this parameter in all OVX rats treated with different substances (except with FU 200). After memory impairment (Figure 4(d)), a significant decrease in the spontaneous alternations was observed in normal rats (SHAM 2 + SCOP) as well as in ovariectomized rats (OVX + SCOP) as compared to the age-matched normal rats (SHAM 1). Apart from the 50 mg/kg dose of *F. umbellata* aqueous extract, all treatments induced a significant increase in the percentage of spontaneous alternations as compared to ovariectomized rats (OVX + SCOP).

3.4. Effect of 7-Methoxycoumarin and F. umbellata Extract on Long-Term Memory. The radial arm maze test was performed for 8 days, from the 14th to the 21st days of treatment. It was noted that before the scopolamine-induced memory impairment, the ovariectomized rats (OVX) showed more working (Figure 5(a)) and spatial reference memory (Figure 5(b)) errors as compared to normal rats (SHAM 2), but the difference was not statistically significant. After scopolamine administration, normal (SHAM 2) and ovariectomized rats displayed more ($p < 0.001$) working and spatial reference memory errors as compared to normal rats, which did not receive scopolamine (SHAM 1). The ovariectomized rats treated with *F. umbellata* aqueous extract (50 and 200 mg/kg) as well as MC (1 mg/kg) showed a significant ($p < 0.001$) reduction of working memory and spatial reference memory errors as compared to the OVX group.

The variations of the scanning time in the radial maze with different groups are depicted in Figure 5(c). It can be observed that ovariectomized rats (OVX) are faster in the radial arm maze before scopolamine injection as compared to all other groups. Moreover, the time required to collect all the baits in the radial arm maze gradually decreased from day 1 to day 7 in rats treated with the *F. umbellata* aqueous extract at both doses as well as with MC. Scopolamine administration on day 8 significantly ($p < 0.01$) increased the time taken to collect all baits by ovariectomized (OVX + SCOP) and normal (SHAM 2 + SCOP) rats as compared to the normal control group (SHAM 1). However, ovariectomized rats treated with *F. umbellata* aqueous extract (200 mg/kg) and MC (1 mg/kg) showed a significant ($p < 0.01$) reduction in this parameter as compared to OVX rats.

3.5. Effect of 7-Methoxycoumarin and F. umbellata Extract on Anxiety Parameters. It can be observed in Figures 6(a) and 6(c) that ovariectomy induced a significant increase in the number of rearing ($p < 0.01$) and grooming ($p < 0.001$) as compared to normal rats. There was a significant decrease in the number of rearing with piracetam ($p < 0.05$), *F. umbellata* at the dose of 200 mg/kg ($p < 0.001$), and MC ($p < 0.001$),

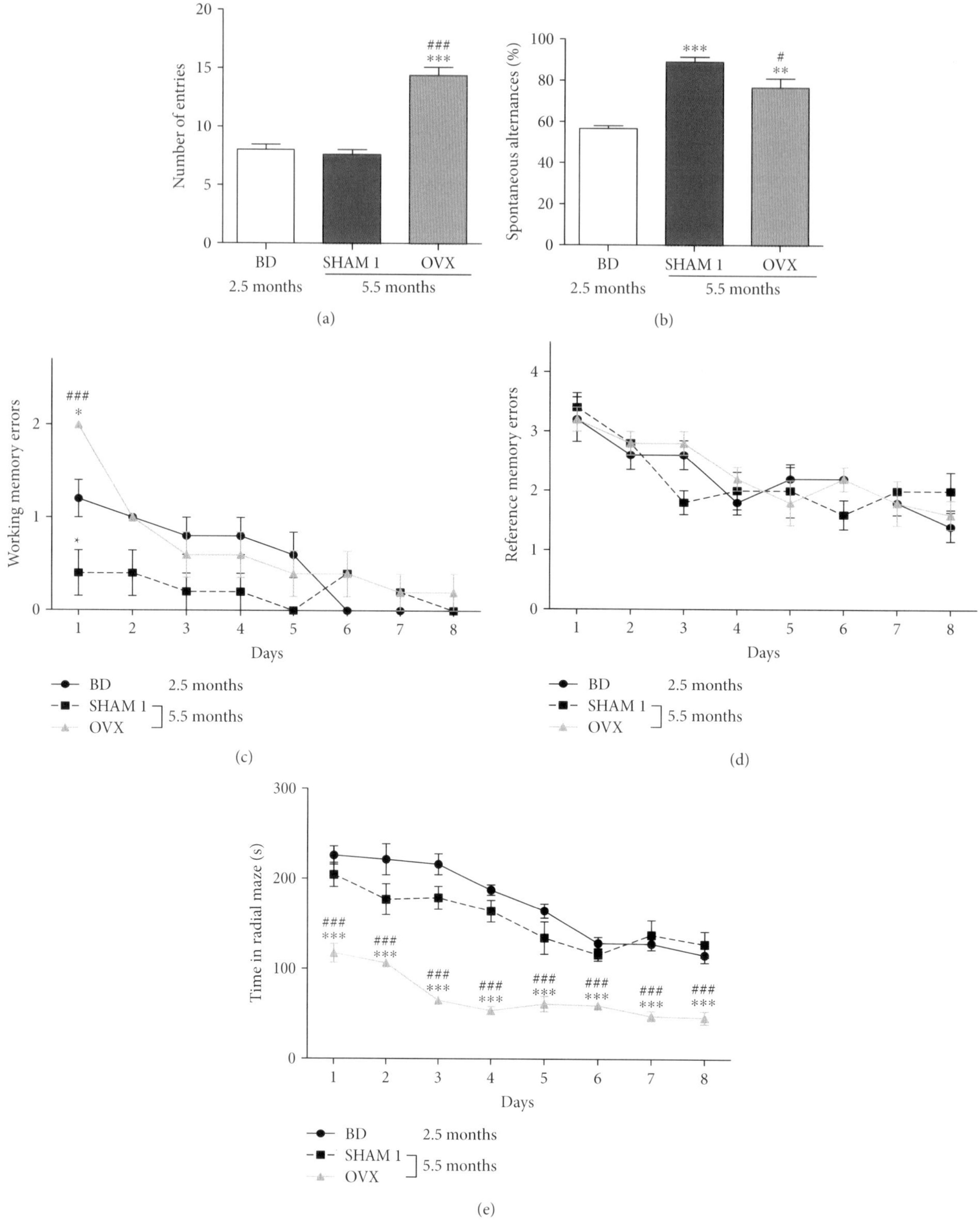

FIGURE 2: Effects of age and ovariectomy on number of entries (a), spontaneous alternances (b), working memory (c) and spatial reference memory (d) errors, and the time past in radial maze (e). OVX = ovariectomized rat aged 5.5 months; BD = nonovariectomized rats aged 2.5 months which served as basic data; SHAM 1 = nonovariectomized rats aged 5.5 months. $^{*}p < 0.05$, $^{**}p < 0.01$, and $^{***}p < 0.001$ as compared to control BD. $^{\#}p < 0.05$ and $^{\#\#\#}p < 0.001$ as compared to the NOR group.

whereas the number of grooming was significantly reduced with piracetam ($p < 0.01$), estradiol ($p < 0.001$), *F. umbellata* 50 mg/kg ($p < 0.001$) and 200 mg/kg ($p < 0.01$), and MC ($p < 0.01$) treatment. Following the administration of scopolamine, there was a significant ($p < 0.001$) increase in the number of rearing as well as grooming in normal rats

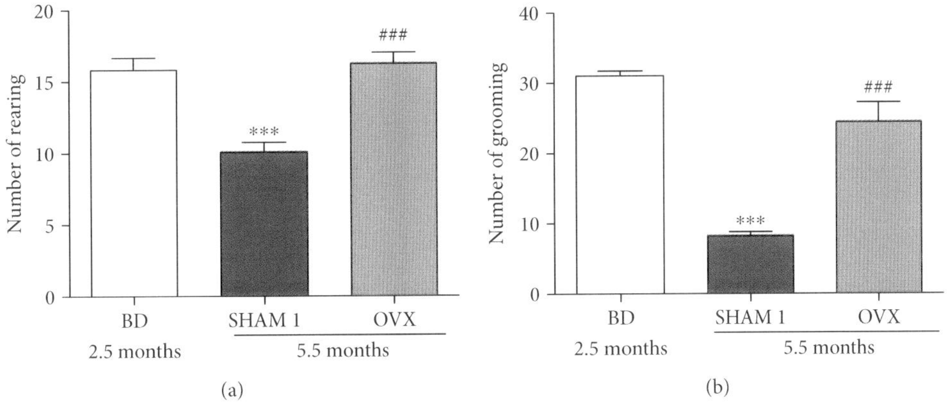

FIGURE 3: Effects of age and ovariectomy on number of rearing (a) and the number of grooming (b) of rats in the Y-maze. OVX = ovariectomized rat aged 5.5 months; BD = nonovariectomized rats aged 2.5 months which served as basic data; SHAM 1 = nonovariectomized rats aged 5.5 months. $^{***}p < 0.001$ as compared to control BD. $^{\#\#\#}p < 0.001$ as compared to the NOR group.

(SHAM 2 + SCOP) and ovariectomized (OVX + SCOP) rats as compared to normal rats (Figures 6(b) and 6(d)) which did not receive scopolamine (SHAM 1). Piracetam, *F. umbellata* aqueous extract at all tested doses, and MC significantly decreased the number of rearing and grooming. E2V (1 mg/kg) induced a significant reduction only in the number of grooming as compared to the OVX group.

3.6. Effects on the Weight and the Microarchitecture of the Brain. A significant ($p < 0.01$) decrease in the brain wet weight was observed in ovariectomized rats as compared to normal rats (Figure 7(a)). However, no significant changes were noted following treatment with the different tested substances in this parameter. No alterations in the microarchitecture of hippocampal brain regions were noted in this work (Figure 7(b)).

3.7. Effects on Oxidative Stress Parameters. Figure 8 depicts the effects of treatments on MDA and GSH levels in the brain's homogenate. A decrease in GSH level ($p < 0.01$) and an increase in MDA level ($p < 0.05$) were observed in the OVX group as compared to the sham-operated group following scopolamine administration. All treated groups prevented a decrease in GSH and an increase in MDA, but only the MC group reached statistical significant level ($p < 0.05$ for GSH and $p < 0.01$ for MDA).

4. Discussion

When women achieve menopause, they are challenged by the effects of estrogen loss on energy, mood, cognitive function, and memory. These stresses are compounded by increased risks for cardiovascular diseases, osteoporosis, cancer, and neurodegenerative diseases [1]. One of the most common diseases among the elderly population is AD, which is classified as a highly complex and progressive neurodegenerative disease [5]. AD is the main cause of dementia worldwide and is characterized by memory decrease and cognitive dysfunction [30]. Two main hypotheses explain the morphological and biochemical changes in AD patients: amyloid and cholinergic hypothesis [31]. The "cholinergic hypothesis" is characterized by a decrease in acetylcholine (ACh) in cholinergic neurons present in the hippocampus and cerebral cortex [32]. The scopolamine-induced memory impairment rat model, which mimics certain aspects of AD-related cognitive impairment and dementia, is based on the cholinergic hypothesis. In fact, scopolamine is a nonselective antagonist of the muscarinic receptor which is capable of blocking cholinergic transmission causing cognitive and memory dysfunction, leading to learning and memory deficits [26, 33]. Scopolamine-induced AD-like conditions in ovariectomized rats have long been used to demonstrate the neuroprotective effects of xenobiotic substances [34, 35]. However, none of these studies lasted 84 days after ovariectomy, which is known to be the required time for the setup of postmenopause-like conditions in rats [19–21].

In this study, we demonstrated that subchronic treatment with *F. umbellata* aqueous extract and 7-methoxycoumarin significantly improved memory and decreased rearing and grooming in scopolamine-demented ovariectomized rats. The Y-maze and the radial arm maze are well-characterized hippocampus-dependent spatial memory tasks used in this study. The Y-maze task is a specific and sensitive test of spatial recognition memory in rodents, which is suitable for evaluating memory as it highlights the ability of rodents to explore a novel environment using their hippocampi mainly [36, 37]. Short-term memory was then assessed through spontaneous alternation behavior in the Y-maze as previously described [23, 27, 38]. In the first set of tests, the percentage of spontaneous alternations was found to increase with age. Moreover, a 3-month endogenous estrogen depletion following ovariectomy significantly decreased the percentage of spontaneous alternations. These results suggest that rats gaining insurance with age are more stable in the maze. On the other hand, anxiety parameters significantly decreased with age, but increased with ovariectomy in the Y-maze. The aforementioned results suggest that ovariectomy negatively impacts locomotor activity in rats, making them display anxious behavior. Curiously, ovariectomized rats were quite rapid in the collection of baits in the radial maze, but this performance was accompanied with a high number of working memory errors which decreased with habituation. This can be explained by the great appetite that

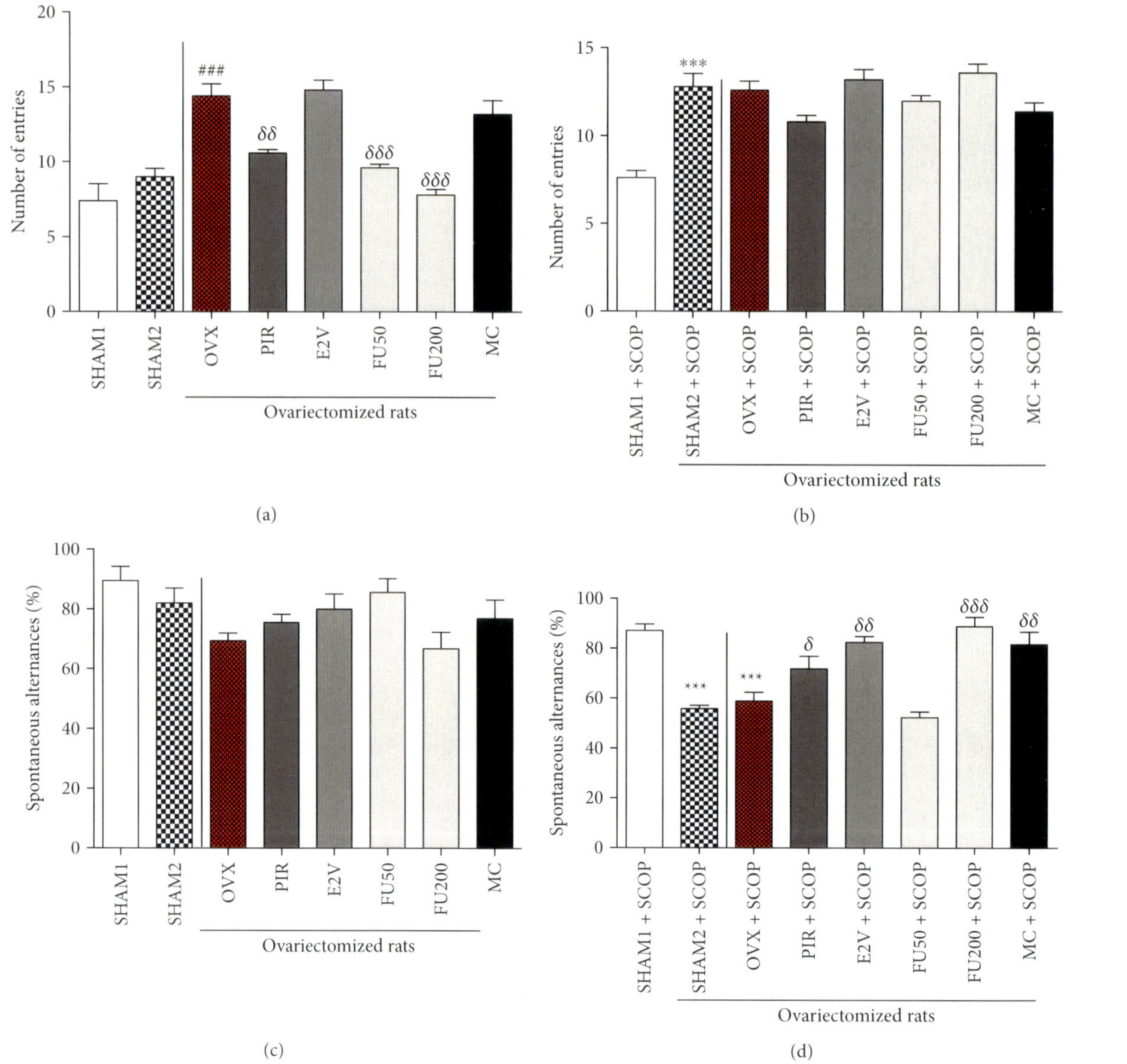

FIGURE 4: Graphic representation of the number of entries (a and b) and percentage of spontaneous alternances (c and d) before and after scopolamine exposition in rats treated with different substances into the Y-maze. SHAM 1 = sham-operated rats treated with vehicle as normal control 1; SHAM 2 = sham-operated rats treated with vehicle as normal control 2; OVX = ovariectomized rats treated with vehicle as negative control; PIR = ovariectomized rats treated with piracetam at the dose of 1.5 mg/kg BW as positive control 1; E2V = ovariectomized rats treated with estradiol valerate at the dose of 1 mg/kg BW as positive control 2; FU 50 and 200 = ovariectomized rats treated with *F. umbellata* aqueous extract at the doses of 50 and 200 mg/kg BW, respectively; MC = ovariectomized rats treated with 7-methoxycoumarin at the dose of 1 mg/kg BW. SCOP = animal that received a single dose of scopolamine (2 mg/kg BW). $^{***}p < 0.001$ as compared to the SHAM 1 group; $^{\#\#\#}p < 0.001$ as compared to the SHAM 2 group; $^{\delta}p < 0.01$, $^{\delta\delta}p < 0.01$, and $^{\delta\delta\delta}p < 0.001$ as compared to the OVX group.

sets up with ovariectomy. These results are consistent with those of Fader et al. [34], who reported that ovariectomy increased the number of working memory errors in the radial arm maze. Studies on both humans and animals indicate that estrogens may also improve memory in women with Alzheimer's disease and reduce the incidence rate of the disease [39]. Moreover, thirty minutes after scopolamine injection, the number of entries increased while the percentage of spontaneous alternations decreased in rats as compared to normal rats which did not receive scopolamine. *F. umbellata* aqueous extract on the other hand is effective on memory deficits induced by ovariectomy; it loses its promnesic efficacy when ovariectomy is coupled to muscarinic neurotransmission failure. This suggests that the *F. umbellata* extract active components could act upon muscarinic receptors to enhance memory. The failure to do so was due to the presence of scopolamine acting as an antagonist.

The 8-arm radial maze task is widely used in evaluating the effect of drugs, stress, and various other environmental factors on learning and memory [40]. Visual cues set up at

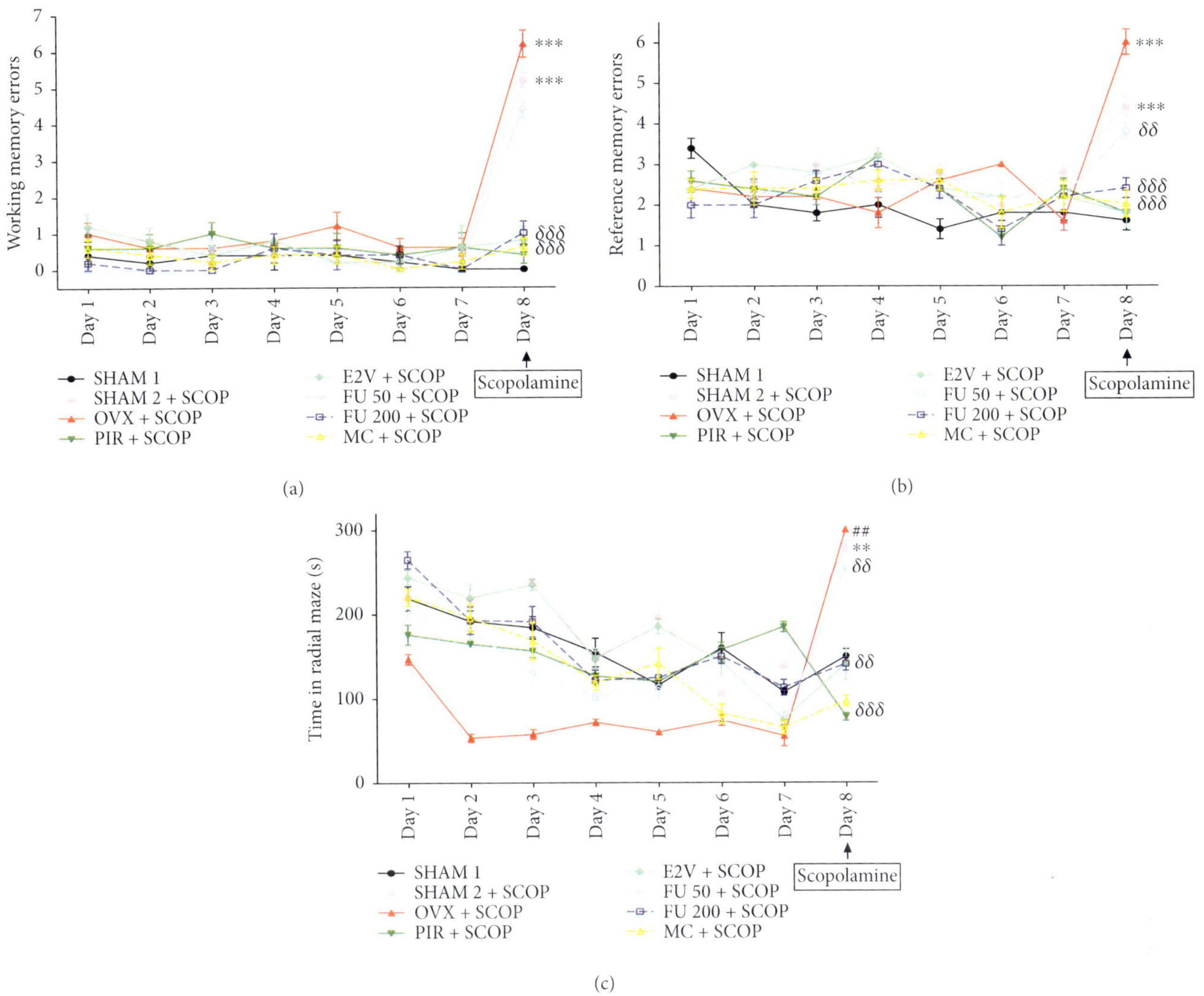

FIGURE 5: Graphic representation of the working memory (a) and spatial reference memory (b) errors as well as the time past in radial maze (c) before and after scopolamine exposition in rats treated with different substances into the Y-maze. SHAM 1 = sham-operated rats treated with vehicle as normal control 1; SHAM 2 = sham-operated rats treated with vehicle as normal control 2; OVX = ovariectomized rats treated with vehicle as negative control; PIR = ovariectomized rats treated with piracetam at the dose of 1.5 mg/kg BW as positive control 1, E2V = ovariectomized rats treated with estradiol valerate at the dose of dose 1 mg/kg BW as positive control 2; FU 50 and 200 = ovariectomized rats treated with *F. umbellata* aqueous extract at the doses of 50 and 200 mg/kg BW, respectively; MC = ovariectomized rats treated with 7-methoxycoumarin at the dose of 1 mg/kg BW. SCOP = animal that received a single dose of scopolamine (2 mg/kg BW). $^{**}p < 0.01$ and $^{***}p < 0.001$ as compared to the SHAM 1 group; $^{\#\#}p < 0.01$ as compared to the SHAM 2 group; $^{\delta\delta}p < 0.01$ and $^{\delta\delta\delta}p < 0.001$ as compared to the OVX group.

the same position throughout the radial maze task acted as spatial references as they are associated with long-term memory and allow the animals to remember the location of the baited arms in the maze. The short-term memory associated with the hippocampus can keep records only for a few seconds to minutes. Memory contents can be transferred, particularly through exercises in the long-term memory [41, 42]. In the second set of tests, working memory errors significantly reduced with age, whereas ovariectomy increased this parameter. It appears from these results that ovariectomy negatively affects the short-term memory by causing anterograde amnesia [41]. Treatment with *F. umbellata* aqueous extract at the dose of 200 mg/kg as well as MC at the dose of 1 mg/kg protected rats against scopolamine-induced memory impairment as evidenced by significantly increased spontaneous alternations, reflecting an improvement in short-term memory. These results suggest that *F umbellata* and its major compound are endowed with neuroprotective activities given that working memory and reference memory are variables that report the physiological status of the brain [42]. It has been reported that estrogen administered to ovariectomized rats improves working memory performance during acquisition of the radial arm maze task with four arms baited and prevents the disruptive effects of scopolamine on that task [34]; these findings are consistent with ours. The prevention by estrogen of impairments in working memory

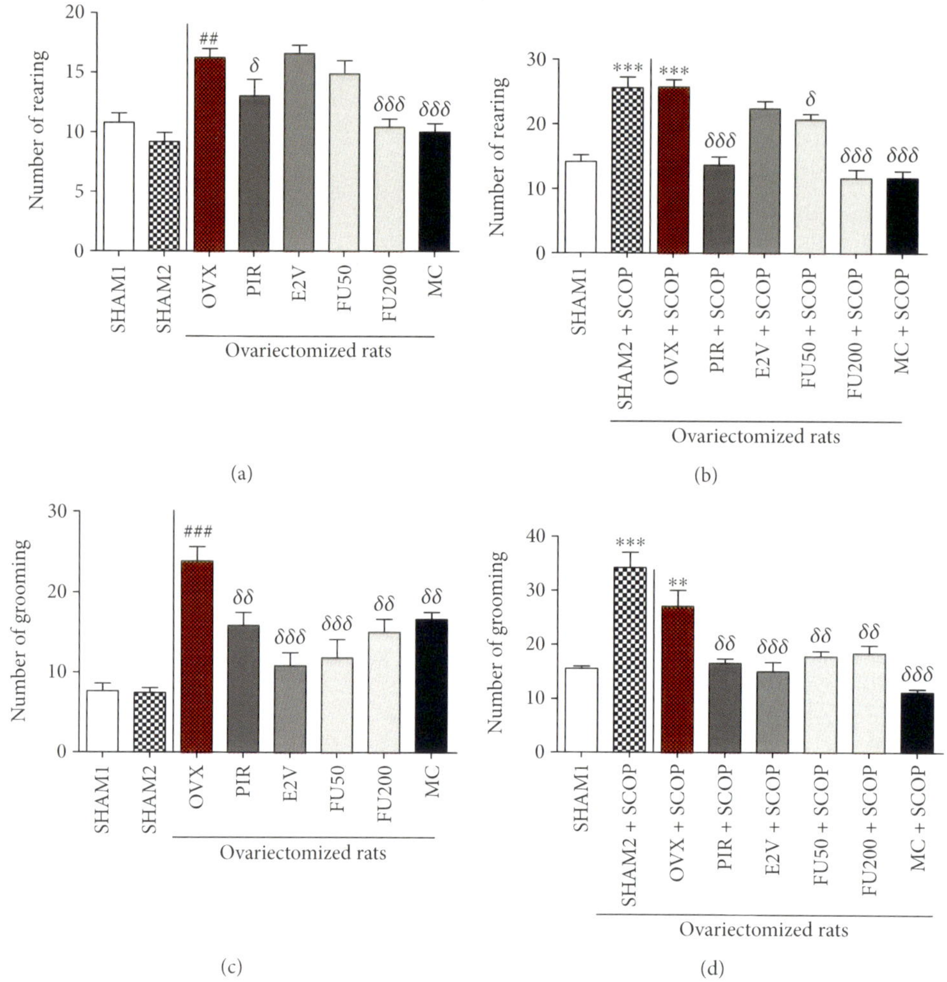

FIGURE 6: Graphic representation of the number of rearing (a and b) and grooming (c and d) of rats in the Y-maze before and after scopolamine exposition in rats treated with different substances into the Y-maze. SHAM 1 = sham-operated rats treated with vehicle as normal control 1; SHAM 2 = sham-operated rats treated with vehicle as normal control 2; OVX = ovariectomized rats treated with vehicle as negative control; PIR = ovariectomized rats treated with piracetam at the dose of 1.5 mg/kg BW as positive control 1; E2V = ovariectomized rats treated with estradiol valerate at the dose of 1 mg/kg BW as positive control 2; FU 50 and 200 = ovariectomized rats treated with *F. umbellata* aqueous extract at the doses of 50 and 200 mg/kg BW, respectively; MC = ovariectomized rats treated with 7-methoxycoumarin at the dose of 1 mg/kg BW. SCOP = animal that received a single dose of scopolamine (2 mg/kg BW). $^{**}p < 0.01$ and $^{***}p < 0.001$ as compared to the SHAM 1 group; $^{\#\#}p < 0.01$ and $^{\#\#\#}p < 0.001$ as compared to the SHAM 2 group; $^{\delta}p < 0.05$, $^{\delta\delta}p < 0.01$, and $^{\delta\delta\delta}p < 0.001$ as compared to the OVX group.

performance following scopolamine administration has been attributed to the ability of estrogen to bolster cholinergic functioning in the hippocampus by increasing the activity of choline acetyltransferase [43]. Authors also hypothesized that estrogen may act as growth factors for cholinergic neurons [44] to facilitate reactive fiber growth in hippocampi of ovariectomized rats [45]. Since *F. umbellata* contains phytoestrogens, it can act like estrogen in hippocampi and then counteract the effects of scopolamine. *F. umbellata* aqueous extract components could protect rats against memory impairment by binding on estrogen receptors (ERα and ERβ) found in several brain regions including the hippocampus, thereby inhibiting cholinesterase increase induced by scopolamine [46]. The UHPLC-MS performed with this extract revealed that *F. umbellata* contains genistein and biochanin A, well-characterized phytoestrogens [18]. Indeed, previous scientific reports showed that soy isoflavones (daidzein and genistein) improved learning ability and memory of rodents [47, 48] as well as humans [49, 50]. These activities were attributed to the ability of soy isoflavones to mimic the effects of endogenous estrogens through estrogen receptor β in the brain [51]. So far, 7-methoxycoumarin failed to transactivate ERβ such as *F. umbellata* extracts in HEK293T cells stably transfected with ERβ in a reporter gene assay [17]; it induced its estrogenicity via a nongenomic pathway [18]. The observed neuroprotective effects of *F. umbellata* might be due to the presence of genistein or related chemicals in this plant. Although MC failed to transactivate ERβ; coumarins are well known as selective inhibitors of acetylcholinesterase [52, 53]. MC could therefore pass through a nongenomic pathway in the brain to increase acetylcholine concentration, thereby increasing nerve impulses [54]. Anxiety is a parameter that negatively affects learning and memory. The injection of scopolamine helps to accentuate the

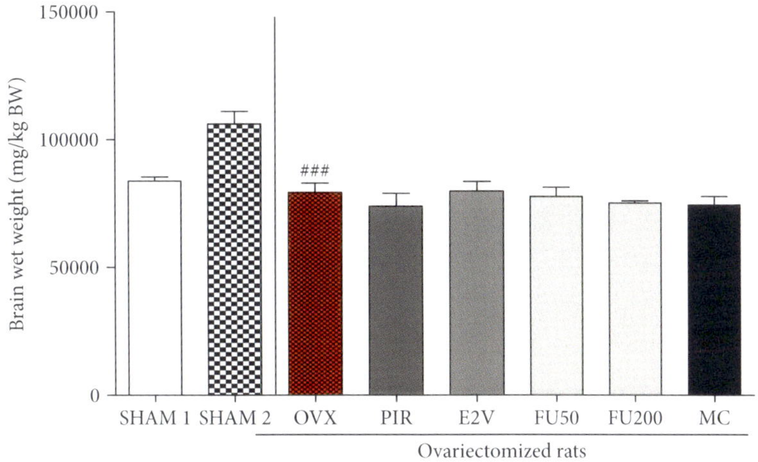

(a)

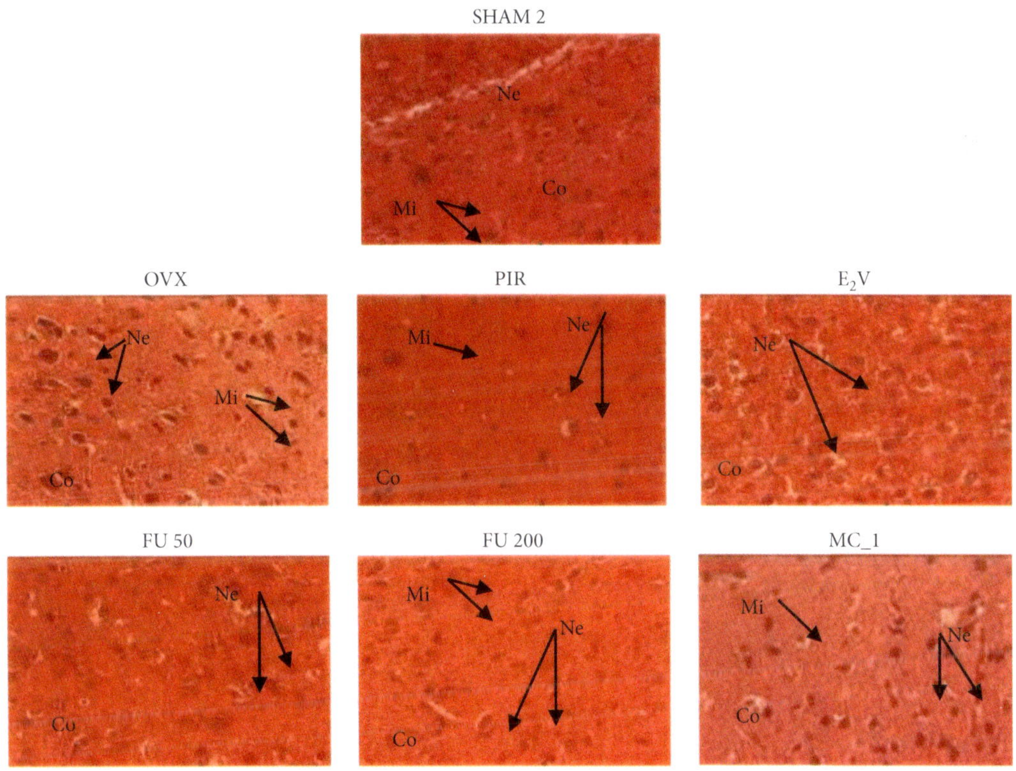

(b)

FIGURE 7: Graphical representation of brain wet weight (a) and microphotographs of HE-stained sections (400x) of the hippocampal region of the brain (b) from different experimental rat groups in postmenopause-like conditions after 3 weeks of treatment. SHAM 1 = sham-operated rats treated with vehicle as normal control 1; SHAM 2 = sham-operated rats treated with vehicle as normal control 2; OVX = ovariectomized rats treated with vehicle as negative control; PIR = ovariectomized rats treated with piracetam at the dose of 1.5 mg/kg BW as positive control 1; E2V = ovariectomized rats treated with estradiol valerate at the dose of dose 1 mg/kg BW as positive control 2; FU 50 and 200 = ovariectomized rats treated with *F. umbellata* aqueous extract at the doses of 50 and 200 mg/kg BW, respectively; MC = ovariectomized rats treated with 7-methoxycoumarin at the dose of 1 mg/kg BW. Mi = microglia; Ne = neurons; Co = cortex. $^{###}p < 0.001$ as compared to SHAM 2 group.

disorder in rats. The treatments with *F. umbellata* aqueous extract at doses of 50 and 200 mg/kg as well as MC decreased the number of rearing as well as grooming in rats. A chemical messenger widespread in the brain is GABA, which reduces activity of neurons. Some researchers believe that GABA would serve among other things to control the fear or anxiety manifested by neuronal excitation [55]. Scopolamine-induced memory deficits are accompanied with changes in acetylcholinesterase activity [56]. *F. umbellata* aqueous extract and MC exhibited anxiolytic properties and act as GABA agonists that bind to receptor GABAergic neurons and modulating the activity of the nervous system [55].

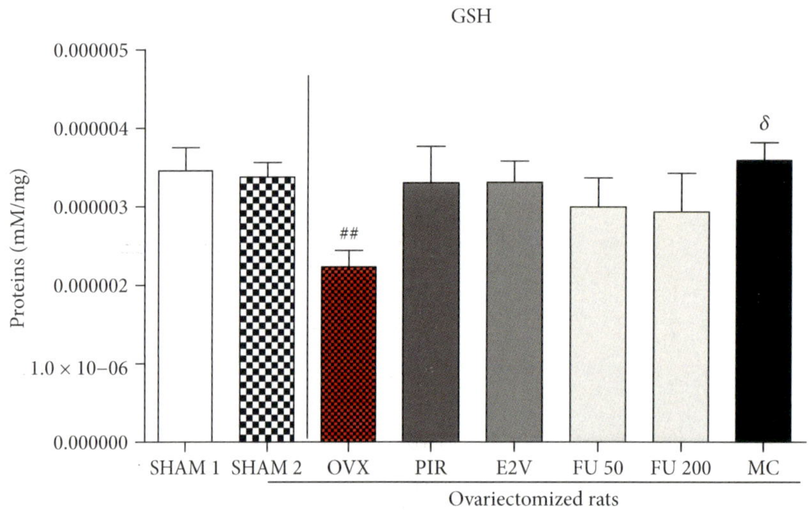

(a)

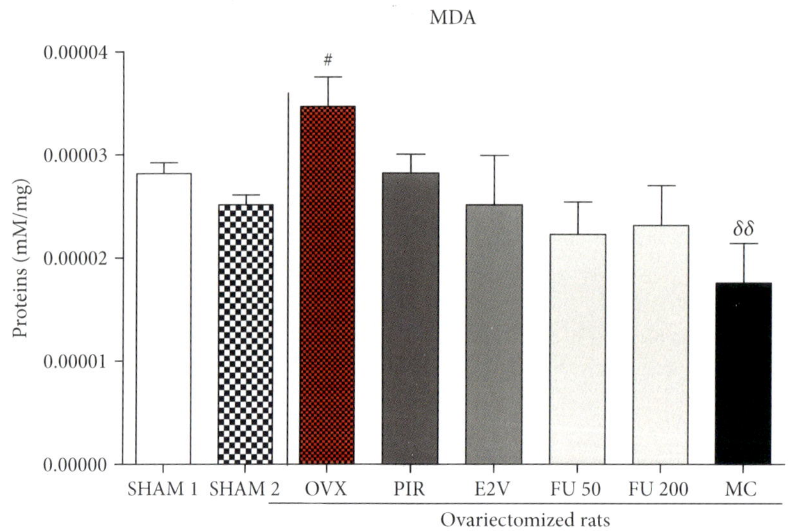

(b)

Figure 8: Reduction in glutathione-GSH (a) and malondialdehyde-MDA (b) after scopolamine exposition in rats treated with different substances. SHAM 1 = sham-operated rats treated with vehicle as normal control 1; SHAM 2 = sham-operated rats treated with vehicle as normal control 2; OVX = ovariectomized rats treated with vehicle as negative control; PIR = ovariectomized rats treated with piracetam at the dose of 1.5 mg/kg BW as positive control 1; E2V = ovariectomized rats treated with estradiol valerate at the dose of dose 1 mg/kg BW as positive control 2; FU 50 and 200 = ovariectomized rats treated with *F. umbellata* aqueous extract at the doses of 50 and 200 mg/kg BW, respectively; MC = ovariectomized rats treated with 7-methoxycoumarin at the dose of 1 mg/kg BW. $^{\#}p < 0.05$ as compared to SHAM 1; $^{\#\#}p < 0.01$ as compared to the SHAM 2 group; $^{\delta}p < 0.05$ and $^{\delta\delta}p < 0.01$ as compared to the OVX group.

It is well known that scopolamine-induced memory deficits are accompanied with oxidative damage [57]. A decrease in GSH level and an increase in MDA level in OVX rats were observed after scopolamine administration as compared to sham-operated rats. GSH is an important intracellular radical scavenger, a substrate of many xenobiotic elimination reactions, and participates in the elimination of reactive intermediates by reducing hydroperoxides [58, 59]. The depletion of GSH levels leads to the increase in oxidative stress. MC prevented the scopolamine-induced accumulation of hydroperoxides by increasing GSH levels. In addition, MDA levels are a lipid peroxidation biomarker. The main target of reactive oxygen species (ROS) is the polyunsaturated fatty acid in cell membranes. They cause lipid peroxidation and formation of MDA, which may lead to damage of cell structure and function [60]. MC reduced MDA levels as compared to the OVX group in this study. These results suggest a reduction of LDL peroxidation. From this result, the neuroprotective effects of MC may be attributable to its possible antioxidant activity.

5. Conclusion

As *F. umbellata* aqueous extract, 7-methoxycoumarin significantly increased spontaneous alternation and decreased the working and spatial reference memory errors, the time taken to collect the baits in the 8-arm radial maze, and the rearing and grooming in ovariectomized rats. Taken altogether, the aforementioned results suggest that 7-methoxycoumarin is endowed with potential neuroprotective effects in rats. In addition, MC showed an antioxidant activity, which could account for its neuroprotective effects. 7-Methoxycoumarin is responsible at least in part for the neuroprotective effects of *F. umbellata*.

Abbreviations

C-hex: Cyclohexane
CPC: Centrifugal partition chromatography
DCM: Dichloromethane
DMSO: Dimethylsulfoxide
ER: Estrogen receptor
F: Fraction
CNH: Cameroon National Herbarium
HPLC: High-performance liquid chromatography
MC: 7-Methoxycoumarin
MeOH: Methanol
NMR: nuclear magnetic resonance.

Ethical Approval

Housing of animals and all experiments were approved by the Cameroon Institutional National Ethic Committee, which adopted all procedures recommended by the European Union on the protection of animals used for scientific purposes (CEE Council 86/609; reg. no. FWA-IRD 0001954).

Authors' Contributions

Stéphane Zingue, Harquin Simplice Foyet, and Dieudonné Njamen designed the experiments. Stéphane Zingue, Harquin Simplice Foyet, Sefirin Djiogue, Yannick Ezo'o Ezo'o, and Hervé Hervé Ngatanko Abaïssou carried out the *in vivo* part of the study. Stéphane Zingue, Harquin Simplice Foyet, and Hervé Hervé Ngatanko Abaïssou wrote the manuscript. Dieudonné Njamen supervised the work. All authors read and approved the final manuscript.

Acknowledgments

Dr. Foyet Harquin Simplice Foyet was supported by The World Academy of Sciences grant (no. 12-132 RG/BIO/AF/AC_G) and United Nations Educational, Scientific and Cultural Organization FR (12-132 RG/BIO/AF/AC_G of August 2013). The authors also thank Alexander von Humboldt Foundation for the material support offered to Dieudonné Njamen.

References

[1] M.-A. Arevalo, I. Azcoitia, and L. M. Garcia-Segura, "The neuroprotective actions of oestradiol and oestrogen receptors," *Neuroscience*, vol. 16, no. 1, pp. 17–29, 2015.

[2] I. Azcoitia, C. Fernandez-Galaz, A. Sierra, and L. M. Garcia-Segura, "Gonadal hormones affect neuronal vulnerability to excitotoxin-induced degeneration," *Journal of Neurocytology*, vol. 28, no. 9, pp. 699–710, 1999.

[3] C. R. Overk, P. Y. Lu, Y. T. Wang et al., "Effects of aromatase inhibition versus gonadectomy on hippocampal complex amyloid pathology in triple transgenic mice," *Neurobiology of Disease*, vol. 45, no. 1, pp. 479–487, 2012.

[4] F. Ding, J. Yao, L. Zhao, Z. Mao, S. Chen, and R. D. Brinton, "Ovariectomy induces a shift in fuel availability and metabolism in the hippocampus of the female transgenic model of familial Alzheimer's," *PLoS One*, vol. 8, no. 3, article e59825, 2013.

[5] A. S. Morrison and C. Lyketsos, "A review on the pathophysiology of Alzheimers disease and directions in treatment," *Advances Study in Nursing*, vol. 3, no. 8, pp. 256–270, 2005.

[6] Alzheimer's Disease International (ADI), *The Global Impact of Dementia. An Analys of Prevalence, Incidence, Cost and Trends*, World Alzheimer Report, London, UK, 2015.

[7] V. Haroutunian, M. Schnaider-Beeri, J. Schmeidler et al., "Role of the neuropathology of Alzheimer disease in dementia in the oldest-old," *Archives of Neurology*, vol. 65, no. 9, pp. 1211–1217, 2008.

[8] Alzheimer's Association, "2015 Alzheimer's disease facts and figures," *Alzheimer's & Dementia*, vol. 11, no. 3, pp. 332–384, 2015.

[9] E. Scott, Q. G. Zhang, R. Wang, R. Vadlamudi, and D. Brann, "Estrogen neuroprotection and the critical period hypothesis," *Frontiers in Neuroendocrinology*, vol. 33, no. 1, pp. 85–104, 2012.

[10] B. B. Sherwin, "Estrogen and cognitive functioning in women," *Endocrine Reviews*, vol. 24, no. 2, pp. 133–151, 2003.

[11] J. E. Rossouw, G. L. Anderson, R. L. Prentice et al., "Risks and benefits of estrogen plus progestin in healthy postmenopausal women: principal results from the Women's Health Initiative randomized controlled trial," *Journal of the American Medical Association*, vol. 288, no. 3, pp. 321–333, 2002.

[12] Million Women Study Collaborators, "Breast cancer and hormone-replacement therapy in the Million Women Study," *The Lancet*, vol. 362, no. 9382, pp. 419–427, 2003.

[13] Million Women Study Collaborators, "Endometrial cancer and hormone-replacement therapy in the Million Women Study," *The Lancet*, vol. 365, no. 9470, pp. 1543–1551, 2005.

[14] J. Pitkin, "Alternative and complementary therapies for the menopause," *Menopause International*, vol. 18, no. 1, pp. 20–27, 2012.

[15] M. Arbonnier, *Arbres, arbustes et lianes des zones sèches d'Afrique de l'Ouest*, 2009, Editions Quæ RD 10; F- 78026 Versailles Cedex, France; Muséum National d'histoire Naturelle (MNHN) ; Service des publications scientifiques, 57 Rue Cuvier, F-75005 Paris, France.

[16] K. Babu, S. G. Shankar, and S. Rai, "Comparative pharmacognostic studies on the barks of four Ficus species," *Turkish Journal of Botany*, vol. 34, no. 3, pp. 215–224, 2010.

[17] S. Zingue, T. Michel, J. Tchatchou et al., "Estrogenic effects of Ficus umbellata Vahl. (Moraceae) extracts and their ability to alleviate some menopausal symptoms induced by ovariectomy in Wistar rats," *Journal of Ethnopharmacology*, vol. 179, no. 1, pp. 332–344, 2016.

[18] S. Zingue, T. Michel, C. B. M. Nde et al., "Estrogen-like and tissue-selective effects of 7-methoxycoumarin from Ficus umbellata (Moraceae): an in vitro and in vivo study," *BMC Complementary and Alternative Medicine*, vol. 17, no. 1, pp. 383–396, 2017.

[19] D. Njamen, C. B. Magne Ndé, Z. Tanee Fomum, and J. C. Mbanya, "Preventive effects of an extract of Erythrina Lysistemon (Fabaceae) on some menopausal problems: studies on the rat," *Journal of Complementary and Integrative Medicine*, vol. 4, no. 1, 2007.

[20] M. E. Basha, S. Chang, L. J. Burrows et al., "Effect of estrogen on molecular and functional characteristics of the rodent vaginal muscularis," *The Journal of Sexual Medicine*, vol. 10, no. 5, pp. 1219–1230, 2013.

[21] D. D. Paul Désiré, M. N. Yolande Sandrine, B. Danielle Claude et al., "In vivo estrogenic-like activities of Gouania longipetala Hemsl. (Rhamnaceae) bark extracts in a post-menopause-like model of ovariectomized Wistar rats," *Journal of Ethnopharmacology*, vol. 168, no. 1, pp. 122–128, 2015.

[22] R. J. Wurtman, S. G. Magil, and D. K. Reinstein, "Piracetam diminishes hippocampal acetylcholine levels in rats," *Life Sciences*, vol. 28, no. 10, pp. 1091–1093, 1981.

[23] H. S. Foyet, H. H. Ngatanko Abaïssou, E. Wado, E. Asongalem Acha, and C. Alin, "Emilia coccinae (SIMS) G extract improves memory impairment, cholinergic dysfunction, and oxidative stress damage in scopolamine-treated rats," *BMC Complementary and Alternative Medicine*, vol. 15, no. 1, 2015.

[24] N. G. Hernández-Chan, J. L. Góngora-Alfaro, F. J. Álvarez-Cervera, F. A. Solís-Rodríguez, F. J. Heredia-López, and G. Arankowsky-Sandoval, "Quinolinic acid lesions of the pedunculopontine nucleus impair sleep architecture, but not locomotion, exploration, emotionality or working memory in the rat," *Behavioural Brain Research*, vol. 225, no. 2, pp. 482–490, 2011.

[25] M. D. S. Lapiz-Bluhm, C. O. Bondi, J. Doyen, G. A. Rodriguez, T. Bédard-Arana, and D. A. Morilak, "Behavioural assays to model ′cognitive and affective dimensions of depression and anxiety in rats," *Journal of Neuroendocrinology*, vol. 20, no. 10, pp. 1115–1137, 2008.

[26] L. Hritcu, O. Cioanca, and M. Hancianu, "Effects of lavender oil inhalation on improving scopolamine-induced spatial memory impairment in laboratory rats," *Phytomedicine*, vol. 19, no. 6, pp. 529–534, 2012.

[27] G. J. Beppe, A. B. Dongmo, H. S. Foyet et al., "Memory-enhancing activities of the aqueous extract of Albizia adianthifolia leaves in the 6-hydroxydopamine-lesion rodent model of Parkinson's disease," *BMC Complementary and Alternative Medicine*, vol. 14, no. 1, 2014.

[28] M. Shamnas, R. Ratendra, and U. V. S. Teotia, "Neuroprotective activity of methanol extract of Salvia officinalis flowers in dementia related to Alzheimer disease," *Der Pharmacia Sinica*, vol. 5, no. 2, pp. 29–38, 2014.

[29] M. Padurariu, A. Ciobica, L. Hritcu, B. Stoica, W. Bild, and C. Stefanescu, "Changes of some oxidative stress markers in the serum of patients with mild cognitive impairment and Alzheimer's disease," *Neuroscience Letters*, vol. 469, no. 1, pp. 6–10, 2010.

[30] N. Cortes, R. Alvarez, E. H. Osorio, F. Alzate, S. Berkov, and E. Osorio, "Alkaloid metabolite profiles by GC/MS and acetylcholinesterase inhibitory activities with binding-mode predictions of five Amaryllidaceae plants," *Journal of Pharmaceutical and Biomedical Analysis*, vol. 102, pp. 222–228, 2015.

[31] A. Contestabile, "The history of the cholinergic hypothesis," *Behavioural Brain Research*, vol. 221, no. 2, pp. 334–340, 2011.

[32] D. K. Lahiri, M. R. Farlow, N. H. Greig, and K. Sambamurti, "Current drug targets for Alzheimer's disease treatment," *Drug Development Research*, vol. 56, no. 3, pp. 267–281, 2002.

[33] A. C. G. Souza, C. A. Bruning, C. I. Acker, J. S. S. Neto, and C. W. Nogueira, "2-Phenylethynyl-butyltellurium enhances learning and memory impaired by scopolamine in mice," *Behavioural Pharmacology*, vol. 24, no. 4, pp. 249–254, 2013.

[34] A. J. Fader, P. E. M. Johnson, and G. P. Dohanich, "Estrogen improves working but not reference memory and prevents amnestic effects of scopolamine on a radial-arm maze," *Pharmacology Biochemistry and Behavior*, vol. 62, no. 4, pp. 711–717, 1999.

[35] S. M. R. Wahba, A. S. Darwish, and S. M. Kamal, "Ceria-containing uncoated and coated hydroxyapatite-based galantamine nanocomposites for formidable treatment of Alzheimer's disease in ovariectomized albino-rat model," *Materials Science and Engineering C*, vol. 65, no. 1, pp. 151–163, 2016.

[36] Y. Sadiq, A. B. Alexander, and A. Abdulkarim, "Effect of *Ziziphus mauritiania* (L.) seed extracts on spatial recognition memory of rats as measured by the Y-maze test," *Journal of Natural Products*, vol. 2, no. 1, pp. 31–39, 2009.

[37] M. Bagheri, M.-T. Joghataei, S. Mohseni, and M. Roghani, "Genistein ameliorates learning and memory deficits in amyloid β (1–40) rat model of Alzheimer's disease," *Neurobiology of Learning and Memory*, vol. 95, no. 3, pp. 270–276, 2011.

[38] H. E. Jing, Y.-m. CHEN, J.-h. WANG, and M. A. Yuan-ye, "Effect of co-administration of morphine and cholinergic antagonists on Y-maze spatial recognition memory retrieval and locomotor activity in mice," *Zoological Research*, vol. 29, no. 6, pp. 613–620, 2008.

[39] M.-X. Tang, D. Jacobs, Y. Stern et al., "Effect of oestrogen during menopause on risk and age at onset of Alzheimer's disease," *Lancet*, vol. 348, no. 9025, pp. 429–432, 1996.

[40] M. Mizuno, K. Yamada, A. Olariu, H. Nawa, and T. Nabeshima, "Involvement of brain-derived neurotrophic factor in spatial memory formation and maintenance in a radial arm maze test in rats," *Journal of Neuroscience*, vol. 20, no. 18, pp. 7116–7121, 2000.

[41] T. Myhrer, "Neurotransmitter systems involved in learning and memory in the rat: a meta-analysis based on studies of four behavioral tasks," *Brain Research Reviews*, vol. 41, no. 2-3, pp. 268–287, 2003.

[42] A. D. J. Titus, B. S. Shankaranarayana Rao, H. N. Harsha et al., "Hypobaric hypoxia-induced dendritic atrophy of hippocampal neurons is associated with cognitive impairment in adult rats," *Neuroscience*, vol. 145, no. 1, pp. 265–278, 2007.

[43] M. Singh, E. M. Meyer, W. J. Millard, and J. W. Simpkins, "Ovarian steroid deprivation results in a reversible learning impairment and compromised cholinergic function in female Sprague–Dawley rats," *Brain Research*, vol. 644, no. 2, pp. 305–312, 1994.

[44] H. Honjo, T. Tamura, Y. Matsumoto et al., "Estrogen as a growth factor to central nervous cells," *The Journal of Steroid*

Biochemistry and Molecular Biology, vol. 41, no. 3–8, pp. 633–635, 1992.

[45] S. W. Scheff, J. K. Morse, and S. T. DeKosky, "Neurotrophic effects of steroids on lesion-induced growth in the hippocampus. I. The asteroidal condition," *Brain Research*, vol. 457, no. 2, pp. 246–250, 1988.

[46] M. Hosseini, T. Mohammadpour, R. Karami, Z. Rajaei, H. Reza Sadeghnia, and M. Soukhtanloo, "Effects of the hydro-alcoholic extract of Nigella sativa on scopolamine-induced spatial memory impairment in rats and its possible mechanism," *Chinese Journal of Integrative Medicine*, vol. 21, no. 6, pp. 438–444, 2015.

[47] A. M. Duncan, W. R. Phipps, and M. S. Kurzer, "Phyto-oestrogens," *Best Practice & Research Clinical Endocrinology & Metabolism*, vol. 17, no. 2, pp. 253–271, 2003.

[48] Y. H. Huang, X. Y. Xin, and Y. Q. Chen, "Effects of genistein and 17β estradiol on the spatial learning and memory in ovariecomized rats," *Journal of Fourth Military Medical University*, vol. 25, no. 1, pp. 46–49, 2004.

[49] S. File, N. Jarrett, E. Fluck, R. Duffy, K. Casey, and H. Wiseman, "Eating soya improves human memory," *Psychopharmacology*, vol. 157, no. 4, pp. 430–436, 2001.

[50] L. Zhao and R. D. Brinton, "WHI and WHIMS follow-up and human studies of soy isoflavones on cognition," *Expert Review of Neurotherapeutics*, vol. 7, no. 11, pp. 1549–1564, 2007.

[51] Y. B. Lee, H. J. Lee, and H. S. Sohn, "Soy isoflavones and cognitive function," *The Journal of Nutritional Biochemistry*, vol. 16, no. 11, pp. 641–649, 2005.

[52] F. Leonetti, M. Catto, O. Nicolotti et al., "Homo- and hetero-bivalent edrophonium-like ammonium salts as highly potent, dual binding site AChE inhibitors," *Bioorganic & Medicinal Chemistry*, vol. 16, no. 15, pp. 7450–7456, 2008.

[53] L. G. de Souza, M. N. Rennó, and J. D. Figueroa-Villar, "Coumarins as cholinesterase inhibitors: a review," *Chemico-Biological Interactions*, vol. 254, no. 1, pp. 11–23, 2016.

[54] X.-M. Peng, G. L. V. Damu, and C. H. Zhou, "Current developments of coumarin compounds in medicinal chemistry," *Current Pharmaceutical Design*, vol. 19, no. 21, pp. 3884–3930, 2013.

[55] I. Gauthier and P. Nuss, "Anxiety disorders and GABA neurotransmission: a disturbance of modulation," *Neuropsychiatric Disease and Treatment*, 2015.

[56] R. Kaur, S. Parveen, S. Mehan, D. Khanna, and S. Kalra, "Neuroprotective effect of Ellagic acid against chronically scopolamine induced Alzheimer's type memory and cognitive dysfunctions: possible behavioural and biochemical evidences," *International Journal of Preventive Medicine*, vol. 1, no. 2, pp. 45–64, 2015.

[57] Y. K. Lee, D. Y. Yuk, T. I. Kim et al., "Protective effect of the ethanol extract of *Magnolia officinalis* and 4-O-methylhonokiol on scopolamine-induced memory impairment and the inhibition of acetylcholinesterase activity," *Journal of Natural Medicines*, vol. 63, no. 3, pp. 274–282, 2009.

[58] Z. Gregus, T. Fekete, E. Halaszi, and C. D. Klaassen, "Lipoic acid impairs glycine conjugation of benzoic acid and renal excretion of benzoylglycine," *Drug Metabolism and Disposition*, vol. 24, no. 6, pp. 682–688, 1996.

[59] P. Nicotera and S. Orrenius, "Role of thiols in protection against biological reactive intermediates," *Advances in Experimental Medicine and Biology*, 1986.

[60] H. Kuper, A. Tzonou, E. Kaklamani et al., "Tobacco smoking alcohol consumption and their interaction in the causation of hepatocellular carcinoma," *International Journal of Cancer*, vol. 85, no. 4, pp. 498–502, 2000.

10

Xiao-Xu-Ming Decoction Reduced Mitophagy Activation and Improved Mitochondrial Function in Cerebral Ischemia and Reperfusion Injury

Rui Lan,[1] **Yong Zhang**,[2] **Tao Wu**,[1] **Yun-Zhi Ma**,[1] **Bao-Qi Wang**,[3] **Hai-Zhong Zheng**,[3] **Ya-Na Li**,[1] **Yan Wang**,[1] **Chun-Qing Gu**,[1] **and Ji-Tao Wu**[1]

[1]*Encephalopathy Hospital, The First Affiliated Hospital of Henan University of Chinese Medicine, Henan 450000, China*
[2]*Cerebral Palsy Rehabilitation Department, The Third Affiliated Hospital of Zhengzhou University, Henan 450000, China*
[3]*Henan University of Chinese Medicine, Henan 450000, China*

Correspondence should be addressed to Ji-Tao Wu; wujitao1345@126.com

Academic Editor: Anatol Manaenko

We investigated whether Xiao-Xu-Ming decoction reduced mitophagy activation and kept mitochondrial function in cerebral ischemia-reperfusion injury. Rats were randomly divided into 5 groups: sham, ischemia and reperfusion (IR), IR plus XXMD (60 g/kg/day) (XXMD60), IR plus cyclosporin A (10 mg/kg/day) (CsA), and IR plus vehicle (Vehicle). Focal cerebral ischemia and reperfusion models were induced by middle cerebral artery occlusion (MCAO). Cerebral infarct areas were measured by triphenyl tetrazolium chloride staining. Cerebral ischemic injury was evaluated by hematoxylin and eosin staining (HE) and Nissl staining. Ultrastructural features of mitochondria and mitophagy in the penumbra of the ischemic cortex were observed by transmission electron microscopy. Mitophagy was detected by immunofluorescence labeled with LC3B and VDAC1. Autophagy lysosome formation was observed by immunofluorescence labeled with LC3B and Lamp1. The expression of LC3B, Beclin1, and Lamp1 was analyzed by Western blot. The rats subjected to MCAO showed worsened neurological score and cell ischemic damage. These were all significantly reversed by XXMD or CsA. Moreover, XXMD/CsA notably downregulated mitophagy and reduced the increase in LC3, Beclin1, and Lamp1 expression induced by cerebral ischemia and reperfusion. The findings demonstrated that XXMD exerted neuroprotective effect via downregulating LC3, Beclin1, Lamp1, and mitochondrial p62 expression level, thus leading to the inhibition of mitophagy.

1. Introduction

Mitochondria play crucial roles in energy production, programmed cell death, calcium homeostasis, reactive oxidative phosphorylation, and cell cycle regulation [1]. Autophagy is a vital conserved process for the bulk degradation and recycling of unnecessary proteins and organelle by the lysosomal degradation pathway. Starvation [2], hypoxia [3], and endoplasmic reticulum stress [4] notably activated autophagy. The roles of autophagy in the cerebral ischemia injury have been widely studied. Recent reports have found that autophagy [5–7] is widely evoked following cerebral ischemia-reperfusion injury. The findings have clarified that autophagy can be destructive [8] or protective [9]. Mitophagy, as one type of selective autophagy, is extremely important for maintaining mitochondrial homeostasis by removing damaged mitochondria [10]. Mitophagy which regulates the mitochondrial number in response to metabolic demand is a form of quality control to eliminate damaged mitochondria [11]. A large body of evidence has indicated the specific events containing endoplasmic reticulum (ER) stress, oxidative stress, and excitotoxicity involved in the cerebral ischemic brain initiate mitophagy [12]. Mitophagy is mainly evident in neurons [5] and astrocytes [13] subjected to cerebral ischemia. The role of mitophagy in cerebral ischemia is still controversial. Enhanced mitophagy attenuates mitochondrial dysfunction after cerebral ischemia [14, 15]. Other studies have suggested that deleterious autophagic processes lead to cell death and attenuated mitophagy may protect neurons from cerebral injury [16, 17]. It is generally accepted that failure to adequately remove damaged mitochondria or excessive degradation will lead to cell death [10].

Xiao-Xu-Ming decoction has been widely used to treat stoke and has notable effects [18]. Our previous studies have revealed that XXMD alleviates BBB disruption and protects neurovascular unit and mitochondria from cerebral injury induced by cerebral ischemia and reperfusion [19–21]. However, whether XXMD could regulate mitophagy following cerebral ischemia and reperfusion has not been studied yet. Therefore, the present study was aimed at exploring the effect of XXMD treatment on mitophagy and mitochondrial function after cerebral ischemia and reperfusion.

2. Methods and Materials

2.1. Animals. All experiments were performed on adult male Sprague-Dawley rats (Experimental Animal Center and Central Lab, Henan Province Hospital of Chinese Medicine, China) weighing 250~280 g. 92 rats were housed in temperature- and humidity-controlled (55 ± 5%) rooms with a 12 h light-dark cycle on a 12 : 12 h light. All animals were allowed to move and feed freely. The experimental protocols and animal handling procedures were approved by the Animal Care and Use Committee (ACUC) of the First Affiliated Hospital of Henan University of Chinese Medicine.

2.2. Preparation of XXMD. The crude drugs were purchased from Traditional Chinese Medicine Pharmacy of the First Affiliated Hospital of Henan University of Chinese Medicine. XXMD was prepared as previously reported [19–21]. The first decoction lasted for 1 h in a drug (1) : distilled water (10) ratio (*w* : *v*), and then the suspension was collected. The above process was repeated three times. The collected herbs were soaked with 75% ethanol for 24 h, and the liquid was gained. The above mixed suspension from three decoctions was centrifuged at 2000 ×g for 20 min, and the supernatant was obtained. Ethanol was slowly added to the suspension and kept stirred until the concentration reached 75% ethanol (*v*/*v*). Mixed suspension and the liquid obtained from the gruffs were centrifuged at 2000 ×g for 20 min and then concentrated at the final concentration of 2 g/ml (*w*/*v*). Eventually, the liquid was stored for the study.

2.3. Groups and Drug Administration. We previously examined the effects of different dosages of XXMD on cerebral ischemic injury and found that 60 g/kg/day gave maximal protective effects in the treatment of cerebral ischemic injury [19]. Previous studies have demonstrated that the immunosuppressor cyclosporin A (CsA, Solarbio Life Science, Beijing, China) reduces brain damage induced by cerebral ischemia in rats [22, 23]. It is well known that CsA could inhibit mitochondrial permeability transition, mitochondrial swelling [24, 25], and mitophagy [26, 27]. It has been reported that CsA suppresses cytochrome C efflux to the cytoplasm [28]. In the current study, we designed CsA as a control treatment in this study. In addition, evidence has determined that the dose of 10 mg/kg CsA is the optimal dose for neuroprotective effects in ischemic brain injury [28, 29]. In the study, rats were randomly divided into five groups: sham control (Sham) group, ischemia and reperfusion (IR) group, ischemia and reperfusion plus XXMD (60 g/kg/day, XXMD60) group, ischemia and reperfusion plus cyclosporin A (10 mg/kg, CsA) group, and ischemia and reperfusion plus dimethyl sulfoxide and ethanol (Vehicle) group.

The drug administrations were performed twice a day at 8:00 and 18:00 for 3 days before the induction of ischemia and lasted until the conclusion of the experiment. The rats in the XXMD60 group were orally administered XXMD. Others in the Sham and IR groups were given the same volume of distilled water. The rats in the CsA group were intraperitoneally injected with CsA, which was dissolved in polyethoxylated castor oil and 95% ethanol and further diluted with saline at a dosage of 10 mg/kg. The same solution lacking CsA was used for vehicle treatment.

2.4. Focal Cerebral Ischemia and Reperfusion Model. Focal cerebral ischemia and reperfusion was performed as described previously [19–21]. Briefly, the rats were anesthetized with 10% chloral hydrate (350 mg/kg, i.p.), and the left common carotid artery (CCA) was exposed. A unified nylon monofilament (Beijing Sunbio Biotech, Beijing, China), with a diameter of 0.26 mm and a length of 40 mm with its tip rounded, was inserted about 20 mm from the CCA bifurcation to block the origin of the middle cerebral artery (MCA). Reperfusion was initiated by withdrawal of the suture until the tip cleared the lumen of the ECA after 90 min of occlusion. In the current study, the rats in the IR, XXMD60, CsA, and Vehicle groups subjected to cerebral ischemia followed by reperfusion. Animals in the Sham group only underwent the same surgical procedure, but the suture was not inserted. Examination of neurological deficits was performed at 24 h after reperfusion. The neurological deficits were scored on a four-point scale described by Hara et al. [30], and the rats that underwent MCAO without any detectable neurological deficits were excluded from the further investigations

2.5. Neurological Deficit Score. Examination of neurological deficits was performed at 24 h after reperfusion. The neurological deficits were scored on a four-point scale described by Hara et al. [30] with a minor modification: 0—no neurological deficit, 1—mild focal neurological deficit (animal showed forelimb flexion), 2—moderate focal neurological deficit (decreased resistance to lateral push and forelimb flexion without circling), and 3—severe focal deficit (decreased resistance to lateral push and forelimb flexion with circling). In the present study, the rats subjected to MCAO without any detectable neurological deficits were excluded from the following investigations and analyses to exclude operative failures.

2.6. Cerebral Infarct Area. The rats were sacrificed under deep anesthesia and perfused transcardially with normal saline. The brains were sectioned into coronal slices from rostral to caudal and stained with 1% 2,3,5-triphenyl tetrazolium chloride staining for 15 min at 37°C away from light.

Then, the brain tissues were differentiated according to the white-colored infarct area and the red-purple noninfarct area. Cerebral infarct areas were calculated according to the previous study [20].

2.7. General Histology. The rats were anesthetized with 10% chloral hydrate (350 mg/kg, i.p.) and perfused transcardially with normal saline followed by 4% paraformaldehyde (0.1 M phosphate-buffered saline, pH 7.4) at 24 h after reperfusion. Then, the brain tissues were postfixed in the above fixative for 24 h and processed routinely for paraffin embedding. A series of 5 μm thick sections were cut on a rotary microtome for hematoxylin and eosin (HE) staining and Nissl staining as previously described [20, 21]. And the number of intact cells in the penumbra of the ischemic cortex by Nissl staining was counted throughout five lesion regions randomly.

2.8. Electron Microscopy. Transmission electron microscopy was used to investigate the morphology of mitochondria and mitophagy after ischemia and reperfusion. At 24 h after reperfusion, the rats were perfused transcardially with cold 0.9% saline, followed by 4% paraformaldehyde and 1% glutaraldehyde. 1.0 mm^3 of coronal sections located in peri-infarct areas of the ipsilateral cortex was postfixed in 2% osmium for 90 min, dehydrated, and embedded in Epon 812 Resin (TAAB, Berks, UK). Ultrathin (60 nm) sections were cut with a diamond knife, stained with uranyl acetate and lead citrate, and observed with an electron microscope (JEM-1400, Tokyo, Japan).

2.9. ATP Content Measurement. Purified mitochondria were extracted with a tissue mitochondrial isolation kit according to the manufacturer's instructions (Jiancheng Bioengineering Inc., Nanjing, China). Briefly, fresh brain cortical tissue was homogenized in 1 : 10 (*w*/*v*) ice-cold homogenization buffer plus 1 mM PMSF and centrifuged at 600*g* for 5 min at 4°C. The supernatants were centrifuged at 11,000*g* for 10 min at 4°C. The isolated mitochondrial fraction was collected for malonaldehydes (MDA, markers of oxidative damage), ATP assay, and Western blot. The ATP level was assessed with an ATP assay kit (Jiancheng Bioengineering Inc., Nanjing, China) according to the manufacturer's instructions and a previous study [14]. Mitochondrial fraction was centrifuged at 10,000*g* for 10 min, and then the supernatant was collected for the following assay. ATP reagents were added into a microwell for 5 min at 37°C, and samples were added and mixed for 10 s and measured by a Synergy HT multimode microplate reader. Results were expressed as nmol per mg protein calculated against a standard curve.

2.10. MDA Level Measurement. The MDA levels were examined with a MDA assay kit (Jiancheng Bioengineering Inc., Nanjing, China) according to the manufacturer's protocol and a previous study [14]. Briefly, the MDA reagent was incubated with the supernatant of mitochondrial lysis for 40 min at 95°C and then was detected with a Synergy HT multimode microplate reader at 532 nm absorbance. Results were expressed as nmol per mg protein.

2.11. Immunofluorescence Staining. The brain sections were dewaxed followed by the antigen repair method and then washed three times with PBS. The sections were blocked with 5% normal goat serum for 1 h at room temperature and incubated with a primary antibody at 4°C overnight. After washing with PBS, sections were incubated with an appropriate secondary antibody for 1 h at room temperature. Sections were stained with DAPI (Beyotime, Haimen, Jiangsu, China) for 15 min and observed with a fluorescence microscope (Olympus/BX51) after three 5 min washes with PBS. For double immunofluorescence, sections were incubated consecutively with pairs of primary and secondary antibodies. Sections were examined under a fluorescence microscope (Olympus/BX51, Tokyo, Japan). Double-stained cells of different groups were counted throughout five lesion regions randomly in the penumbra of the ischemic cortex.

2.12. Immunohistochemistry Staining. For immunohistochemistry, the brain slices were deparaffinized by xylene, the gradient alcohol was rehydrated, and the antigen was repaired. The slices were incubated with 0.3% H_2O_2 in PBS. After blocking with 5% normal goat serum, the sections were incubated with a mouse monoclonal Beclin1 antibody at appropriate concentration at 4°C overnight. After washing in PBS, the sections were incubated with the secondary antibody conjugated with horseradish peroxidase (Hua'an Biotechnology, Hangzhou, China) for 1 h at 37°C and then visualized using a general SP immunohistochemical kit (Solarbio Life Science, Beijing, China). The sections were photographed and observed with a light microscope (Olympus/BX51, Tokyo, Japan).

2.13. Western Blot. Equal qualities of protein solutions were separated by electrophoresis of appropriate concentrations of polyacrylamide gels and transferred to the polyvinylidene fluoride membranes (Millipore, Bedford, MA, USA). After blocking with 5% skim milk in Tris-buffered saline containing 0.1% Tween-20 (TBST) for 2 h at room temperature, the membranes were probed with primary antibodies at 4°C overnight. After washing with TBST three times for 10 min each, the membranes were incubated with the secondary antibody conjugated with horseradish peroxidase. Eventually, the targeted antigens were detected by standard chemical luminescence methods (Millipore, Bedford, MA, USA) on the Bio-Rad ChemiDoc™ MP imaging system. Band intensities were measured with Quantity One software (Bio-Rad Laboratories, Hercules, CA, USA).

2.14. Statistical Analysis. Data are presented as the means ± standard error of the mean (SEM). Statistical significance was determined by one-way ANOVA followed by Tukey's multiple comparison test or unpaired Student's *t*-tests using SPSS 11.5 for Windows (Chicago, IL, USA). All were considered statistically significant for $p < 0.05$.

3. Results

3.1. XXMD Reduced Cerebral Infarct Areas and Ameliorated Neurological Deficits. Cerebral infarct areas and neurological deficits induced by cerebral ischemia and reperfusion were

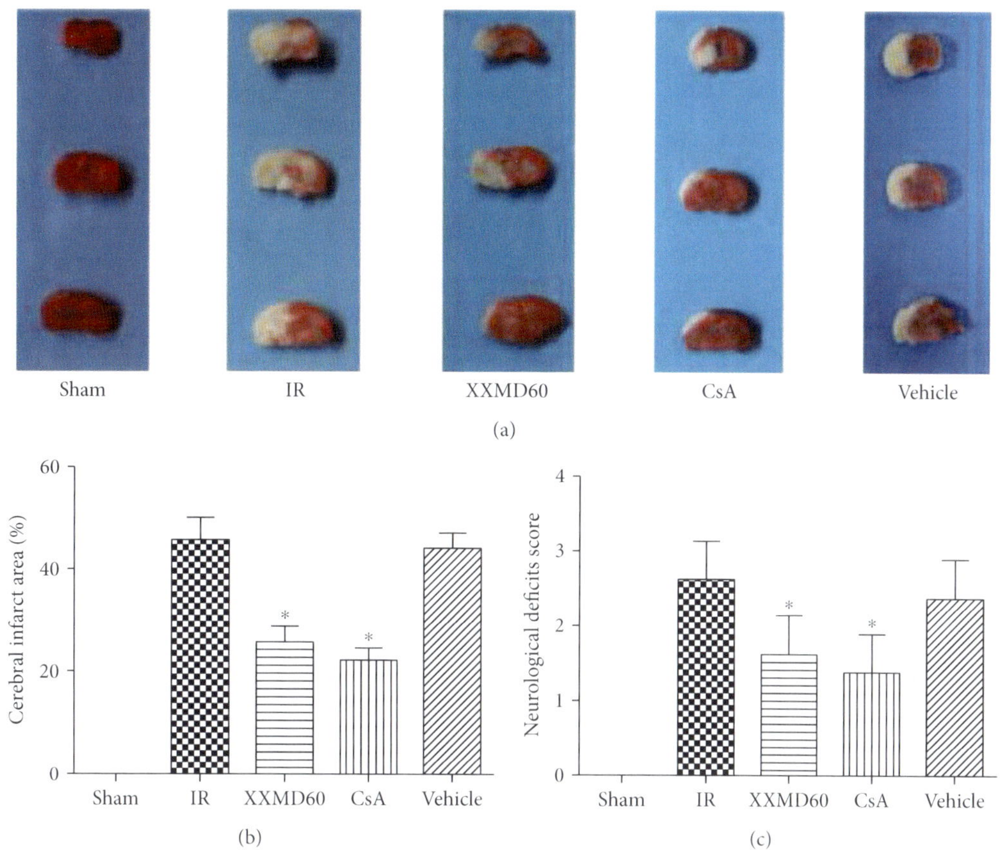

FIGURE 1: Cerebral infarct areas and neurological deficit score at 24 h after reperfusion. (a) Representative images of TTC-stained brain slices. The infarct area appeared white, whereas noninfarct areas were stained red-purple. (b) Quantitative analysis of cerebral infarct areas. (c) Effect of XXMD on the neurological deficit score. XXMD/CsA treatment significantly improved the neurological deficit score. Data are reported as the means ± SEM. $n = 4$ for TTC staining and $n = 8$ for the neurological deficit score. $^*p < 0.05$ versus the IR group.

evaluated by TTC staining and Hara's scores, respectively. The rats in the Sham group showed no neurological deficits and cerebral infarct areas. XXMD (60 g/kg/day) and CsA (10 mg/kg/day) treatment significantly reduced infarct areas in the territory of the middle cerebral artery compared to the IR group ($p < 0.05$). The rats subjected to ischemia and reperfusion showed severe neurological deficits; however, XXMD or CsA treatment significantly reduced neurological deficit scores compared with the IR group ($p < 0.05$) (Figure 1).

3.2. XXMD Alleviated Cell Injury. Cell injury was estimated by HE staining and Nissl staining. The images of HE staining showed that the cells with the abundant cytoplasm and clear nuclei were arranged orderly in the Sham group. After 90 min of ischemia and 24 h of reperfusion, most neurons in the ischemic penumbra of the cerebral cortex appeared shrunken and deep stained in the IR group. In contrast to the IR group, residual neuron structures were improved with visible membranes and nuclei and more intact neurons in the XXMD60 and CsA groups. The characteristics of ischemic injury in the Vehicle group were similar to those in the IR group. Nissl staining found that most cells were shrunk with an enlarged intercellular space and had deep color staining in the IR and Vehicle group. However, these characteristic changes were improved by XXMD and CsA treatment. Furthermore, there were more intact cells in the penumbra of the ischemic cortex in the XXMD-treated or CsA-treated rats compared to the IR group ($p < 0.05$) (Figure 2).

3.3. XXMD Reduced the Formation of Mitophagy in the Ischemic Cortex Penumbra. The characteristics of neuronal mitophagy in the ischemic penumbra were observed by electron microscopy. Healthy mitochondria and nuclei were observed in the Sham group (Figure 3(a)). After 24 h of reperfusion, neurons displayed mitochondrial swelling, loss of matrix density, and the formation of vacuoles. Some partially degraded mitochondria and numerous autophagic vacuoles were detected in the IR group and Vehicle group (Figures 3(b) and 3(e)). A higher magnification showed double-membraned autophagosomes containing damaged mitochondria (Figures 3(g), 3(i), and 3(j)). In contrast, mitochondria with some slight swelling and nearly normal matrix density were detected in the XXMD-treated group and CsA group (Figures 3(c) and 3(d)). Autophagosomes were frequently observed and were more abundant than in the IR and Vehicle groups. Typical autolysosomes were observed in neurons in the CsA group (Figure 3(h)).

3.4. XXMD Improved Mitochondrial Function. Levels of ATP and MDA were determined to assess mitochondrial function after 24 h of reperfusion. MDA levels in the IR and Vehicle

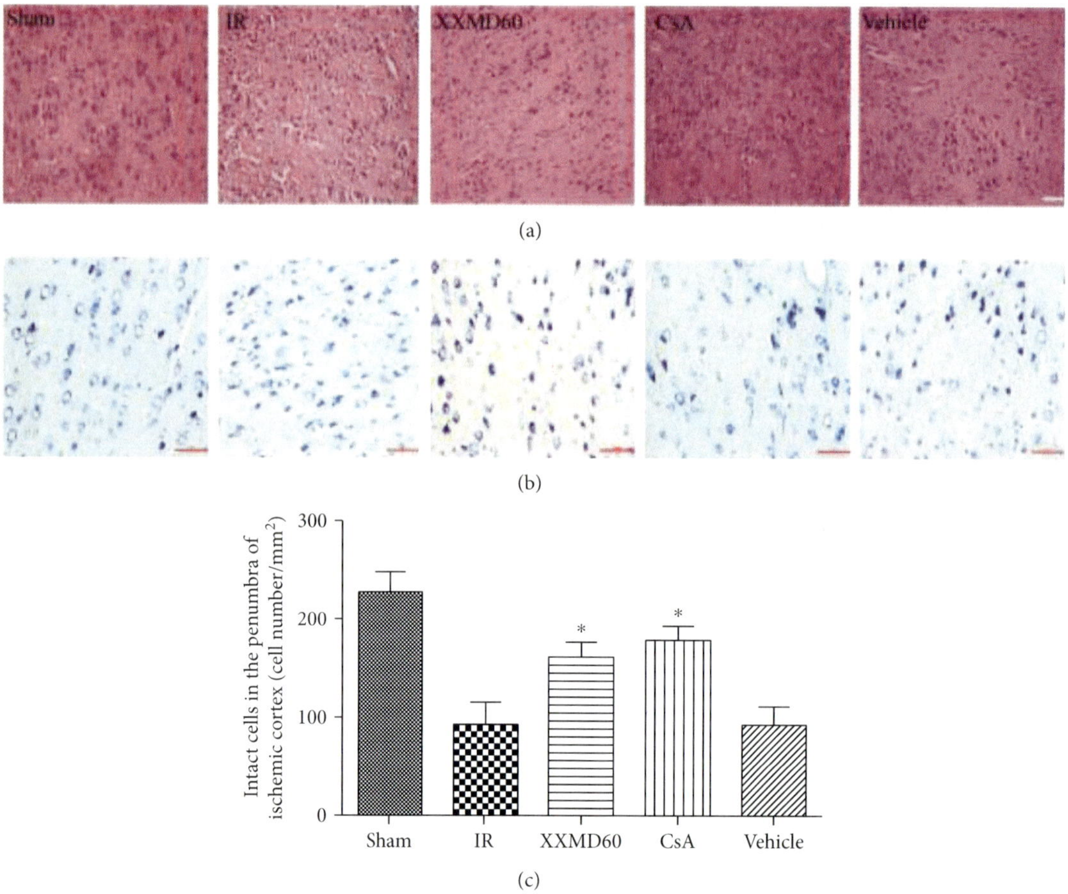

FIGURE 2: Histological changes of the penumbra of the ischemic cortex by groups. (a) HE images of cortical sections in different groups. (b) Representative images of Nissl staining in different groups. (c) Analysis of intact cells in the penumbra of the ischemic cortex. The number of intact cells in the XXMD60 group and CsA group was significantly higher than that in the IR group. Data are reported as the means ± SEM. $n = 5$; $^*p < 0.05$ versus the IR group. Scale bar = 50 μm.

groups were significantly increased compared with those in the sham rats ($p < 0.05$), while treatment with 60 g/kg/day XXMD or 10 mg/kg/day CsA dramatically suppressed the production of MDA in the rats subjected to cerebral ischemia compared with that in the IR group ($p < 0.05$). In addition, we found the significant decrease in the ATP level after cerebral ischemia and reperfusion ($p < 0.05$), and XXMD or CsA treatment notably prevented the decrease in ATP levels compared with the IR group ($p < 0.05$) (Figure 4).

3.5. XXMD Downregulated Mitophagy in the Penumbra of the Ischemic Cortex. Immunofluorescent staining of microtubule-associated protein 1 light chain 3B (LC3B, autophagic marker) and voltage-dependent anion-selective channel 1 (VDAC1, mitochondrial marker) was used to determine mitophagy. The nuclei were stained by 4′,6-diamidino-2-phenylindole (DAPI). The immunoreactive products for LC3B were distributed in the cytoplasm. In sham-operated animals, cortical cells displayed diffuse and weak staining for LC3B in the cytoplasm. The morphology of positive cells with the shrunken cytoplasm was changed following cerebral ischemia and reperfusion in the IR and Vehicle groups. After being irritated by this stimulus, intense LC3B staining was mainly observed in the ischemic penumbra and appeared granular in the cytoplasm. LC3B (red) that colocalized with VDAC1 (green) in the cytoplasm showed that increased mitophagy (yellow) occurred in cortical neurons, suggesting that ischemia and reperfusion significantly promoted mitophagy ($p < 0.05$). Immunointensity of mitophagy was reduced in samples from the XXMD-treated or CsA-treated groups, and the inhibitory effect of CsA treatment on mitophagy was more obvious ($p < 0.05$) (Figure 5).

3.6. XXMD Reduced Autolysosome Formation in the Penumbra of the Ischemic Cortex. Autophagosomes fused with lysosomes and formed autolysosomes to degrade proteins and organelles and then complete the course of autophagy. Immunofluorescent staining of LC3B (autophagic marker) and lysosomal-associated membrane protein 1 (Lamp1, lysosome marker) was used to determine autolysosome formation in different groups. The positive cells labeled with Lamp1 were notably increased in the rats subjected to MCAO compared with the rats in the Sham group ($p < 0.05$). LC3B (red) that colocalized with Lamp1 (green) in the cytoplasm showed autophagy lysosomes, and the images suggested that ischemia and reperfusion activated the

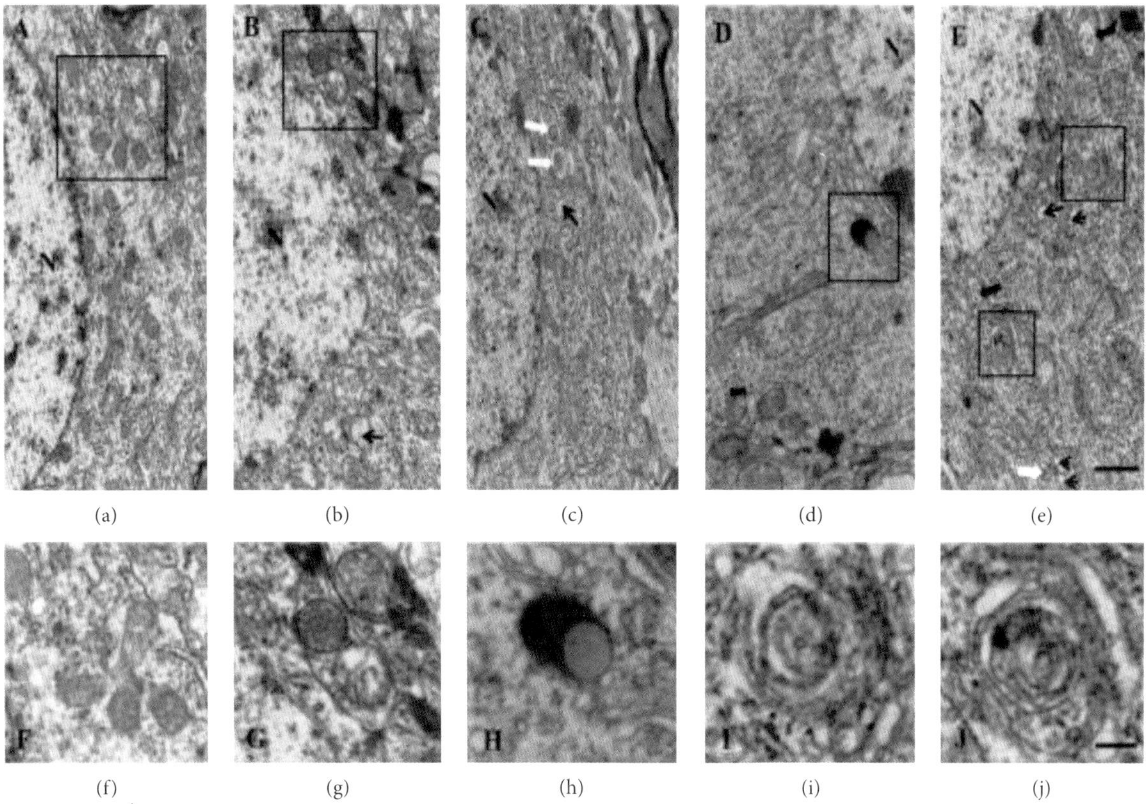

FIGURE 3: Representative electron microphotographs of neuronal mitophagy in the ischemic penumbra of the cerebral cortex at 24 h after the reperfusion. (a) The Sham group with normal mitochondrial ultrastructures. (f) Enlargement of the boxed area in (a). (b) Typical mitophagy structure and swollen mitochondria were revealed in the IR group. (c) Autophagy structure (white arrow) and autophagic vacuoles (small black arrow) were also shown in the XXMD60 group. (d) Autolysosomes were observed in neurons in the CsA group. High magnifications revealed autolysosome (h). (e) The characteristics of autophagy structure (white arrow), autophagic vacuoles (small black arrow), and swollen mitochondria (big black arrow) were observed in the Vehicle group. High magnifications revealed typical mitophagy structure (i and j). N: nuclear, $n = 3$, scale bar = 1 μm (a–e), scale bar = 0.5 μm (f–j).

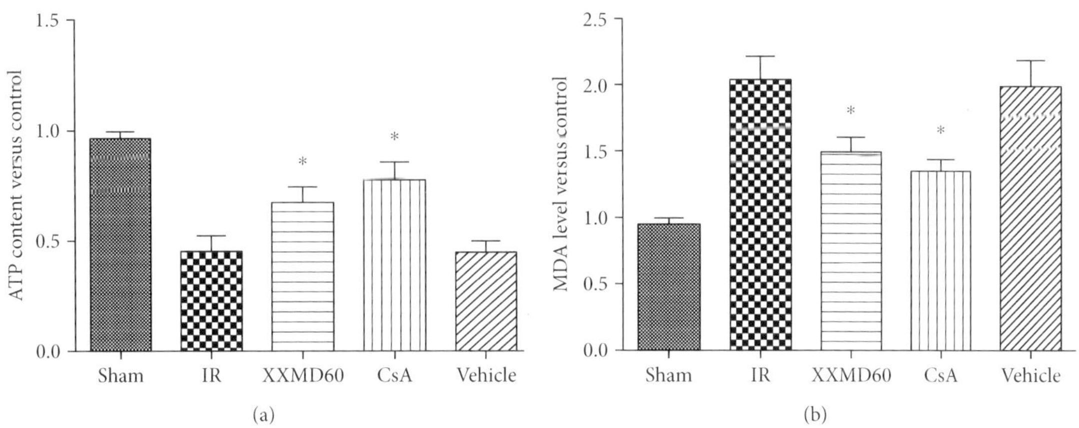

FIGURE 4: XXMD improved mitochondrial function at 24 h after reperfusion. (a) ATP content of different groups. (b) MDA levels of different groups. Data are reported as the means ± SEM. $n = 5$, $^*p < 0.05$ versus the IR group.

significant increases in autophagy lysosome formation ($p < 0.05$). However, the increase was sharply suppressed in samples from the XXMD-treated or CsA-treated groups ($p < 0.05$). Additionally, the greatest lower effect on autophagy lysosome formation was exerted by CsA ($p < 0.05$) (Figure 6).

3.7. XXMD Regulated Mitophagy-Related Protein Expression and p62 Translocation to the Mitochondria. To investigate the effects of XXMD on mitophagy and the activity of the lysosomal pathway, we detected expression of mitophagy-related proteins including LC3B, Beclin1, and Lamp1 in the ischemic cortex 24 h after reperfusion by Western blot and

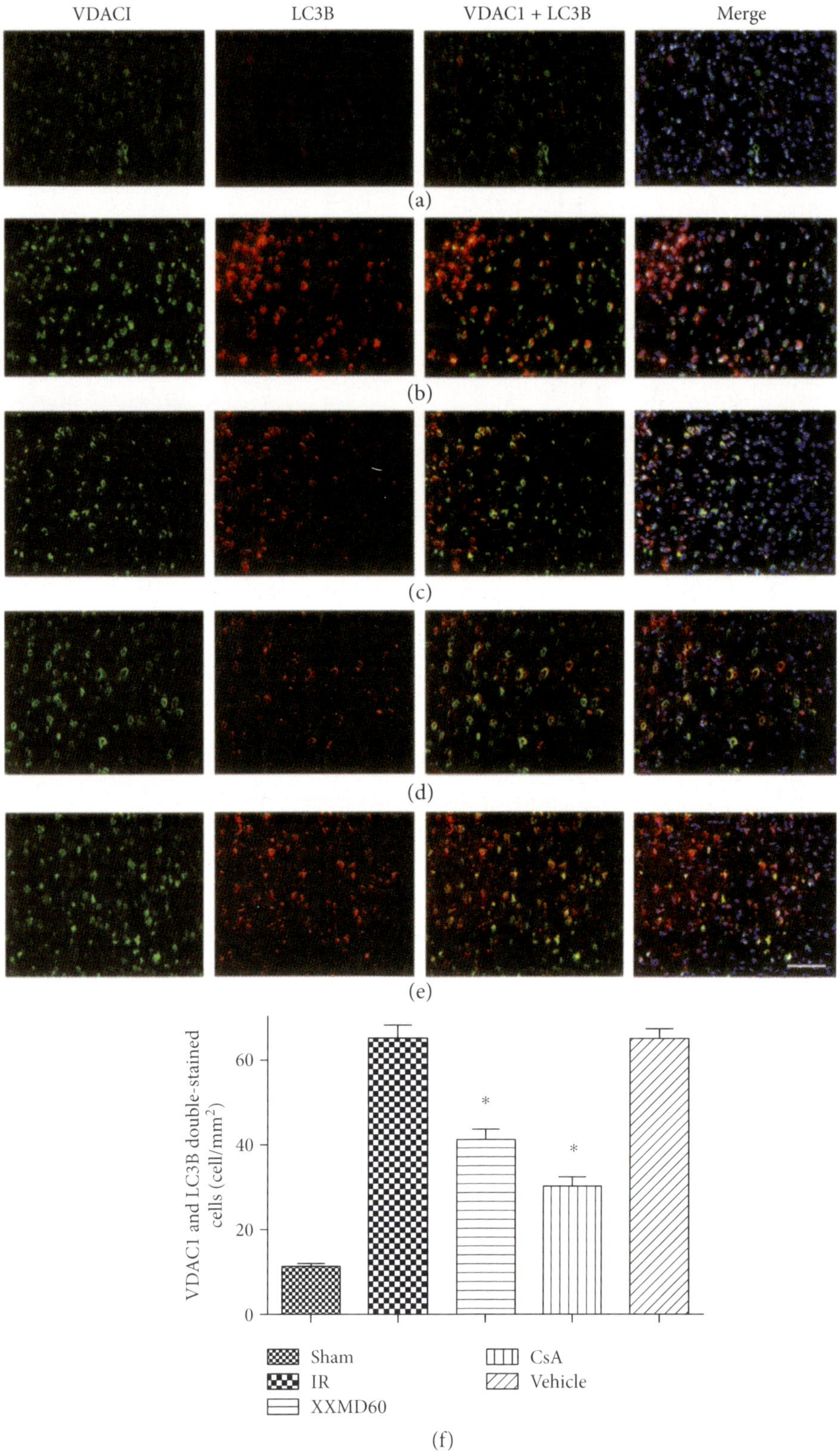

FIGURE 5: Double immunofluorescence staining for VDAC1 and LC3B in the penumbra of the ischemic cortex at 24 h after reperfusion. VDAC1 and LC3B double-stained cells (yellow) indicated mitophagy. (a) Representative microphotographs of rats in the Sham group. (b) Representative microphotographs of rats in the IR group. (c) Representative microphotographs of rats in the XXMD60 group. (d) Representative microphotographs of rats in the CsA group. (e) Representative microphotographs of rats in the Vehicle group. The images indicated that LC3B-positive cells were significantly detected in the peri-infarct area. Overlapping images showed that LC3B partly colocalized with VDAC1. (f) Quantification of VDAC1 and LC3B double-stained cells. $n = 4$, scale bar = 50 μm. $^{*}p < 0.05$ versus the IR group.

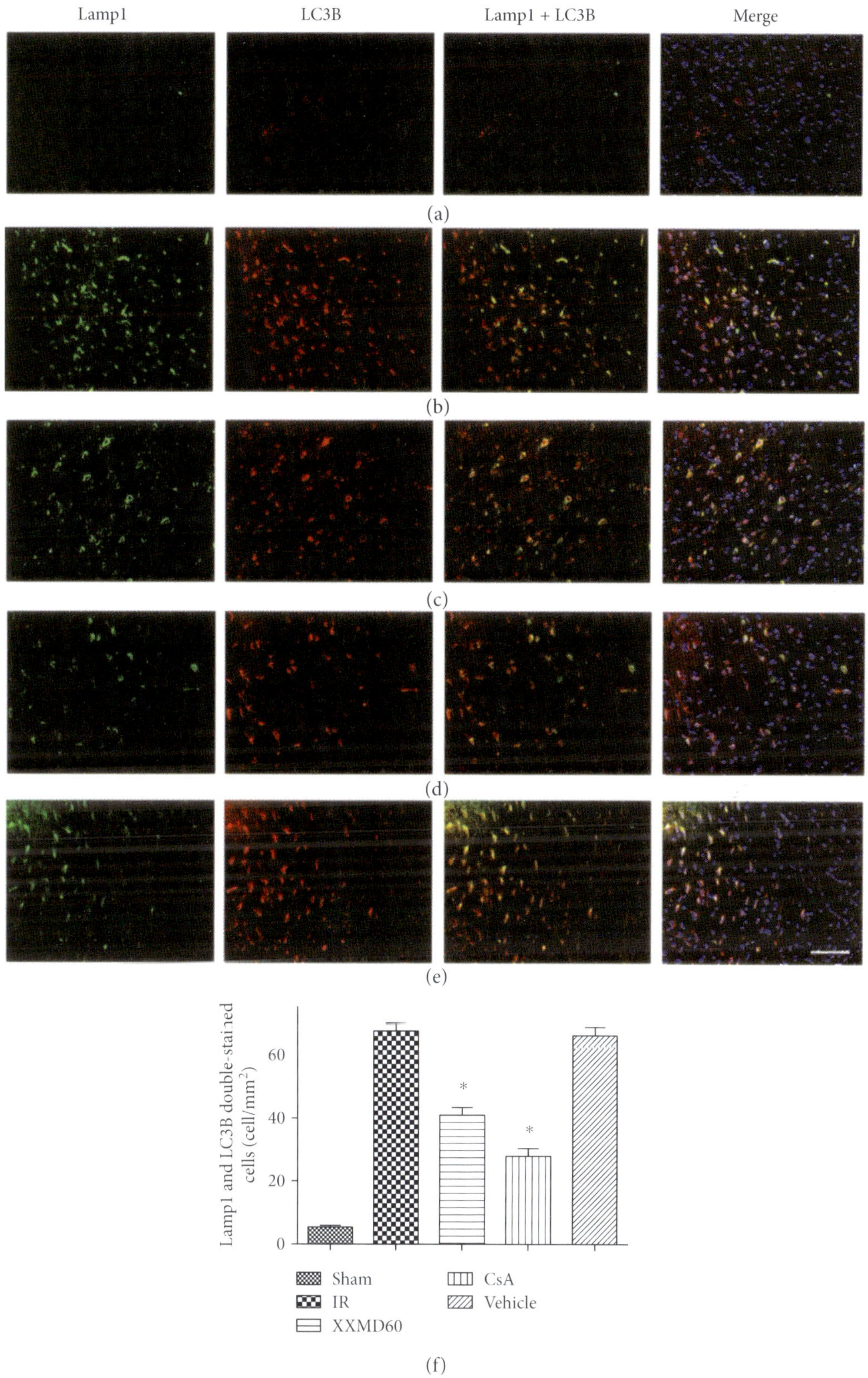

FIGURE 6: Double immunofluorescence staining for LC3B and Lamp1 of different groups in the penumbra of the ischemic cortex at 24 h after reperfusion. LC3B (red) immunostaining that colocalized in Lamp1-positive cells (green) indicating autophagic lysosomes. (a) Representative microphotographs of rats in the Sham group. (b) Representative microphotographs of rats in the IR group. (c) Representative microphotographs of rats in the XXMD60 group. (d) Representative microphotographs of rats in the CsA group. (e) Representative microphotographs of rats in the Vehicle group. (f) Quantification of Lamp1 and LC3B double-stained cells. $n = 4$, scale bar = 50 μm. $^*p < 0.05$ versus the IR group.

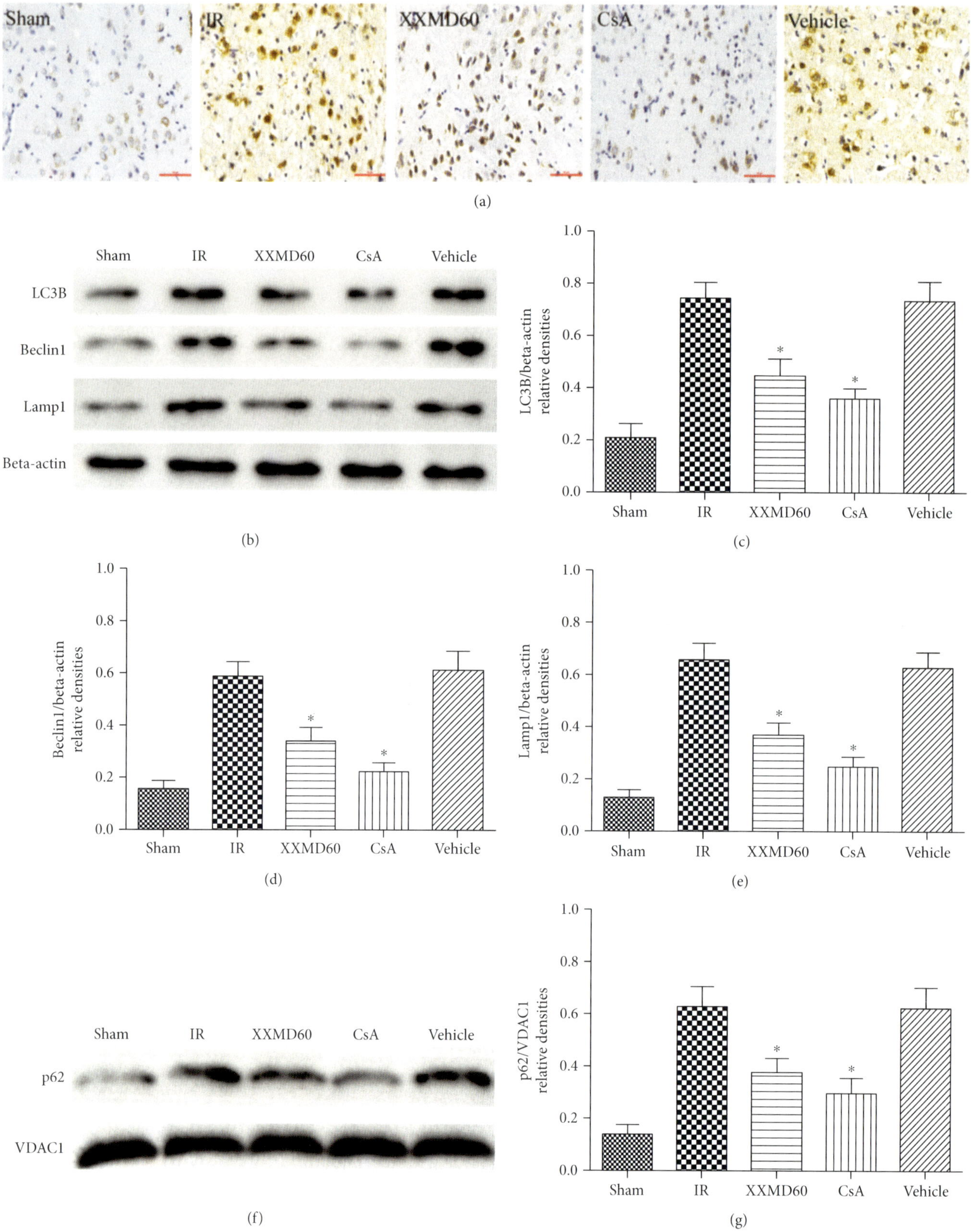

FIGURE 7: Beclin1 immunohistochemistry and expression levels of LC3, Beclin1, Lamp1, and mitochondrial p62 at 24 h after reperfusion following 90 min of cerebral ischemia. (a) Representative microphotographs of immunohistochemistry for Beclin1. (b) Western blots of LC3, Beclin1, and Lamp1. Beta-actin bands were the internal control. (c) Quantitative evaluation of LC3B. (d) Quantitative evaluation of Beclin1. (e) Quantitative evaluation of Lamp1. (f) Western blot of p62 in the mitochondrial fraction. VDAC1 bands were the internal control. (g) Quantitative evaluation of mitochondrial p62. Data are reported as the means ± SEM. $n = 4$, $^{*}p < 0.05$ versus the IR group.

immunohistochemistry. The results of Western blots were consistent with immunohistochemistry staining for Beclin1 and immunofluorescence staining for LC3B and Lamp1. The findings showed that cerebral ischemia and reperfusion resulted in a significant increase in LC3B, Beclin1, and Lamp1 expression compared with the Sham group ($p < 0.05$). Treatment with XXMD or CsA markedly downregulated LC3B, Beclin1, and Lamp1 expression after 90 min of ischemia and 24 h of reperfusion compared with the IR group ($p < 0.05$). p62 can bind to ubiquitinated mitochondria to direct phagophores through a LC3-binding domain [14, 31, 32]. We further examined p62 expression levels in mitochondrial fractions by Western blot. As shown in Figures 7(f) and 7(g), a significant increase in p62 expression was detected in the mitochondrial fractions after ischemia and reperfusion in contrast to the rats in the Sham group ($p < 0.05$). These results also showed that XXMD/CsA treatment reduced p62 translocation to mitochondria, demonstrating that XXMD/CsA significantly decreased mitophagy ($p < 0.05$) (Figure 7).

4. Discussion

In present study, the rats treated with XXMD/CsA showed markedly decreased brain damage at 24 h after reperfusion following 90 min of cerebral ischemia. XXMD treatment significantly suppressed mitophagy activation, and reduced mitophagy may play a vital role in brain injury following ischemia and reperfusion.

Cerebral ischemia and reperfusion injury is a complex pathological process. Necrosis, apoptosis, and autophagic cell death, as three different types of cell death, are considered to involve in neural tissue damage [33]. Plenty of evidence has indicated that mitophagy, characterized by abnormal mitochondria within autophagosomes or fused with autophagic vesicles in the ischemic penumbra area, is activated [14, 34]. Insufficient or excessive mitophagy can result in cellular death, caused by damaged mitochondrial accumulation or removal of indispensable mitochondria, respectively [17, 35]. Our previous findings have demonstrated that XXMD could protect mitochondria from ischemic injury and inhibit apoptosis through the mitochondrial p53 pathway [21]. However, whether XXMD involves in modulating mitophagy in brain injury was unknown. In this study, we further explored mitophagy induced by cerebral ischemia and reperfusion and the effects of XXMD treatment on mitophagy and mitochondrial function after cerebral ischemia and reperfusion. Electron microscopy showed that swollen or vacuolated mitochondria with fragmented cristae and activated mitophagy appeared following ischemia and reperfusion. Nevertheless, mitochondrial damage was alleviated indicating relative integrity of cristae structure, and a few structures of autophagy and mitophagy appeared in the XXMD- or CsA-treated group. Mitochondria are those essential organelles for generation and action of reactive oxygen species (ROS) in brain cells [36]. Damaged mitochondria following ischemia and reperfusion could result in the increase in ROS, and meanwhile, mitochondrial ATP levels are considered an indicator of cell death [14]. The present results demonstrated that treatment with 60 g/kg/day XXMD or 10 mg/kg CsA dramatically prevented the decrease in ATP content and reduced MDA levels, suggesting that inhibition in ROS production and protection of mitochondrial function may also have a role in protective effects of XXMD.

LC3B, the most widely used marker for revealing the presence of autophagosomes during autophagy activation, is attached to the autophagosome membrane, suggesting that the amount of LC3B closely correlates with the number of autophagosome [36, 37]. The results showed that increased LC3B immunoreactivity was mainly located in the cytoplasm of cells in the penumbra of the ischemic cortex and XXMD treatment downregulated LC3B expression. VDAC1, the abundant mitochondrial outer membrane protein, forms a cylindrical channel [38]. Moreover, we detected mitophagy using double immunofluorescence labeling with anti-LC3B and VDAC1 antibodies. LC3B colocalized with VDAC1 in the cytoplasm, suggesting that ischemia and reperfusion promoted significantly mitophagy. There is a significant decrease in LC3B/VDAC1 colabeling in the ipsilateral hemisphere in XXMD-treated and CsA-treated groups. Beclin1, a component of the class 3 phosphoinositide 3-kinase (PI3K) complex, is required for autophagy and LC3, and Beclin1 is involved in the early stages of autophagosome formation [33, 36]. The data showed that LC3B and Beclin1 expression was increased after 24 h of reperfusion, whereas XXMD or CsA treatment robustly prevented ischemia-reperfusion-induced upregulation of LC3B and Beclin1 expression. Additionally, marked upregulation of the lysosomal marker Lamp1 further supported the notion that mitophagic/lysosomal pathway was activated in cerebral ischemia and reperfusion. XXMD or CsA treatment downregulated Lamp1 expression. In addition, p62, a sensitive marker for mitophagy, recruits phagophores through an LC3-binding domain to degrade the damaged mitochondria [31, 32]. We further demonstrated that XXMD downregulated p62 translocation to mitochondria in response to ischemia-reperfusion injury. Based on the above findings, we hypothesized that XXMD modulated selective mitochondrial autophagy formation in the penumbra of the ischemic cortex following ischemia and reperfusion in the rat brain.

The evidence presented in this study indicated that XXMD treatment may exert protective effects on cerebral ischemia-reperfusion injury partly by the regulating mitophagy. This may shed lights on a novel mechanism of XXMD treatment against focal cerebral ischemia and reperfusion injury.

5. Conclusion

In conclusion, the present study demonstrated that mitophagy was increased in the penumbra of the ischemic cortex after cerebral ischemia and reperfusion. Additionally, XXMD/CsA downregulated LC3B, Beclin1, and Lamp1 expression and reduced p62 translocation to mitochondria, which may be related to attenuated mitochondrial dysfunction and suppressed mitophagy after stroke.

Authors' Contributions

Rui Lan and Yong Zhang contributed equally to this work.

Acknowledgments

This work was supported by the National Natural Science Foundation of China (Grant no. 81503422).

References

[1] P. S. Vosler, S. H. Graham, L. R. Wechsler, and J. Chen, "Mitochondrial targets for stroke: focusing basic science research toward development of clinically translatable therapeutics," *Stroke*, vol. 40, no. 9, pp. 3149–3155, 2009.

[2] A. Kuma, M. Hatano, M. Matsui et al., "The role of autophagy during the early neonatal starvation period," *Nature*, vol. 432, no. 7020, pp. 1032–1036, 2004.

[3] W. Balduini, S. Carloni, and G. Buonocore, "Autophagy in hypoxia-ischemia induced brain injury: evidences and speculations," *Autophagy*, vol. 5, no. 2, pp. 221–223, 2009.

[4] T. Yorimitsu, U. Nair, Z. Yang, and D. J. Klionsky, "Endoplasmic reticulum stress triggers autophagy," *Journal of Biological Chemistry*, vol. 281, no. 40, pp. 30299–30304, 2006.

[5] X. Zhang, H. Yan, Y. Yuan et al., "Cerebral ischemia-reperfusion-induced autophagy protects against neuronal injury by mitochondrial clearance," *Autophagy*, vol. 9, no. 9, pp. 1321–1333, 2013.

[6] Y. D. Wen, R. Sheng, L. S. Zhang et al., "Neuronal injury in rat model of permanent focal cerebral ischemia is associated with activation of autophagic and lysosomal pathways," *Autophagy*, vol. 4, no. 6, pp. 762–769, 2008.

[7] R. Sheng, L. S. Zhang, R. Han, X. Q. Liu, B. Gao, and Z. H. Qin, "Autophagy activation is associated with neuroprotection in a rat model of focal cerebral ischemic preconditioning," *Autophagy*, vol. 6, no. 4, pp. 482–494, 2010.

[8] M. Koike, M. Shibata, M. Tadakoshi et al., "Inhibition of autophagy prevents hippocampal pyramidal neuron death after hypoxic-ischemic injury," *The American Journal of Pathology*, vol. 172, no. 2, pp. 454–469, 2008.

[9] S. Carloni, S. Girelli, C. Scopa, G. Buonocore, M. Longini, and W. Balduini, "Activation of autophagy and Akt/CREB signaling play an equivalent role in the neuroprotective effect of rapamycin in neonatal hypoxia-ischemia," *Autophagy*, vol. 6, no. 3, pp. 366–377, 2010.

[10] Y. C. Tang, H. X. Tian, T. Yi, and H. B. Chen, "The critical roles of mitophagy in cerebral ischemia," *Protein & Cell*, vol. 7, no. 10, pp. 699–713, 2016.

[11] D. Yu, M. Li, B. Ni, J. Kong, and Z. Zhang, "Induction of neuronal mitophagy in acute spinal cord injury in rats," *Neurotoxicity Research*, vol. 24, no. 4, pp. 512–522, 2013.

[12] Y. Yuan, X. Zhang, Y. Zheng, and Z. Chen, "Regulation of mitophagy in ischemic brain injury," *Neuroscience Bulletin*, vol. 31, no. 4, pp. 395–406, 2015.

[13] E. Motori, J. Puyal, N. Toni et al., "Inflammation-induced alteration of astrocyte mitochondrial dynamics requires autophagy for mitochondrial network maintenance," *Cell Metabolism*, vol. 18, no. 6, pp. 844–859, 2013.

[14] Q. Li, T. Zhang, J. Wang et al., "Rapamycin attenuates mitochondrial dysfunction via activation of mitophagy in experimental ischemic stroke," *Biochemical and Biophysical Research Communications*, vol. 444, no. 2, pp. 182–188, 2014.

[15] W. Zuo, S. Zhang, C. Y. Xia, X. F. Guo, W. B. He, and N. H. Chen, "Mitochondria autophagy is induced after hypoxic/ischemic stress in a Drp1 dependent manner: the role of inhibition of Drp1 in ischemic brain damage," *Neuropharmacology*, vol. 86, pp. 103–115, 2014.

[16] S. H. Baek, A. R. Noh, K. A. Kim et al., "Modulation of mitochondrial function and autophagy mediates carnosine neuroprotection against ischemic brain damage," *Stroke*, vol. 45, no. 8, pp. 2438–2443, 2014.

[17] R. Y. Shi, S. H. Zhu, V. Li, S. B. Gibson, X. S. Xu, and J. M. Kong, "BNIP3 interacting with LC3 triggers excessive mitophagy in delayed neuronal death in stroke," *CNS Neuroscience & Therapeutics*, vol. 20, no. 12, pp. 1045–1055, 2014.

[18] D. L. Fu, L. Lu, W. Zhu et al., "Xiaoxuming decoction for acute ischemic stroke: a systematic review and meta-analysis," *Journal of Ethnopharmacology*, vol. 148, no. 1, pp. 1–13, 2013.

[19] R. Lan, J. Xiang, G. H. Wang et al., "*Xiao-Xu-Ming* decoction protects against blood-brain barrier disruption and neurological injury induced by cerebral ischemia and reperfusion in rats," *Evidence-Based Complementary and Alternative Medicine*, vol. 2013, Article ID 629782, 12 pages, 2013.

[20] R. Lan, J. Xiang, Y. Zhang et al., "PI3K/Akt pathway contributes to neurovascular unit protection of *Xiao-Xu-Ming* decoction against focal cerebral ischemia and reperfusion injury in rats," *Evidence-Based Complementary and Alternative Medicine*, vol. 2013, Article ID 459467, 16 pages, 2013.

[21] R. Lan, Y. Zhang, J. Xiang et al., "Xiao-Xu-Ming decoction preserves mitochondrial integrity and reduces apoptosis after focal cerebral ischemia and reperfusion via the mitochondrial p53 pathway," *Journal of Ethnopharmacology*, vol. 151, no. 1, pp. 307–316, 2014.

[22] Y. Shiga, H. Onodera, Y. Matsuo, and K. Kogure, "Cyclosporin A protects against ischemia-reperfusion injury in the brain," *Brain Research*, vol. 595, no. 1, pp. 145–148, 1992.

[23] H. Uchino, E. Elmer, K. Uchino et al., "Amelioration by cyclosporin A of brain damage in transient forebrain ischemia in the rat," *Brain Research*, vol. 812, no. 1-2, pp. 216–226, 1998.

[24] A. P. Halestrap, C. P. Connern, E. J. Griffiths, and P. M. Kerr, "Cyclosporin A binding to mitochondrial cyclophilin inhibits the permeability transition pore and protects hearts from ischaemia/reperfusion injury," *Molecular and Cellular Biochemistry*, vol. 174, no. 1/2, pp. 167–172, 1997.

[25] X. Wei, Y. Qi, X. Zhang et al., "Cadmium induces mitophagy through ROS-mediated PINK1/Parkin pathway," *Toxicology Mechanisms and Methods*, vol. 24, no. 7, pp. 504–511, 2014.

[26] I. Kim, S. Rodriguez-Enriquez, and J. J. Lemasters, "Selective degradation of mitochondria by mitophagy," *Archives of Biochemistry and Biophysics*, vol. 462, no. 2, pp. 245–253, 2007.

[27] S. Rodriguez-Enriquez, I. Kim, R. T. Currin, and J. J. Lemasters, "Tracker dyes to probe mitochondrial autophagy (mitophagy) in rat hepatocytes," *Autophagy*, vol. 2, no. 1, pp. 39–46, 2006.

[28] K. Domanska-Janik, L. Buzanska, J. Dluzniewska, H. Kozlowska, A. Sarnowska, and B. Zablocka, "Neuroprotection by cyclosporin A following transient brain ischemia corre-

lates with the inhibition of the early efflux of cytochrome *C* to cytoplasm," *Brain Research Molecular Brain Research*, vol. 121, no. 1-2, pp. 50–59, 2004.

[29] T. Yoshimoto and B. K. Siesjö, "Posttreatment with the immunosuppressant cyclosporin A in transient focal ischemia," *Brain Research*, vol. 839, no. 2, pp. 283–291, 1999.

[30] H. Hara, P. L. Huang, N. Panahian, M. C. Fishman, and M. A. Moskowitz, "Reduced brain edema and infarction volume in mice lacking the neuronal isoform of nitric oxide synthase after transient MCA occlusion," *Journal of Cerebral Blood Flow & Metabolism*, vol. 16, no. 4, pp. 605–611, 1996.

[31] G. Bjorkoy, T. Lamark, A. Brech et al., "p62/SQSTM1 forms protein aggregates degraded by autophagy and has a protective effect on huntingtin-induced cell death," *Journal of Cell Biology*, vol. 171, no. 4, pp. 603–614, 2005.

[32] S. Pankiv, T. H. Clausen, T. Lamark et al., "p62/SQSTM1 binds directly to Atg8/LC3 to facilitate degradation of ubiquitinated protein aggregates by autophagy," *Journal of Biological Chemistry*, vol. 282, no. 33, pp. 24131–24145, 2007.

[33] A. Rami, A. Langhagen, and S. Steiger, "Focal cerebral ischemia induces upregulation of Beclin 1 and autophagy-like cell death," *Neurobiology of Disease*, vol. 29, no. 1, pp. 132–141, 2008.

[34] T. G. Demarest, E. L. Waite, T. Kristian et al., "Sex-dependent mitophagy and neuronal death following rat neonatal hypoxia–ischemia," *Neuroscience*, vol. 335, pp. 103–113, 2016.

[35] A. Ordureau and J. W. Harper, "Cell biology: balancing act," *Nature*, vol. 510, no. 7505, pp. 347-348, 2014.

[36] K. Liu, Y. Sun, Z. Gu, N. Shi, T. Zhang, and X. Sun, "Mitophagy in ischaemia/reperfusion induced cerebral injury," *Neurochemical Research*, vol. 38, no. 7, pp. 1295–1300, 2013.

[37] F. Tian, K. Deguchi, T. Yamashita et al., "In vivo imaging of autophagy in a mouse stroke model," *Autophagy*, vol. 6, no. 8, pp. 1107–1114, 2010.

[38] S. Geisler, K. M. Holmstrom, D. Skujat et al., "PINK1/Parkin-mediated mitophagy is dependent on VDAC1 and p62/SQSTM1," *Nature Cell Biology*, vol. 12, no. 2, pp. 119–131, 2010.

11

Pediatric Multiple Sclerosis and Cognition: A Review of Clinical, Neuropsychologic, and Neuroradiologic Features

Ozgul Ekmekci

Department of Neurology, Faculty of Medicine, Ege University, Izmir, Turkey

Correspondence should be addressed to Ozgul Ekmekci; ozgul.ekmekci@ege.edu.tr

Academic Editor: Lambros Messinis

Multiple sclerosis (MS) is an inflammatory demyelinating and neurodegenerative disease. Although cognitive impairment has been well established in adult patients with MS, its occurrence in patients with pediatric-onset MS has recently been reported. In this review, I discuss the main features of cognitive impairment in pediatric MS as determined by long-term follow-up studies, neuropsychiatric test batteries, and the results of neuroradiological imaging studies that investigated the pathogenesis of pediatric MS. The most commonly affected cognitive domains in adults are attention, processing speed, and visuomotor skills; language and intelligence are also affected in pediatric MS. A young age at disease onset is the strongest risk factor for these impairments, which may be due to the effect of inflammatory demyelination and neurodegeneration on the developing central nervous system and neural networks in children. Cognitive impairment has long-term effects on patients' academic life and the quality of their social life. Therefore, all patients with pediatric MS should be screened and monitored for cognitive impairment. This review also highlights the need for neuropsychological test batteries that assess different cognitive domains in children and adolescents with multiple sclerosis and for cognitive rehabilitation programs to improve the quality of their academic and social life.

1. Introduction

Multiple sclerosis (MS) is an autoimmune-mediated neurodegenerative and demyelinating disorder of the central nervous system primarily affecting young adults. Approximately 2–5% of MS patients have onset before age 18 [1, 2]. The International Pediatric Multiple Sclerosis Study Group defined diagnostic criteria for pediatric MS [3]. MS can cause both physical and cognitive disability. The occurrence of cognitive impairment is well established in adult patients with MS, occurring in approximately 45–65% of these patients [4]. The cognitive domains that are most commonly affected in adult MS patients are complex attention, information processing speed, episodic memory, visuospatial abilities, and executive functions [5]. Cognitive impairment in pediatric MS patients has been described with different studies reporting cognitive impairment in 30–50% of cases [5–8]. Cognitive impairment in pediatric multiple sclerosis differs from that in adults in terms of the cognitive domains involved. Factors such as age, maturation of the central nervous system, and cognitive reserve have different effects on cognition in childhood. The maturation status of the central nervous system at the time of MS onset is a long-term prognostic factor, and it is crucial to develop appropriate neuropsychological test batteries that assess different cognitive domains in children and adolescents with MS. Moreover, cognitive rehabilitation to improve the quality of academic and social life in pediatric MS patients has not yet been well studied. In this review, I discuss the main features of cognitive impairment in pediatric MS, long-term follow-up findings, neuropsychiatric test batteries, and the result of neuroradiological imaging studies that investigated the pathogenesis of pediatric MS.

2. The Main Features of Cognitive Impairment in Pediatric MS Patients

Banwell and Anderson were the first to use a neuropsychological battery to systematically investigate a cohort of patients with pediatric MS. They assessed cognitive functions in 10 children with MS and identified deficits in general cognition, language, visuomotor integration, and verbal and visual memory. Children with longer disease duration demonstrated deficits in executive functions, information processing speed, and working memory, suggesting that children with longer disease duration and a younger age at onset are at higher risk for cognitive impairment [6].

MacAllister et al. evaluated 37 children and adolescents with MS and reported significant cognitive impairment in 35% of these patients. The most common impairment was in complex attention. They also found receptive language problems and poor naming in many patients, whereas verbal fluency was unaffected. Immediate verbal memory was impaired in only one patient; however, delayed recall was impaired in seven patients. The researchers suggested that, in these patients, the effect of MS on attention and memory was similar to that in adults with MS, but visuospatial functions were less affected. They found a strong relationship between cognitive impairment and Expanded Disability Status Scale (EDSS) score, total number of relapses, and disease duration [7].

In a multicenter study, Amato and colleagues assessed the frequency, pattern, and clinical correlates of cognitive impairment in childhood and adolescent MS cases and compared these characteristics with those in healthy controls. The researchers used a neuropsychological battery to assess intelligence quotient (IQ), memory, attention/concentration, executive functions, and language. They found significant cognitive impairment in 31% of the patients with MS, and 53% of the cases failed at least two tests. Both verbal and performance IQ scores were lower in MS patients than in healthy controls. The most frequently affected cognitive domains were memory, particularly visuospatial memory, complex attention, verbal comprehension, and executive functions. In this study, EDSS and number of relapses were not adequate descriptors of cognitive condition; cognitive impairments were found also in patients with low disability levels. In this cohort, there was a significant correlation between cognitive impairment and low IQ scores. Low IQ score was also significantly associated with younger age at disease onset [8].

In a study of the magnetic resonance imaging (MRI) correlates of cognitive impairment in pediatric MS patients, Till et al. found impairments in attention and processing speed, visuomotor integration, and expressive language. They observed cognitive impairment in 29.4% of the MS patients. Full-scale IQ and verbal IQ were significantly reduced in children with MS and a higher IQ was associated with a shorter disease duration and an older age at disease onset. Moreover, a higher full-scale IQ was correlated with a lower EDSS score, and patients with cognitive impairment tended to be male. Finally, cognitive impairment was associated with a longer disease duration and a younger age at onset [9].

In a large multicenter study, Julian et al. examined cognitive function in 231 pediatric patients with MS ($n = 187$) or clinically isolated syndrome ($n = 44$). The cognitive impairment was noted in 35% of patients with MS and 18% of patients with clinically isolated syndrome. The cognitive areas that were most frequently affected were fine motor coordination (54%), visuomotor integration (50%), and information processing speed (35%). EDSS score was the only variable that was significantly and independently associated with reduced cognitive function [10].

The methods and results of these cross-sectional studies are shown in Table 1. Although these studies used different neuropsychological tests and different definitions of cognitive impairment, they found similar rates of cognitive impairment. The rate of cognitive impairment in pediatric MS ranged from 29.4% to 35%. Full-scale IQ and verbal and performance IQ were lower in children with MS. Low IQ scores were associated with higher EDSS score and young age at disease onset [8, 9]. The relationship of cognitive impairment with young age at onset and disease duration was similar in many studies [6–9]. However, the relationship between EDSS score and cognitive impairment varied between these studies. For example, Julian et al. and Banwell and Anderson found that EDSS score was associated with cognitive impairment but other studies did not [6, 10]. These studies suggested that cognitive impairment affected academic and social activities negatively and impaired the quality of life [6–8].

In summary, similar to adult patients, pediatric MS patients experience deficits in attention, information processing speed, memory, executive functions, and visuomotor integration. Additionally, unlike in adults, MS affects language functions and intelligence occurs in particularly young children. The relationship between cognitive dysfunction and disease duration, disability scores, and relapse frequency is unclear. The strongest predictor is a younger age at disease onset. Although the relationship between motor disability and cognitive disability is controversial, cognitive impairment could occur independently from motor disability. Cognitive impairment affects academic and social activities and quality of life. Monitoring of cognitive impairment in pediatric MS patients is important to enable optimal treatment and rehabilitation for prevention of further cognitive disability.

Another factor affecting MS-induced cognitive functions is cognitive reserve. The cognitive reserve theory states that individual differences in how tasks are processed or neural networks are used can allow some people to cope better with brain pathology than others [11]. It has been shown that both heritable (brain reserve) and environmental (greater intellectual enrichment) factors may attenuate the negative effects of MS on cognitive status in adults [12]. The role of cognitive reserve in pediatric MS is unclear. Pastò et al. assessed the potential impact of cognitive reserve on cognition in a cohort of pediatric MS patients. A total of 48 pediatric MS patients and 57 healthy controls were included in this study, and patients were followed up for 4.7 ± 0.4 years. Cognitive reserve was estimated by measuring the IQ at baseline, and cognitive impairment was defined as failure in $\geqslant 3$ tests of an extensive neuropsychological battery that included the Selective Reminding Test (SRT) and Selective Reminding Test-Delayed (SRT-D), the 10/36 Spatial Recall Test (SPART), the 10/36 Spatial Recall Test-Delayed, the Symbol Digit Modalities Test (SDMT), the Trail Making tests (TMT-A and TMT-B), a Semantic and Phonemic Verbal Fluency Test, an Oral Denomination Test from the Aachener Aphasia Test, the Token Test, the Indication of Pictures from the Neuropsychological Examination for Aphasia, and Phrase Comprehension Test from the Battery for the

Table 1: Methods and results of cross-sectional studies.

Authors	MS sample size	Control sample size	Cognitive impairment definition	Neuropsychological tests	Impaired cognitive domains	Impairment rate
Banwell and Anderson [6]	10	—	Each individual's performance on each measure was scored relative to age norms.	Full-Scale IQ, Verbal IQ, Performance IQ, Verbal Comprehension Index, Perceptual Organization Index, Freedom from Distractibility Index, Processing Speed Index, CELF, COWAT, CELF formulated sentences, TLC Ambiguous sentences, VMI, Rey-O Figure, Grooved Pegboard, Vigilance subtest, CMS, CAVLT, WJRTA, WRAT	Language, visuomotor integration, verbal and visual memory, information processing speed, working memory and executive functions, general cognition	
MacAllister et al. [7]	37	—	Scores > 1.5 SDs below the published normative means on least 2 cognitive tasks	TMT, COWAT, Boston Naming Test, CELF-3rd edition, two subtests of the WRAML: Verbal Learning and Visual Learning, VMI	Complex attention receptive language, naming, memory	35%
Amato et al. [8]	63	57	Scoring less than the 5th percentile of healthy control performance on least 3 tests	WISC-R, SRT and SRT-D from the Rao's BRB, SPART and SPART-D from the BRB, SDMT from the BRB, TMT A and B, Modified Card Sorting Test, Semantic and Phonemic Verbal Fluency Test, and Oral Denomination Test from the Aachener Aphasia Test	Complex attention, visual and verbal memory, executive functions, language function	31%
Till et al. [9]	35	33	Three or more test scores 1.5 SDs below the normative values on the test battery	WASI, TMT-A and B, SDMT-Oral version, Visual Matching from the Woodcock–Johnson III (WJ-III) Test of Cognitive Abilities, Rapid Picture Naming from the WJ-III Test of Cognitive Abilities, Conner's Continuous Performance Test—5th edition, WSR, WMI-5th edition, Verbal Fluency subtest from the Delis–Kaplan Executive Function System, Picture Vocabulary from WJ-III Tests of Academic Achievement, Vocabulary and Similarities subtests from the WASI, WCST	Attention, information processing speed, expressive language, visuomotor integration	29.4%

Table 1: Continued.

Authors	MS sample size	Control sample size	Cognitive impairment definition	Neuropsychological tests	Impaired cognitive domains	Impairment rate
Julian et al. [10]	187 (MS) 44 (CIS)	—	≥33% of test scores < 1 SD below normative data	WASI Full 2, Wechsler Individual Achievement Test II Pseudoword Decoding, Expressive One-Word Picture Vocabulary Test, Digit Span test, Wechsler Intelligence Scale for Children Coding Test, Contingency Naming Test, Delis Kaplan Executive Function System Trail Making Test, California Verbal Learning Test-Child version or II, WMI-6th edition, Wechsler Abbreviated Scale of Intelligence Matrix Reasoning, Grooved Pegboard Test	Fine motor speed, visuomotor integration, information processing speed	35% (MS) 18% (CIS)

BRB: Rao's Brief Repeatable Battery; CAVLT: children's auditory verbal learning test; CELF: clinical evaluation of language fundamentals; CMS: children's memory scale; COWAT: controlled oral word association test; Rey-O: Rey–Osterreith complex figure; SDMT: Symbol Digit Modalities Test; SRT Selective Reminding Test; SRT-D: Selective Reminding Test-Delayed; SPART: Spatial Recall Test; SPART-D: Spatial Recall Test-Delayed; TMT: Trail Making Test; TLC: test of language competence; VMI: Beery–Buktenica visual motor integration test; WASI: Wechsler Abbreviated Scale of Intelligence; WCST: Wisconsin card sorting test; WISC-R: Wechsler Intelligence Scale for Children-Revised; WJ: Woodcock Johnson; WJRTA: Woodcock Johnson-revised tests of achievement; WRAML: wide range assessment of memory and learning test; WRAT: wide range achievement test; WSR: word selective reminding.

Analysis of Aphasic Deficits. The reliable change index (RCI) method was used to assess changes in neuropsychological performance. Cognitive impairment was found in 29.2% of patients with pediatric onset MS at baseline. Deterioration in cognitive performance was detected using the RCI method in 37.6% patients with pediatric onset MS. A higher cognitive reserve predicted stable or improving performance, whereas a lower reserve was associated with deteriorating performance at follow-up [13]. In other studies, on traumatic brain injury, higher cognitive reserve was associated with higher performance and a greater resistance to the development cognitive deficits [13–15]. Thus, measurement of cognitive reserve can be used to identify patients at high risk for cognitive impairment. Alternatively, cognitive reserve can be used to develop cognitive-protective approaches and cognitive rehabilitation programs.

Compared to adults, children are better able to compensate for brain damage because of the greater neural plasticity of the developing brain. Pediatric MS occurs during periods of brain growth, myelination, and neural network maturation; therefore, longitudinal follow-up studies are important to understanding the interactions between progressive brain pathology and maturation, neural plasticity, and compensatory abilities. During 2- and 5-year follow-ups of childhood and adolescent MS cases in their multicenter study, Amato et al. used the same neuropsychological battery as that used at baseline, with alternative versions of the tests to assess memory, attention/concentration, executive functions, and language. At the 2-year follow-up, 70% of patients failed at least three tests, and overall, 75% of the cases were classified as having deteriorating cognitive performance. Failure was more prominent in tests of verbal memory, complex attention, verbal fluency, and receptive language. An individual cognitive change index was also calculated to assess the direction of change in cognition over the follow-up period. At the 2-year follow-up, cognitive deterioration was observed in 75% of the patients, while 25% of the cases were classified as stable or improving. At the 5-year follow-up, the cognitive impairment index decreased in 56% of the patients, improved in 25%, and remained stable in 18.8%. Cognitive deterioration was associated with male sex, younger age at disease onset, and lower educational level. The cognitive domains with the most tendencies toward deterioration were visuospatial learning and expressive language [16, 17].

In a small cohort of patients with pediatric MS, MacAllister et al. assessed cognitive function longitudinally and found deficits in attention, executive functions, and memory. Their findings suggested that neurological impairment early in the course of the disease was predictive of cognitive decline over time. There was no strong association between duration of disease and cognitive decline. The results suggested that, in patients with pediatric MS, cognition might deteriorate over time relative to that of their peers and their baseline performance [18].

In a longitudinal study, Charvet et al. evaluated cognitive function in 62 patients with pediatric MS and five with clinically isolated syndrome. The researchers evaluated cognition at baseline and at follow-up, with a mean follow-up time of 1.64 ± 0.63 years. Cognitive impairment was detected in 37% of patients at baseline and 33% of patients at follow-up. The most commonly impaired cognitive functions included visuomotor integration, information processing speed, and attention. The researchers indicated that cognitive performance might remain stable, or even improve, over a short period of time [19].

In another longitudinal study, Hosseini et al. investigated how the age at disease onset and cognitive reserve may affect cognitive maturation in children and adolescents with pediatric MS. They used two standardized and widely used neuropsychological measures (SDMT and TMT) to assess visual scanning, information processing speed, and working memory. Cognitive reserve capacity was assessed using the patient's baseline full-scale IQ and parental social status. They used growth curve analysis to evaluate cognitive maturation over childhood and adolescence. Their results showed that a younger age at disease onset was associated with decreased performance on neuropsychological measures (SDMT and TMT). A younger age of disease onset was also associated with lower developmental gain on the neuropsychological measures. Cognitive reserve, including baseline full-scale IQ and parental social status, did not protect against cognitive deterioration [20].

Till et al. investigated the extent, pattern, and correlates of change in cognitive functioning over an approximately 15-month interval in 28 patients with pediatric MS and compared their findings with data from 26 healthy controls. The RCI was used to determine individual differences on test scores over time in this prospective longitudinal study. Participants were categorized as showing either "decline" or "improvement" if changes in scores exceeded the RCI on three or more tests. They observed that healthy controls were more likely to show improvement across multiple domains of function than patients with pediatric MS were. When cognitive change was examined on an individual basis, cognitive deterioration was observed in seven of 28 patients with pediatric MS and only one of 26 healthy controls. Clinically significant improvement on three or more of the neuropsychological tests was detected in 69.2% of healthy controls compared with only 17.9% of pediatric MS patients. Patients with pediatric MS showed decline mainly on tests of information processing speed and attention, visuomotor integration, verbal fluency, abstract visual memory, calculation, and spelling. An association was found between disease duration and deterioration in visuomotor integration. The results showed that patients who were classified as having declined cognitive function (n : 7) did not differ from those with stable/improved cognitive function (n : 21) with regard to age at testing, age at disease onset, disease duration, sex, mood-related symptoms, baseline IQ, and EDSS scores. The researchers reported that patients with pediatric MS failed to demonstrate age-expected improvements in several domains of cognitive performance [21].

In a study investigating long-term outcomes in adult patients with pediatric-onset MS, SDMT scores were lower in patients with pediatric onset than adult onset both in unadjusted analysis and after adjustment for disease duration. The researchers suggested that, in adulthood, pediatric-onset MS may result in greater impairment in processing speed and that further investigation of other cognitive domains was warranted in this group of patients [22].

The methods and results of longitudinal follow-up studies are shown in Table 2. The duration of follow-up in these studies varied between 1 and 5 years. In Amato et al.'s study, most of the patients (75%) showed deteriorating performance between baseline and year 2; however, comparing baseline and 5-year testing, cognitive impairment index deterioration was observed in 56% of the patients, improvement in 25%, and stability in 18.8% [16, 17]. Charvet et al. emphasized that most of the cases had a stable cognitive function in the mean 1.6-year follow-up [19]. Till et al. found that 75% of the cases showed stabilization or improvement in cognitive function at 15 months follow-up, but the improvement rate was less than that of healthy controls [21]. The variations in the results of the studies may be related to the differences in follow-up periods and evaluation methods used.

The reason for the improvements observed in children may be the ongoing development in the brain and neural plasticity. Brain development and neural plasticity may be involved in the success of cognitive rehabilitation and cognitive reserve enhancement approaches. Alternatively, cognitive performance in patients with pediatric MS may deteriorate in the long term relative to their baseline performance and the performance of their peers. This worsening cognitive state can be explained by impairment of the maturation and development of the immature central nervous system by demyelinating and neurodegenerative processes.

3. Social Cognition

Social cognition, a distinct area of cognitive function, refers to "the mental operations that underlie social interactions, including perceiving, interpreting, and generating responses to the intentions, dispositions, and behaviors of others" [23]. The theory of mind is an essential domain of social cognition, defined as the ability to infer other people's mental states, including beliefs, desires, knowledge, and intentions, hence explaining and predicting their behavior [24]. Social cognitive impairment has been studied in autism, psychiatric disorders, and developmental and neurodegenerative diseases. However, studies on social cognition in pediatric MS are very limited, with only one study published in the literature. Charvet and colleagues examined social cognition in 28 patients with pediatric-onset MS and 38 healthy controls. They used the SDMT and all three theories of mind tasks: reading the mind in the eyes test, the faux pas test, and the false-belief task. Patients with pediatric-onset MS performed worse than healthy controls on all theories of mind tasks, including both affective (eyes test) and cognitive (faux pas test and false-belief task) measures. Information processing speed, which was measured by SDMT, was slower in the pediatric-onset MS group (38%) than in the healthy control group (6%). However, when logistic regression analysis was performed to assess the influence of information processing speed on the theory of mind tasks, they suggested that information processing speed had no influence on the theory of mind [25]. Social cognitive impairment has been reported in adult patients with MS who were otherwise cognitively intact [26, 27]. Social cognition is important for the ability to form and maintain personal relationships. The effect of MS on social cognition is particularly important in patients with pediatric-onset MS since their social cognition skills are still undergoing development [25–27]. More studies on social cognition in pediatric MS are needed for the identification and prevention of social adjustment problems in these patients.

4. Neuropsychological Test Batteries for Pediatric MS

The aforementioned studies applied neuropsychological tests developed for adults to pediatric patients with MS. There is a need for a standardized, well-approved neuropsychological battery to detect MS-related deficits in pediatric patients. It is important to establish neuropsychological test batteries for evaluating cognitive domains that appear more frequently in children than adults and for assessing cognitive maturation in this age group. Several studies have attempted to establish such a neuropsychological test battery and to measure the sensitivity of presently available tests.

In an Italian multicenter study, Portaccio et al. validated a brief neuropsychological battery that they derived from the extensive battery used by Amato and colleagues. The researchers aimed to develop a Brief Neuropsychological Battery for Children (BNBC) with MS. The extensive neuropsychological battery involved the Wechsler Intelligence Scale for Children-Revised (WISC-R), the Selective Reminding Test (SRT, SRT-Delayed) from Rao's Brief Repeatable Battery (BRB), the Spatial Recall Test (SPART, SPART-D) from the BRB, the Symbol Digit Modalities Test (SDMT) from the BRB, Trail Making Test (TMT-A and TMT-B), Modified Card Sorting Test, Semantic Verbal Fluency Test (SVFT), Phonemic Verbal Fluency Test (PVFT), the Oral Denomination Test from the Aachener Aphasia Test, Token Test, the Indication of Pictures from the Neuropsychological Examination for Aphasia, and the Phrase Comprehension Test from the Battery for the Analysis of Aphasic Deficits (Table 3). Cognitive functions were assessed in 61 patients with childhood and juvenile MS and in 58 healthy controls. In this study, cognitive impairment was found in 41% of MS patients. Verbal and spatial memory (SRT and SPART), attention and concentration (SDMT and TMT), and language abilities (SVFT and Token Test) were the most frequently affected cognitive domains. Discriminant function analysis showed that the SDMT, the TMT-B, the Selective Reminding Test-Consistent Long-Term Retrieval (SRT-CLTR), and the vocabulary test from the WISC had higher discriminating ability. Therefore, using these tests, the researchers created the BNBC, which had a sensitivity of 96% and a specificity of 76% [28]. (Table 4).

Smerbeck et al. investigated the sensitivity and validity of two visual processing tests in 43 children with pediatric MS and 45 healthy controls: the Brief Visuospatial Memory Test-Revised (BVMT-R) and the SDMT. Previous large cross-sectional studies had demonstrated the sensitivity of

Table 2: Methods and results of longitudinal follow-up studies.

Authors	MS sample size at follow-up	Healthy controls sample size at follow-up	Duration of follow-up	Neuropsychological tests	Rate of decline in MS sample	Impaired cognitive domains
Amato et al. [16]	56	—	2 years	SRT, SRT-D, SPART, SPART-D, SDMT, TMT-A, TMT-B, Tower of London Test, Semantic and Phonemic Verbal Fluency Test, Oral Denomination Test from the Aachener Aphasia Test	70% (failure on at least 3 tests) (change in CCI between baseline and 2 years) Deteriorating: 75% Stable: 11.5% Improving: 13.5%	Verbal memory, complex attention, verbal fluency, receptive language
Amato et al. [17]	48	—	5 years	SRT, SRT-D, SPART, SPART-D, SDMT, TMT-A, TMT-B, Tower of London Test, Semantic and Phonemic Verbal Fluency Test, Oral Denomination Test from the Aachener Aphasia Test	38% (failure on at least 3 tests) (change in CCI between baseline and 5 years) Deteriorating: 56% Stable: 18.8% Improving: 25% (change in CCI between years 2 and 5) Deteriorating: 22.9% Stable: 10.4% Improving: 66.7%	Visual–spatial learning, expressive language
MacAllister et al. [18]	12	—	21.58 ± 9.3 months	TMT, COWAT, Boston Naming Test, CELF 3rd edition, WRAML, WMI	5/12 (cognitive decline assessed using the criteria of more tests showing impaired at the time of the 2nd test than at the baseline) 7/12 (cognitive decline assessed using the criteria of decline in *z*-score composite from the baseline to the time of the 2nd test)	Attention, executive functions, memory
Charvet et al. [19]	62 (MS) 5 (CIS)	—	1.64 ± 0.63 years	WASI, WASI-II, CVLT-C, CVLT-II, EOWPVT, WIAT-II, VMI, Digit Span subtest from WISC-IV, WAIS-IV, TMT	Rate of impairment was 37% at baseline and 33% at follow-up Most participants showed no change while $n = 4$ (6%) declined on two or more tasks and $n = 6$ (9%) improved on 2 or more tasks	Visuomotor integration, information processing speed, attention

Table 2: Continued.

Authors	MS sample size at follow-up	Healthy controls sample size at follow-up	Duration of follow-up	Neuropsychological tests	Rate of decline in MS sample	Impaired cognitive domains
Hosseini et al. [20]	35	—	Neuropsychological evaluations were conducted at baseline and up to four more assessments, with each evaluation separated by a minimum of 1 year.	SDMT, TMT, WASI, WISC-III	This study examined changes in cognitive maturation in a cohort of pediatric-onset MS patients as a function of age at disease onset and cognitive reserve factors (baseline IQ and parental social status) Younger age at disease onset was associated with a greater likelihood of cognitive decline on both the TMT-B ($p = 0.001$) and SDMT ($p = 0.005$)	Younger age at disease-onset increases the vulnerability for disrupted performance on measures of information processing, visual scanning, perceptual/motor speed, and working memory
Till et al. [21]	28	26	13–16 months (mean: 15 months)	WASI, Visual Matching from the WJ Tests of Cognitive Abilities, TMT A-B, SDMT, Conner's Continuous Performance Test (5th edition)–number of omission errors, Vocabulary and Similarities subtests of the WASI, WJ Tests of Achievement, Verbal Fluency Test from DKEFS, VMI, Block Design and Matrix Reasoning subtests from the WASI, TOMAL-2, WSR, Grooved Pegboard test	Improving: 18% in MS group, 86% in control group The RCI method results showed that the majority of patients remained stable or improved over time (21 of 28; 75%), with only seven of 28 patients (25%) demonstrating decline on three or more of the neuropsychological tests. Only 1 of 26 controls (3.8%) showed cognitive deterioration ($p < 0.05$).	Attention, information processing speed, visuomotor integration, verbal fluency, visual memory, calculation, spelling ability

CCI: cognitive change index; CVLT: California Verbal Learning Test; DKEFS: Delis–Kaplan executive function system; EOWPVT: Expressive One-Word Picture Vocabulary Test; RCI: reliable change index; TOMAL-2: test of memory and learning-2nd edition; WAIS-IV: Wechsler adult intelligence scale 4th edition; WIAT-II: Wechsler Individual Achievement Test-2nd edition.

TABLE 3: Neuropsychological tests.

Neuropsychological test	Cognitive domain
WISC-R (Wechsler Intelligence Scale for Children)	IQ (intelligence quotient)
SRT-LTS (Selective Reminding Test-Long-Term Storage) SRT-CLTR (Selective Reminding Test-Consistent Long-Term Retrieval) SRT-D (Selective Reminding Test-Delayed) SPART (Spatial Recall Test) SPART-D (Spatial Recall Test-Delayed)	Memory
MCST (Modified Card Sorting Test)	Abstract/conceptual reasoning
SDMT (Symbol Digit Modalities Test) TMT-A/ B (Trail Making Test A/B)	Attention/concentration
SVFT (Semantic Verbal Fluency Test) PVFT (Phonemic Verbal Fluency Test) IPT (Indication of Pictures Test) PCT (Phrase Comprehension Test) Token Test ODT (Oral Denomination Test)	Language

TABLE 4: Brief Neuropsychological Battery for Children (BNBC).

(i) SRT
(ii) SDMT
(iii) TMT
(iv) Vocabulary test from the WISC-R

Duration: 30 minutes. Sensitivity (96%), specificity (76%).

these tests in adults. They found statistically significant differences between children with MS and healthy controls on BVMT-R Total Learning, BVMT-R Delayed Recall, and SDMT. These findings indicated that two relatively brief measures of visual-cognitive processing could be successfully applied to the pediatric population and could be useful in detecting and monitoring significant cognitive impairment [29].

Charvet et al. evaluated the SDMT as a screening tool for identifying pediatric onset MS patients at risk for cognitive impairment. The SDMT showed 77% sensitivity and 81% specificity for detecting neuropsychological impairment when administered within 1 year. Age and EDSS score were negatively correlated with SDMT score. The researchers concluded that these results support the use of the SDMT as a screening tool for cognitive function in pediatric MS [30].

5. Neuroradiologic Studies and Anatomic Correlation of Cognitive Impairment in Pediatric MS Patients

Several neuroradiologic studies have reported a correlation between deficits in executive function and atrophy of the thalamus and frontal lobes, as well as the correlation of a decrease in cognitive speed and mathematical performance with corpus callosum damage [31–33].

To normalize total and regional brain volumes for head size in their MRI correlations, Till and colleagues calculated cortical gray matter, thalamic, and global brain volumes using a scaling factor computed using the normalization of atrophy method. In addition, they also calculated T1- and T2-weighted lesion volumes in MS patients. Thirty-five pediatric-onset MS patients and 33 healthy controls were included in the study. Thalamic volume, corpus callosum area, normalized brain volume, and normalized gray matter volume were significantly lower in patients with MS than in healthy controls. Thalamic volume was strongly and positively correlated with an index global intellectual function in MS patients. MS patients with cognitive impairment did not differ from MS patients without cognitive impairment with regard to T1 or T2 lesion volume, normalized grey matter volume, or normalized brain volume. Neuropsychologic test performance was highly correlated with global and regional brain volume and less strongly correlated with T1 and T2 lesion volumes. The researchers suggested that cognitive impairment was related to the neurodegenerative component of MS [9].

The cerebellum is another anatomical area associated with cognitive function. It is a strategic node in various networks such as coordination and cognitive-behavioral loops [34]. Weier et al. examined associations between cognitive outcomes and cerebellar volume independent of cerebral volume in patients with pediatric MS. Twenty-eight pediatric-onset MS patients and 33 age- and sex-matched healthy controls were included in this study. All subjects underwent structural MRI and neuropsychological evaluation to assess intelligence, attention, information processing speed, language, visuomotor integration, and fine-motor dexterity. Neuropsychological battery included the Wechsler Abbreviated Scale of Intelligence (WASI), the TMT-B, the SDMT-oral version, Beery Visual Motor Integration, the vocabulary subtest of the WASI, and the Grooved Pegboard test. Cognitive performance in patients with MS was reduced relative to that in the healthy controls in the domains of attention, information processing speed, expressive language, visuomotor integration, and fine motor dexterity. Cerebellar volumes did not differ between MS group and healthy controls; however, cerebellar posterior lobe volume and infratentorial lesion volume accounted for extra variance in cognitive measures of information processing (SDMT) and vocabulary within MS patients in regression analysis. The researchers suggested that in addition to cerebral volume, the cerebellar volume was another correlate of cognitive function in children and adolescents with MS [35].

In a neuroradiologic study, Rocca and colleagues performed a structural and functional MRI examination to investigate the mechanisms responsible for the presence and severity of cognitive impairment in pediatric patients with MS. A total of 35 pediatric patients with MS and 16 sex- and age-matched healthy controls were included in the study. The researchers used voxel-based analysis with advanced structural MRI techniques to determine the patterns of regional involvement of white and gray matter according to patient's cognitive profile. They also used functional MRI to quantify the resting-state functional connectivity of the default mode network (DMN). The BNBC was used to assess participants' cognitive function, and subjects with abnormal performance in two tests were classified as cognitively impaired. Among the patients with MS, 45% were classified as cognitively impaired. Spatial and verbal memory abilities, language, attention, and concentration were the most significantly involved cognitive areas. The results showed that cognitively impaired patients with MS had a higher occurrence of T2 lesions and white and gray matter damage, including atrophy and diffusivity abnormalities in the posterior region of the parietal lobes close to midline (precuneus, posterior cingulum, and corpus callosum). Reduced resting-state functional connectivity in the precuneus was observed in cognitively impaired patients, whereas cognitively preserved patients showed increased resting-state functional connectivity in the anterior cingulate cortex. The researchers concluded that the presence and severity of cognitive impairment were associated with structural and functional abnormalities of the posterior core regions of the DMN in pediatric patients with MS [36].

In these neuroradiological studies, researchers used different parameters such as global brain volume, thalamic volume, gray matter volume, T1-T2 lesion volume, and cerebellar volume. Cognitive impairment has been related to T2 hyperintense lesions, diffuse white matter damage, and cortical and deep gray matter atrophy in adult MS patients [37]. Neuropathologic findings have revealed that MS affects regions that are functionally or anatomically involved in cognitive processes, such as cortical and deep gray matter, hippocampus, white matter, including normal appearing white matter in adult patients [38]. Consistent with the findings in adult patients, studies in pediatric MS patients suggest that a relationship exists between cognitive impairment and gray matter atrophy, white matter atrophy, and global and regional brain volume [9, 36].

6. Conclusions

A third of the pediatric MS patients experience cognitive impairment. In pediatric cases, the influence of demyelination on the developing central nervous system and neural network affects cognitive function negatively; on the other hand, neural plasticity and ability of compensation can have a positive effect on cognitive functions. Unlike in adults, intelligence and language functions are affected in pediatric MS. Young age at disease onset increases the risk of cognitive impairment. Although varying findings have been reported for the relationship between motor disability and cognitive disability, cognitive impairment may also occur independently from motor disability. Cognitive reserve is important both for the detection of patients with high risk and for the development of cognitive-protective approaches and rehabilitation. Knowledge about social cognition is limited in pediatric MS. Cognitive impairment in pediatric MS is a critical problem that has long-term effects on patients' academic and social quality of life; thus, the development of appropriate neuropsychological test batteries is important for screening patients who are at risk. Current studies have shown that SDMT and Brief Neuropsychological Battery for Children (BNBC) could be effectively used for screening cognitive functions in pediatric MS.

MRI studies have suggested that cognitive impairment in pediatric MS can be related to both gray matter atrophy and white matter atrophy and global and regional brain volume. More longitudinal studies with standardized neuropsychological batteries and advanced MRI techniques are needed to explore the mechanism of cognitive impairments and predict high-risk group. Understanding the pathogenesis of impaired cognition and the involvement of specific cognitive areas in pediatric MS will guide the development of treatment and rehabilitation, including cognitive rehabilitation, about which limited data are available in pediatric MS patients.

Assessment of cognitive function is also important for the evaluation of response to treatment. While defining the response to treatment and disease activity in pediatric MS, preservation of age-expected global and regional brain growth and age-expected cognitive maturation and function should be assessed, as well as the number of relapses, disability progression, and MR findings such as new, enlarging, or enhancing lesions.

References

[1] P. Duquette, T. J. Murray, J. Pleines et al., "Multiple sclerosis in childhood: clinical profile in 125 patients," *The Journal of Pediatrics*, vol. 111, no. 3, pp. 359–363, 1987.

[2] A. Ghezzi, V. Deplano, J. Faroni et al., "Multiple sclerosis in childhood: clinical features of 149 cases," *Multiple Sclerosis Journal*, vol. 3, no. 1, pp. 43–46, 1997.

[3] L. B. Krupp, M. Tardieu, M. P. Amato et al., "International Pediatric Multiple Sclerosis Study Group criteria for pediatric multiple sclerosis and immune-mediated central nervous system demyelinating disorders: revisions to the 2007 definitions," *Multiple Sclerosis Journal*, vol. 19, no. 10, pp. 1261–1267, 2013.

[4] S. M. Rao, "Neuropsychology of multiple sclerosis," *Current Opinion in Neurology*, vol. 8, no. 3, pp. 216–220, 1995.

[5] J. A. Bobholz and S. M. Rao, "Cognitive dysfunction in multiple sclerosis: a review of recent developments," *Current Opinion in Neurology*, vol. 16, no. 3, pp. 283–288, 2003.

[6] B. L. Banwell and P. E. Anderson, "The cognitive burden of multiple sclerosis in children," *Neurology*, vol. 64, no. 5, pp. 891–894, 2005.

[7] W. S. MacAllister, A. L. Belman, M. Milazzo et al., "Cognitive functioning in children and adolescents with multiple sclerosis," *Neurology*, vol. 64, no. 8, pp. 1422–1425, 2005.

[8] M. P. Amato, B. Goretti, A. Ghezzi et al., "Cognitive and psychosocial features of childhood and juvenile MS," *Neurology*, vol. 70, no. 20, pp. 1891–1897, 2008.

[9] C. Till, R. Ghassemi, B. Aubert-Broche et al., "MRI correlates of cognitive impairment in childhood-onset multiple sclerosis," *Neuropsychology*, vol. 25, no. 3, pp. 319–332, 2011.

[10] L. Julian, D. Serafin, L. Charvet et al., "Cognitive impairment occurs in children and adolescents with multiple sclerosis: results from a United States network," *Journal of Child Neurology*, vol. 28, no. 1, pp. 102–107, 2013.

[11] Y. Stern, "Cognitive reserve," *Neuropsychologia*, vol. 47, no. 10, pp. 2015–2028, 2009.

[12] J. F. Sumowski and V. M. Leavitt, "Cognitive reserve in multiple sclerosis," *Multiple Sclerosis Journal*, vol. 19, no. 9, pp. 1122–1127, 2013.

[13] L. Pastò, E. Portaccio, B. Goretti et al., "The cognitive reserve theory in the setting of pediatric-onset multiple sclerosis," *Multiple Sclerosis Journal*, vol. 22, no. 13, pp. 1741–1749, 2016.

[14] S. R. Kesler, H. F. Adams, C. M. Blasey, and E. D. Bigler, "Premorbid intellectual functioning, education, and brain size in traumatic brain injury: an investigation of the cognitive reserve hypothesis," *Applied Neuropsychology*, vol. 10, no. 3, pp. 153–162, 2003.

[15] J. E. Farmer, S. M. Kanne, J. S. Haut, J. Williams, B. Johnstone, and K. Kirk, "Memory functioning following traumatic brain injury in children with premorbid learning problems," *Developmental Neuropsychology*, vol. 22, no. 2, pp. 455–469, 2002.

[16] M. P. Amato, B. Goretti, A. Ghezzi et al., "Cognitive and psychosocial features in childhood and juvenile MS two-year follow-up," *Neurology*, vol. 75, no. 13, pp. 1134–1140, 2010.

[17] M. P. Amato, B. Goretti, A. Ghezzi et al., "Neuropsychological features in childhood and juvenile multiple sclerosis five-year follow-up," *Neurology*, vol. 83, no. 16, pp. 1432–1438, 2014.

[18] W. S. MacAllister, C. Christodoulou, M. Milazzo, and L. B. Krupp, "Longitudinal neuropsychological assessment in pediatric multiple sclerosis," *Developmental Neuropsychology*, vol. 32, no. 2, pp. 625–644, 2007.

[19] L. E. Charvet, E. H. O'Donnell, A. L. Belman et al., "Longitudinal evaluation of cognitive functioning in pediatric multiple sclerosis: report from the US pediatric multiple sclerosis network," *Multiple Sclerosis Journal*, vol. 20, no. 11, pp. 1502–1510, 2014.

[20] B. Hosseini, D. B. Flora, B. L. Banwell, and C. Till, "Age of onset as a moderator of cognitive decline in pediatric-onset multiple sclerosis," *Journal of the International Neuropsychological Society*, vol. 20, no. 08, pp. 796–804, 2014.

[21] C. Till, N. Racine, D. Araujo et al., "Changes in cognitive performance over a 1-year period in children and adolescents with multiple sclerosis," *Neuropsychology*, vol. 27, no. 2, pp. 210–219, 2013.

[22] N. F. Baruch, E. H. O'Donnell, B. I. Glanz et al., "Cognitive and patient-reported outcomes in adults with pediatric-onset multiple sclerosis," *Multiple Sclerosis Journal*, vol. 22, no. 3, pp. 354–361, 2016.

[23] M. F. Green, D. L. Penn, R. Bentall et al., "Social cognition in schizophrenia: an NIMH workshop on definitions, assessment, and research opportunities," *Schizophrenia Bulletin*, vol. 34, no. 6, pp. 1211–1220, 2008.

[24] R. Adolphs, "Cognitive neuroscience: cognitive neuroscience of human social behavior," *Nature Reviews Neuroscience*, vol. 4, no. 3, pp. 165–178, 2003.

[25] L. E. Charvet, R. E. Cleary, K. Vazquez, A. Belman, and L. B. Krupp, "Social cognition in pediatric-onset multiple sclerosis (MS)," *Multiple Sclerosis Journal*, vol. 20, no. 11, pp. 1478–1484, 2014.

[26] M. Jehna, C. Langkammer, M. Wallner-Blazek et al., "Cognitively preserved MS patients demonstrate functional differences in processing neutral and emotional faces," *Brain Imaging and Behavior*, vol. 5, no. 4, pp. 241–251, 2011.

[27] J. Cotter, J. Firth, C. Enzinger et al., "Social cognition in multiple sclerosis, a review and meta-analysis," *Neurology*, vol. 87, no. 16, pp. 1727–1736, 2016.

[28] E. Portaccio, B. Goretti, S. Lori et al., "The brief neuropsychological battery for children: a screening tool for cognitive impairment in childhood and juvenile multiple sclerosis," *Multiple Sclerosis Journal*, vol. 15, no. 5, pp. 620–626, 2009.

[29] A. M. Smerbeck, J. Parrish, D. Serafin et al., "Visual-cognitive processing deficits in pediatric multiple sclerosis," *Multiple Sclerosis Journal*, vol. 17, no. 4, pp. 449–456, 2011.

[30] L. E. Charvet, R. Beekman, N. Amadiume, A. L. Belman, and L. B. Krupp, "The symbol digit modalities test is an effective cognitive screen in pediatric onset multiple sclerosis (MS)," *Journal of the Neurological Sciences*, vol. 341, no. 1-2, pp. 79–84, 2014.

[31] C. Till, C. Ho, A. Dudani, D. García-Lorenzo, D. L. Collins, and B. L. Banwell, "Magnetic resonance imaging predictors of executive functioning in patients with pediatric-onset multiple sclerosis," *Archives of Clinical Neuropsychology*, vol. 27, no. 5, pp. 495–509, 2012.

[32] A. Bethune, V. Tipu, J. G. Sled et al., "Diffusion tensor imaging and cognitive speed in children with multiple sclerosis," *Journal of the Neurological Sciences*, vol. 309, no. 1-2, pp. 68–74, 2011.

[33] C. Till, A. Deotto, V. Tipu et al., "White matter integrity and math performance in pediatric multiple sclerosis: a diffusion tensor imaging study," *NeuroReport*, vol. 22, no. 18, pp. 1005–1009, 2011.

[34] D. Timmann, J. Drepper, M. Frings et al., "The human cerebellum contributes to motor, emotional and cognitive associative learning. A review," *Cortex*, vol. 46, no. 7, pp. 845–857, 2010.

[35] K. Weier, C. Till, V. Fonov et al., "Contribution of the cerebellum to cognitive performance in children and adolescents with multiple sclerosis," *Multiple Sclerosis Journal*, vol. 22, no. 5, pp. 599–607, 2016.

[36] M. A. Rocca, M. Absinta, M. P. Amato et al., "Posterior brain damage and cognitive impairment in pediatric multiple sclerosis," *Neurology*, vol. 82, no. 15, pp. 1314–1321, 2014.

[37] F. Paul, "Pathology and MRI: exploring cognitive impairment in MS," *Acta Neurologica Scandinavica*, vol. 134, Supplement 200, pp. 24–33, 2016.

[38] G. C. DeLuca, R. L. Yates, H. Beale, and S. A. Morrow, "Cognitive impairment in multiple sclerosis: clinical, radiologic and pathologic insights," *Brain Pathology*, vol. 25, pp. 79–98, 2015.

12

Comparing Sensitivity and Specificity of Addenbrooke's Cognitive Examination-I, III and Mini-Addenbrooke's Cognitive Examination in Parkinson's Disease

Tivadar Lucza,[1] Zsuzsanna Ascherman,[2] Márton Kovács,[2,3] Attila Makkos,[2,3] Márk Harmat,[2,3] Annamária Juhász,[2,4] József Janszky,[2,4] Sámuel Komoly,[2] Norbert Kovács,[2,4] Krisztina Dorn,[5] and Kázmér Karádi[1]

[1]*Institute of Behavioral Sciences, University of Pécs, Pécs, Hungary*
[2]*Department of Neurology, University of Pécs, Pécs, Hungary*
[3]*Doctoral School of Clinical Neuroscience, University of Pécs, Pécs, Hungary*
[4]*MTA-PTE Clinical Neuroscience MR Research Group, Pécs, Hungary*
[5]*Pediatric Clinic, University of Pécs, Pécs, Hungary*

Correspondence should be addressed to Norbert Kovács; kovacsnorbert06@gmail.com and Kázmér Karádi; karadikazmer@gmail.com

Academic Editor: Barbara Picconi

Background. Parkinson's disease (PD) is the second most common neurodegenerative disorder characterized by numerous motor and nonmotor symptoms. Neurocognitive disorders (NCD) are one of the most troublesome problems and their diagnosis is often challenging. *Methods.* We compared the sensitivity and specificity of several versions of Addenbrooke Cognitive Examination (ACE, ACE-III, and Mini-ACE) on 552 subjects with PD. Normal cognition, mild and major NCD were judged in accordance with the respective criteria of the Diagnostic and Statistical Manual of Mental Disorders 5th edition. Subsequently, we applied the receiver operation characteristic (ROC) analysis in comparison of different education levels. *Results.* For subjects with education level 0–8 and 9–12 years, the ACE-III had the best discriminating capabilities for mild NCD (cut-off scores: 83.5 and 85.5 points, respectively), while Mini-ACE was the best for subjects having education > 12 years (cut-off score: 25.5 points). For detecting major NCD, ACE-III had the best diagnostic accuracy in all levels of education (cut-off scores: 70.5, 77.5, and 78.5 points for subjects having education level 0–8, 9–12, and >12 years, respectively). *Conclusion.* ACE-III and its nested version, the Mini-ACE, had the best screening abilities for detecting mild and major NCD in PD.

1. Introduction

Parkinson's disease (PD) is the second most common neurodegenerative disorder characterized by both motor and nonmotor symptoms [1]. Besides the well-known motor symptoms including bradykinesia, resting tremor, and rigidity, numerous nonmotor symptoms (NMS) exist [2]. Among the NMSs, fatigue, autonomic disturbances, sleep disorders, depression, apathy, behavioral disturbances, and cognitive impairments are the most frequent and troublesome [3, 4]. Although some cognitive deficits do exist in the early stages of the disease interfering executive functions, working memory, and visuospatial functioning [5, 6], more pronounced neurocognitive disorders (NCDs) may develop as the disease progresses [7, 8]. These neuropsychological deficits are partly related to the dysfunction of dopaminergic frontostriatal circuits [9, 10].

NCDs are characterized by a decline from a previously attained level of cognitive functioning. This decline should be both clinically relevant in manner and objectively measurable in order to establish the diagnosis. In the clinical practice, basically, two diagnostic frameworks exist for diagnosing NCDs in PD.

The Task Forces and Committees of the International Parkinson's Disease and Movement Disorders Society (IPDMDS) established the criteria for mild cognitive impairment in PD (PD-MCI) [11] and the Parkinson's disease dementia (PDD) [12]. Although PD-MCI might develop in the early stages of PD [13], it is more characteristic of later phases. PD-MCI is defined as a stage between dementia and normal cognitive functioning with subjective concern and objective decline of cognitive functioning, without major impairment in the everyday functions [11, 14]. In addition to executive dysfunction, there is an alteration of posterior cortical functions in PD-MCI [15]. Prevalence of PD-MCI is increased by age, disease duration, and disease severity [11, 14]. Diagnosing PD-MCI is an important issue because PD-MCI predicts the development of dementia [16]. The establishment of the diagnosis of the PD-MCI is based on abbreviated (Level-I) and comprehensive (Level-II) assessments [11]. In accordance with the IPDMDS Task Force Guidelines, in PD-MCI, the cognitive functions (memory, executive function) are 1 to 2 standard deviations below the average level. PDD has more severe cortical dysfunctions compared with PD-MCI [12, 15]. Cortical profile of PDD represents an impairment of memory and language skill, while subcortical profile has a decline in attention, executive and visuospatial functions [17, 18]. PDD usually develops several years after the onset of motor symptoms [12]. The prevalence of PDD is approximately 20–40% [19–21]. The IPDMDS Task Force Guidelines provides a guideline for a diagnostic procedure for determining PDD [19, 22]. The diagnostic procedure also consists of abbreviated (Level-I) and comprehensive (Level-II) assessment as it is shown in PD-MCI. Detecting PDD is extremely important in the treatment of PD and in screening appropriate candidates for deep brain stimulation.

The fifth edition of the Diagnostic and Statistical Manual of Mental Disorders (DSM-5) also provides a common framework for the diagnosis of neurocognitive disorders, first by describing the main cognitive syndromes and then defining criteria to delineate specific etiological subtypes. The DSM-5 defines the mild and major NCDs in PD, which largely overlap with the PD-MCI and PDD terminology.

Diagnosing dementia in Parkinson's disease patient population poses significant challenges. The screening procedure includes several tests for the abbreviated assessment of PDD. These screening tools may represent short (Mini-Mental State Examination (MMSE) and Montreal Cognitive Examination [23] (MoCA)) and "longer" test batteries (e.g., Mattis Dementia Rating Scale and the Addenbrooke's Cognitive Examination) [19, 22, 24, 25].

The Addenbrooke's Cognitive Examination (ACE), a screening tool, has had substantial and rapid development over the years. The original version of ACE (ACE-I) was developed to differentiate Alzheimer's disease from frontotemporal dementia and to detect the early stages of these dementia syndromes [26]. The maximum score of ACE-I is 100, and higher numbers represent better functioning. ACE-I assesses six cognitive domains, where the maximum scores are 10 points for orientation, 8 points for attention, 35 points for memory, 14 points for verbal fluency, 28 points for language skills, and 5 points for visuospatial ability. ACE-I also includes the nested version of MMSE. The Spanish version of ACE-I was able to detect dementia in PD, and it could discriminate PDD from Alzheimer's dementia but not from frontotemporal dementia [27].

The Addenbrooke's Cognitive Examination-Revised (ACE-R) was developed soon after the publication of ACE-I considering the strengths and weaknesses of ACE-I [28] and had been translated into many languages [29–33]. While ACE-I has only one version, the ACE-R includes three alternative versions, allowing multiple testing over extended time. Significant changes were made in the language and visuospatial parts. ACE-R has five subscores representing various cognitive domains: attention/orientation (18 points), memory (26 points), verbal fluency (14 points), language skills (26 points), and visuospatial abilities (16 points). The maximum score is 100 in ACE-R. Recently, ACE-R has been used extensively worldwide [29, 32–34].

The newest version of the ACE test family is the Addenbrooke's Cognitive Examination-III (ACE-III) [35]. Its maximum score is also 100 points. Compared to ACE-R, ACE-III has some modifications in the attention domain, the syntactical and semantical complexity of language skill, and visuospatial ability items to accommodate removal of MMSE items. ACE-III assesses the domain of attention (18 points), memory (26 points), verbal fluency (14 points), language (26 points), and visuospatial (16 points) functions. ACE-III cognitive subscores correlate with the scores of comprehensive neuropsychological tests, and ACE-III has similar sensitivity and specificity for detecting Alzheimer's disease and frontotemporal dementia as ACE-R.

One of the most important differences is that the ACE-III does not provide the score of MMSE anymore. Therefore, a short form, the Mini-Addenbrooke's Cognitive Examination (Mini-ACE), was derived from ACE-III [36]. The administration time of ACE-III is 15–20 minutes, whereas Mini-ACE takes about 5 minutes to complete. Mini-ACE consists of only five items (attention: 4 points; memory: 7 points; verbal fluency: 7 points; clock drawing: 5 points; recall: 7 points) with a maximum score of 30. The Mini-ACE can be assessed as a stand-alone screening instrument or as a nested version in the ACE-III. Although several language validations of ACE-III and Mini-ACE exist [37–40], the diagnostic accuracy of ACE-III or Mini-ACE in the diagnosis of PD-MCI and PDD has not been investigated.

In the present study, we aimed to compare the sensitivity and specificity of the different ACE variants available in Hungarian (ACE-I, ACE-III, and Mini-ACE) for detecting mild and major NCD in PD in accordance with the DSM-5 criteria.

2. Materials and Methods

Five hundred and seventy-nine consecutive PD patients were recruited for the study. Patients were treated at the Department of Neurology, University of Pécs. Each patient fulfilled the clinical diagnostic criteria for PD [41] and gave written informed consent according to the approval of the Regional Ethical Board of the University of Pécs.

History of alcoholism, cerebrovascular disease, and other conditions known to impair mental status served as exclusion criteria for participation. Each patient had a routine brain MRI (or brain CT if the MRI examination was contraindicated). Patients with focal abnormalities on neuroimaging studies, abnormalities in thyroid hormone levels, or uncompensated systemic diseases (i.e., diabetes, hypertension, and heart failure) were also excluded. According to the above-mentioned criteria, twenty-seven patients were excluded from the study.

Patients were evaluated using the Hungarian version of Mini-Mental State Examination (MMSE) [42], Addenbrooke Cognitive Examination I (ACE-I) [22] and III (ACE-III), Mini-Addenbrooke Cognitive Examination (Mini-ACE), Montgomery-Asberg Depression Rating Scale (MADRS) [43], and the Lille Apathy Rating Scale (LARS) [44, 45]. The severity of Parkinsonian symptoms was evaluated by the Hoehn-Yahr stage (HYS) [46], the Movement Disorders Society-sponsored Unified Parkinson's Disease Rating Scale (MDS-UPDRS) [47], and the Unified Dyskinesia Rating Scale (UDysRS) [48] if motor complications were present.

Subsequently, PD patients were divided into three groups based on the DSM-5 criteria: patients with major neurocognitive disorder (major NCD group), mild neurocognitive disorder (mild NCD group), and patients without any NCD (normal cognition) [24, 25].

Statistical analysis was performed using *IBM SPSS* (version 19, a SPSS Inc. IBM) and *R for Windows* 3.1.2 statistical software. Because data did not follow a normal distribution, Kruskal-Wallis nonparametric test was applied. Since HY and sex are dichotomous and categorical variables, Pearson's chi-square and Kendall-tau tests were applied to these variables. Receiver operating characteristic curve statistics for MMSE, ACE-I, ACE-III, and Mini ACE were calculated in SPSS software.

3. Results

A total of 27 patients were excluded for the further analyses because of the presence of clinically severe depression and/or anxiety judged by the neuropsychological examination or abnormalities present on the neuroimaging. Out of 552 evaluated PD patients, 277 had normal cognition, 165 had mild NCD, and 110 had major NCD according to DSM-5 classification. Table 1 shows the demographic and clinical characteristics of these groups. Except for levodopa equivalent dose (LED, mg) and sex, all demographic and clinical variables showed significant differences. There were significant differences in the total scores and the subscores of ACE-I, ACE-III, Mini-ACE, and MMSE between normal, mild, and major NCD groups.

Table 2 shows the results of the ROC analysis of detecting mild NCD based on the different levels of education years. According to Youden's index, ACE-III has the best diagnostic accuracy in individuals having 0–8 years of education (sensitivity: 93%; specificity: 64%, area under curve (AUC) area: 73%, cut-off score: 83.5 points) and 9–12 years of education (sensitivity: 80%, specificity: 78%, AUC area: 77%, cut-off score: 85.5 points). However, the Mini-ACE test has the best performance among subjects with >12 years of education (sensitivity: 71%, specificity: 79%, AUC area: 82%, cut-off score: 25.5 points).

For detecting major NCD (Table 3), ACE-III test has a best diagnostic accuracy across all levels of education. Among subjects with 0–8 years of education, its sensitivity and specificity was 80% and 90%, respectively (AUC: 89%, the cut-off score was 70.5 points). In PD patients with 9–12 years of formal education, the specificity and sensitivity of ACE-III was 90% and 74%, respectively (AUC area: 92% and the cut-off score: 77.5 points). In individuals having more than 12 years of education, its sensitivity and sensitivity was 95% and 92%, respectively (AUC: 97%, and the cut-off score: 78.5 points).

4. Discussion

Cognitive impairment influences the quality of life of Parkinson's patients and is detectable in newly diagnosed patients [6, 45, 49]. The diagnosis of PD-MCI is important because it could influence the therapeutic decisions and it also could be the harbinger of PDD [13, 50]. The frequency of PD-MCI and dementia in PD may be about 30% depending on the age, disease duration, and comorbidities. Based on its clinical relevance, it is critical to identify mild and major neurocognitive disorders in PD. Therefore, reliable, valid, and accurate screening tests are warranted in the clinical practice.

The three different variants of the Addenbrooke's Cognitive Examination may help establish the Level-I diagnosis [19]. The ACE test was originally developed for the discrimination of Alzheimer's disease from frontotemporal dementia [26]. Reyes et al. demonstrated 92% sensitivity and 91% specificity of ACE-I (cut-off score: 83) in the detection of dementia of a small number of patients with Parkinson's disease [51]. In a small group of Hungarian subjects with Parkinson's disease, the ACE-I sensitivity and specificity in detecting dementia were 74% and 78.1% with 80 point cut-off score of [22]. Lucza et al. demonstrated 83.5 point cut-off score of ACE-I (sensitivity: 87.1%, specificity: 79.7%) in differentiating mild neurocognitive disorder in PD, and 80.5 points (sensitivity: 86.9%, specificity: 73.7%) in PD with major neurocognitive disorder [24, 25].

The next version of the Addenbrooke's test family, the ACE-R, has never been formally translated and validated in Hungary. Therefore, in this study, we could not evaluate its discriminative capabilities. However, it has been utilized internationally for screening PD-MCI and PDD. The sensitivity and specificity of ACE-R detecting PD-MCI are 69% and 84% with 89 point cut-off score of [52]. ACE-R was also used to differentiate cognitive functions in PD from Parkinsonian syndromes [53]. This study demonstrated the usefulness of verbal fluency subscore in the differential diagnosis of PDD from Parkinsonism. ACE-R has 85.5 point cut-off score (sensitivity: 68%, specificity: 91%) in discriminating PD-MCI from PD with normal cognition and 82.5 points (sensitivity:

Table 1: Demographic and clinical characteristics of Parkinson's disease patients with normal cognition, mild and major neurocognitive disorder.

	Normal cognition ($N = 277$)					Mild neurocognitive disorder ($N = 165$)					Major neurocognitive disorder ($N = 110$)					
	Median	Percentile 25	Percentile 75	Mean	Standard deviation	Median	Percentile 25	Percentile 75	Mean	Standard deviation	Median	Percentile 25	Percentile 75	Mean	Standard deviation	p value
Age	64	56	68	61.80	9.80	69	65	74	68.81	7.73	73	66	78	71.84	7.70	0.000
Education	13	11	16	13.63	2.98	12	11	13	11.97	2.85	11	8	12	11.01	3.39	0.000
Sex (M/F)[a]	157/120					94/71					66/44					0.82
Disease onset	57	48	64	55.36	11.55	61	53	69	61.21	10.73	65	56	74	63.73	12.22	0.000
Disease duration	5	2	9	6.36	6.04	6	2	11	7.57	6.28	6	2	13	8.06	7.06	0.04
MDS UPDRS part1	10	6	15	10.76	6.33	14	9	19	14.44	6.77	19	13	24	18.97	6.65	0.000
MDS UPDRS part2	10	5	17	11.17	7.60	14	9	20	14.75	7.72	20	12	27	19.61	8.82	0.000
MDS UPDRS part3	26	18	35	27.97	13.20	35	27	42	35.63	12.82	47	39	56	48.13	13.45	0.000
MDS UPDRS part4	4	1	5	3.89	3.20	4	2	6	4.30	3.33	4	4	6	5.11	3.27	0.003
Hoehn-Yahr stage[a]	2	2	2	2.25	.72	2	2	3	2.62	.85	3	3	4	3.27	.86	0.000
LED (mg)	480	150	920	616.29	582.09	680	200	1020	732.89	621.08	522	150	950	639.25	556.31	0.091
MADRS total score	8	4	13	8.8	6.3	12	7	17	12.7	6.9	17	12	20	17.0	6.6	0.000
MMSE total score	29	28	30	28.72	1.32	28	26	29	27.41	1.76	25	22	27	24.20	3.12	0.000
ACE-I total score	92	87	95	90.31	5.91	83	77	87	82.26	6.83	69	63	75	68.55	8.79	0.000
ACE-I orientation	10	10	10	9.92	.32	10	10	10	9.76	.63	10	9	10	9.05	1.46	0.000
ACE-I attention	8	8	8	7.83	.53	8	7	8	7.48	.95	7	5	8	6.33	1.73	0.000
ACE-I memory	31	28	33	30.33	4.05	27	22	30	25.96	4.99	19	16	24	19.62	5.39	0.000
ACE-I verbal fluency	11	9	12	10.39	2.05	9	7	10	8.38	2.34	6	4	7	5.53	2.41	0.000

Table 1: Continued.

	Normal cognition (N = 277)					Mild neurocognitive disorder (N = 165)					Major neurocognitive disorder (N = 110)					
	Median	Percentile 25	Percentile 75	Mean	Star dard deviation	Median	Percentile 25	Percentile 75	Mean	Standard deviation	Median	Percentile 25	Percentile 75	Mean	Standard deviation	p value
ACE-I language	28	27	28	27.53	.76	27	27	28	27.04	1.11	26	25	27	25.65	1.94	0.000
ACE-I spatial visual	5	4	5	4.30	.9[illegible]	4	3	5	3.65	1.13	2	1	3	2.37	1.31	0.000
ACE-III total score	91	86	95	90.08	6.0[illegible]	83	77	87	81.92	6.48	68	60	76	66.99	9.91	0.000
ACE-III attention	18	17	18	17.37	1.02	17	16	18	16.63	1.47	14	13	17	14.55	2.46	0.000
ACE-III memory	23	21	25	22.56	3.15	20	17	22	19.44	3.99	14	12	18	14.45	4.53	0.000
ACE-III verbal fluency	11	9	12	10.36	2.09	9	7	10	8.42	2.31	5	4	7	5.40	2.44	0.000
ACE-III language	26	25	26	25.09	1.42	24	23	25	23.88	1.96	22	20	24	21.58	3.08	0.000
ACE-III spatial visual	15	14	16	14.69	1.52	14	12	15	13.55	1.88	11	9	13	11.01	2.73	0.000
Mini-ACE total score	27	25	29	26.4	2.9	23	20	25	22.4	3.4	16	13	19	15.8	4.3	0.000

ACE-I: Addenbrooke's Cognitive Examination version I; ACE-III: Addenbrooke's Cognitive Examination version III; Mini-ACE: Mini Addenbrooke's Cognitive Examination; MMSE: Mini Mental State Examination; MDS UPDRS: Movement Disorders Society Unified Parkinson's Disease Rating Scale (Pearson chi-square and Kendall-tau).

Table 2: Diagnostic accuracy of ACE-I, ACE-III, Mini-ACE, and MMSE for detecting mild neurocognitive disorder in the respect of education years.

Mild neurocognitive disorder		Best cut-off score	Sensitivity	Specificity	Youden's index	Positive likelihood ratio	Negative likelihood ratio	AUC area
ACE-I	0–8	84.5	0.862	0.571	0.433	2.011	0.241	0.713
	9–12	86.5	0.850	0.614	0.464	2.204	0.244	0.787
	>12	90.5	0.847	0.626	0.473	2.263	0.244	0.819
ACE-III	0–8	83.5	0.931	0.643	0.574	2.607	0.107	0.733
	9–12	85.5	0.805	0.786	0.511	2.917	0.477	0.771
	>12	88.5	0.765	0.744	0.509	2.985	0.316	0.838
Mini-ACE	0–8	23.5	0.793	0.714	0.507	2.776	0.290	0.749
	9–12	24.5	0.850	0.514	0.364	1.750	0.292	0.746
	>12	25.5	0.718	0.798	0.516	3.553	0.354	0.820
MMSE	0–8	26.5	0.414	0.857	0.271	2.897	0.684	0.602
	9–12	27.5	0.575	0.743	0.318	2.236	0.572	0.723
	>12	28.5	0.612	0.714	0.326	2.141	0.544	0.696

Table 3: Diagnostic accuracy of ACE-I, ACE-III, Mini-ACE, and MMSE for detecting major neurocognitive disorder in the respect of education years.

Major neurocognitive disorder		Best cut-off score	Sensitivity	Specificity	Youden's index	Positive likelihood ratio	Negative likelihood ratio	AUC area
ACE-I	0–8	74.5	0.821	0.744	0.565	3.207	0.241	0.871
	9–12	76.5	0.848	0.773	0.622	3.743	0.196	0.915
	>12	80.5	0.903	0.927	0.881	13.076	0.050	0.974
ACE-III	0–8	70.5	0.805	0.907	0.702	8.545	0.226	0.895
	9–12	77.5	0.909	0.740	0.649	3.497	0.123	0.926
	>12	78.5	0.957	0.927	0.894	12.439	0.100	0.972
Mini-ACE	0–8	17.5	0.718	0.791	0.509	3.430	0.357	0.833
	9–12	20.5	0.833	0.747	0.580	3.289	0.223	0.894
	>12	21.5	0.907	0.917	0.824	10.884	0.101	0.968
MMSE	0–8	25.5	0.744	0.860	0.604	5.329	0.298	0.866
	9–12	26.5	0.803	0.780	0.583	3.650	0.253	0.868
	>12	27.5	0.814	0.809	0.623	4.262	0.230	0.903

70%, specificity: 73%) in discriminating PD-MCI from PDD in Czech PD population (a sample of 69 persons) [54].

The newest versions of the ACE test batteries, the ACE-III and Mini-ACE, have never been tested previously for the detection of mild and major NCD in PD (PubMed search using the keywords "Parkinson's disease" AND "ACE-III" OR "Parkinson's disease" AND "ACE III", performed on July 29, 2018). In our cohort of patients, ACE-III had better discriminative abilities than ACE-I had. Moreover, ACE-III was also better in screening for mild and major NCD than the MMSE. Generally, the discriminative accuracy of Mini-ACE was between those of ACE and ACE-III with the exception of screening for mild NCD in PD among subjects having > 12 years of formal education.

As far as the authors are aware of, this is the first validation study of ACE-III and Mini-ACE for detecting mild and major NCDs in PD. In the present study, we demonstrated that ACE has an acceptable sensitivity for detecting both mild and major NCD; however, its specificity was below the expectation in the group of patients having low education levels (up to and including 8 years of education). One of the strengths of our study was that we could establish valid and reliable discriminative thresholds for different education levels. Although we have included a large pool of patients with wide age distribution and various disease severity stages to improve the consistency of our data, we are also aware of some limitations. Despite of measuring the MADRS, we did not use these scores for excluding patients with depression.

Because the symptoms of depression are largely overlapping with numerous features of PD (e.g., slowness of thinking, sexual disturbances, and changes in appetite) and many subjects experience nonmotor fluctuations (e.g., having depressed mood or anxiety in OFF state while not having such phenomena in the ON periods), they might have higher MADRS scores without clinically significant depression. Therefore, we decided to exclude only those patients who had severe depression diagnosed by the neuropsychologists ($n = 27$) but not based on the MADRS values alone.

Abbreviations

ACE:	Addenbrooke's Cognitive Examination
AUC:	Area under the curve
Mini-ACE:	Mini Addenbrooke's Cognitive Examination
MMSE:	Mini-Mental State Examination
MADRS:	Montgomery-Asberg Depression Rating Scale
DSM-5:	Diagnostic and Statistical Manual of Mental Disorders 5th edition
LED:	Levodopa equivalent dosage
MCI:	Mild cognitive impairment
NCD:	Neurocognitive disorder
ROC:	Receiver operating characteristic
HYS:	Hoehn-Yahr stage
MDS-UPDRS:	Movement Disorders Society Sponsored version of Unified Parkinson's Disease Rating Scale
PD:	Parkinson's disease
PD-MCI:	Mild cognitive impairment in Parkinson's disease.

Disclosure

ZA received <1000 EUR consultation fees from Hungarian subsidiaries of Novartis, GlaxoSmithKline, UCB, and Teva Pharmaceutical Industries Ltd. MK reported no financial disclosure. AM reported no financial disclosure. MH reported no financial disclosure. AJ reported no financial disclosure. JJ received <1000 EUR consultation fees from Hungarian subsidiaries of UCB, Valeant, and Eisai. SK received <1000 EUR consultation fees from Hungarian subsidiaries of Biogen, TEVA, Astellas, Pfizer, and Novartis. NK received <1000 EUR consultation fees from Hungarian subsidiaries of Medtronic, Boehringer Ingelheim, Novartis, GlaxoSmithKlin, UCB, Krka, and Abbvie. KK reported no financial disclosure.

Authors' Contributions

LT participated in the research project (conception, organization, and execution), statistical analysis (design, execution, and review and critique), and manuscript (writing of the first draft and review and critique). ZA participated in the research project (organization), statistical analysis (review and critique), and manuscript (review and critique). MK participated in the research project (execution), statistical analysis (execution), and manuscript (review and critique). AM participated in the research project (execution), statistical analysis (execution), and manuscript (review and critique). MH participated in the research project (organization), statistical analysis (review and critique), and manuscript (review and critique). SK participated in the research project (organization), statistical analysis (review and critique), and manuscript (review and critique). GD participated in the research project (organization), statistical analysis (review and critique), and manuscript (review and critique). JJ participated in the research project (conception), statistical analysis (review and critique), and manuscript (review and critique). NK participated in the research project (conception), research project (organization), statistical analysis (review and critique), and manuscript (writing of the first draft and review and critique). KD participated in the research project (conception and organization) and manuscript (writing of the first draft and review and critique). KK participated in the research project, statistical analysis, and manuscript.

Acknowledgments

This study was supported by the Hungarian Brain Research Program (2017-1.2.1-NKP-2017-00002, NKFIH EFOP-3.6.2-16-2017-00008, NKFIH SNN125143, and ÚNKP-17-4-I.-PTE-311) government-based funds. Our research was partly financed by the Higher Education Institutional Excellence Program of the Ministry of Human Capacities in Hungary, within the framework of the 5th thematic program of the University of Pécs, Hungary (20765-3/2018/FEKUTSTRAT).

References

[1] A. J. Lees, J. Hardy, and T. Revesz, "Parkinson's disease," *Lancet*, vol. 373, no. 9680, pp. 2055–2066, 2009.

[2] R. F. Pfeiffer, "Non-motor symptoms in Parkinson's disease," *Parkinsonism & Related Disorders*, vol. 22, Supplement 1, pp. S119–S122, 2016.

[3] T. Simuni, C. Caspell-Garcia, C. S. Coffey et al., "Baseline prevalence and longitudinal evolution of non-motor symptoms in early Parkinson's disease: the PPMI cohort," *Journal of Neurology, Neurosurgery, and Psychiatry*, vol. 89, no. 1, pp. 78–88, 2018.

[4] K. R. Chaudhuri, P. Odin, A. Antonini, and P. Martinez-Martin, "Parkinson's disease: the non-motor issues," *Parkinsonism & Related Disorders*, vol. 17, no. 10, pp. 717–723, 2011.

[5] A. A. Kehagia, R. A. Barker, and T. W. Robbins, "Neuropsychological and clinical heterogeneity of cognitive impairment and dementia in patients with Parkinson's disease," *Lancet neurology.*, vol. 9, no. 12, pp. 1200–1213, 2010.

[6] K. Karádi, T. Lucza, Z. Aschermann et al., "Visuospatial impairment in Parkinson's disease: the role of laterality," *Laterality*, vol. 20, no. 1, pp. 112–127, 2014.

[7] W. G. J. Reid, M. A. Hely, J. G. L. Morris, C. Loy, and G. M. Halliday, "Dementia in Parkinson's disease: a 20-year neuro-

psychological study (Sydney multicentre study)," *Journal of Neurology, Neurosurgery, and Psychiatry*, vol. 82, no. 9, pp. 1033–1037, 2011.

[8] M. A. Hely, J. G. L. Morris, W. G. J. Reid, and R. Trafficante, "Sydney multicenter study of Parkinson's disease: non-L-dopa-responsive problems dominate at 15 years," *Movement Disorders*, vol. 20, no. 2, pp. 190–199, 2005.

[9] A. A. Kehagia, R. A. Barker, and T. W. Robbins, "Cognitive impairment in Parkinson's disease: the dual syndrome hypothesis," *Neuro-degenerative Diseases*, vol. 11, no. 2, pp. 79–92, 2013.

[10] J. Blatt, A. Vellage, B. Baier, and N. G. Muller, "The contribution of acetylcholine and dopamine to subprocesses of visual working memory – what patients with amnestic mild cognitive impairment and Parkinson's disease can tell us," *Neuropsychologia*, vol. 61, pp. 89–95, 2014.

[11] I. Litvan, D. Aarsland, C. H. Adler et al., "MDS Task Force on mild cognitive impairment in Parkinson's disease: critical review of PD-MCI," *Movement Disorders*, vol. 26, no. 10, pp. 1814–1824, 2011.

[12] M. Emre, D. Aarsland, R. Brown et al., "Clinical diagnostic criteria for dementia associated with Parkinson's disease," *Movement Disorders*, vol. 22, no. 12, pp. 1689–1707, 2007, quiz 837.

[13] G. Santangelo, C. Vitale, M. Picillo et al., "Mild cognitive impairment in newly diagnosed Parkinson's disease: a longitudinal prospective study," *Parkinsonism & Related Disorders*, vol. 21, no. 10, pp. 1219–1226, 2015.

[14] D. Aarsland, K. Bronnick, C. Williams-Gray et al., "Mild cognitive impairment in Parkinson disease: a multicenter pooled analysis," *Neurology*, vol. 75, no. 12, pp. 1062–1069, 2010.

[15] R. Biundo, L. Weis, S. Facchini et al., "Cognitive profiling of Parkinson disease patients with mild cognitive impairment and dementia," *Parkinsonism & Related Disorders*, vol. 20, no. 4, pp. 394–399, 2014.

[16] E. Mamikonyan, P. J. Moberg, A. Siderowf et al., "Mild cognitive impairment is common in Parkinson's disease patients with normal Mini-Mental State Examination (MMSE) scores," *Parkinsonism & Related Disorders*, vol. 15, no. 3, pp. 226–231, 2009.

[17] A. Robillard, "Clinical diagnosis of dementia," *Alzheimer's & dementia : the journal of the Alzheimer's Association.*, vol. 3, no. 4, pp. 292–298, 2007.

[18] K. S. Santacruz and D. Swagerty, "Early diagnosis of dementia," *American Family Physician*, vol. 63, no. 4, pp. 703–713, 2001.

[19] B. Dubois, D. Burn, C. Goetz et al., "Diagnostic procedures for Parkinson's disease dementia: recommendations from the movement disorder society task force," *Movement Disorders*, vol. 22, no. 16, pp. 2314–2324, 2007.

[20] K. Dujardin, B. Dubois, F. Tison et al., "Parkinson's disease dementia can be easily detected in routine clinical practice," *Movement Disorders*, vol. 25, no. 16, pp. 2769–2776, 2010.

[21] W. Poewe, S. Gauthier, D. Aarsland et al., "Diagnosis and management of Parkinson's disease dementia," *International journal of clinical practice.*, vol. 62, no. 10, pp. 1581–1587, 2008.

[22] B. Kaszás, N. Kovács, I. Balás et al., "Sensitivity and specificity of Addenbrooke's Cognitive Examination, Mattis Dementia Rating Scale, Frontal Assessment Battery and Mini Mental State Examination for diagnosing dementia in Parkinson's disease," *Parkinsonism & Related Disorders*, vol. 18, no. 5, pp. 553–556, 2012.

[23] C. Zadikoff, S. H. Fox, D. F. Tang-Wai et al., "A comparison of the mini mental state exam to the Montreal cognitive assessment in identifying cognitive deficits in Parkinson's disease," *Movement Disorders*, vol. 23, no. 2, pp. 297–299, 2008.

[24] T. Lucza, K. Karádi, J. Kállai et al., "Screening mild and major neurocognitive disorders in Parkinson's disease," *Behavioural Neurology*, vol. 2015, Article ID 983606, 10 pages, 2015.

[25] T. Lucza, K. Karádi, S. Komoly et al., "Neurokognitív zavarok diagnosztizálási és kezelési lehetőségei Parkinson-kórban," *Orvosi Hetilap*, vol. 156, no. 23, pp. 915–926, 2015.

[26] P. S. Mathuranath, P. J. Nestor, G. E. Berrios, W. Rakowicz, and J. R. Hodges, "A brief cognitive test battery to differentiate Alzheimer's disease and frontotemporal dementia," *Neurology*, vol. 55, no. 11, pp. 1613–1620, 2000.

[27] A. Chade, M. Roca, T. Torralva et al., "Detecting cognitive impairment in patients with Parkinson's disease with a brief cognitive screening tool: the Addenbrooke's Cognitive Examination (ACE)," *Dementia & Neuropsychologia*, vol. 2, no. 3, pp. 197–200, 2008.

[28] E. Mioshi, K. Dawson, J. Mitchell, R. Arnold, and J. R. Hodges, "The Addenbrooke's Cognitive Examination Revised (ACE-R): a brief cognitive test battery for dementia screening," *International Journal of Geriatric Psychiatry*, vol. 21, no. 11, pp. 1078–1085, 2006.

[29] V. A. Carvalho and P. Caramelli, "Brazilian adaptation of the Addenbrooke's Cognitive Examination-Revised (ACE-R)," *Dementia & Neuropsychologia*, vol. 1, no. 2, pp. 212–216, 2007.

[30] C. Gonçalves, M. S. Pinho, V. Cruz et al., "The Portuguese version of Addenbrooke's Cognitive Examination-Revised (ACE-R) in the diagnosis of subcortical vascular dementia and Alzheimer's disease," *Aging, Neuropsychology and Cognition*, vol. 22, no. 4, pp. 473–485, 2015.

[31] M. Siciliano, S. Raimo, D. Tufano et al., "The Addenbrooke's Cognitive Examination Revised (ACE-R) and its sub-scores: normative values in an Italian population sample," *Neurological Sciences*, vol. 37, no. 3, pp. 385–392, 2016.

[32] T. Torralva, M. Roca, E. Gleichgerrcht, A. Bonifacio, C. Raimondi, and F. Manes, "Validation of the Spanish version of the Addenbrooke's Cognitive Examination-Revised (ACE-R)," *Neurologia*, vol. 26, no. 6, pp. 351–356, 2011.

[33] H. Yoshida, S. Terada, H. Honda et al., "Validation of the revised Addenbrooke's Cognitive Examination (ACE-R) for detecting mild cognitive impairment and dementia in a Japanese population," *International Psychogeriatrics*, vol. 24, no. 1, pp. 28–37, 2012.

[34] A. J. Larner, "Addenbrooke's Cognitive Examination-Revised (ACE-R) in day-to-day clinical practice," *Age and Ageing*, vol. 36, no. 6, pp. 685-686, 2007.

[35] S. Hsieh, S. Schubert, C. Hoon, E. Mioshi, and J. R. Hodges, "Validation of the Addenbrooke's Cognitive Examination III in frontotemporal dementia and Alzheimer's disease," *Dementia and Geriatric Cognitive Disorders*, vol. 36, no. 3-4, pp. 242–250, 2013.

[36] S. Hsieh, S. McGrory, F. Leslie et al., "The Mini-Addenbrooke's Cognitive Examination: a new assessment tool for dementia,"

Dementia and Geriatric Cognitive Disorders, vol. 39, no. 1-2, pp. 1–11, 2015.

[37] B. Peixoto, M. Machado, P. Rocha et al., "Validation of the Portuguese version of Addenbrooke's Cognitive Examination III in mild cognitive impairment and dementia," *Advances in Clinical and Experimental Medicine*, vol. 27, no. 6, pp. 781–786, 2018.

[38] D. Bruno, A. Slachevsky, N. Fiorentino et al., "Argentinian/Chilean validation of the Spanish-language version of Addenbrooke's Cognitive Examination III for diagnosing dementia," *Neurologia*, 2017.

[39] B. R. Wang, Z. Ou, X. H. Gu, C. S. Wei, J. Xu, and J. Q. Shi, "Validation of the Chinese version of Addenbrooke's Cognitive Examination III for diagnosing dementia," *International Journal of Geriatric Psychiatry*, vol. 32, no. 12, pp. e173–e179, 2017.

[40] J. A. Matias-Guiu, R. Fernández de Bobadilla, G. Escudero et al., "Validation of the Spanish version of Addenbrooke's Cognitive Examination III for diagnosing dementia," *Neurologia*, vol. 30, no. 9, pp. 545–551, 2015.

[41] I. Litvan, K. P. Bhatia, D. J. Burn et al., "Movement Disorders Society Scientific Issues Committee report: SIC Task Force appraisal of clinical diagnostic criteria for Parkinsonian disorders," *Movement Disorders*, vol. 18, no. 5, pp. 467–486, 2003.

[42] A. Egerhazi, "The early diagnosis and differential diagnosis of Alzheimer's disease with clinical methods," *Orvosi Hetilap*, vol. 149, no. 51, pp. 2433–2440, 2008.

[43] S. A. Montgomery and M. Asberg, "A new depression scale designed to be sensitive to change," *The British Journal of Psychiatry*, vol. 134, no. 4, pp. 382–389, 1979.

[44] R. Weintraut, K. Karádi, T. Lucza et al., "Lille Apathy Rating Scale and MDS-UPDRS for screening apathy in Parkinson's disease," *Journal of Parkinsons Disease*, vol. 6, no. 1, pp. 257–265, 2016.

[45] M. Kovacs, A. Makkos, Z. Aschermann et al., "Impact of sex on the nonmotor symptoms and the health-related quality of life in Parkinson's disease," *Parkinson's Disease*, vol. 2016, Article ID 7951840, 12 pages, 2016.

[46] M. M. Hoehn and M. D. Yahr, "Parkinsonism: onset, progression and mortality," *Neurology*, vol. 17, no. 5, pp. 427–442, 1967.

[47] K. Horváth, Z. Aschermann, P. Ács et al., "Validation of the Hungarian MDS-UPDRS: why do we need a new Parkinson scale?," *Ideggyogyaszati szemle*, vol. 67, no. 3-4, pp. 129–134, 2014.

[48] K. Horvath, Z. Aschermann, P. Acs et al., "Az Egységesített Dyskinesia-Pontozóskála magyar nyelvi validációja," *Ideggyogyaszati szemle*, vol. 68, no. 5-6, pp. 183–188, 2015.

[49] M. F. B. Sousa, R. L. Santos, C. Arcoverde et al., "Quality of life in dementia: the role of non-cognitive factors in the ratings of people with dementia and family caregivers," *International Psychogeriatrics*, vol. 25, no. 7, pp. 1097–1105, 2013.

[50] I. Leroi, H. Pantula, K. McDonald, and V. Harbishettar, "Neuropsychiatric symptoms in Parkinson's disease with mild cognitive impairment and dementia," *Parkinson's Disease*, vol. 2012, article 308097, 10 pages, 2012.

[51] M. A. Reyes, S. P. Lloret, E. R. Gerscovich, M. E. Martin, R. Leiguarda, and M. Merello, "Addenbrooke's Cognitive Examination validation in Parkinson's disease," *European Journal of Neurology*, vol. 16, no. 1, pp. 142–147, 2009.

[52] P. McColgan, J. R. Evans, D. P. Breen, S. L. Mason, R. A. Barker, and C. H. Williams-Gray, "Addenbrooke's Cognitive Examination-Revised for mild cognitive impairment in Parkinson's disease," *Movement Disorders*, vol. 27, no. 9, pp. 1173–1177, 2012.

[53] T. Rittman, B. C. Ghosh, P. McColgan et al., "The Addenbrooke's Cognitive Examination for the differential diagnosis and longitudinal assessment of patients with parkinsonian disorders," *Journal of Neurology, Neurosurgery, and Psychiatry*, vol. 84, no. 5, pp. 544–551, 2013.

[54] D. Berankova, E. Janousova, M. Mrackova et al., "Addenbrooke's Cognitive Examination and individual domain cut-off scores for discriminating between different cognitive subtypes of Parkinson's disease," *Parkinson's Disease*, vol. 2015, article 579417, 7 pages, 2015.

13

Ceftriaxone Treatment for Neuronal Deficits: A Histological and MEMRI Study in a Rat Model of Dementia with Lewy Bodies

Ying-Jui Ho,[1] Jun-Cheng Weng,[2,3] Chih-Li Lin,[4] Mei-Shiuan Shen,[1] Hsin-Hua Li,[4] Wen-Chieh Liao,[5,6] Nu-Man Tsai,[7] Ching-Sui Hung,[8] Te-Jen Lai,[9,10] and I-Yen Lee[11]

[1]*Department of Psychology, Chung Shan Medical University Hospital, Chung Shan Medical University, Taichung 402, Taiwan*
[2]*Department of Medical Imaging and Radiological Sciences, Chang Gung University, Taoyuan 33302, Taiwan*
[3]*Department of Psychiatry, Chang Gung Memorial Hospital, Chiayi 613, Taiwan*
[4]*Institute of Medicine, Chung Shan Medical University, Taichung 402, Taiwan*
[5]*Department of Anatomy, Faculty of Medicine, Chung Shan Medical University, Chung Shan Medical University Hospital, Taichung 402, Taiwan*
[6]*Department of Pediatrics, Chung Shan Medical University Hospital, Taichung 402, Taiwan*
[7]*School of Medical Laboratory and Biotechnology, Chung Shan Medical University, Taichung 402, Taiwan*
[8]*Occupational Safety and Health Office, Taipei City Hospital, Taipei 10341, Taiwan*
[9]*Department of Psychiatry, Chung Shan Medical University Hospital, Chung Shan Medical University, Taichung 402, Taiwan*
[10]*Institute of Medicine, Chung Shan Medical University, Taichung 402, Taiwan*
[11]*Division of Urology, Department of Surgery, Tungs' Taichung Metroharbor Hospital, Taichung 43503, Taiwan*

Correspondence should be addressed to Ying-Jui Ho; joshuayjho@gmail.com, Ching-Sui Hung; bessyhung@gmail.com, Te-Jen Lai; tejenlai@hotmail.com, and I-Yen Lee; homer9001065@gmail.com

Academic Editor: Barbara Picconi

Dementia with Lewy bodies (DLB) is characterized by neuronal deficits and α-synuclein inclusions in the brain. Ceftriaxone (CEF), a β-lactam antibiotic, has been suggested as a therapeutic agent in several neurodegenerative disorders for its abilities to counteract glutamate-mediated toxicity and to block α-synuclein polymerization. By using manganese-enhanced magnetic resonance imaging (MEMRI) and immunohistochemistry, we measured the effects of CEF on neuronal activity and α-synuclein accumulation in the brain in a DLB rat model. The data showed that CEF corrected neuronal density and activity in the hippocampal CA1 area, suppressed hyperactivity in the subthalamic nucleus, and reduced α-synuclein accumulation, indicating that CEF is a potential agent in the treatment of DLB.

1. Introduction

Dementia with Lewy bodies (DLB) is a common neurodegenerative dementia, accounting for approximately 10%–25% of the dementia population. DLB patients show progressive cognitive decline and motor dysfunction. Psychiatric symptoms are reported in 99.2% of patients with DLB. DLB patients show higher subscores in the items of delusions, hallucinations, agitation, anxiety, irritation, and aberrant motor behavior, compared to the patients with Parkinson's disease dementia, which seriously affects their quality of life and social activities [1]. There is currently no rat model suitable for searching for more effective medications. In addition to the symptoms of progressive dementia and parkinsonism, accumulation of Lewy bodies in the central nervous system is the hallmark of DLB [2, 3]. Lewy bodies are cytoplasmic eosinophilic protein inclusions of α-synuclein (α-syn) [4–6]. β-Amyloid (Aβ) suppresses the clearance of α-syn [7, 8] and accelerates oligomerization of α-syn and its toxicity, leading to the deterioration caused by α-syn [9]. Moreover, direct or indirect interactions of α-syn and Aβ promote their mutual aggregation and accumulation, disturb the function of mitochondria, cause excessive glutamate release in the synapse, and eventually result in excitotoxicity and cell death in the brain [8]. That is, Aβ aggravates the neurotoxicity of α-syn in the brain [10].

Viral vectors carrying the *SNCA* gene can constantly express α-syn in the host. Some studies have injected these vectors into the hippocampus, cortex, and striatum of rats to model the pathological changes seen in DLB [9, 11]. The advantages of using viral vectors are low cost, fast model establishment, and high expression of genes. Additionally, specific regions of the brain that are of research interest may be targeted [12]. Although viral vectors can deliver specific genes to the brain tissues of the host, the use of the method to transfer genes to larger brain regions, such as the cortex, remains a challenge [13, 14]. In the present study, the α-syn gene vector was injected into the lateral ventricle of rats, which diffused with the flow of the cerebrospinal fluid, facilitated α-syn expression throughout the regions of the brain, and contributed to the establishment of a rat model for DLB.

There is currently no specific medicine for treating DLB. Because of the cognitive dysfunction in patients with DLB, memantine, an antagonist of N-methyl-D-aspartate (NMDA) receptors, is used to alleviate this symptom. This indicates the involvement of glutamatergic hyperactivity in the disease. Rothstein and colleagues found that ceftriaxone (CEF) increases the expression of glutamate transporter-1 (GLT-1), which can remove excessive glutamate released in the synaptic cleft, reduce excitotoxicity, and yield neuroprotective effects [15]. We have demonstrated that CEF treatment prevents the decrease of neuronal activity [16] and loss of neuronal density in the nigrostriatal system and in the hippocampus in a Parkinson's disease (PD) rat model [17, 18]. Moreover, an *in vitro* model of PD revealed that CEF binds with high affinity to α-syn and blocks its polymerization [19].

Manganese-enhanced magnetic resonance imaging (MEMRI) is a valuable imaging tool for directly measuring activity-dependent neuronal events in a living animal [20]. Manganese ion (Mn^{2+}) may enter neurons through voltage-gated calcium (Ca^{2+}) channels [21] where it is retained there with a biological half-life of 51–74 days according to a study of adult rats' brains [22]. Before MR imaging, the animal was injected intraperitoneally (i.p.) with $MnCl_2$, and its neurons took up Mn^{2+} when activated. A quantitative analysis indicated that Mn^{2+} accumulates in neurons according to their activity, because Ca^{2+} elevation is related to the firing activity in excitatory neurons [23]. In addition, its paramagnetic feature enables Mn^{2+} to shorten the longitudinal relaxation time (T1) of water protons and thus enhance the T1-weighted MR signal that is specific to the tissues where Mn^{2+} has accumulated [24], thus rendering it an excellent MRI-detectable contrast agent [25]. Therefore, tissue contrast in Mn^{2+}-induced T1 signal intensity in MEMRI may be contingent upon the differential accumulation of Mn^{2+} in active and silent brain regions in which topography can be absolutely quantified by measuring the absolute T1 (or $R1 = T1^{-1}$) value [23, 26].

When combined with pharmacological manipulation, MEMRI can be used to detect changes in neuronal activities that are produced by the treatment. However, whether changes of neuronal activity are accompanied by a loss of neurons in the DLB rat model remains unclear. The purpose of this study was to elucidate the effects of CEF (100 mg/kg/day) on neuronal density and activity in the brain of the DLB rat model using immunohistochemistry and MEMRI.

2. Materials and Methods

2.1. Animals. Twelve-week-old male Wistar rats (420 ± 30 g; $n = 25$; BioLASCO Taiwan Co Ltd., ROC) were randomly assigned to groups of 3 or 4 and housed in acrylic cages ($35 \times 56 \times 19\ cm^3$) in a temperature-controlled animal room (21–25°C) with free access to food and water. Photoperiods in rodent rooms were controlled using an automatic timer set to provide 12 h of light (from 7:00 to 19:00) and 12 h of dark (from 19:00 to 7:00). To minimize defensive behaviors and stress response to the experimenter, prior to the start of the experiment, all animals were handled for 5 min/day on 2 consecutive days. All experimental procedures were performed according to the NIH Guide for the Care and Use of Laboratory Animals and were approved by the Animal Care Committee of Chung Shan Medical University (IACUC approval number 1455). All efforts were made to minimize animal suffering and to reduce the number of animals used [27].

2.2. General Procedures. For inducing DLB in the rat model, rats were randomly divided into three groups and underwent stereotaxic brain surgery on day 0 as described in our previous reports [8, 27]. Briefly, the rats were anesthetized by an i.p. injection of Zoletil (20 mg/kg; Virbac, Carros, France) and mounted in a stereotaxic frame. To overexpress α-syn, recombinant adeno-associated viral (rAAV) vector containing human α-syn gene, *SNCA*, (10 μg/10 μL/rat) was injected into the left lateral cerebral ventricle using the following coordinates adapted from the rat brain atlas: AP: −0.8 mm, ML: −1.5 mm, and DV: −3.6 mm from the bregma, midline, and skull surface, respectively. The $A\beta_{1-42}$ solution (5 μg/2.5 μL/side × 2 sides/rat) was bilaterally infused in the prefrontal cortex using the following stereotaxic coordinates: AP: 1.6 mm, ML: ±2.0 mm, and DV: −2 mm from the bregma, midline, and skull surface, respectively. During the 5 days after surgery, the rats were housed individually in plastic cages and 10% sucrose solution was provided ad libitum to prevent weight loss after surgery and reduce mortality.

Starting from the next day after the surgery (day 1), the animals received the following treatments: the "sham + saline" group ($n = 5$) and "DLB + saline" group ($n = 7$) were injected with saline (1 mL/kg/day, i.p.), and the "DLB + CEF" group ($n = 6$) was injected with ceftriaxone (CEF) (100 mg/kg/day, i.p.) (Roche, Kaiseraugst, Switzerland) for 27 days.

Hydrated manganese chloride ($MnCl_2 \cdot 4H_2O$, Sigma Aldrich, UK) was dissolved in saline at a concentration of 100 μmol/mL (20 mg/mL). On day 26, all rats received two 1 mL/kg i.p. injections of $MnCl_2$ solution separated by 1 h (total dose 40 mg/kg) [28]. Twenty-four hours later (day 27), when Mn^{2+}-induced signal enhancement reached a stable asymptotic level [28], the rats were transported to the MR center for MR imaging, anesthetized during imaging, and transported back to the animal room.

On day 28, rats were euthanized by exposure to CO_2, transcardially perfused with phosphate-buffered saline (PBS) followed by 4% paraformaldehyde in PBS. The brain was then immediately removed and postfixed in PBS containing 30% sucrose and 4% paraformaldehyde at 4°C until use.

2.3. MEMRI Data Acquisition. Brain images were acquired on a 7T MRI system (Bruker BioSpec, Karlsruhe, Germany), as described in our previous paper [16]. Briefly, rats were initially anesthetized with 5% isoflurane vapor in oxygen at a flow rate of 500 mL/min. T2-weighted contrast of anatomical images was acquired using the turbo rapid acquisition with relaxation enhancement sequence. T1-weighted images were acquired using a multislice spin-echo sequence. To improve detection sensitivity over the full extent of Mn^{2+} concentrations, R1 images were acquired using a rapid acquisition with relaxation enhancement with variable time of repetition. Six sets of images corresponding to six TRs (ranging from 500 to 3500 ms) were taken during the recovery of the longitudinal magnetization to perform R1 mapping. The R1 maps shown in the paper are representations of the distribution of Mn^{2+} uptake in the region of interest (ROI) that were manually defined in the hippocampus and subthalamic nucleus (STN) in the coronal images. The mean signal intensity for all voxels in the ROIs, averaged for both hemispheres, was used to compare R1 differences between the groups.

2.4. Histological Assessment. For histological assessment, frozen coronal sections of the brain (25 μm thick) were cut and mounted on gelatinized slides and maintained in PBS until staining. The regions seen in the stained brain sections were identified according to the rat brain atlas [29] and used for image analysis to measure histological changes, as described previously [17, 28, 30–34]. The ROI was defined in the hippocampus (bregma −2.76 mm to −4.20 mm).

Nissl staining, which is used to identify pyramidal cells in the hippocampus, was performed as described in our previous reports [16, 17, 32]. α-Syn staining was used to evaluate the density of α-syn immune-positive cells in the brain sections [8, 35]. The coronal sections were rinsed (3×5 min each) with 0.05 M Tris buffer (TB), incubated for 20 min at room temperature with 0.3% hydrogen peroxide to block endogenous peroxidase activity, and blocked by incubation for 1 h at room temperature in 100% normal goat serum dissolved in TB containing 10% Triton-100. They were then incubated overnight at 4°C with polyclonal rabbit anti-α-syn antibody (1 : 100; GeneTex, USA) and incubated sequentially for 2 h at room temperature with HRP-conjugated goat anti-rabbit IgG (1 : 200; GeneTex, USA), followed by 5 min at room temperature with 3,3′-diaminobenzidine tetrachloride (DAB; Sigma, USA) before being dehydrated in ethanol and xylene. The stained sections of images were acquired using a microscope (ZEISS AXioskop 2, Germany). The density of neurons and α-syn-positive cells (number/mm^2) in the brain sections were counted using the Image Pro Plus Software 6.0 (Media Cybernetics, CA, USA) as described in our previous paper [16].

2.5. Data Analysis. SPSS 17.0 statistical software was used for data analysis. Analysis of variance (ANOVA) and the least-significant difference (LSD) post hoc test were used to analyze the data. All results are expressed as the mean ± standard error of the mean (SEM). The level of significance was defined as $P < 0.05$.

3. Results

3.1. Image Analysis. One-way ANOVA revealed significant differences in brain MRI images between the groups. Compared with the sham + saline group, the DLB + saline group showed decreased R1, Mn^{2+} uptake level in the hippocampal CA1 area ($F(2,17) = 3.79$, $P = 0.05$) (LSD post hoc test, P value = 0.03). However, normal Mn^{2+} uptake in the hippocampal CA1 area was seen after CEF treatment because no difference between the sham + saline and DLB + CEF groups was found (Figure 1). One-way ANOVA revealed significant differences in STN MRI images between the groups ($F(2,17) = 5.57$, $P = 0.016$). The LSD post hoc test revealed a higher Mn^{2+} uptake and neuronal activity in the DLB + saline group, compared with the sham + saline group ($P < 0.05$). The rats receiving CEF treatment showed the same neural activity in the STN as did the controls (Figure 2).

3.2. Histological Assay

3.2.1. Density of Pyramidal Neurons in the Hippocampal CA1. The ANOVA revealed that density of pyramidal neurons in the hippocampal CA1 showed a significant difference ($F(2,14) = 56.69$, $P < 0.001$), and post hoc analysis showed that rats in the DLB + saline group had a significantly lower neuronal density than did those in the sham + saline group ($P < 0.001$). The DLB + CEF group showed a higher neuronal density than the DLB + saline group ($P < 0.001$) (Figure 3).

3.2.2. Density of α-Syn in the Dentate Gyrus. The ANOVA revealed significant differences in the density of α-syn-positive cells in the hippocampal dentate gyrus (DG) ($F(2,14) = 3.91$, $P < 0.05$) (partial eta squared = 0.638), and post hoc analysis showed that rats in the DLB + saline group (152 ± 56 number/mm^2) had a significantly higher density of α-syn-positive cells compared with the sham + saline group (23 ± 10 number/mm^2) ($P < 0.05$). The DLB + CEF group (90 ± 32 number/mm^2) showed no difference in the density of α-syn-positive cells compared with the sham + saline group (Figure 4).

4. Discussion

In the DLB rat model, we found an accumulation of α-syn in the hippocampal DG and lowered neuronal density and activity in the hippocampal CA1 of the DLB + saline group compared with the sham + saline group. In addition, hyperactivity in the STN was also observed in DLB + saline rats. Treatment with CEF at a dose of 100 mg/kg corrected these

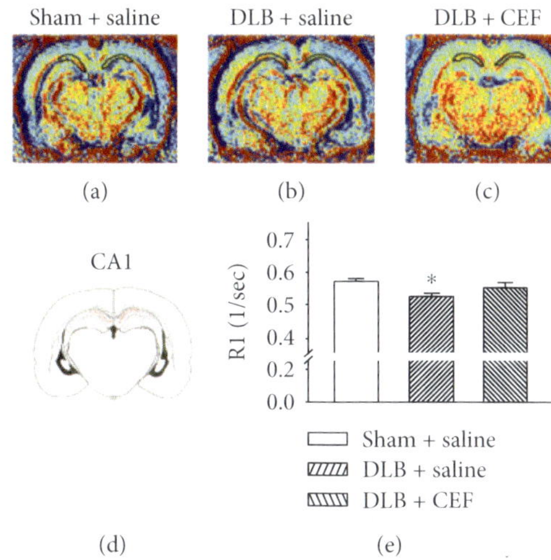

FIGURE 1: Effect of treatment with ceftriaxone (CEF) on neuronal activity in the hippocampal CA1 area of the DLB rat model. The rats were bilaterally infused with $A\beta_{1-42}$ in the prefrontal cortex and unilaterally infused with viral vectors with the *SNCA* gene in the left lateral ventricle to model DLB in rats. The sham + saline group and DLB + saline group were injected with saline (1 mL/kg/day, i.p.), and the DLB + CEF group was injected with CEF (100 mg/kg/day, i.p.) for 27 days. (a–c) Coronal R1 maps of the rat brain. The regions of interest used for quantitative analysis of Mn^{2+}-induced signal enhancement in the hippocampal CA1 area are indicated by the outlines on the schematic (d). (e) Quantitative results. Data are expressed as the mean ± SEM. $^{*}P < 0.05$, compared with the sham + saline group.

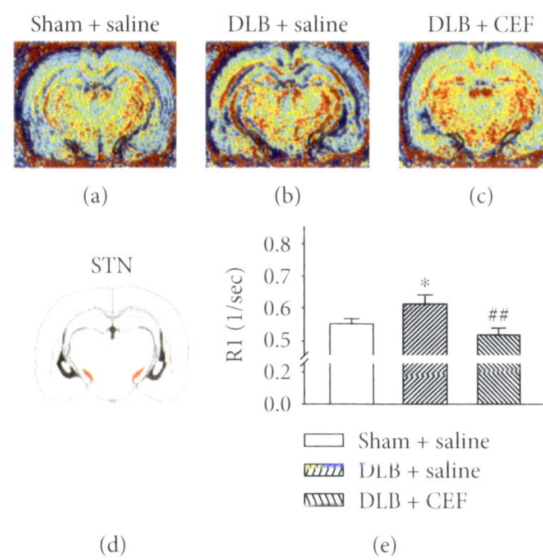

FIGURE 2: Effect of treatment with ceftriaxone (CEF) on neuronal activity in the subthalamic nucleus (STN) in the DLB rat model. The group names are the same as those in Figure 1. (a–c) Coronal R1 maps of the rat brain. The regions of interest used for quantitative analysis of Mn^{2+}-induced signal enhancement in the STN are indicated by the outlines on the schematic (d). (e) Quantitative results. Data are expressed as the mean ± SEM. $^{*}P < 0.05$, compared with the sham + saline group; $^{\#\#}P < 0.01$, compared with the DLB + saline group.

neuronal deficits. CEF was previously found to increase GLT-1 expression, resulting in sequestration of excess synaptic glutamate and protection of hippocampal neurons from excitotoxicity [36]. It has been reported that treatment with CEF prevented neurodegeneration in the hippocampus and nigrostriatal system, increasing neuronal activity [16] and improving cognitive function in an MPTP-induced PD rat model [17, 18]. We have previously reported that CEF, at the dosages of 100 and 200 mg/kg, per se did not affect motor function, cognitive behavior, and neuronal density in the hippocampus in healthy rats [17]. These results suggest that CEF can prevent DLB-related neuronal deficits in the brain.

The present study revealed that the injection of $A\beta$ and viral vectors with the *SNCA* gene into the brain caused an accumulation of α-syn, neuronal loss, and lowered neuronal activity in the hippocampus, suggesting that this method can induce a useful model of DLB. The pathophysiology of DLB is related to the aggregation of Lewy bodies and Lewy neurites that are formed by α-syn accumulation [37, 38], resulting in neurotoxicity and cell loss in the limbic system, brainstem, and cortical regions [5, 39, 40]. Although α-syn accumulation is the core pathological feature of DLB, the deposition of extracellular $A\beta$ is also observed in the brains of up to 80% of DLB patients [7]. Direct and indirect

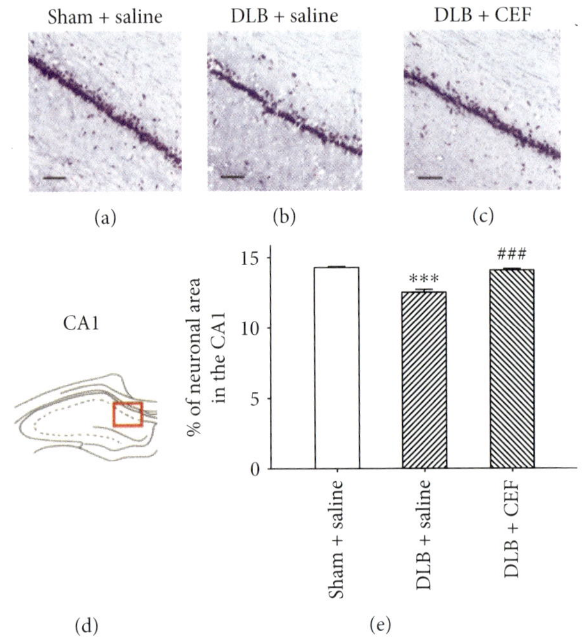

Figure 3: Effect of ceftriaxone (CEF) on the neuronal density in the hippocampal CA1 area of DLB rats. The treatment and group names are the same as those in Figure 1. (a–c) Coronal brain sections of the hippocampal CA1 area; pyramidal cells are revealed through Nissl staining. Magnification, 200x; bar, 100 μm. (d) CA1 region of the hippocampus. (e) Quantitative results. Data are expressed as mean ± SEM. $^{***}P < 0.001$, compared with the sham + saline group; $^{\#\#\#}P < 0.001$, compared with the DLB + saline group.

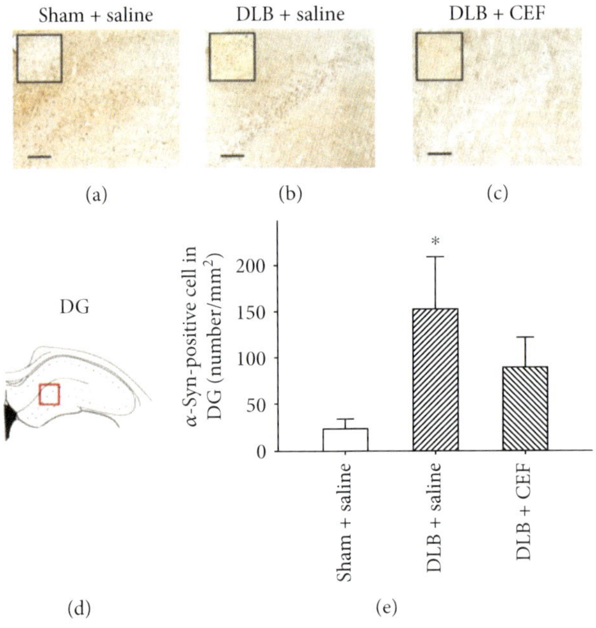

Figure 4: Effect of ceftriaxone (CEF) on the density of α-synuclein- (α-syn-) positive cells in the DG of DLB rats. The treatment and group names are the same as those in Figure 1. (a–c) Coronal sections in the DG. α-Syn-positive cells are indicated by anti-α-syn labeling in representative coronal sections. Magnification, 200x; bar, 100 μm. High magnification images (1000x) of α-syn-positive cells are shown in the insets. (d) The DG of the hippocampus. (e) Quantitative results. Data are expressed as the mean ± SEM. $^{*}P < 0.05$, compared with the sham + saline group.

interaction between α-syn and Aβ has been reported to promote α-syn aggregation [8]. Aβ increases the toxicity of α-syn [8] and aggravates the relevant defects triggered by α-syn, causing neurodegeneration [41]. Thus, in addition to injecting the α-syn gene vector into the rat's lateral ventricle, Aβ was also injected into the bilateral prefrontal cortex to more accurately model the pathological characteristics of DLB. In this study, the α-syn gene vector was injected into the lateral ventricle of rats, which diffused with the flow of the cerebrospinal fluid and facilitated the expression of

α-syn throughout the regions of the brain. A high level of α-syn accumulation was observed in the hippocampal DG area of DLB + saline rats, which may be involved in lower density of pyramidal neurons in the hippocampal CA1 because the abnormal accumulation of α-syn in the limbic system leads to cell loss and dysfunction in the hippocampus [42]. Reportedly, CEF binds to α-syn [19] and may thus block polymerization of α-syn and exert neuroprotective effects *in vitro* [19], which may underlie the effects of CEF on reducing α-syn accumulation and restoring neuronal density and activity in the hippocampus of DLB rats. The subject number in the study is relatively small. The level of α-syn in the DG of the hippocampus in the DLB + CEF group may be only partially reversed. To increase statistical power and to provide convincing treatment effect, further study using a larger number of subject is needed.

Aβ oligomers have been reported to play a pivotal role in synaptic impairment and neuronal degeneration [43]. Based on this amyloid hypothesis, the formation of soluble species of Aβ can directly interfere with memory formation and cause synaptic degradation, excitotoxicity, and cell death [44], leading to cognitive decline. Glutamate is one of the main excitatory neurotransmitters in the central nervous system, is involved in synaptic plasticity, memory, and learning, and plays a substantial role in the pathogenesis from the early stages of neurodegenerative diseases. To bind Aβ peptides, NMDA receptors have attracted considerable interest because of their toxic effects and involvement in neurodegeneration [45]. Aβ oligomers interfere with glutamatergic transmission. Under pathological conditions, elevation of Aβ levels blocks glutamate uptake at the synaptic cleft, leading to increased glutamate levels, stimulation of NMDA receptors [46], and activation of extrasynaptic NR2B-enriched NMDA receptors [45], causing an increase of intracellular calcium levels and the activation of metabolic pathways responsible for neuronal shrinkage, synaptic loss, and neurodegeneration [47]. Moreover, Aβ oligomers form complexes with alpha7-nicotinic receptors at presynaptic sites, causing increased levels of glutamate release, and they are involved in synaptic plasticity [48]. These factors indicate that Aβ is responsible for impairments of synaptic plasticity, cell loss, and neuronal death.

Glutamatergic hyperactivity can cause neurodegeneration [49, 50] and may thus be involved in the parkinsonism of DLB. STN neurons express glutamate, innervate the substantia nigra (SNc), and are hyperactivated in PD. Modulation of STN activity by deep brain stimulation improves parkinsonism, indicating that STN hyperactivity is associated with the development of parkinsonian features [51, 52]. STN hyperactivation increases glutamate release, causing excitotoxicity of dopaminergic neurons in the SNc [53]. In the present MEMRI-based study, we observed hyperactivity in the STN in the DLB + saline rats and found that this change was prevented with CEF treatment. This was consistent with our previous findings that CEF prevents dopaminergic and hippocampal degeneration in a PD rat model [17, 18]. We therefore suggest that CEF treatment reduced STN hyperactivity by increasing GLT-1 expression and glutamate reuptake and thus blocked neurodegeneration in the DLB rat model.

The risk of developing dementia in patients with DLB may increase with hippocampal cell loss, because the decline in cognitive function is associated with hippocampal degeneration [54]. Since that hippocampal CA1 is reported to be involved in working memory and cognition [55] and that neurogenesis is observed in the DG [56], dysfunction of the hippocampus may result in impairments of memory and recognition [57, 58]. The hippocampus shows vulnerability of excitotoxic damage due to rich of glutamatergic synapses [36]; excessive glutamate release and excitotoxicity-induced neurodegeneration in this region may lead to memory and recognition impairment, as seen in patients with DLB. The present study revealed hippocampal lesions in the CA1 of DLB rats, which was accompanied by lowered neuronal activity, as measured using MEMRI. Our another study found impairments in cognitive behaviors, for example, object recognition and avoidance learning, in the DLB rats, where deficits were improved after CEF treatment. (Data have been submitted for publication.) Regarding the clinical features of patients with DLB, in addition to cognitive dysfunction, motor impairment is also observed. However, in the experiment, the DLB rats did not exhibit motor dysfunction (data not shown). According to the "1-year rule," the consensus guidelines to distinguish DLB and PD dementia [59], if cognitive impairment occurs within 1 year following the onset of motor impairment or if cognitive impairment occurs earlier than motor impairment, DLB is diagnosed. Lack of motor impairment in the present study may be due to the short experimental period (only 28 days). The present histological findings showing increased α-syn-positive cells in the hippocampus of DLB rats are in line with that α-syn pathologies observed in the hippocampus of patients with DLB, which is associated with memory impairment [60]. Furthermore, increasing evidence supports that α-syn aggregates may be the real culprit, causing deficits in neurotransmission and neurogenesis in the hippocampus, which is considered to be involved in mechanisms for the hippocampal dysfunctions and associated neuropsychiatric manifestations in synucleinopathy [61]. CEF treatment prevented decreased neuronal density and activity in the area, indicating that CEF may have the potential for treating neurodegeneration and dementia in patients with DLB [17].

Increase of GLT-1 expression may be involved in the CEF-induced prevention of the loss of neuronal function in DLB rats. Excessive release of glutamate and hyperactivity of the glutamatergic system play a critical role in neuronal and behavioral symptoms in neurodegenerative diseases [62, 63]. GLT-1 is responsible for glutamate clearance [64–67] and thus prevents glutamate excitotoxicity [68–70]. In previous studies [17, 18], we found that CEF treatment caused a dose-dependent increase in GLT-1 expression in the brain, had a neuroprotective effect in the hippocampus and nigrostriatal dopaminergic system, and improved cognitive function. We thus suggest that upregulation of GLT-1 and reduction of excitotoxicity may underlie the neuronal protective effect of CEF. Further studies are needed to elucidate the downstream molecular pathway of CEF that modulates glutamate transmission and their neuroprotective effects.

MEMRI data associated with Mn^{2+} uptake are used to quantitatively evaluate neural activity, where R1 value represents the accumulation of Mn^{2+} in neurons [23]. Consistently, our data showed that MEMRI R1 values in the hippocampus reflect cell loss in the DLB rats and treatment effects of CEF against the disease [16]. Higher neuronal activities in the STN of the DLB + saline group indicated similar clinical and pathological characteristics associated with parkinsonism and neurodegeneration [71]. Elevation of STN activities (i.e., a burst pattern of neuronal firing) is also observed in patients with PD [72]. Our previous study found a significant positive correlation between MEMRI R1 and neuronal density in the hippocampus [16], indicating that R1 values in the hippocampus may serve as an indicator of neuronal density of the hippocampus in the DLB rat model. Although the present data revealed hippocampal lesions with abnormal neuronal activity 4 weeks after the surgery, it would be of interest to measure the changes long after the surgery, which would provide evidence to elucidate whether the DLB rat model shares the same progressive features as in patients with DLB.

In conclusion, the results demonstrated that CEF treatment prevented the loss of neuronal density and activity in the hippocampus and also normalized the hyperactivity of the STN in the DLB rat model. Treatment with CEF prevented the accumulation of α-syn in the hippocampus. Moreover, the MEMRI R1 value may serve as a suitable indicator for DLB severity and treatment effect. Our data provide support for the use of CEF as a potential therapeutic agent to prevent dementia in patients with DLB.

Disclosure

Some of the data in this paper have been presented as conference posters.

Acknowledgments

This work was supported by grants from the Ministry of Science and Technology (106-2410-H-040-003-MY2, 104-2923-H-040-001-MY3, 104-2314-B-040-007-MY2, 104-2628-E-040-001-MY2, 106-2320-B-040-021-MY3, and 104-2628-E-182-004-MY2), Chung Shan Medical University Hospital (CSH-2017-C-007), Taipei City Government, Taiwan (10501-62-046). The authors appreciate Dr. Pai-Yi Chiu's contribution of critical review of this paper. Microscopy and cryosectioning were performed in the Instrument Center of Chung Shan Medical University, which is supported by the MOST, Ministry of Education, and Chung Shan Medical University. The authors appreciate the full support from the Instrumentation Center and Department of Electrical Engineering, National Taiwan University, Taiwan.

References

[1] P. Y. Chiu, C. T. Tsai, P. K. Chen, W. J. Chen, and T. J. Lai, "Neuropsychiatric symptoms in Parkinson's disease dementia are more similar to Alzheimer's disease than dementia with Lewy bodies: a case-control study," *PLoS One*, vol. 11, no. 4, article e0153989, 2016.

[2] H. Oda, Y. Yamamoto, and K. Maeda, "Neuropsychological profile of dementia with Lewy bodies," *Psychogeriatrics*, vol. 9, no. 2, pp. 85–90, 2009.

[3] J. Macijauskienė and V. Lesauskaitė, "Dementia with Lewy bodies: the principles of diagnostics, treatment, and management," *Medicina*, vol. 48, no. 1, pp. 1–8, 2012.

[4] M. G. Spillantini, R. A. Crowther, R. Jakes, M. Hasegawa, and M. Goedert, "α-Synuclein in filamentous inclusions of Lewy bodies from Parkinson's disease and dementia with Lewy bodies," *Proceedings of the National Academy of Sciences of the United States of America*, vol. 95, no. 11, pp. 6469–6473, 1998.

[5] W. S. Kim, K. Kågedal, and G. M. Halliday, "Alpha-synuclein biology in Lewy body diseases," *Alzheimer's Research & Therapy*, vol. 6, no. 5-8, p. 73, 2014.

[6] K. Beyer, M. Domingo-Sabat, and A. Ariza, "Molecular pathology of Lewy body diseases," *International Journal of Molecular Sciences*, vol. 10, no. 3, pp. 724–745, 2009.

[7] S. E. Marsh and M. Blurton-Jones, "Examining the mechanisms that link β-amyloid and α-synuclein pathologies," *Alzheimer's Research & Therapy*, vol. 4, no. 2, p. 11, 2012.

[8] C.-L. Lin, Y.-S. Cheng, H.-H. Li et al., "Amyloid-β suppresses AMP-activated protein kinase (AMPK) signaling and contributes to α-synuclein-induced cytotoxicity," *Experimental Neurology*, vol. 275, Part 1, pp. 84–98, 2016.

[9] C. R. Overk, A. Cartier, G. Shaked et al., "Hippocampal neuronal cells that accumulate α-synuclein fragments are more vulnerable to Aβ oligomer toxicity via mGluR5 – implications for dementia with Lewy bodies," *Molecular Neurodegeneration*, vol. 9, no. 1, p. 18, 2014.

[10] C.-C. Chang, H.-H. Li, Y.-T. Chang et al., "Aβ exacerbates α-synuclein-induced neurotoxicity through impaired insulin signaling in α-synuclein-overexpressed human SK-N-MC neuronal cells," *CNS Neuroscience & Therapeutics*, vol. 24, no. 1, pp. 47–57, 2018.

[11] Y. Lim, V. M. Kehm, E. B. Lee et al., "α-Syn suppression reverses synaptic and memory defects in a mouse model of dementia with Lewy bodies," *Journal of Neuroscience*, vol. 31, no. 27, pp. 10076–10087, 2011.

[12] H. Mochizuki, M. Yamada, and Y. Mizuno, "α-Synuclein overexpression model," *Journal of Neural Transmission Supplementa*, vol. 70, pp. 281–284, 2006.

[13] P. Aldrin-Kirk, M. Davidsson, S. Holmqvist, J. Y. Li, and T. Björklund, "Novel AAV-based rat model of forebrain synucleinopathy shows extensive pathologies and progressive loss of cholinergic interneurons," *PLoS One*, vol. 9, no. 7, article e100869, 2014.

[14] M. F. Chesselet, "In vivo alpha-synuclein overexpression in rodents a useful model of Parkinson's disease," *Experimental Neurology*, vol. 209, no. 1, pp. 22–27, 2008.

[15] J. D. Rothstein, S. Patel, M. R. Regan et al., "β-Lactam antibiotics offer neuroprotection by increasing glutamate transporter expression," *Nature*, vol. 433, no. 7021, pp. 73–77, 2005.

[16] J. C. Weng, M. A. Tikhonova, J. H. Chen et al., "Ceftriaxone prevents the neurodegeneration and decreased neurogenesis seen in a Parkinson' disease rat model: an immunohistochemical and MRI study," *Behavioural Brain Research*, vol. 305, pp. 126–139, 2016.

[17] C. Y. Hsu, C. S. Hung, H. M. Chang, W. C. Liao, S. C. Ho, and Y. J. Ho, "Ceftriaxone prevents and reverses behavioral and neuronal deficits in an MPTP-induced animal model of Parkinson's disease dementia," *Neuropharmacology*, vol. 91, pp. 43–56, 2015.

[18] S. C. Ho, C. C. Hsu, C. R. Pawlak et al., "Effects of ceftriaxone on the behavioral and neuronal changes in an MPTP-induced Parkinson's disease rat model," *Behavioural Brain Research*, vol. 268, pp. 177–184, 2014.

[19] P. Ruzza, G. Siligardi, R. Hussain et al., "Ceftriaxone blocks the polymerization of α-synuclein and exerts neuroprotective effects in vitro," *ACS Chemical Neuroscience*, vol. 5, no. 1, pp. 30–38, 2013.

[20] Y. J. Lin and A. P. Koretsky, "Manganese ion enhances T1-weighted MRI during brain activation: an approach to direct imaging of brain function," *Magnetic Resonance in Medicine*, vol. 38, no. 3, pp. 378–388, 1997.

[21] A. Takeda, "Manganese action in brain function," *Brain Research Reviews*, vol. 41, no. 1, pp. 79–87, 2003.

[22] A. Takeda, J. Sawashita, and S. Okada, "Biological half-lives of zinc and manganese in rat brain," *Brain Research*, vol. 695, no. 1, pp. 53–58, 1995.

[23] S. Kikuta, Y. Nakamura, Y. Yamamura et al., "Quantitative activation-induced manganese-enhanced MRI reveals severity of Parkinson's disease in mice," *Scientific Reports*, vol. 5, no. 1, article 12800, 2015.

[24] O. Eschenko, S. Canals, I. Simanova, M. Beyerlein, Y. Murayama, and N. K. Logothetis, "Mapping of functional brain activity in freely behaving rats during voluntary running using manganese-enhanced MRI: implication for longitudinal studies," *NeuroImage*, vol. 49, no. 3, pp. 2544–2555, 2010.

[25] A. C. Silva and N. A. Bock, "Manganese-enhanced MRI: an exceptional tool in translational neuroimaging," *Schizophrenia Bulletin*, vol. 34, no. 4, pp. 595–604, 2008.

[26] J. C. Weng, J. H. Chen, P. F. Yang, and W. Y. I. Tseng, "Functional mapping of rat barrel activation following whisker stimulation using activity-induced manganese-dependent contrast," *NeuroImage*, vol. 36, no. 4, pp. 1179–1188, 2007.

[27] M. J. Castelhano-Carlos and V. Baumans, "The impact of light, noise, cage cleaning and in-house transport on welfare and stress of laboratory rats," *Laboratory Animals*, vol. 43, no. 4, pp. 311–327, 2009.

[28] S. J. Jackson, R. Hussey, M. A. Jansen et al., "Manganese-enhanced magnetic resonance imaging (MEMRI) of rat brain after systemic administration of $MnCl_2$: hippocampal signal enhancement without disruption of hippocampus-dependent behavior," *Behavioural Brain Research*, vol. 216, no. 1, pp. 293–300, 2011.

[29] G. Paxinos and C. Watson, *The Rat Brain in Stereotaxic Coordinates*, Academic Press, London, 2nd edition, 1986.

[30] A. L. Wang, Y. M. Liou, C. R. Pawlak, and Y. J. Ho, "Involvement of NMDA receptors in both MPTP-induced neuroinflammation and deficits in episodic-like memory in Wistar rats," *Behavioural Brain Research*, vol. 208, no. 1, pp. 38–46, 2010.

[31] H. N. Sy, S. L. Wu, W. F. Wang et al., "MPTP-induced dopaminergic degeneration and deficits in object recognition in rats are accompanied by neuroinflammation in the hippocampus," *Pharmacology, Biochemistry, and Behavior*, vol. 95, no. 2, pp. 158–165, 2010.

[32] M. H. Hsieh, S. C. Ho, K. Y. Yeh et al., "Blockade of metabotropic glutamate receptors inhibits cognition and neurodegeneration in an MPTP-induced Parkinson's disease rat model," *Pharmacology, Biochemistry, and Behavior*, vol. 102, no. 1, pp. 64–71, 2012.

[33] M. H. Hsieh, S. L. Gu, S. C. Ho et al., "Effects of MK-801 on recognition and neurodegeneration in an MPTP-induced Parkinson's rat model," *Behavioural Brain Research*, vol. 229, no. 1, pp. 41–47, 2012.

[34] M. A. Tikhonova, S. C. Ho, A. A. Akopyan et al., "Neuroprotective effects of ceftriaxone treatment on cognitive and neuronal deficits in a rat model of accelerated senescence," *Behavioural Brain Research*, vol. 330, pp. 8–16, 2017.

[35] L.-K. Song, K.-L. Ma, Y.-H. Yuan et al., "Targeted overexpression of α-synuclein by rAAV2/1 vectors induces progressive nigrostriatal degeneration and increases vulnerability to MPTP in mouse," *PLoS One*, vol. 10, no. 6, article e0131281, 2015.

[36] S. K. Hota, K. Barhwal, K. Ray, S. B. Singh, and G. Ilavazhagan, "Ceftriaxone rescues hippocampal neurons from excitotoxicity and enhances memory retrieval in chronic hypobaric hypoxia," *Neurobiology of Learning and Memory*, vol. 89, no. 4, pp. 522–532, 2008.

[37] B. C. V. Campbell, Q.-X. Li, J. G. Culvenor et al., "Accumulation of insoluble α-synuclein in dementia with Lewy bodies," *Neurobiology of Disease*, vol. 7, no. 3, pp. 192–200, 2000.

[38] W. J. Schulz-Schaeffer, "The synaptic pathology of alpha-synuclein aggregation in dementia with Lewy bodies, Parkinson's disease and Parkinson's disease dementia," *Acta Neuropathologica*, vol. 120, no. 2, pp. 131–143, 2010.

[39] J. Burre, M. Sharma, and T. C. Sudhof, "Definition of a molecular pathway mediating α-synuclein neurotoxicity," *Journal of Neuroscience*, vol. 35, no. 13, pp. 5221–5232, 2015.

[40] M. Ingelsson, "Alpha-synuclein oligomers neurotoxic molecules in Parkinson's disease and other Lewy body disorders," *Frontiers in Neuroscience*, vol. 10, p. 408, 2016.

[41] M. Colom-Cadena, E. Gelpi, S. Charif et al., "Confluence of α-synuclein, tau, and β-amyloid pathologies in dementia with Lewy bodies," *Journal of Neuropathology & Experimental Neurology*, vol. 72, no. 12, pp. 1203–1212, 2013.

[42] E. Iseki, N. Takayama, W. Marui, K. Uéda, and K. Kosaka, "Relationship in the formation process between neurofibrillary tangles and Lewy bodies in the hippocampus of dementia with Lewy bodies brains," *Journal of the Neurological Sciences*, vol. 195, no. 1, pp. 85–91, 2002.

[43] Z. Esposito, L. Belli, S. Toniolo, G. Sancesario, C. Bianconi, and A. Martorana, "Amyloid β, glutamate, excitotoxicity in Alzheimer's disease: are we on the right track?," *CNS Neuroscience & Therapeutics*, vol. 19, no. 8, pp. 549–555, 2013.

[44] D. J. Selkoe, "Soluble oligomers of the amyloid beta-protein impair synaptic plasticity and behavior," *Behavioural Brain Research*, vol. 192, no. 1, pp. 106–113, 2008.

[45] G. Rammes, A. Hasenjäger, K. Sroka-Saidi, J. M. Deussing, and C. G. Parsons, "Therapeutic significance of NR2B-containing NMDA receptors and mGluR5 metabotropic glutamate receptors in mediating the synaptotoxic effects of β-amyloid

oligomers on long-term potentiation (LTP) in murine hippocampal slices," *Neuropharmacology*, vol. 60, no. 6, pp. 982-990, 2011.

[46] L. Texidó, M. Martín-Satué, E. Alberdi, C. Solsona, and C. Matute, "Amyloid β peptide oligomers directly activate NMDA receptors," *Cell Calcium*, vol. 49, no. 3, pp. 184–190, 2011.

[47] W. Danysz and C. G. Parsons, "Alzheimer's disease, β-amyloid, glutamate, NMDA receptors and memantine - searching for the connections," *British Journal of Pharmacology*, vol. 167, no. 2, pp. 324-352, 2012.

[48] R. Gray, A. S. Rajan, K. A. Radcliffe, M. Yakehiro, and J. A. Dani, "Hippocampal synaptic transmission enhanced by low concentrations of nicotine," *Nature*, vol. 383, no. 6602, pp. 713–716, 1996.

[49] R. Lee Mosley, E. J. Benner, I. Kadiu et al., "Neuroinflammation, oxidative stress, and the pathogenesis of Parkinson's disease," *Clinical Neuroscience Research*, vol. 6, no. 5, pp. 261–281, 2006.

[50] A. Plaitakis and P. Shashidharan, "Glutamate transport and metabolism in dopaminergic neurons of substantia nigra: implications for the pathogenesis of Parkinson's disease," *Journal of Neurology*, vol. 247, Supplement 2, pp. II25–II35, 2000.

[51] P. Limousin, P. Krack, P. Pollak et al., "Electrical stimulation of the subthalamic nucleus in advanced Parkinson's disease," *New England Journal of Medicine*, vol. 339, no. 16, pp. 1105–1111, 1998.

[52] L. Capus, A. Melatini, M. Zorzon et al., "Chronic bilateral electrical stimulation of the subthalamic nucleus for the treatment of advanced Parkinson's disease," *Neurological Sciences*, vol. 22, no. 1, pp. 57-58, 2001.

[53] M. Luquin, L. Saldise, J. Guillen et al., "Does increased excitatory drive from the subthalamic nucleus contribute to dopaminergic neuronal death in Parkinson's disease?," *Experimental Neurology*, vol. 201, no. 2, pp. 407–415, 2006.

[54] H. Hall, S. Reyes, N. Landeck et al., "Hippocampal Lewy pathology and cholinergic dysfunction are associated with dementia in Parkinson's disease," *Brain*, vol. 137, no. 9, pp. 2493–2508, 2014.

[55] M. R. Hunsaker, J. A. Thorup, T. Welch, and R. P. Kesner, "The role of CA3 and CA1 in the acquisition of an object-trace-place paired-associate task," *Behavioral Neuroscience*, vol. 120, no. 6, pp. 1252–6, 2006.

[56] H. A. Cameron and R. D. G. Mckay, "Adult neurogenesis produces a large pool of new granule cells in the dentate gyrus," *The Journal of Comparative Neurology*, vol. 435, no. 4, pp. 406–417, 2001.

[57] W. N. Zhang, H. H. J. Pothuizen, J. Feldon, and J. N. P. Rawlins, "Dissociation of function within the hippocampus: effects of dorsal, ventral and complete excitotoxic hippocampal lesions on spatial navigation," *Neuroscience*, vol. 127, no. 2, pp. 289–300, 2004.

[58] N. J. Broadbent, L. R. Squire, and R. E. Clark, "Spatial memory, recognition memory, and the hippocampus," *Proceedings of the National Academy of Sciences of the United States of America*, vol. 101, no. 40, pp. 14515–14520, 2004.

[59] I. G. McKeith, D. W. Dickson, J. Lowe et al., "Diagnosis and management of dementia with Lewy bodies: third report of the DLB consortium," *Neurology*, vol. 65, no. 12, pp. 1863–1872, 2005.

[60] D. H. Adamowicz, S. Roy, D. P. Salmon et al., "Hippocampal α-synuclein in dementia with Lewy bodies contributes to memory impairment and is consistent with spread of pathology," *The Journal of Neuroscience*, vol. 37, no. 7, pp. 1675–1684, 2017.

[61] W. Yang and S. Yu, "Synucleinopathies: common features and hippocampal manifestations," *Cellular and Molecular Life Sciences*, vol. 74, no. 8, pp. 1485–1501, 2017.

[62] G. Battaglia, C. L. Busceti, G. Molinaro et al., "Endogenous activation of mGlu5 metabotropic glutamate receptors contributes to the development of nigro-striatal damage induced by 1-methyl-4-phenyl-1,2,3,6-tetrahydropyridine in mice," *The Journal of Neuroscience*, vol. 24, no. 4, pp. 828–835, 2004.

[63] L. Chen, J. Liu, U. Ali et al., "Blockade of mGluR5 reverses abnormal firing of subthalamic nucleus neurons in 6-hydroxydopamine partially lesioned rats," *The Chinese journal of physiology*, vol. 54, no. 5, pp. 303–309, 2011.

[64] N. J. Maragakis, J. Dietrich, V. Wong et al., "Glutamate transporter expression and function in human glial progenitors," *Glia*, vol. 45, no. 2, pp. 133–143, 2004.

[65] A. Furuta, J. D. Rothstein, and L. J. Martin, "Glutamate transporter protein subtypes are expressed differentially during rat CNS development," *The Journal of Neuroscience*, vol. 17, no. 21, pp. 8363–8375, 1997.

[66] O. Bar-Peled, H. Ben-Hur, A. Biegon et al., "Distribution of glutamate transporter subtypes during human brain development," *Journal of Neurochemistry*, vol. 69, no. 6, pp. 2571–2580, 1997.

[67] K. Kim, S. G. Lee, T. P. Kegelman et al., "Role of excitatory amino acid transporter-2 (EAAT2) and glutamate in neurodegeneration: opportunities for developing novel therapeutics," *Journal of Cellular Physiology*, vol. 226, no. 10, pp. 2484–2493, 2011.

[68] J. D. Rothstein, M. Dykes-Hoberg, C. A. Pardo et al., "Knockout of glutamate transporters reveals a major role for astroglial transport in excitotoxicity and clearance of glutamate," *Neuron*, vol. 16, no. 3, pp. 675–686, 1996.

[69] Y. Kanai and M. A. Hediger, "The glutamate and neutral amino acid transporter family: physiological and pharmacological implications," *European Journal of Pharmacology*, vol. 479, no. 1–3, pp. 237–247, 2003.

[70] S. S. Huang, J. He, D. M. Zhao, X. Y. Xu, H. P. Tan, and H. Li, "Effects of mutant huntingtin on mGluR5-mediated dual signaling pathways: implications for therapeutic interventions," *Cellular and Molecular Neurobiology*, vol. 30, no. 7, pp. 1107–1115, 2010.

[71] D. Neef and A. D. Walling, "Dementia with Lewy bodies: an emerging disease," *American Family Physician*, vol. 73, no. 7, pp. 1223–1229, 2006.

[72] S.-T. Tsai, W.-Y. Chuang, C.-C. Kuo et al., "Dorsolateral subthalamic neuronal activity enhanced by median nerve stimulation characterizes Parkinson's disease during deep brain stimulation with general anesthesia," *Journal of Neurosurgery*, vol. 123, no. 6, pp. 1394–1400, 2015.

14

Altered Small-World Networks in First-Episode Schizophrenia Patients during Cool Executive Function Task

Zongya Zhao, [1,2] **Yaqing Cheng**, [3] **Zhenxin Li**, [1,2] **and Yi Yu** [1,2]

[1] *School of Biomedical Engineering, Xinxiang Medical University, Xinxiang 453003, China*
[2] *Key Lab of Neurosense and Control, Xinxiang Medical University, Xinxiang 453003, China*
[3] *Department of Computer Technology, Henan Information Engineering School, Zhengzhou 450000, China*

Correspondence should be addressed to Zongya Zhao; zhaozongya_paper@126.com and Yi Yu; 203691831@qq.com

Academic Editor: Fabio M. Macciardi

At present, little is known about brain functional connectivity and its small-world topologic properties in first-episode schizophrenia (SZ) patients during cool executive function task. In this paper, the Trail Making Test-B (TMT-B) task was used to evaluate the cool executive function of first-episode SZ patients and electroencephalography (EEG) data were recorded from 14 first-episode SZ patients and 14 healthy controls during this cool executive function task. Brain functional connectivity between all pairs of EEG channels was constructed based on mutual information (MI) analysis. The constructed brain functional networks were filtered by three thresholding schemes: absolute threshold, mean degree, and a novel data-driven scheme based on orthogonal minimal spanning trees (OMST), and graph theory was then used to study the topographical characteristics of the filtered brain graphs. Results indicated that the graph theoretical measures of the theta band showed obvious difference between SZ patients and healthy controls. In the theta band, the characteristic path length was significantly longer and the cluster coefficient was significantly smaller in the SZ patients for a wide range of absolute threshold T. However, the cluster coefficient showed no significant changes, and the characteristic path length was still significantly longer in SZ patients when calculated as a function of mean degree K. Interestingly, we also found that only the characteristic path length was significantly longer in SZ patients compared with healthy controls after using the OMST scheme. Pearson correlation analysis showed that the characteristic path length was positively correlated with executive time of TMT-B for the combined SZ patients and healthy controls ($r = 0.507$, $P = 0.006$), but not for SZ patients alone ($r = 0.072$, $P = 0.612$). The above results suggested a less optimal organization of the brain network and could be useful for understanding the pathophysiologic mechanisms underlying cool executive dysfunction in first-episode SZ patients.

1. Introduction

Schizophrenia (SZ), one of the most serious mental disorders, usually causes many aspects of cognitive dysfunction, including memory, attention, and executive function [1]. And executive dysfunction is considered to be one of the most critical cognitive dysfunctions [2]. Generally, executive function is involved in a range of higher-level cognitive processes including anticipation, goal selection, planning, behavior's choice, inhibition, self-control, and self-monitoring [3, 4]. At present, a large number of studies have shown that patients with schizophrenia are accompanied by severe executive dysfunction [5–8].

It has been demonstrated that the cognitive dysfunction or other symptoms of SZ can be interpreted in terms of altered brain functional connectivity among different brain regions [9]. A large number of electroencephalography (EEG) and functional magnetic resonance imaging (fMRI) studies have confirmed dysfunctional connectivity in SZ patients [10–16]. Among the usually applied methods to study functional connectivity, such as coherence and correlation coefficient, mutual information (MI) has been widely applied in many studies to investigate the information communication and connectivity among different brain regions [11, 17, 18]. MI is based on information theory [19] and can be used to measure the amount of information that can be obtained about one variable from the measurement of another. Different from the traditional correlation coefficient which only measures linear dependence between time series, MI takes account of both linear and nonlinear dependencies, which makes MI a superior method for studying dynamical coupling or information transmission between EEG data. Some researchers tried to use MI to study schizophrenia, but the results do not seem consistent [11, 17, 20].

In recent years, graph theory analysis has been widely applied to study the topologic characteristics of brain functional networks. Previous studies have implied that the small-world network is considered to be one of the most appropriate models to balance local segregation and integration in the human brain [21, 22]. The small-world network is characterized by a higher cluster coefficient compared to a random network and a shorter path length compared to a regular network, which allows for more efficient information transfer among distant brain regions. Previous EEG studies have indicated that SZ patients showed a disrupted small-world network in the rest state [23, 24], during working memory task [25–27], during oddball paradigm task [28, 29], and in processing local contextual information [30]. For example, Shim et al. [28] found that reduced cluster coefficients and increased path lengths appeared in SZ patients during an oddball task. Therefore, we hypothesized that the disrupted small-world network would also appear in SZ patients during a cool executive function task.

Because executive function impairment is considered to be one of the most critical cognitive dysfunctions, it is of importance to investigate the brain functional networks in SZ patients during an executive function task. Zelazo and Müller [31] divided executive function into cool executive function and hot executive function. The hot executive function is related to emotional involvement and needs flexible evaluation about the emotional significance of the stimulus, whereas the cool executive function is unrelated to emotional involvement and often caused by decontextualized tasks, because the cool executive function is not involved in emotional arousal and clinical observations have shown that emotional reactions of SZ patients usually do not match their inner experience [32]. At present, some cool executive function tasks including Trail Making Test-A (TMT-A) and Trail Making Test-B (TMT-B) have been applied to evaluate the cool executive function of schizophrenia patients [33, 34]. However, little is known about the brain functional connectivity and its small-world topologic properties in first-episode schizophrenia patients during a cool executive function task.

By taking all these considerations into account, the aim of the present study was to combine functional connectivity based on MI with graph theory analysis to investigate the brain functional network in first-episode SZ patients during a cool executive function task. In this paper, the functional connectivity matrixes were constructed by using MI analysis between all pairs of EEG channels in different frequency bands. Then, the constructed brain functional networks were filtered by three thresholding schemes: absolute threshold, mean degree, and a novel data-driven scheme based on orthogonal minimal spanning trees (OMST), and graph theoretical measures were calculated. The differences between SZ patients and healthy controls were evaluated by statistical analysis. Finally, Pearson's correlation was used to evaluate the relationship between cluster coefficient C or path length L and task performance.

2. Materials and Methods

2.1. Subjects. 14 first-episode SZ patients (9 male and 5 female) were recruited from the Henan Psychiatric Hospital of China according to the Structured Clinical Interview for DSM-IV, and any patients with a history of medication treatment, drug abuse/dependence, electroconvulsive therapy, or other psychiatric and neurological diseases were excluded. The mean age of the 14 SZ patients was 28.21 ± 6.94 years, the mean duration of illness was 18.26 ± 7.03 months, and all patients are right-handed. For healthy controls, a group of 14 subjects matched for sex, age, and dominant side was recruited (9 male and 5 female; mean age: 25.13 ± 3.75; all right-handed), and any healthy controls with a past or current psychiatric illness, drug dependence, neurological disorders, or severe somatic diseases were excluded. The study was approved by the ethics committee of Henan Psychiatric Hospital of China, and an informed consent form was signed by all participants before the experiment.

2.2. EEG Recordings and MI Computation. The EEG data were recorded from all participants when they were performing a cool executive function task, that is, the TMT-B task. As for the TMT-B task that evaluates quick visual search, visual space sorting, and cognitive set transfer functions, the participants were asked to connect numbers (1–13) and letters (A–M) using a pen on a paper according to an alternating sequence as fast as possible, and the pen tip cannot leave the paper during this process. The execution time to complete this task and the error number that is the number of incorrectly linked numbers and letters were used to evaluate the task performance of the participants.

The EEG data were recorded at a sampling rate of 1000 Hz from 24 channels (FP1, FPz, FP2, AF3, AF4, F7, F5, F3, F1, Fz, F2, F4, F6, F8, T7, C3, C4, T8, P7, P3, P4, P8, O1, and O2) that were mounted on the scalp with a 64-channel EEG cap according to the 10-20 standard system. And the impedance of all electrodes was below 10 kΩ.

Offline EEG preprocessing was carried out by using Matlab 7.7.0 R2010a software (Mathworks Inc., USA) equipped with the EEGLAB toolbox [35]. Firstly, a 0.5–30 Hz zero-phase bandpass filter was applied. Then, ocular and prominent muscle artifacts were removed by means of independent component analysis (ICA), and the average number of artifactual independent components was 3.1 $\pm$ 0.8 (mean $\pm$ std) and 3.4 $\pm$ 0.7 (mean $\pm$ std) for healthy controls and SZ patients, respectively. Subsequently, the EEG data were divided into 10-second epochs and recomputed against the average reference. Finally, the following 4 frequency bands were obtained using a zero-phase bandpass filter: delta (0.5–3 Hz), theta (4–7 Hz), alpha (8–13 Hz), and beta (13–30 Hz).

MI is based on information theory and can be used to measure the amount of information that can be obtained about one variable from the measurement of another. The main advantage of MI is that it takes account of both linear and nonlinear dependencies. The detailed calculation method of MI was described in some previously published literature [11, 17, 18, 36]. Briefly, given two random variables X and Y, the pairwise MI is defined as

$$\mathrm{MI}(X,Y)=\sum_{x,y}P_{XY}(x,y)\log_2\frac{P_{XY}(x,y)}{P_X(x)P_Y(y)}, \quad (1)$$

where $P_X(x)$ is the probability that x is drawn from X and $P_{XY}(x,y)$ is the joint probability density function for the measurements of X and Y that produce the values x and y.

MI is estimated from a finite number of samples, and the probability densities, $P_X(x)$ and $P_{XY}(x,y)$, are approximated by histogram (using bin size of 100). For a fair comparison across subjects and frequency bands, here we computed the normalized MI as

$$\text{Normalized MI}(X,Y)=\frac{MI(X,Y)}{H(X)+H(Y)}, \quad (2)$$

where $H(X)$ and $H(X)$ are the entropies and $H(X)$ is defined as $\sum_x P_X(x)\log_2 P_X(x)$. The normalized MI is in the range of [0, 1]. Here, the data are separated into 10-second epochs for MI computation in order to increase the sample size as well as to enhance the stationarity and consistency of the MI computation.

MI between all pairs of EEG channels was computed, resulting in a 24×24 matrix (24 is the number of EEG channels). For each epoch, the MI matrix was computed, and an average MI matrix for each subject was obtained by averaging the MI matrixes calculated from all epochs. According to the above process, the MI matrixes for the above-mentioned four frequency bands (delta: 0.5–3 Hz, theta: 4–7 Hz, alpha: 8–13 Hz, and beta: 13–30 Hz) were computed.

2.3. Graph Theoretical Analysis. In this paper, the MI matrix was converted into an undirected binary graph by applying three network filtering schemes: absolute threshold T, mean degree K, and OMST method. Because there is no optimal way to select T, here the range of $0.15 < T < 0.45$ (in step of 0.005) was selected for the four bands. It is well-known that the edge number in a graph has a great relationship with the values of L and C, and the edge number in the 2 graphs (SZ patients and healthy controls) will be different by applying a certain T. Therefore, in order to eliminate this effect, the L and C were calculated as a function of degree K ($2 < K < 8$, in step of 0.1).

Recently, Dimitriadis et al. [37, 38] proposed a novel data-driven topological filtering scheme based on OMST, which filters brain connectivity networks based on the optimization between the global efficiency of the network and the cost preserving its wiring. Here, we tried using the OMST method to filter the constructed brain networks and recomputed graph theoretical measures. After the MI matrix was converted into an undirected binary graph, the graph theoretical measures, such as characteristic path length L and cluster coefficient C, were computed. Detailed descriptions and calculation methods for L and C could be found in some previously published literature [39, 40].

The small-world network is characterized by a similar path length and higher cluster coefficient compared to a random network, that is, $\gamma = C_{\mathrm{real}}/C_{\mathrm{random}} > 1$, $\lambda = L_{\mathrm{real}}/L_{\mathrm{random}} \approx 1$. And the small-world index could be defined as $\sigma = \gamma/\lambda$. For the small-world network, the σ is greater than 1. Here, in order to compute small-world indexes of experimental networks (SZ patients and healthy controls), after applying the OMST filtering scheme, 300 random networks were generated for each experimental network by using the Markov-chain algorithm [41, 42]. As a result, the mean small-world index σ of experimental networks (SZ patients and healthy controls) was computed.

2.4. Statistical Analysis. All statistical analyses were carried out using SPSS version 21.0 software (SPSS Inc., Chicago, IL). The Shapiro-Wilk test was used to test for normality of distribution. Task performance, such as execution time and error number, was statistically compared between SZ patients and healthy controls by using independent sample t-test. The differences of C and L between SZ patients and healthy controls for each value over a range of T or degree K were compared by using the Mann–Whitney U test. In addition, Pearson correlation analysis was applied to explore whether there existed correlation between C or L and task performance. $P < 0.05$ showed that a significant difference existed.

3. Results

The mean executive times of the TMT-B task for SZ patients and healthy controls were 123.85 ± 27.11 s and 75.93 ± 17.79 s, respectively. Independent sample t-test was used to analyze their statistical difference, and results indicated that the mean executive time of SZ patients was significantly longer than that of healthy controls ($P = 0.000$). The mean error numbers during TMT-B for SZ patients and healthy controls were 1.46 ± 1.98 and 0.31 ± 0.84, respectively, and statistical analysis implied that the mean error number of SZ patients was significantly larger than that of healthy controls ($P = 0.001$). We believed that the above behavioral results were mainly due to the cool executive dysfunction of SZ patients.

Figure 1 showed the computed mean cluster coefficient C and characteristic path length L for SZ patients and healthy controls as a function of threshold T in the delta band (Figure 1(a)), theta band (Figure 1(b)), alpha band (Figure 1(c)), and beta band (Figure 1(d)). In all frequency bands, it was found that the mean cluster coefficient C decreased almost linearly with the increase of T. This was because more and more connectivity between the nodes in the graph was lost when threshold T increased. In addition, when T values were small, the characteristic path length L increased almost linearly with the increase of T, and this was because more and more connectivity between the nodes

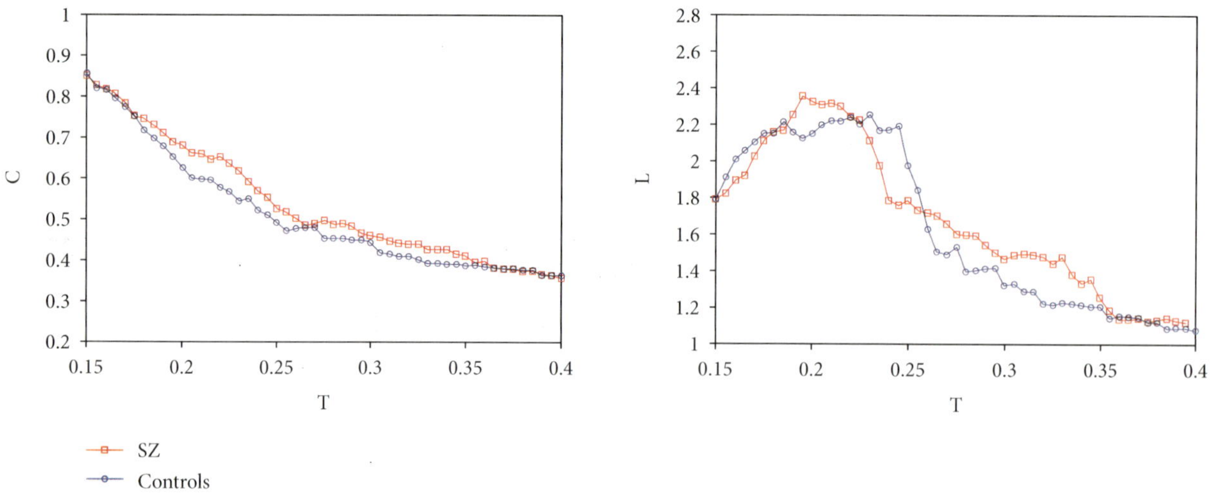

(a) Delta band

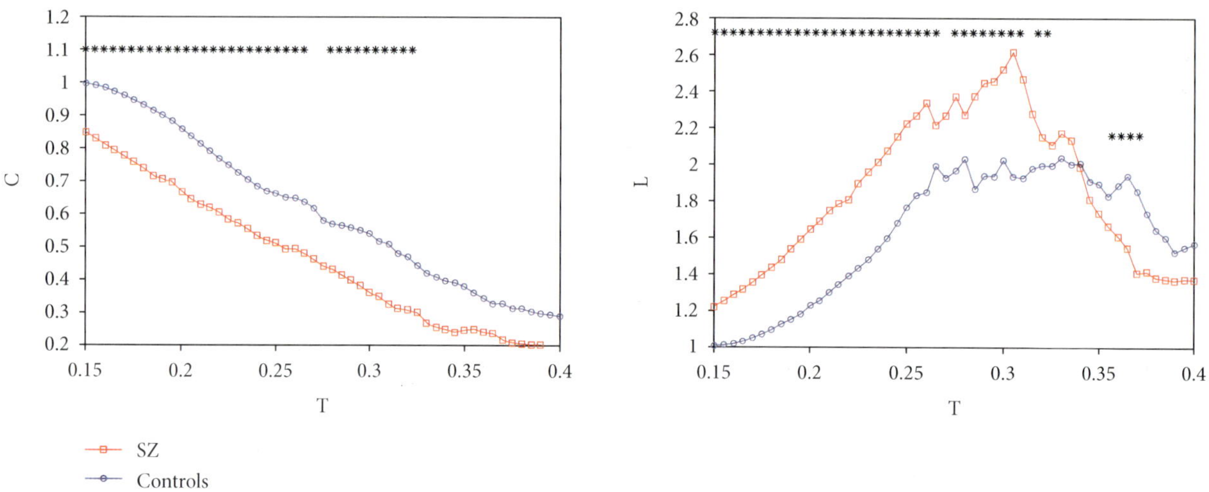

(b) Theta band

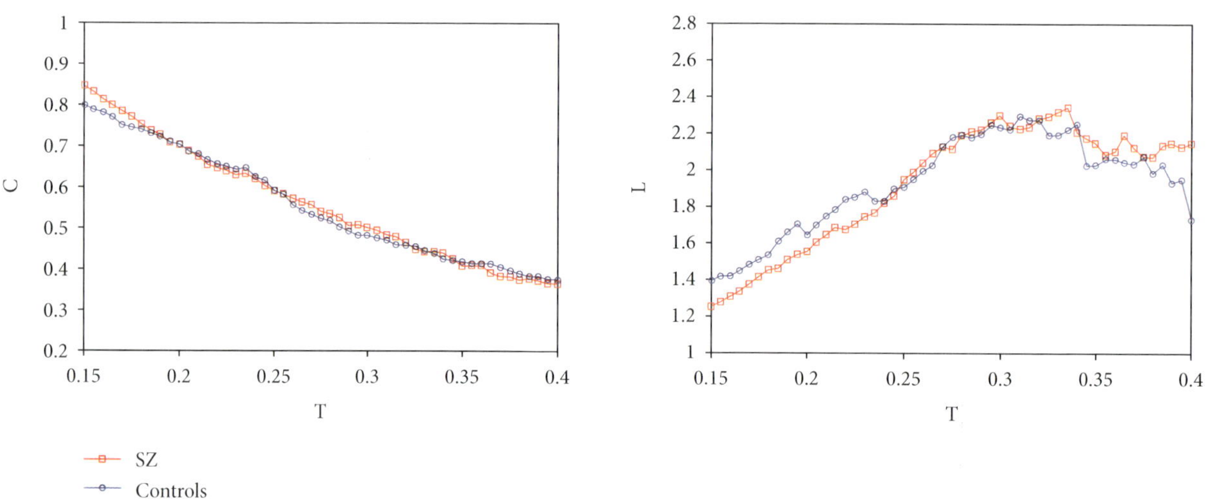

(c) Alpha band

Figure 1: Continued.

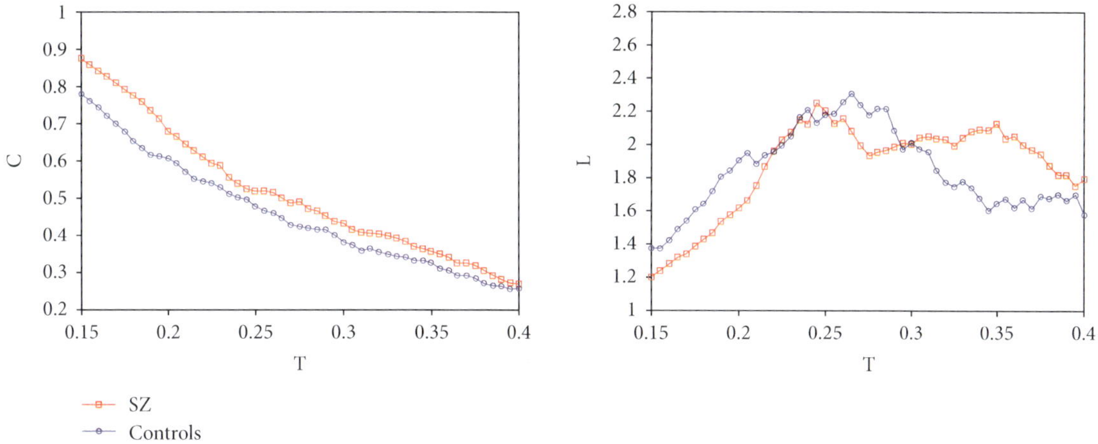

(d) Beta band

Figure 1: Mean cluster coefficient C and characteristic path length L for SZ patients (square) and healthy controls (circle) as a function of T in the delta band (a), theta band (b), alpha band (c), and beta band (d). The asterisks showed significant difference between SZ patients and healthy controls ($P < 0.05$).

dropped out when threshold T increased, which increased the average path length between randomly selected nodes. When the threshold T reached a certain value, the characteristic path length L started to decrease. This phenomenon could be explained by the fact that the graph was divided into more than 2 subgraphs when T further increased and the resulted subgraphs were smaller than the original graph, which led to the decrease of mean L.

As shown in Figures 1(a), 1(c), and 1(d), there existed no significant difference between SZ patients and healthy controls for C and L in the delta, alpha, and beta bands in the range of $0.15 < T < 0.45$ (in step of 0.005). As indicated in Figure 1(b), for a wide range of T ($0.15 < T < 3.3$), there always existed significant differences between SZ patients and healthy controls for C and L in the theta band. And the most significant difference for C and L occurred at $T = 0.195$ (Mann–Whitney U test, $U = 40.000$, $W = 145.000$, $P = 0.008$) and 0.305 (Mann–Whitney U test, $U = 27.000$, $W = 132.000$, $P = 0.001$), respectively.

As shown in Figure 2, the mean cluster coefficient C and characteristic path length L for SZ patients and healthy controls were computed as a function of degree K in the delta band (Figure 2(a)), theta band (Figure 2(b)), alpha band (Figure 2(c)), and beta band (Figure 2(d)). For all frequency bands, it was found that the mean cluster coefficient C increased almost linearly with the increase of K. For the delta (Figure 2(a)), alpha (Figure 2(c)), and beta (Figure 2(d)) bands, there was no significant difference between SZ patients and healthy controls for C and L. As shown in Figure 2(b), there existed significant difference for L between SZ patients and healthy controls for wide ranges of $2.2 < K < 2.8$ and $4.0 < K < 5.8$ ($P < 0.05$), and the most significant difference occurred at $K = 4.1$ (Mann–Whitney U test, $U = 37.000$, $W = 142.000$, $P = 0.005$). However, there was no significant difference for C between SZ patients and healthy controls for the whole range of K.

The above two network thresholding schemes (absolute threshold and mean degree) are arbitrary thresholding schemes that might add bias for group and task comparisons and reduce the possibility of the reproducibility of the findings across studies from different research groups. So recently, Dimitriadis et al. [37, 38] proposed a novel data-driven topological filtering scheme based on OMST, which filters brain connectivity networks based on the optimization between the global efficiency of the network and the cost preserving its wiring. Here, the graph theoretical measures were recomputed by applying the OMST filtering scheme. As shown in Figure 3, the mean cluster coefficient C (Figure 3(a)) and characteristic path length L (Figure 3(b)) for SZ patients and healthy controls were computed based on the OMST scheme in the four bands. It is obvious that there was no significant difference for C between SZ patients and healthy controls in the four bands. However, significant difference existed only in the theta band for L between SZ patients and healthy controls (Mann–Whitney U test, $U = 30.500$, $W = 135.500$, $P = 0.002$), which was consistent with that of the mean degree K scheme (Figure 2(b)).

The small-world index could be defined as $\sigma = \gamma/\lambda$, where $\gamma = C_{\text{real}}/C_{\text{random}}$ and $\lambda = L_{\text{real}}/L_{\text{random}}$. After applying the OMST filtering scheme for experimental networks (SZ patients and healthy controls), 300 random networks were generated for each experimental network by using the Markov-chain algorithm [41, 42], and the corresponding γ, λ, and σ were computed. Results indicated that the small-world indexes of SZ patients and healthy controls were 3.148 ± 1.263 and 2.892 ± 1.475, respectively, and the small-world indexes of both groups were greater than 1, indicating that both groups had small-world network characteristics during the TMT-B task. However, it was found that there was no significant difference for the small-world index between the two groups (Mann–Whitney U test, $U = 64.000$, $W = 169.000$, $P = 0.118$).

Pearson correlation analysis was applied to explore whether there existed correlation between C or L and the task performance (executive time). As indicated in Figure 4(a), the correlation coefficient between executive time and C

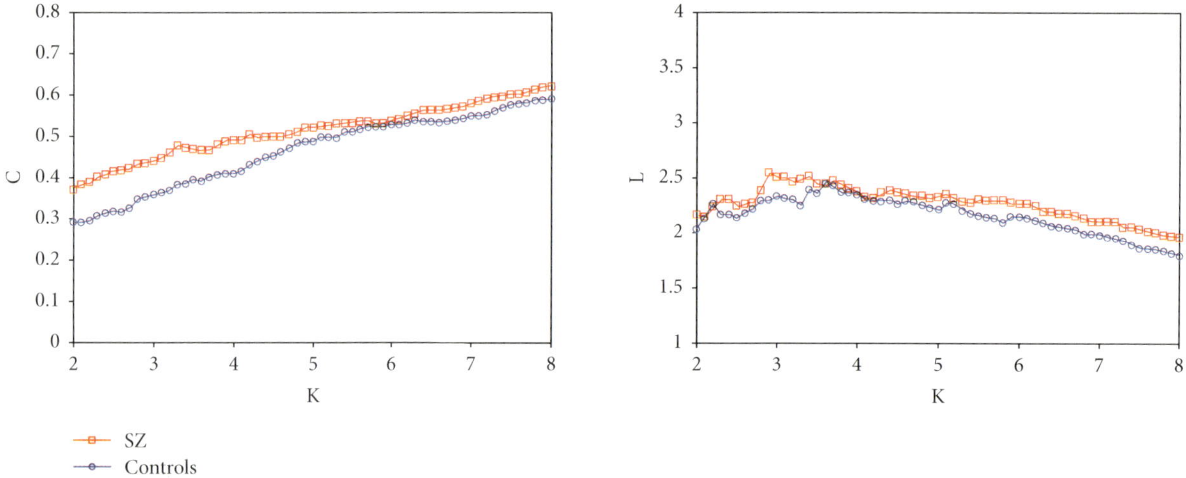

(a) Delta band

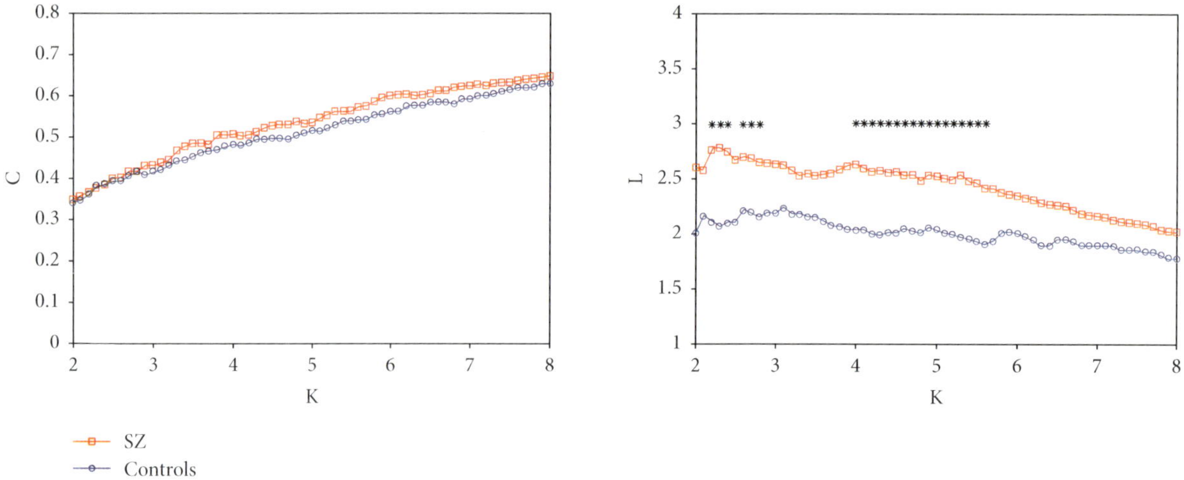

(b) Theta band

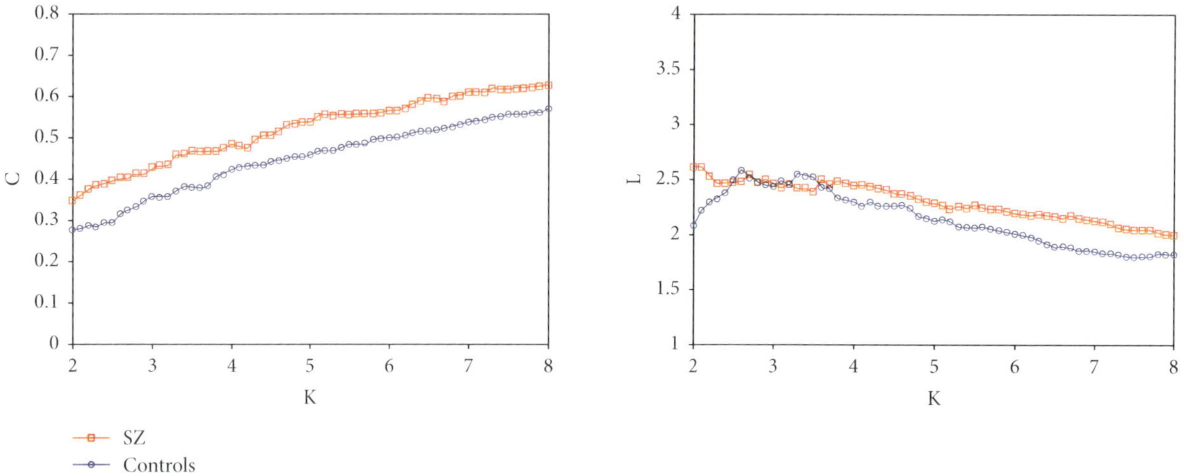

(c) Alpha band

Figure 2: Continued.

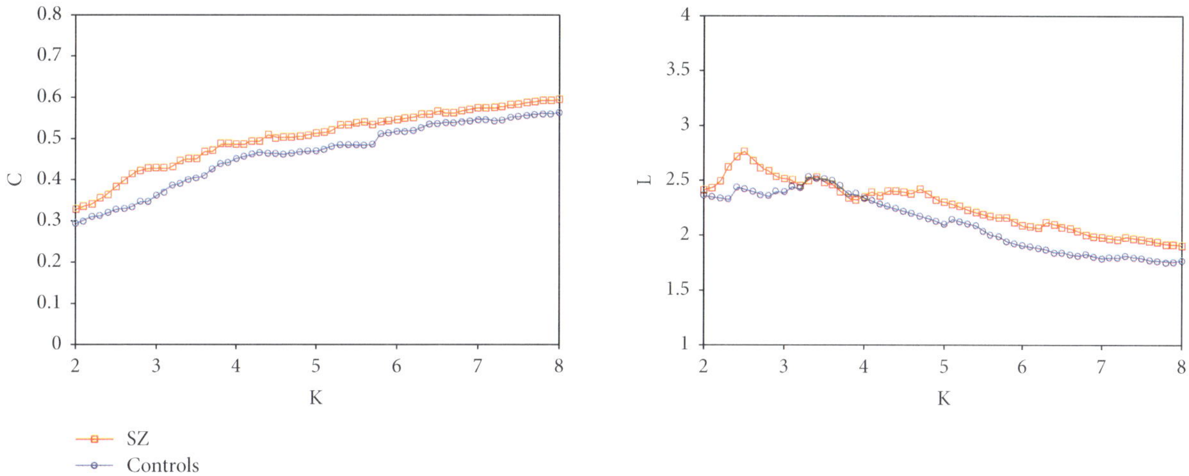

(d) Beta band

FIGURE 2: Mean cluster coefficient C and characteristic path length L for SZ patients (square), healthy controls (circle), ordered network (cross), and random network (triangle) as a function of K in the delta band (a), theta band (b), alpha band (c), and beta band (d). The asterisks showed significant difference between SZ patients and healthy controls ($P < 0.05$).

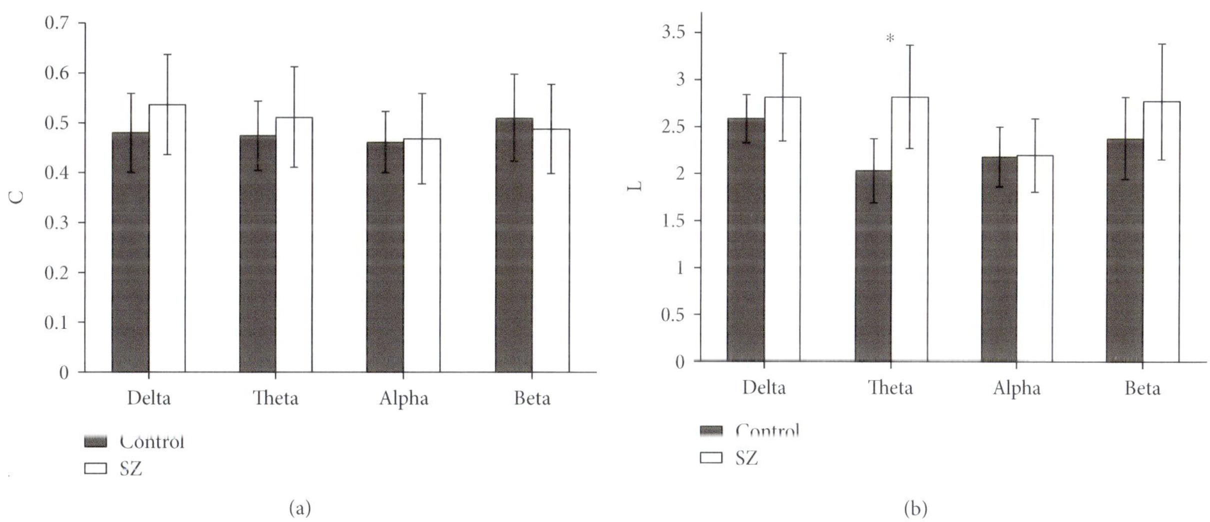

FIGURE 3: Mean cluster coefficient C (a) and characteristic path length L (b) in the four bands for SZ patients and healthy controls based on the OMST filtering scheme. The asterisk showed significant difference between SZ patients and healthy controls ($P < 0.05$).

was not significant for the combined SZ patients and healthy controls ($r = 0.146$, $P = 0.448$) or SZ patients alone ($r = -0.186$, $P = 0.521$). Figure 4(b) showed that the L were positively correlated with executive times for the combined SZ patients and healthy controls ($r = 0.507$, $P = 0.006$), but not for SZ patients alone ($r = 0.072$, $P = 0.412$).

4. Discussion

Here, we studied the brain functional connectivity and its small-world topologic properties underlying cool executive dysfunction in first-episode SZ patients for the first time. We observed that changes of small-world network properties mainly appeared in the theta band, not in the delta, alpha, or beta band, and the SZ group was characterized by a longer characteristic path length L (having significant difference compared with the healthy group) and relatively higher cluster coefficient C (no significant difference compared with the healthy group) in the theta band, suggesting a less optimal organization of the brain network in SZ patients.

It was well-known that the characteristic path length L is defined as the average shortest paths for all possible pairs of nodes and stands for global efficiency of information integration across different brain areas. Our results showed that in the theta band, the L of SZ patients was significantly longer than that of healthy controls over a wide range of threshold T (Figure 1(b)), and this pattern was still present when L was calculated as a function of degree K

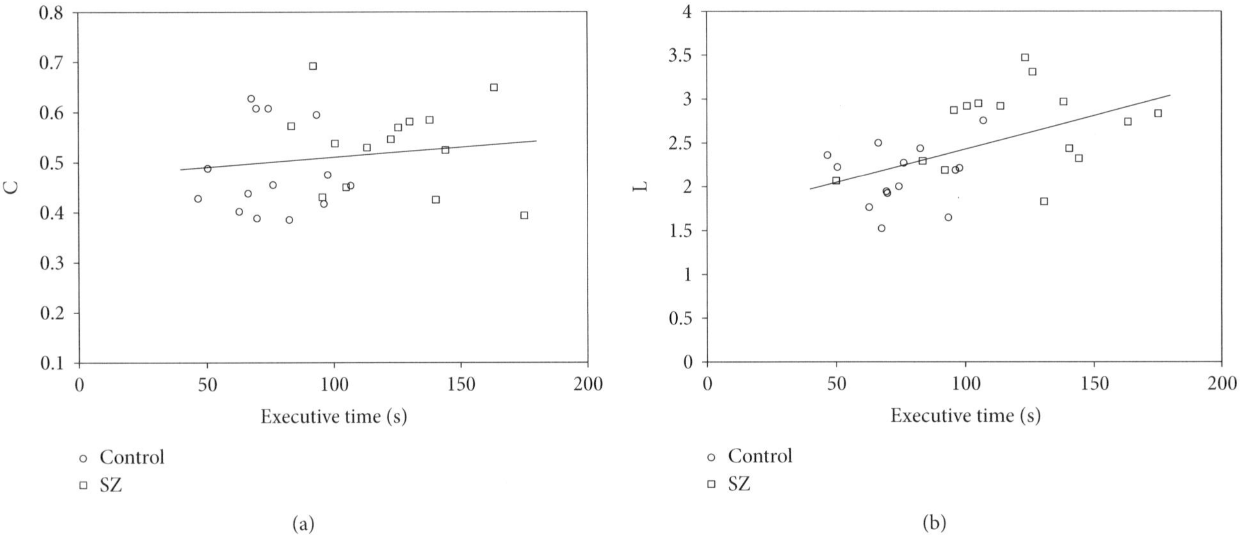

FIGURE 4: Pearson correlation analysis between C (a) or L (b) and task performance (executive time) in the theta band for SZ patients (square) and healthy controls (circle).

(Figure 2(b)) or by using the OMST filtering scheme (Figure 3(b)), suggesting a more effective information integration and communication across different brain regions in healthy controls compared with SZ patients. In addition, some fMRI studies have reported fewer hubs (i.e., highly connected nodes) in SZ patients [43, 44], and such reduction in the number of highly connected nodes may explain the longer L for SZ patients in our study. Moreover, the cluster coefficient C was considered as a metric of the network segregation and of the local efficiency of information communication. It was indicated that the C of SZ patients was significantly smaller than that of healthy controls over the whole range of T (Figure 1(a)), suggesting that the local connections of networks in SZ patients were relatively spared. However, no significant difference for C occurred between SZ patients and healthy controls when C was calculated as a function of degree K (Figure 2(a)) or by applying the OMST filtering scheme (Figure 3(a)). It was well-known that the edge number in a graph has a great relationship with the values of L and C, and the edge number in the two graphs (SZ patients and healthy controls) will be different by applying a certain T. Therefore, it was necessary to compute L and C as a function of degree K, which ensured the same edge number in the two groups, and the resulted differences in L and C between the two groups would represent the differences of network configuration.

Although the above two network thresholding schemes (absolute threshold and mean degree) have been widely applied to threshold brain networks, they might add bias for group and task comparisons and reduce the possibility of the reproducibility of the findings across studies from different research groups. Therefore, in order to test the reproducibility of our results, we applied a novel data-driven topological filtering scheme based on the OMST proposed by Dimitriadis et al. [37, 38] to filter our constructed brain networks. Interestingly, we also found that significant difference existed only in the theta band for L between SZ patients and healthy controls (Figure 3(b)), which was consistent with that of the mean degree K scheme (Figure 2(b)). As described above, no matter which filtering scheme is used, our results always showed that SZ patients showed a significantly longer L compared to healthy controls. Therefore, the longer L in SZ patients cannot be due to the influence of other factors in the two groups and reflects a true disturbance in the brain network organization of this illness, which was consistent with some previously published literature [27–29].

We applied the OMST scheme to threshold experimental networks (SZ patients and healthy controls), and corresponding random networks were generated to compute the small-world index. For a small-world network, the C should be much larger than that of the random network and L should be close to that of a random network. Interestingly, the calculated small-world indexes of both groups were greater than 1, suggesting that both groups had small-world network characteristics in the theta band. However, the small-world index of SZ patients was larger than that of healthy controls, but no significant difference existed.

We also studied the correlations between C (Figure 4(a)) or L (Figure 4(b)) of the theta-band brain network and task performance (executive time). Previous literatures have reported that SZ patients need to spend more time to finish some executive tasks due to their executive dysfunction [3, 45], and our results indicated that the mean executive time of TMT-B task for SZ patients was significantly longer than that of healthy controls, which was consistent with these literatures. Figure 4(b) showed that the L was positively correlated with executive times for the combined SZ patients and healthy controls, suggesting that the longer L would lead to the longer executive time of the TMT-B task. It was well-known that L reflects the global efficiency of information integration across different brain areas, and the L of SZ patients was significantly longer than that of healthy controls (Figure 3(b)). By taking all these considerations into account, we could infer that increased L, suggesting reduced global information integration ability, eventually led to increased executive time in SZ patients.

In recent years, a large number of studies have found that abnormal theta oscillation was closely related to SZ [46]. Increased theta activity was often observed in SZ patients during the rest state [47], whereas many studies showed reduced theta activity in SZ patients during various tasks [48]. In addition, the altered theta-band brain functional connectivity among different brain regions in SZ patients also has been confirmed in many literatures [10, 49]. The theta band was considered to play a key role in large-scale functional integration by combining the activities of various brain regions together [46, 50], and executive function that is involved in a range of higher-level cognitive processes relies on the integration of different brain areas for proper functioning [49]. The present study showed that there existed significant difference for small-world topologic properties between the two groups during the cool executive task only in the theta band, not in the other frequency bands, which supported the above-mentioned results. However, our study indicated that there was no significant difference for the small-world index in the theta band between first-episode SZ patients and healthy controls during the cool executive function task, which was in contrast with the study of Jhung et al. [26] in which the small-world index in the theta band of first-episode SZ patients during working memory task significantly decreased compared with that of healthy controls. This might suggest that the impairment degree of the cold executive function is much less than that of working memory function in first-episode SZ patients.

The present study has certain limitations. Firstly, in order to get more reliable conclusions, the sample size of subjects must be increased. Secondly, we studied the small-world topologic properties of SZ patients during only one cool executive task, that is, the TMT-B task, but it is not clear whether task difficulty influences the small-world topologic properties of SZ patients. Therefore, it is necessary and interesting to design cool executive tasks with different difficulty to study this issue in future work. Moreover, from a methodological point of view, our study converted functional connectivity based on MI into a binary graph, which would result in the loss of part of the information compared to the weighted graph.

5. Conclusions

Our results indicated that a less-optimal organization of the brain functional network in the theta band occurred in first-episode SZ patients compared with healthy controls. SZ patients owned a significantly longer characteristic path length L in the theta band no matter which filtering scheme is used, which suggested a disturbance in globally efficient communication between different brain areas in SZ patients. The present study combining functional connectivity and graph theory analysis provided helpful findings to reveal the pathophysiologic mechanisms underlying cool executive dysfunction in first-episode SZ patients.

Acknowledgments

This work was supported by the support project for the Disciplinary Group of Psychology and Neuroscience in Xinxiang Medical University (no. 2016PN-KFKT-19), the Aid Project for the Leading Young Teachers in Henan Provincial Institutions of Higher Education of China (no. 2014GGJS-096), the Doctoral Scientific Research Foundation of Xinxiang Medical University (no. XYBSKYZZ201718), the open project of the School of Biomedical Engineering in Xinxiang Medical University (no. 2018-BME-KFKT-07), the Scientific and Technological Project of Henan Province (no. 182102310555), and the Key Scientific Research Project of Henan Province (no. 14B416010).

References

[1] J. M. Haro, C. Altamura, R. Corral et al., "Understanding the impact of persistent symptoms in schizophrenia: cross-sectional findings from the pattern study," *Schizophrenia Research*, vol. 169, no. 1–3, pp. 234–240, 2015.

[2] A. K. Martin, B. Mowry, D. Reutens, and G. A. Robinson, "Executive functioning in schizophrenia: unique and shared variance with measures of fluid intelligence," *Brain and Cognition*, vol. 99, pp. 57–67, 2015.

[3] J. M. Gavilán and J. E. García-Albea, "Executive dysfunction in schizophrenia and its association with mentalizing abilities," *Revista de Psiquiatría y Salud Mental*, vol. 8, no. 3, pp. 119–129, 2015.

[4] E. Neill and S. L. Rossell, "Executive functioning in schizophrenia: the result of impairments in lower order cognitive skills?," *Schizophrenia Research*, vol. 150, no. 1, pp. 76–80, 2013.

[5] A. Adan, M. . M. Capella, G. Prat, D. A. Forero, S. López-Vera, and J. F. Navarro, "Executive functioning in men with schizophrenia and substance use disorders. Influence of lifetime suicide attempts," *Plos One*, vol. 12, no. 1, article e0169943, 2017.

[6] D. Sasabayashi, Y. Takayanagi, S. Nishiyama et al., "Increased frontal gyrification negatively correlates with executive function in patients with first-episode schizophrenia," *Cerebral Cortex*, vol. 27, no. 4, pp. 2686–2694, 2016.

[7] E. Theochari, E. Tsaltas, and D. Kontis, "Obsessive compulsive symptoms, social functioning and executive functions in chronic schizophrenia," *European Psychiatry*, vol. 41, article S386, Supplement, 2017.

[8] Z. Zhou, Y. Zhu, J. Wang, and H. Zhu, "Risperidone improves interpersonal perception and executive function in patients with schizophrenia," *Neuropsychiatric Disease and Treatment*, vol. 13, pp. 101–107, 2017.

[9] C. Andreou, G. Leicht, G. Nolte et al., "Resting-state theta-band connectivity and verbal memory in

schizophrenia and in the high-risk state," *Schizophrenia Research*, vol. 161, no. 2-3, pp. 299–307, 2015.

[10] D. Shreekantiah Umesh, S. K. Tikka, N. Goyal, S. H. Nizamie, and V. K. Sinha, "Resting state theta band source distribution and functional connectivity in remitted schizophrenia," *Neuroscience Letters*, vol. 630, pp. 199–202, 2016.

[11] E. Carlino, M. Sigaudo, R. Rosato, S. Vighetti, and P. Rocca, "Electroencephalographic connectivity analysis in schizophrenia," *Neuroscience Letters*, vol. 604, pp. 145–150, 2015.

[12] G. Di Lorenzo, A. Daverio, F. Ferrentino et al., "Altered resting-state EEG source functional connectivity in schizophrenia: the effect of illness duration," *Frontiers in Human Neuroscience*, vol. 9, p. 234, 2015.

[13] C. Andreou, G. Nolte, G. Leicht et al., "Increased resting-state gamma-band connectivity in first-episode schizophrenia," *Schizophrenia Bulletin*, vol. 41, no. 4, pp. 930–939, 2015.

[14] J. A. Hadley, N. V. Kraguljac, D. M. White, L. ver Hoef, J. Tabora, and A. C. Lahti, "Change in brain network topology as a function of treatment response in schizophrenia: a longitudinal resting-state fMRI study using graph theory," *npj Schizophrenia*, vol. 2, no. 1, article 16014, 2016.

[15] M. Schneider, H. Walter, C. Moessnang et al., "Altered DLPFC-hippocampus connectivity during working memory: independent replication and disorder specificity of a putative genetic risk phenotype for schizophrenia," *Schizophrenia Bulletin*, vol. 43, no. 5, pp. 1114–1122, 2017.

[16] L. Zhang, B. Li, H. Wang et al., "Decreased middle temporal gyrus connectivity in the language network in schizophrenia patients with auditory verbal hallucinations," *Neuroscience Letters*, vol. 653, pp. 177–182, 2017.

[17] S. H. Na, S. H. Jin, S. Y. Kim, and B. J. Ham, "EEG in schizophrenic patients: mutual information analysis," *Clinical Neurophysiology*, vol. 113, no. 12, pp. 1954–1960, 2002.

[18] J. Jeong, J. C. Gore, and B. S. Peterson, "Mutual information analysis of the EEG in patients with Alzheimer's disease," *Clinical Neurophysiology*, vol. 112, no. 5, pp. 827–835, 2001.

[19] J. A. Vastano and H. L. Swinney, "Information transport in spatiotemporal systems," *Physical Review Letters*, vol. 60, no. 18, pp. 1773–1776, 1988.

[20] A. Fernández, C. Gómez, R. Hornero, and J. J. López-Ibor, "Complexity and schizophrenia," *Progress in Neuro-Psychopharmacology and Biological Psychiatry*, vol. 45, pp. 267–276, 2013.

[21] M. Bolaños, E. M. Bernat, B. He, and S. Aviyente, "A weighted small world network measure for assessing functional connectivity," *Journal of Neuroscience Methods*, vol. 212, no. 1, pp. 133–142, 2013.

[22] W. Li, Y. Lin, and Y. Liu, "The structure of weighted small-world networks," *Physica A: Statistical Mechanics and its Applications*, vol. 376, no. 1, pp. 708–718, 2007.

[23] M. Jalili and M. G. Knyazeva, "EEG-based functional networks in schizophrenia," *Computers in Biology and Medicine*, vol. 41, no. 12, pp. 1178–1186, 2011.

[24] M. Rubinov, S. A. Knock, C. J. Stam et al., "Small-world properties of nonlinear brain activity in schizophrenia," *Human Brain Mapping*, vol. 30, no. 2, pp. 403–416, 2009.

[25] S. Schinkel, G. Zamora-López, O. Dimigen, W. Sommer, and J. Kurths, "Functional network analysis reveals differences in the semantic priming task," *Journal of Neuroscience Methods*, vol. 197, no. 2, pp. 333–339, 2011.

[26] K. Jhung, S. H. Cho, J. H. Jang et al., "Small-world networks in individuals at ultra-high risk for psychosis and first-episode schizophrenia during a working memory task," *Neuroscience Letters*, vol. 535, no. 1, pp. 35–39, 2013.

[27] S. Micheloyannis, E. Pachou, C. J. Stam et al., "Small-world networks and disturbed functional connectivity in schizophrenia," *Schizophrenia Research*, vol. 87, no. 1-3, pp. 60–66, 2006.

[28] M. Shim, D. W. Kim, S. H. Lee, and C. H. Im, "Disruptions in small-world cortical functional connectivity network during an auditory oddball paradigm task in patients with schizophrenia," *Schizophrenia Research*, vol. 156, no. 2-3, pp. 197–203, 2014.

[29] J. Gomez-Pilar, A. Lubeiro, J. Poza et al., "Functional EEG network analysis in schizophrenia: evidence of larger segregation and deficit of modulation," *Progress in Neuro-Psychopharmacology and Biological Psychiatry*, vol. 76, pp. 116–123, 2017.

[30] N. Fogelson, L. Li, Y. Li, M. Fernandez-del-Olmo, D. Santos-Garcia, and A. Peled, "Functional connectivity abnormalities during contextual processing in schizophrenia and in Parkinson's disease," *Brain and Cognition*, vol. 82, no. 3, pp. 243–253, 2013.

[31] P. D. Zelazo and U. Müller, "Executive function in typical and atypical development," in *Blackwell Handbook of Childhood Cognitive Development*, U. Goswami, Ed., pp. 445–469, Blackwell Publishers Ltd, 2002.

[32] P. Marsh, T. P. Beauchaine, and B. Williams, "Dissociation of sad facial expressions and autonomic nervous system responding in boys with disruptive behavior disorders," *Psychophysiology*, vol. 45, no. 1, pp. 100–110, 2008.

[33] Y. Yu, Y. Zhao, Y. Si et al., "Estimation of the cool executive function using frontal electroencephalogram signals in first-episode schizophrenia patients," *Biomedical Engineering Online*, vol. 15, no. 1, p. 131, 2016.

[34] N. Ojeda, J. Peña, P. Sánchez et al., "Efficiency of cognitive rehabilitation with REHACOP in chronic treatment resistant Hispanic patients," *NeuroRehabilitation*, vol. 30, no. 1, pp. 65–74, 2012.

[35] A. Delorme and S. Makeig, "EEGLAB: an open source toolbox for analysis of single-trial EEG dynamics including independent component analysis," *Journal of Neuroscience Methods*, vol. 134, no. 1, pp. 9–21, 2004.

[36] Z. Jane Wang, P. Pamela, and M. J. McKeown, "A novel segmentation, mutual information network framework for EEG analysis of motor tasks," *Biomedical Engineering Online*, vol. 8, no. 1, p. 9, 2009.

[37] S. I. Dimitriadis, C. Salis, I. Tarnanas, and D. E. Linden, "Topological filtering of dynamic functional brain networks unfolds informative chronnectomics: a novel data-driven thresholding scheme based on orthogonal minimal spanning trees (OMSTs)," *Frontiers in Neuroinformatics*, vol. 11, p. 28, 2017.

[38] S. I. Dimitriadis, M. Antonakakis, P. Simos, J. M. Fletcher, and A. C. Papanicolaou, "Data-driven topological filtering based on orthogonal minimal spanning trees: application to multigroup magnetoencephalography resting-state connectivity," *Brain Connectivity*, vol. 7, no. 10, pp. 661–670, 2017.

[39] Y. Liu, M. Liang, Y. Zhou et al., "Disrupted small-world networks in schizophrenia," *Brain*, vol. 131, no. 4, pp. 945–961, 2008.

[40] T. Liu, Y. Chen, P. Lin, and J. Wang, "Small-world brain functional networks in children with attention-deficit/

hyperactivity disorder evealed by EEG synchrony," *Clinical EEG and Neuroscience*, vol. 46, no. 3, pp. 183–191, 2014.

[41] O. Sporns and J. D. Zwi, "The small world of the cerebral cortex," *Neuroinformatics*, vol. 2, no. 2, pp. 145–162, 2004.

[42] R. Milo, S. Shen-Orr, S. Itzkovitz, N. Kashtan, D. Chklovskii, and U. Alon, "Network motifs: simple building blocks of complex networks," *Science*, vol. 298, no. 5594, pp. 824–827, 2002.

[43] C.-Y. Z. Lo, T.-W. Su, C.-C. Huang et al., "Randomization and resilience of brain functional networks as systems-level endophenotypes of schizophrenia," *Proceedings of the National Academy of Sciences of the United States of America*, vol. 112, no. 29, pp. 9123–9128, 2015.

[44] S. Ma, V. D. Calhoun, T. Eichele, W. Du, and T. Adalı, "Modulations of functional connectivity in the healthy and schizophrenia groups during task and rest," *NeuroImage*, vol. 62, no. 3, pp. 1694–1704, 2012.

[45] E. C. Chiu, S. C. Lee, C. J. Kuo, F. W. Lung, I. P. Hsueh, and C. L. Hsieh, "Development of a performance-based measure of executive functions in patients with schizophrenia," *Plos One*, vol. 10, no. 11, article e0142790, 2015.

[46] P. J. Uhlhaas, C. Haenschel, D. Nikolic, and W. Singer, "The role of oscillations and synchrony in cortical networks and their putative relevance for the pathophysiology of schizophrenia," *Schizophrenia Bulletin*, vol. 34, no. 5, pp. 927–943, 2008.

[47] L. V. Moran and L. E. Hong, "High vs low frequency neural oscillations in schizophrenia," *Schizophrenia Bulletin*, vol. 37, no. 4, pp. 659–663, 2011.

[48] E. Başar and B. Güntekin, "Review of delta, theta, alpha, beta, and gamma response oscillations in neuropsychiatric disorders," *Supplements to Clinical Neurophysiology*, vol. 62, p. 303, 2013.

[49] B. Griesmayr, B. Berger, R. Stelzig-Schoeler, W. Aichhorn, J. Bergmann, and P. Sauseng, "EEG theta phase coupling during executive control of visual working memory investigated in individuals with schizophrenia and in healthy controls," *Cognitive, Affective, & Behavioral Neuroscience*, vol. 14, no. 4, pp. 1340–1355, 2014.

[50] A. von Stein and J. Sarnthein, "Different frequencies for different scales of cortical integration: from local gamma to long range alpha/theta synchronization," *International Journal of Psychophysiology*, vol. 38, no. 3, pp. 301–313, 2000.

15

Increased Risk of Dementia in Patients with Antidepressants: A Meta-Analysis of Observational Studies

Yao-Chin Wang,[1,2,3] Po-An Tai,[4] Tahmina Nasrin Poly,[1,3] Md Mohaimenul Islam,[1,3] Hsuan-Chia Yang,[1,4] Chieh-Chen Wu,[1,3] and Yu-Chuan (Jack) Li[1,3,5,6]

[1]*Graduate Institute of Biomedical Informatics, College of Medical Science and Technology, Taipei Medical University, Taipei, Taiwan*
[2]*Department of Emergency, Min-Sheng General Hospital, Taoyuan City, Taiwan*
[3]*International Center for Health Information Technology (ICHIT), Taipei Medical University, Taipei, Taiwan*
[4]*Department of Surgery, School of Medicine, Buddhist Tzu Chi University, Hualien, Taiwan*
[5]*Department of Dermatology, Wan Fang Hospital, Taipei, Taiwan*
[6]*TMU Research Center of Cancer Translational Medicine, Taipei, Taiwan*

Correspondence should be addressed to Yu-Chuan (Jack) Li; jaak88@gmail.com

Academic Editor: Shinro Matsuo

Antidepressants are the most commonly and widely used medication for its effectiveness in the treatment of anxiety and depression. A few epidemiological studies have documented that antidepressant is associated with increased risk of dementia so far. Here, our aim is to assess the association between antidepressant use and risk of dementia in elderly patients. We searched articles through MEDLINE, EMBASE, Google, and Google Scholar from inception to December 1, 2017, that reported on the association between antidepressant use and dementia risk. Data were collected from each study independently, and study duplication was checked by at least three senior researchers based on a standardized protocol. Summary relative risk (RR) with 95% CI was calculated by using a random-effects model. We selected 9 out of 754 unique abstracts for full-text review using our predetermined selection criteria, and 5 out of these 9 studies, comprising 53,955 participants, met all of our inclusion criteria. The overall pooled RR of dementia was 1.75 (95% CI: 1.033–2.964) for SSRIs whereas the overall pooled RR of dementia was 2.131 (95% CI: 1.427–3.184) for tricyclic use. Also, MAOIs showed a high rate of increase with significant heterogeneity. Our findings indicate that antidepressant use is significantly associated with an increased risk of developing dementia. Therefore, we suggest physicians to carefully prescribe antidepressants, especially in elder patients. Additionally, treatment should be stopped if any symptoms related to dementia are to be noticed.

1. Introduction

Dementia is a neurocognitive disorder characterized by cognitive impairment. As the life expectancy of people has been increasing, and the prevalence of dementia has been increasing dramatically [1], dementia, therefore, has appeared as a major cause of disability and dependence among older people which is triggering huge economic burdens around the world. In 2012, nearly 35.5 million of people had dementia, and this number is expected to be doubled by 2030 and approximately 115 million by 2050 [2, 3]. A few epidemiological studies have found the possible link between late-life depression and consistently an increased risk of dementia so far. These studies also mentioned that several factors like stroke, diabetes mellitus, hypertension, head trauma, and hyperlipidemia might be associated with dementia [4, 5].

Antidepressants are a commonly and widely used medication for its effectiveness in the treatment of anxiety and depression [6]. Despite their benefits in depression, concerns have emerged on their safety and the subsequent risk for dementia, but the results are still inconsistent. Previous studies have demonstrated that antidepressant drugs are responsible for adaptive process disruption. It is basically triggered by serotonin, reduces brain metabolism, and escalates the clinical conversion to dementia risk [7, 8]. Contrary, Schmitt et al. reported that treatment with an antidepressant like SSRIs may help to improve cognitive function in patients with Alzheimer's dementia [9].

Until now, there is no particular meta-analysis on the association between antidepressant use and the risk of dementia among the elderly patients. We therefore conducted a meta-analysis of observational studies to evaluate the relationship between antidepressant use and dementia risk. Finding from our present meta-analysis would assist healthcare providers to improve treatment outcome and improve the existing knowledge about antidepressant therapy. In this meta-analysis, we only included studies that reported patients having exposure to antidepressants for at least one month and included patients' mean age more than 50 years.

2. Methods

This meta-analysis was conducted in accordance with the Preferred Reporting Items for Systematic Reviews and Meta-analyses (PRISMA) (Supplementary Table S1) [10]. We have used similar methods in our previous published three literatures [1, 11, 12].

2.1. Database. In the initial stage, we developed in this study a search strategy by consulting with our senior researchers at the International Center for Health Information Technology lab. Our three senior pharmacists (MMI, TNP, and H-CY) are experts in systematic review and meta-analysis regarding drug-disease and disease-disease associations. We searched for articles on the electronic databases such as PubMed, EMBASE, and Scopus until December 1, 2017, which reported on the possible association between antidepressant use and dementia risk. We used the following search terms as medical subject headlines and keywords: ("Anti-depressant drugs" OR "SSRIs" OR "Tricyclics (TCAs)" OR "Monoamine oxidase inhibitors (MAOIs") And ("Dementia risk") (Supplementary Table S2). To find any missing article in our initial search, we conducted additional searches in the reference lists of all included full text. However, Google Scholar was used to finding academic articles citing eligible articles. After assembling all potential articles, we then used EndNote X7 (Thomson Reuters) to manage and remove the duplicates.

2.2. Eligibility Criteria. Firstly, our authors independently screened all titles and abstracts of all retrieved articles. At the initial stage, they considered all studies published only in English. Additionally, observational study designs such as case-control, cohort, and randomized control trials that reported on antidepressant use and the risk of dementia were considered in our primary search strategy. The following criteria were considered to exclude studies if (1) they published as a letter to the editor, editorial, case study, and short communications; (2) patients had less than 30 days' antidepressant use; and (3) studies had a less than one-year follow-up period.

2.3. Inclusion and Exclusion Criteria. In this stage, two authors (MMI and TNP) retrieved full-text articles and checked the duplication of included studies. We considered only those studies if they met the following criteria:

(1) were published in English

(2) reported an association between antidepressants and dementia risk

(3) having at least 50 participants in both treatment and control groups

(4) having results demonstrated on OR/HR with 95% CI.

(5) having a more than one-year follow-up period

(6) identified dementia patients with ICD-9/biochemical test or other standard procedure

However, they excluded those articles if they were not an observational study and if the participants are not patients with dementia due to antidepressants. If the study met all inclusion criteria at this stage, our two authors (MMI and TNP) further reviewed to ensure the quality of the final analysis. Any disagreements regarding quantitative information (number of participant, dementia identification, duration of therapy, etc.) between two authors (MMI and TNP) were resolved by our main supervisor (YCL) of this study. They also kept some studies for reference, if they provide valuable information regarding their associations.

2.4. Data Extraction and Risk Bias Assessment. We finally included four studies, and those two authors then garnered information from each of these four studies. They collected the following information from four included studies: (a) author name and publication years; (b) study duration, study location, and study design; (c) condition information (i.e., data source, condition definition, and the total number of participants); and (d) odds ratios/hazard ratios with 95% CI for summary calculation.

2.5. Methodological Quality Assessment. The Newcastle-Ottawa Scale (NOS) was used to evaluate the methodological quality of included observational studies (Supplementary Table S3) [13]. We evaluated included studies in three categories: selection (4 stars) and comparability (2 stars) of study groups and assessment of the outcome of interest (3 stars). The star rating system was used to indicate the quality, with 0–6 stars defined as low-quality and 7–9 stars as high-quality.

2.6. Statistical Analysis. In the final analysis, we calculated risk ratios (RRs) with 95% CIs to assess the risk of dementia with antidepressants. Odds ratios are close approximations of RR. We therefore combined odds ratios with HRs, resulting in a common estimate of RR [14]. A risk rate greater than 1 indicates an increased risk of dementia, and a risk rate smaller than 1 indicates a decreased risk of dementia. Statistical significance was evaluated using the 95% CIs. If the 95% CI did not include the neural value 1, we consider the risk statistically significant. In our study, we calculated the risk ratio (RR) from both case-control and cohort studies and used the most adjusted estimate available in each study due to estimation of a valid result.

A random-effects model was used to reduce the heterogeneity among the studies. We used comprehensive

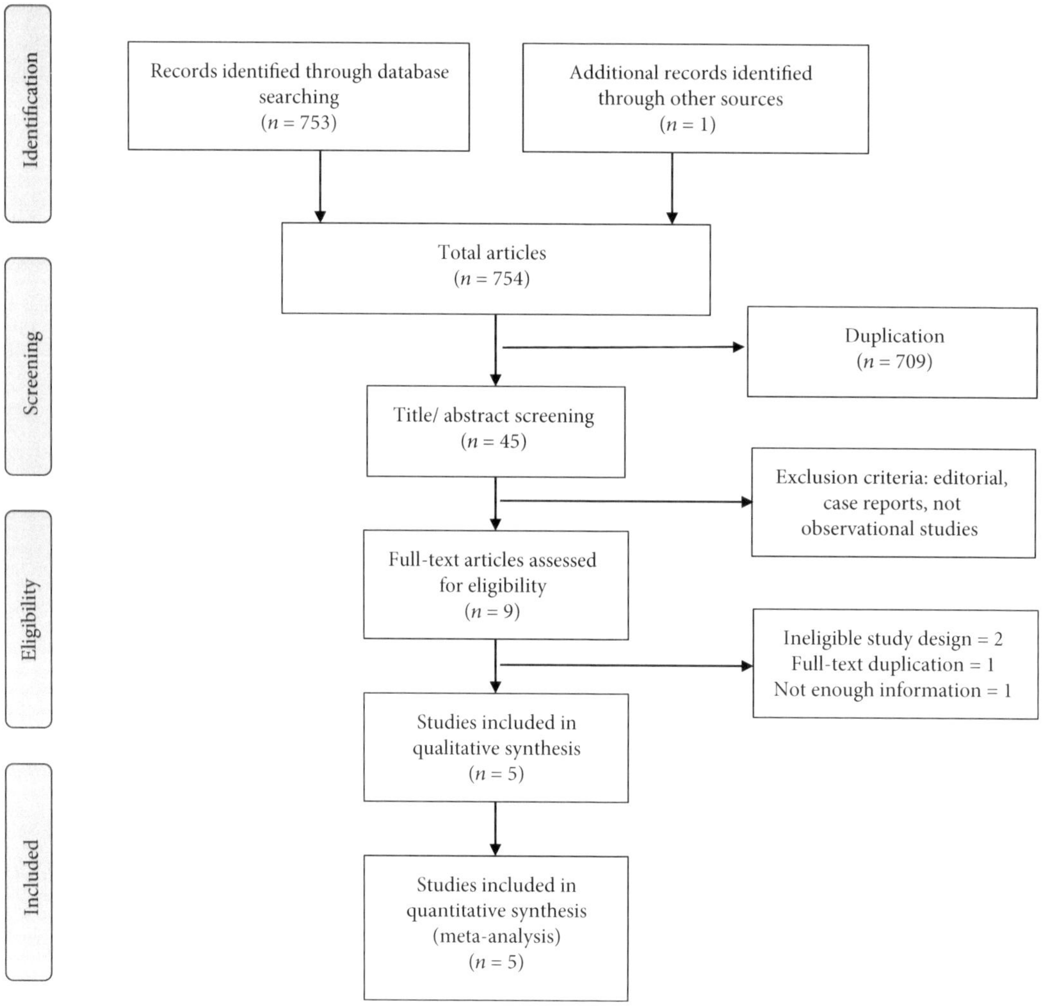

FIGURE 1: Flow chart of study selection. Diagram of study selection, adapted from the PRISMA group 2009 flow diagram.

meta-analysis package (Version 3) to draw forest plots and subgroup estimation. The meta-analysis of proportion uses the binominal distribution for analysis. We quantified heterogeneity of the studies using the I^2 statistic, and its significance was determined based on the accompanying P value in Cochran's Q test. If the I^2 value is 0%, it indicates no heterogeneity, and increasing values represent greater amounts of heterogeneity. The I^2 values of 25%, 50%, and 75% were considered as low, moderate, and high levels of heterogeneity. However, τ^2 values arising from the random-effects models were also used to quantify heterogeneity.

3. Results

3.1. Literature Search. A total of 754 records were identified through our initial database search. Of those, 745 studies were excluded based on our predetermined inclusion and exclusion criteria. We described full details in method parts. We reassessed the full text of the remaining 9 articles. Finally, 5 studies met all our inclusion criteria and were included in the final meta-analysis. A flow chart showing the study selection is presented in Figure 1.

3.2. Study Characteristics. The characteristics of the selected studies are presented in Table 1. The five included observational studies [15–19] were published between 2012 [19] and 2017 [18]. Among these studies, 3 were from Asia and 2 were from North America. Three studies were cohort studies [17–19], and two studies were case-control study designs [15, 16]. Two studies reported that the possible onset age of dementia was over 60 years [17, 19], and three studies reported an age of development of dementia which was below 60 years [15, 16, 18]. Almost every study mentioned antidepressant exposure, and they also evaluated the various classes of antidepressant use and dementia risk. A total of 53,955 study participants were included in our quantitative synthesis of which female patients were higher than male patients. The length of follow-up ranged from 3 to 11 years. All dementia patients were confirmed by checking the medical history, and all of the studies adjusted their results of potential confounding factors.

3.3. Methodological Quality of Included Studies. The Newcastle-Ottawa Scale (NOS) was used to assessed the methodological quality of included observational studies. The mean value for the five studies was 7.8 (Table 2).

Table 1: Characteristics of five included studies regarding antidepressants use and dementia risk.

Author/year	Country	Study duration	Study design	Adjustments	Results
Wei-Sheng Lee-2016 [15]	Taiwan	2005–2011	Case-control	1, 2, 3, 4, 5, 6, 7, 8, 9	For SSRIs, OR = 2.48 (95% CI: 2.27–2.71) For MAOIs, OR = 1.86 (95% CI: 1.47–2.36) For TCAs, OR = 1.44 (95% CI: 1.32–1.57),
Wei-Sheng Lee-2017 [16]	Taiwan	2005–2011	Case-control	1, 2, 3, 4, 5, 6, 7, 8, 9	For SSRIs, OR = 0.58 (95% CI: 0.50–0.69) For TCAs, OR = 1.02 (95% CI: 0.89, 1.17 For NGAs, OR = 4.23 (95% CI: 3.34, 5.37)
Wang 2016 [17]	USA	1991–2010	Cohort	1, 2, 3, 6, 9, 10 , 11, 12, 13, 14, 15, 16, 17, 18	For SSRIs, HR = 1.83 (95% CI) For non-SSRIs, HR = 1.50 (95% CI)
Then 2017 [18]	Taiwan	2003–2006	Cohort	1, 2, 3, 4, 8, 9, 19, 20	For SSRIs, HR = 3.66 (95% CI: 2.62–5.09) For SNRI, HR = 4.73 (95% CI: 2.54–8.80) For TCAs, HR = 3.26 (95% CI: 2.30–4.63) For MAOIs, HR = 4.94 (95% CI: 2.17–11.24)
Goveas 2012 [19]	USA	1996–2007	Cohort	1, 2, 3, 4, 6, 9, 10, 11, 21	For SSRIs, HR = 1.78 (95% CI: 1.01–3.10) For TCAs, HR = 1.78 (95% CI: 0.99–3.21).

(1) age, (2) gender, (3) diabetes, (4) hypertension, (5) stroke, (6) coronary artery disease, (7) head injury, (8) anxiety, (9) depression, (10) smoking, (11) body mass index, (12) cancer, (13) COPD, (14) liver disease, (15) hyperlipidemia, (16) renal disease, (17) thyroid disease, (18) cerebrovascular disease, (19) insomnia, (20) CCI, and (21) history of alcohol consumption.

3.4. Meta-Analysis. In the main analysis, a total of five studies evaluated the risk between selective serotonin reuptake inhibitor (SSRI) use and development of dementia. SSRI use is significantly associated with an increased risk of dementia when compared with nonuse. The overall pooled increase of dementia in patients with SSRI use was RR 1.75 (95% CI: 1.033–2.964) with significant heterogeneity present ($I^2 = 98.553$, tau$^2 = 0.34$) (Figure 2).

Four studies provided the risk estimation of tricyclic (TCA) use and dementia risk. The pooled RR for dementia risk was 2.131 (95% CI: 1.427–3.184) with the patients with TCAs (Figure 3). There was also significant heterogeneity ($I^2 = 96.393$, tau$^2 = 0.378$) among studies.

Two studies evaluated the impact of monoamine oxidase inhibitor (MAOI) therapy and risk of dementia. The overall pooled increase of dementia in patients with MAOI use was RR 2.791 (95% CI: 1.086–7.169) with significant heterogeneity present ($I^2 = 80.019$, tau$^2 = 0.382$) (Figure 4).

3.5. Sensitivity Analysis. Lee et al. [15] evaluated the risk of dementia according to cumulative dose of individual antidepressants. Patients with SSRIs had higher risk of dementia [(HR = 2.04, 95% CI: 1.80–2.31; HR = 2.10, 95% CI: 1.85–2.39; HR = 2.96, 95% CI: 2.60–3.37; and HR = 3.07, 95% CI: 2.69–3.51)] for <840 mg, 841–3000 mg, 3001–10,500 mg, and >10,500 mg. Contrarily, tricyclic was associated with a decreased risk of dementia [(HR = 0.44, 95% CI: 0.38–0.51, HR = 0.26, 95% CI: 0.22–0.30; HR = 0.20, 95% CI: 0.17–0.24; and HR = 0.13, 95% CI: 0.11–0.15)] for <840 mg, 841–3000 mg, 3001–10,500 mg, and >10,500 mg, respectively. Then et al. [18] investigated gender, different age groups, and dementia risk. Males had a higher risk of developing dementia (HR = 3.59, 95% CI: 2.64–4.88) than female patients (HR = 4.45, 95% CI: 3.11–6.37). Additionally, patients aged 45–65 had a higher risk (HR = 8.34, 95% CI: 4.45–15.61) than patients aged ≥65 years (HR = 3.84, 95% CI: 2.98–4.94). Goveas et al. [19] provided information about developing adverse effects such as mild cognitive impairment (HR = 1.70, 95% CI: 1.14–2.54) and probable dementia (HR = 1.24, 95% CI: 0.71–2.17).

3.6. Publication Bias. In our study, we showed the visual interpretation and test for asymmetry of the funnel plot of the publications. However, it is well established that the test of asymmetry will not be reliable when the included study number is not substantial [20]. Figure 5 depicts the funnel plot, indicating the presence of publication bias. Egger's regression test was used to present the funnel asymmetry, and it showed a highly significant publication bias (P value = 0.79).

TABLE 2: Methodological quality assessment of the observational studies using the NOS.

(a)

Case-control study	Selection: Definition adequate	Selection: Representativeness of the cases	Selection: Selection of controls	Selection: Definition of controls	Comparability: Control for important factor or additional factor	Exposure: Ascertainment of exposure	Exposure: Same method of ascertainment for cases and controls	Exposure: Nonresponse rate	Total (0–9)
Wei-Sheng Lee-2017 [16]	*	*	*	*	**	*	*		8
Wei-Sheng Lee-2016 [17]	*	*	*	*	**	*	*		9

Note: a "star (*)" system of the Newcastle-Ottawa Scale (NOS) has been developed for the methodological quality assessment: each study can be awarded a maximum of one star for each numbered item within the selection and exposure categories, while a maximum of two stars can be given for the comparability category.

(b)

Cohort study	Selection: Selection of nonexposed cohort	Selection: Representativeness of the cohort	Selection: Ascertainment of exposure	Selection: Outcome of interest	Comparability: Comparability of cohorts on the basis of the design or analysis	Exposure: Assessment of outcome	Exposure: Follow-up long enough for outcomes to occur	Exposure: Adequacy of follow-up of cohorts	Total (0–9)
Wang 2016 [17]	*	*	*	*	*	*	*		7
Then 2017 [18]	*	*	*	*	**	*	*	*	9
Goveas 2012 [19]	*	*		*	*	*	*		6

Note: a "star (*)" system of the Newcastle-Ottawa Scale (NOS) has been developed for the methodological quality assessment: each study can be awarded a maximum of one star for each numbered item within the selection and exposure categories, while a maximum of two stars can be given for the comparability category.

Study name	Risk ratio	Lower limit	Upper limit	*P* value	Relative weight
W-S Lee 2017	0.580	0.497	0.676	0.000	20.90
W-S Lee 2016	2.480	2.270	2.710	0.000	21.15
Wang 2016	1.830	1.686	1.987	0.000	21.17
Then 2017	3.660	2.626	5.101	0.000	19.62
Goveas 2012	1.780	1.016	3.118	0.044	17.15
	1.750	1.033	2.964	0.037	

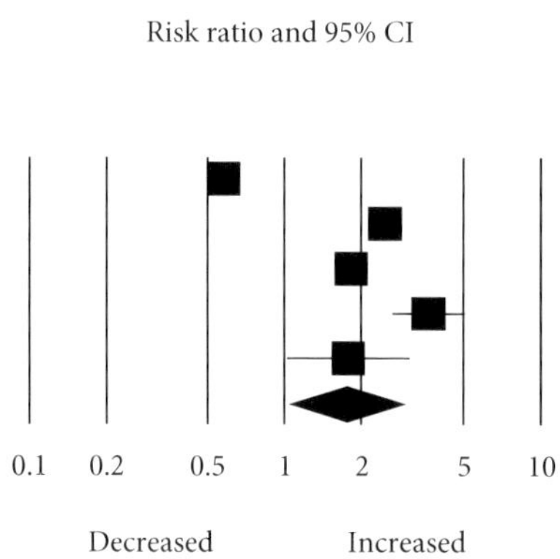

FIGURE 2: Forest plot of studies examining the association between SSRI use and dementia risk.

4. Discussion

4.1. Main Outcome. This current meta-analysis of observational epidemiological studies suggests that use of antidepressants increased a risk of developing dementia among the elderly population when compared with nonusers. Patients with monoamine oxidase inhibitor therapy had a higher risk of developing dementia than those with tricyclic and selective serotonin reuptake inhibitor therapy. Of importance, these findings would make physicians more cautious when they will consider an antidepressant treatment to their patients with depression. However, the

Study name	Risk ratio	Lower limit	Upper limit	P value	Relative weight
W-S Lee 2017	1.440	1.320	1.570	0.000	28.99
W-S Lee 2016	2.480	2.270	2.710	0.000	28.97
Then 2017	3.260	2.298	4.625	0.000	24.02
Goveas 2012	1.780	0.989	3.205	0.055	18.02
	2.131	1.427	3.184	0.000	

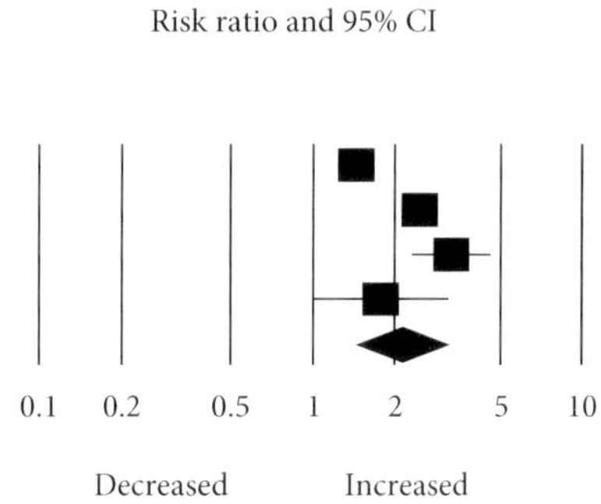

Figure 3: Forest plot of studies examining the association between TCA use and dementia risk.

Study name	Risk ratio	Lower limit	Upper limit	P value	Relative weight
W-S Lee 2016	1.860	1.468	2.357	0.000	58.46
Then 2017	4.940	2.171	11.243	0.000	41.54
	2.791	1.086	7.169	0.033	

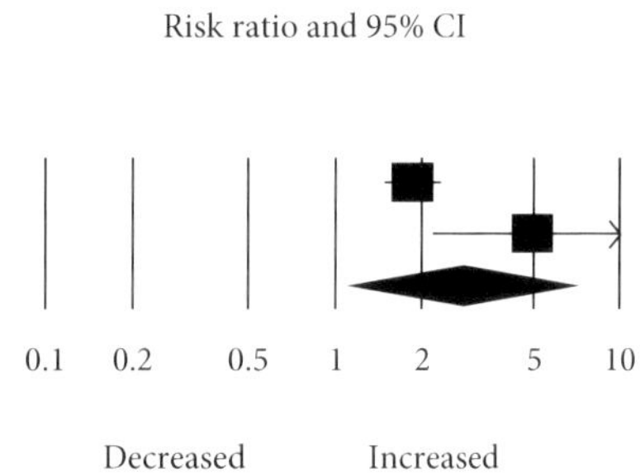

Figure 4: Forest plot of studies examining the association between MAOI use and dementia risk.

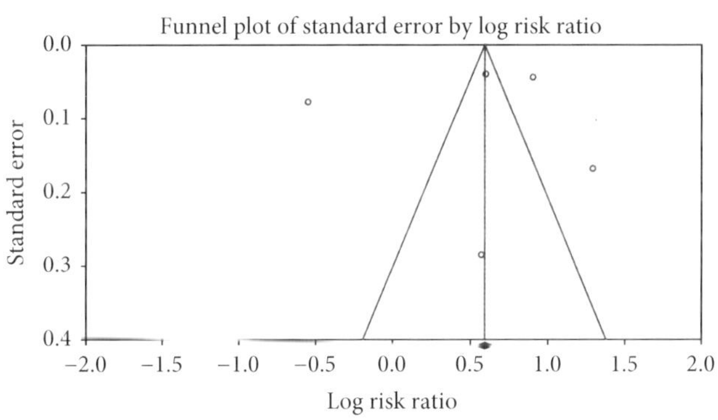

Figure 5: Funnel plot showing the association between antidepressant use and dementia risk.

decision to prescribe antidepressant therapy should be made in the light of the stringent clinical evaluation of benefits and risks, more particularly when physicians will prescribe antidepressants to a patient with depression. If antidepressant therapy is needed, it should be used judiciously and for the shorter period of time. Additionally, healthcare providers should routinely monitor the symptom of dementia risk factors such as memory loss, confusion, and disorientation while initiating or rewriting antidepressants to patients.

4.2. Biological Evidences. The biological mechanisms of the association between antidepressants and risk of developing dementia are still unclear. However, there are various possible ways of explanations for their association. First, the onset of depression before 65 years' age might be linked to the development of dementia and more recent depressive symptoms might link to the prodromal phase of dementia [7, 21]. Several biological studies reported that apolipoprotein (APOE) ε4 is a major known genetic risk factor that synergistically interacts with depression. Their interaction enhances the possibility of dementia risk, but it is not still well established [22, 23]. Second, use of antidepressants might prompt the imbalance of various neurobiological pathways. Therefore, it could help to elevate oxidative and nitrosamine stress as well as inflammation. Additionally, it might promote mitochondrial dysfunction, increased apoptosis, and finally diminished neurotrophic support [24]. Third, Steffens et al. reported that antidepressants increase subclinical cerebrovascular disease risk and promote cognitive decline by elevating potential oxidative stress [25]. Furthermore, to confirm the possible biological mechanism/link, more experimental and biological models are warranted.

4.3. Strengths and Limitations. Our study has several strengths. First, there is an enhanced statistical power to evaluate any association between antidepressant use and dementia risk. Second, this study evaluates the association in great detail and showed an association of different categories of antidepressants. However, our study has several limitations that need to be addressed. First, we included a small number of studies in our analysis. Second, a meta-analysis of epidemiological studies always has some unmeasured or uncontrolled confounding factors from the original studies. Our study findings had some degree of heterogeneity even though we used a random-effects model in our study analysis that helps to reduce publication bias. Third, we did not provide any information regarding dose differential and risk of dementia due to an insufficient amount of information. Fourth, duration of antidepressant and dementia risk were not evaluated because of restrained data. Fifth, types of dementia risk with antidepressant use were not investigated due to lack of information. Sixth, females are more prevalent to depression and anxiety than males are, and females act differently in the metabolism and distribution of antidepressants [26, 27], but we could not categorize dementia risk on the basis of gender. Finally, we were unable to include randomized controlled trials due to the absence of data.

4.4. Recommendation. Till now, no particular treatments are available to improve cognitive and behavioral symptoms of dementia patients. Additionally, antidepressant prescription has been increasing and concerns have been increased due to antidepressant therapy. Therefore, treatment of depression patients with antidepressant therapy should be assessed on a timely basis to reduce any unfavorable effects. If any symptoms are observed, then physicians need to stop antidepressant therapy or treat patients with a low dosage or shorter period of time. It is also indispensable to inform patients or their family about the inauspicious consequence of antidepressant therapy and other treatment options available for their current physical condition. However, to ensure safe and effective treatment, it is high time to provide proper guidelines for patients and healthcare providers.

4.5. Unanswered Questions and Future Direction. Since our study summarized results from several epidemiological studies, this is why we acknowledge that findings from this study could not clarify whether the observed association between antidepressants and dementia risk is the causal effect or other unmeasured confounding variables [28]. Hence, larger long-term prospective randomized control trials and biological studies are warranted to justify a possible biological mechanism which links dementia risk or rebut their association.

5. Conclusion

To our knowledge, this meta-analysis shows the most rigorous and precise analysis regarding antidepressant use and the risk of dementia. Our findings showed a significantly increased risk of dementia with antidepressant therapy. Healthcare providers might preferentially avoid unnecessary prescription of antidepressants to the patients if any symptoms regarding dementia are noticed. Additionally, proper guidelines should be provided for quality and safety treatment.

Acknowledgments

This work was financially supported by the "TMU Research Center of Cancer Translational Medicine" from The Featured Areas Research Center Program within the framework of the Higher Education Sprout Project by the Ministry of Education (MOE) in Taiwan.

References

[1] M. M. Islam, U. Iqbal, B. Walther et al., "Benzodiazepine use and risk of dementia in the elderly population: a systematic review and meta-analysis," *Neuroepidemiology*, vol. 47, no. 3-4, pp. 181–191, 2017.

[2] A. Wimo, L. Jönsson, J. Bond, M. Prince, B. Winblad, and Alzheimer Disease International, "The worldwide economic impact of dementia 2010," *Alzheimer's & Dementia*, vol. 9, no. 1, pp. 1–11.e3, 2013.

[3] C. K. Wu, Y. H. Yang, T. T. Lin et al., "Statin use reduces the risk of dementia in elderly patients: a nationwide data survey and propensity analysis," *Journal of Internal Medicine*, vol. 277, no. 3, pp. 343–352, 2015.

[4] L. A. Profenno, A. P. Porsteinsson, and S. V. Faraone, "Meta-analysis of Alzheimer's disease risk with obesity, diabetes, and related disorders," *Biological Psychiatry*, vol. 67, no. 6, pp. 505–512, 2010.

[5] C. S. Ivan, S. Seshadri, A. Beiser et al., "Dementia after stroke: the Framingham Study," *Stroke*, vol. 35, no. 6, pp. 1264–1268, 2004.

[6] C.-Y. Tsai, H.-C. Yang, M. Islam et al., "Psychotropic medications prescribing trends in adolescents: a nationwide population-based study in Taiwan," *International Journal for Quality in Health Care*, vol. 29, no. 6, pp. 861–866, 2017.

[7] A. L. Byers and K. Yaffe, "Depression and risk of developing dementia," *Nature Reviews Neurology*, vol. 7, no. 6, pp. 323–331, 2011.

[8] C. Shilyansky, L. M. Williams, A. Gyurak, A. Harris, T. Usherwood, and A. Etkin, "Effect of antidepressant treatment on cognitive impairments associated with depression: a randomised longitudinal study," *The Lancet Psychiatry*, vol. 3, no. 5, pp. 425–435, 2016.

[9] J. Schmitt, M. Wingen, J. Ramaekers, E. Evers, and W. Riedel, "Serotonin and human cognitive performance," *Current Pharmaceutical Design*, vol. 12, no. 20, pp. 2473–2486, 2006.

[10] A. Liberati, D. G. Altman, J. Tetzlaff et al., "The PRISMA statement for reporting systematic reviews and meta-analyses of studies that evaluate health care interventions: explanation and elaboration," *PLoS Medicine*, vol. 6, no. 7, article e1000100, 2009.

[11] T. N. Poly, M. M. Islam, B. A. Walther et al., "Exploring the association between statin use and the risk of Parkinson's disease: a meta-analysis of observational studies," *Neuroepidemiology*, vol. 49, no. 3-4, pp. 142–151, 2017.

[12] M. M. Islam, H.-C. Yang, P.-A. Nguyen et al., "Exploring association between statin use and breast cancer risk: an updated meta-analysis," *Archives of Gynecology and Obstetrics*, vol. 296, no. 6, pp. 1043–1053, 2017.

[13] A. Stang, "Critical evaluation of the Newcastle-Ottawa scale for the assessment of the quality of nonrandomized studies in meta-analyses," *European Journal of Epidemiology*, vol. 25, no. 9, pp. 603–605, 2010.

[14] J. P. Higgins and S. Green, *Cochrane Handbook for Systematic Reviews of Interventions version 5.1. 0*, The cochrane collaboration, 2011.

[15] C. Lee, C.-L. Lin, F.-C. Sung, J.-A. Liang, and C.-H. Kao, "Antidepressant treatment and risk of dementia: a population-

based, retrospective case-control study," *The Journal of Clinical Psychiatry*, vol. 77, no. 1, pp. 117–122, 2016, quiz 122.

[16] C. W.-S. Lee, C.-L. Lin, P.-Y. Lin, S. Thielke, K.-P. Su, and C.-H. Kao, "Antidepressants and risk of dementia in migraine patients: a population-based case-control study," *Progress in Neuro-Psychopharmacology and Biological Psychiatry*, vol. 77, pp. 83–89, 2017.

[17] C. Wang, S. Gao, H. C. Hendrie et al., "Antidepressant use in the elderly is associated with an increased risk of dementia," *Alzheimer Disease and Associated Disorders*, vol. 30, no. 2, pp. 99–104, 2016.

[18] C.-K. Then, N.-F. Chi, K.-H. Chung et al., "Risk analysis of use of different classes of antidepressants on subsequent dementia: a nationwide cohort study in Taiwan," *PLoS One*, vol. 12, no. 4, article e0175187, 2017.

[19] J. S. Goveas, P. E. Hogan, J. M. Kotchen et al., "Depressive symptoms, antidepressant use, and future cognitive health in postmenopausal women: the Women's Health Initiative Memory Study," *International Psychogeriatrics*, vol. 24, no. 8, pp. 1252–1264, 2012.

[20] J. P. Higgins and S. Green, *Cochrane Handbook for Systematic Reviews of Interventions*, John Wiley & Sons, 2011.

[21] A. F. Jorm, "History of depression as a risk factor for dementia: an updated review," *Australian & New Zealand Journal of Psychiatry*, vol. 35, no. 6, pp. 776–781, 2016.

[22] I. K. Karlsson, A. M. Bennet, A. Ploner et al., "Apolipoprotein E ε4 genotype and the temporal relationship between depression and dementia," *Neurobiology of Aging*, vol. 36, no. 4, pp. 1751–1756, 2015.

[23] X. Meng and C. D'arcy, "Apolipoprotein E gene, environmental risk factors, and their interactions in dementia among seniors," *International Journal of Geriatric Psychiatry*, vol. 28, no. 10, pp. 1005–1014, 2013.

[24] A. Carvalho, K. Miskowiak, T. Hyphantis et al., "Cognitive dysfunction in depression–pathophysiology and novel targets," *CNS & Neurological Disorders - Drug Targets*, vol. 13, no. 10, pp. 1819–1835, 2014.

[25] D. C. Steffens, H. Chung, K. R. R. Krishnan, W. T. Longstreth, M. Carlson, and G. L. Burke, "Antidepressant treatment and worsening white matter on serial cranial magnetic resonance imaging in the elderly: the cardiovascular health study," *Stroke*, vol. 39, no. 3, pp. 857–862, 2008.

[26] M. M. Islam, U. Iqbal, B. A. Walther et al., "Gender-based personalized pharmacotherapy: a systematic review," *Archives of Gynecology and Obstetrics*, vol. 295, no. 6, pp. 1305–1317, 2017.

[27] R. Keers and K. J. Aitchison, "Gender differences in antidepressant drug response," *International Review of Psychiatry*, vol. 22, no. 5, pp. 485–500, 2010.

[28] M. Kundi, "Causality and the interpretation of epidemiologic evidence," *Ciência & Saúde Coletiva*, vol. 12, no. 2, pp. 419–428, 2007.

16

Apathy is Correlated with Widespread Diffusion Tensor Imaging (DTI) Impairment in Amyotrophic Lateral Sclerosis

Cinzia Femiano,[1] Francesca Trojsi,[1] Giuseppina Caiazzo,[1] Mattia Siciliano,[1,2] Carla Passaniti,[2] Antonio Russo,[1] Alvino Bisecco,[1] Mario Cirillo,[1] Maria Rosaria Monsurrò,[1] Fabrizio Esposito,[3] Gioacchino Tedeschi,[1] and Gabriella Santangelo[2]

[1]*Department of Medical, Surgical, Neurological, Metabolic and Aging Sciences; MRI Research Center SUN-FISM Università degli Studi della Campania "Luigi Vanvitelli", Naples, Italy*
[2]*Department of Psychology, Università degli Studi della Campania "Luigi Vanvitelli", Naples, Italy*
[3]*Department of Medicine, Surgery and Dentistry, Scuola Medica Salernitana, University of Salerno, Baronissi, Salerno, Italy*

Correspondence should be addressed to Francesca Trojsi; francesca.trojsi@unicampania.it

Academic Editor: Giuseppe Bellelli

Apathy is recognized as the most common behavioral change in several neurodegenerative diseases, including amyotrophic lateral sclerosis (ALS), a multisystem neurodegenerative disorder. Particularly, apathy has been reported to be associated with poor ALS prognosis. However, the brain microstructural correlates of this behavioral symptom, reported as the most common in ALS, have not been completely elucidated. Using diffusion tensor imaging (DTI) and tract-based spatial statistics (TBSS), here we aimed to quantify the correlation between brain microstructural damage and apathy scores in the early stages of ALS. Twenty-one consecutive ALS patients, in King's clinical stage 1 or 2, and 19 age- and sex-matched healthy controls (HCs) underwent magnetic resonance imaging and neuropsychological examination. Between-group comparisons did not show any significant difference on cognitive and behavioral variables. When compared to HCs, ALS patients exhibited a decreased fractional anisotropy (FA) [$p < .05$, threshold-free cluster enhancement (TFCE) corrected] in the corpus callosum and in bilateral anterior cingulate cortices. Self-rated Apathy Evaluation Scale (AES) scores and self-rated apathy T-scores of the Frontal Systems Behavior (FrSBe) scale were found inversely correlated to FA measures ($p < .05$, TFCE corrected) in widespread white matter (WM) areas, including several associative fiber tracts in the frontal, temporal, and parietal lobes. These results point towards an early microstructural degeneration of brain areas biologically involved in cognition and behavior regulation in ALS. Moreover, the significant correlations between apathy and DTI measures in several brain areas may suggest that subtle WM changes may be associated with mild behavioral symptoms in ALS even in the absence of overt cognitive and behavioral impairment.

1. Introduction

Apathy is defined as decreased motivation towards goal-directed behaviors [1] and may occur as a symptom of a variety of different psychiatric and neurodegenerative diseases [2, 3]. In particular, several studies have revealed that apathy is the most common behavioral symptom in amyotrophic lateral sclerosis (ALS) [4–6], a multisystem neurodegenerative disease that mainly affects motor areas and exhibits cognitive and behavioral symptoms belonging to the spectrum of frontotemporal lobar degeneration (FTLD) syndrome [7, 8]. Of note, while approximately 5–15% of ALS patients meet the diagnostic criteria for FTLD [9, 10], predominantly developing clinical features typical of the behavioral variant frontotemporal dementia (bvFTD) [10], most patients exhibit behavior and/or cognitive dysfunctions (i.e., ALS with behavioral impairment [ALSbi], with cognitive impairment [ALSci], and with both [ALSbci]), which are not sufficient to diagnose FTLD [8].

From the prognostic point of view, several studies demonstrated that ALS-FTLD patients have a significantly shorter survival than nondemented ones [11–13] and that behavioral impairment rather than dementia or cognitive impairment alone is an important predictor of survival in ALS patients [14]. Among behavioral disturbances, apathy may precede motor symptoms [15], represents an independent (negative) prognostic factor in ALS [16], and may even impact the ability to engage competently in end-of-life decisions [14, 17].

The most common instruments used to detect apathy in ALS patients are the Frontal Systems Behavior (FrSBe) scale, which includes an apathy subscale [18, 19]; the Dimensional Apathy Scale (DAS) [20]; and the Apathy Evaluation Scale (AES) [21]. While FrSBe is not specifically designed for testing patients with physical disability [18, 19], AES is a well-established method for assessing apathy in several neurodegenerative diseases [3, 22]. Both FrSBe and AES allow performing a monodimensional evaluation of apathy. However, this symptom is actually composed of multiple factors related to the cognitive, behavioral, and emotional domains [23], and recent studies employed a factorial analysis of AES scores revealing a triadic or four-factor substructure of the scale in Parkinson's disease [24, 25].

From the neuroanatomical point of view, some structural correlates of behavioral changes have been identified in frontosubcortical circuits in healthy subjects as well as in ALS patients [26, 27] using neuropsychological and advanced magnetic resonance imaging (MRI) evaluations. In this regard, diffusion tensor imaging (DTI) is the advanced MRI method of choice to investigate *in vivo* the integrity of large white matter (WM) tracts in terms of fractional anisotropy (FA) and mean (MD), axial (AD), and radial (RD) diffusivity parameters [28, 29]. Particularly, DTI allowed exploring the structural connectivity in several neurodegenerative diseases, including Alzheimer's disease [30] and the disease spectrum of ALS-FTLD [31–37].

So far, only a few studies have explored the brain structural correlates of apathy in ALS, suggesting that WM abnormalities within anterior cingulum bundle are the most relevant substrates of apathy in ALS [36, 37]. However, in those studies, apathy was only evaluated by the subscale of FrSBe, and patients in early disease stages, according to validated staging systems, were not included.

On this background, using a tract-based spatial statistics (TBSS) DTI approach [38], we aimed to explore the potential association between brain microstructural damage and apathy, using both self- and informant-rated version of the AES, and by the apathy subscale of FrSBe, in the early stages of ALS according to a validated staging system for ALS.

2. Methods

2.1. Case Selection. Twenty-two right-handed patients (13 men, 9 women; mean age 58.19 ± 9.63), 14 with definite ALS and 8 with probable or probable laboratory-supported ALS, according to the revised El Escorial criteria [39], were consecutively recruited at the First Division of Neurology of the University of Campania "Luigi Vanvitelli" (Naples, Italy). Genetic analysis was performed in all patients, exploring *C9ORF72* expansion and mutations of *superoxide dismutase 1* (*SOD1*), *TAR DNA binding protein* (*TARDBP*), and *fused in sarcoma/translocated in liposarcoma* (*FUS/TLS*). Only a woman with familial ALS, carrier of *FUS/TLS* gene mutation (codon 1622 G>A), was not included in the analysis. With regard to clinical phenotypes, according to the ALS subtype classification of Chiò et al. [40], 9 patients had a bulbar onset and 13 a spinal onset; disease phenotypes were classic ($n = 8$), bulbar ($n = 4$), flail arm ($n = 2$), flail leg ($n = 1$), and pyramidal ($n = 7$). Patients were classified according to King's clinical staging system for ALS [41] as follows: Stage 1: involvement of a first region; Stage 2: involvement of a second region; Stage 3: involvement of a third region; and Stage 4: need for gastrostomy or respiratory support (noninvasive ventilation). All the patients enrolled were in King's clinical stage 1 or 2.

As for clinical parameters, we administered the ALS functional rating scale-revised (ALSFRS-R) score, an index of disability status [42], and the Upper Motor Neuron (UMN) score, a measure of pyramidal dysfunction through the evaluation of the number of pathologic reflexes elicited from 16 body sites (i.e., one-sided, glabellum and masseter, and, bilaterally, orbicularis oris, biceps, triceps, finger jerk, knee, ankle, and Babinski responses) [43]. Moreover, we also estimated the disease progression rate according to the following formula: 48 − ALSFRS-R score/months of disease duration [44]. None of the patients had additional neurological diseases or previous mental illnesses.

Nineteen right-handed healthy control subjects (HCs) (9 men, 10 women; mean age 57.53 ± 9.03) were enrolled by "word of mouth" among (nonphysician) employees at the University ($n = 10$) or friends and colleagues of patients' caregivers ($n = 9$). HCs were cognitively normal and had no comorbid neurological, psychiatric, or medical conditions; moreover, they were age-, sex- and education-matched with the enrolled ALS patients (Table 1).

2.2. Neuropsychological Assessment. A 60 min neuropsychological battery, assessing cognitive functioning/ability (global cognitive assessment and executive, memory, and visuospatial abilities) and frontal behavioral disorders, was designed by a team of neurologists and neuropsychologists experienced in the study and management of motor neuron diseases and cognitive decline. Although this neuropsychological battery was not ALS-specific, the tests administered have been widely used in ALS and other movement disorders [45–48]. All tests were administered in the morning following the same sequence to avoid possible interference of the answers of one test over the others [47]. Moreover, if the subject was tired during testing, a further session was scheduled to complete the battery within two weeks from the first one. Considering that respiratory dysfunction may affect cognitive performances [49–51], oxygen saturation and forced vital capacity (FVC) were measured at the time of each examination (i.e., no participants showed oxygen saturation < 92 mmHg and FVC < 80%) [47].

2.2.1. Cognition. The following cognitive domains were evaluated in both ALS patients and HCs: (1) global cognitive impairment by Mini-Mental State Examination (MMSE); (2) executive functions (i.e., the inhibitory control) by the Stroop

Table 1: Detailed patients and controls characteristics of the patients included in the study.

Parameters	ALS patients mean (SD) ($n = 21$)	Controls mean (SD) ($n = 19$)	p (<.05)
	Demographic and clinical measures		
Age	58.4 (9.83)	57.5 (9.03)	.77
Male/female	13/8	9/10	.35
Education	11.3 (4.6)	11.53 (3.94)	.87
Disease duration (months)	18.71 (11.1)	—	
Disease progression rate	.035 (.037)	—	
ALSFRS-R score	41.3 (3.5)	—	
UMN score	6.1 (4.5)	—	
	Neuropsychological parameters		
MMSE	28.9 (1.4)	29.72 (1.18)	.06
Digit span test: forward	5.2 (1.5)	5.53 (1.01)	.4
Digit span test: backward	4.2 (1.3)	4.59 (.8)	.4
Token	33.9 (2.08)	35 (1.2)	.07
Memory prose	12.7 (2.96)	14.3 (2.1)	.06
RCPM	27.1 (4.2)	30 (2.82)	.08
Visual discrimination of scrawls	30.4 (1.5)	30.4 (1.3)	.96
SEF	.3 (.7)	.18 (.53)	.52
	Neurobehavioral variables		
S-AES total score	27.3 (6.7)	25.8 (5.28)	.47
Cognitive factor	12.3 (4.3)	11.5 (2.5)	.51
Behavioral factor	6.9 (1.3)	6.5 (1.5)	.4
Emotional factor	3.4 (1.18)	2.8 (.7)	.09
Other factors	4.6 (1.27)	4.9 (1.4)	.5
I-AES total score	28.6 (7.3)	29.4 (6.3)	.77
Cognitive factor	12.8 (3.6)	13 (2.7)	.9
Behavioral factor	7.2 (1.8)	7.6 (2.7)	.64
Emotional factor	3.5 (1.4)	3.5 (1.5)	.9
Other factors	5 (1.6)	5.2 (1.9)	.78
FrSBe (patient form, total T-score)	49.2 (7.8)	—	—
FrSBe (caregiver form, total T-score)	57.1 (8.7)	—	—
FrSBe (patient form, apathy T-score)	47.9 (9.4)	—	—
FrSBe (caregiver form, apathy T-score)	58.1 (10.8)	—	—
BDI-II	11.6 (5.9)	10.18 (8.04)	.57

ALSFRS-R = Amyotrophic Lateral Sclerosis Functional Rating Scale-Revised; S-, I-AES = self-rated, informant-rated Apathy Evaluation Scale; BDI-II = Beck Depression Inventory II; FrSBe = Frontal Systems Behavior; MMSE = Mini-Mental State Examination; RCPM = Raven's Colored Progressive Matrices; SEF = Stroop Executive Factor; UMN = Upper Motor Neuron.

Color-Word Interference test using the Stroop Executive Factor (SEF) [52], which accounts for motor disability [48], and by the forward and backward digit span tasks [53], assessing working memory and sustained attention; (3) language (i.e., verbal comprehension abilities), by Token Test [54]; (4) long-term verbal memory, by memory prose test [55]; (5) nonverbal abstract reasoning by Raven's Colored Progressive Matrices (RCPM) [56]; and (6) visuo-spatial abilities by visual discrimination (scrawls) test [54].

2.2.2. Neurobehavioral Aspects. Apathy was evaluated by both self-rated and informant-rated versions of the apathy subscale of the FrSBe [18, 19] and AES scales (S-AES and I-AES) [21]. As for FrSBe (score range: 46–230 points for total score; 14–70 points for apathy subscale), the raw scores were converted to T-scores according to gender, age, and years of education [19]. T-Scores were considered as "borderline" impaired when ranging from 60 to 64, while T-scores higher than or equal to 65 reflected pathological changes [57].

As for AES (score range: 18–72 points), we used a cut-off score of 41 for I-AES and 40 for S-AES. These clinical thresholds were estimated using descriptive statistics as reported in Marin et al. [21] and using 2 standard deviations above the mean as critical value. In addition to total score, the AES subscale scores (i.e., cognitive, behavioral, emotional, and other subscales) [21, 25] were employed for the analyses. All subjects completed the Beck Depression Inventory-II (BDI-II) [58], with score range from 0 to 63 points; the standard cut-off ranges were as follows: 0–9 indicated minimal depression, 10–18 indicated mild depression, 19–29 indicated moderate depression, and 30–63 indicated severe depression [58]. Overall, higher scores indicated more severe behavioral symptoms for all these scales.

2.3. Statistical Analysis: Between-Group Comparisons of Demographic, Clinical and Neuropsychological Data. Demographic, clinical, and neuropsychological data were reported for ALS patients and HCs. The Shapiro-Wilk test was used to assess normality and statistical dependency from the distribution of the data; *t*-tests, Mann-Whitney *U* tests, and chi-square tests (all Bonferroni corrected) were used to compare demographic, clinical, neuropsychological, and neurobehavioral scores between ALS patients and HCs. SPSS statistics 21.0 was used to perform all statistical analyses.

For more details about the correlations between apathy scores (i.e., S- and I-AES and apathy subscales of FrSBe) and whole-brain DTI measures, see paragraph on Section 2.6.

2.4. Ethics Statement. The research was conducted according to the principles expressed in the Declaration of Helsinki. Ethical approval was obtained from the Ethics Committee of the University of Campania "Luigi Vanvitelli" of Naples. Patient or family written consent was obtained from each participant.

2.5. Imaging Acquisition. Magnetic-resonance images were acquired on a 3 T scanner equipped with an 8-channel parallel head coil (General Electric Healthcare, Milwaukee, Wisconsin). Whole-brain DTI was performed using a GRE EPI sequence (repetition time = 10,000 ms, echo time = 88 ms, field of view = 320 mm, isotropic resolution = 2.5 mm, b value = 1000 s/mm^2, 32 isotropically distributed gradients, and frequency-encoding RL).

2.6. Diffusion Tensor Imaging (DTI) Analysis. A voxel-based TBSS approach was used for the group analysis of DTI data [38]. DTI data sets were processed with the Functional MRI of the Brain (FMRIB) Software Library (FSL) software package (http://www.fmrib.ox.ac.uk/fsl), according to methods used in our previous studies [59, 60]. Preprocessing included eddy current and motion correction and brain-tissue extraction. After preprocessing, DTI images were averaged and concatenated into 33 (1 B = 0 + 32 B = 1000) volumes, and a diffusion tensor model was fitted at each voxel, generating AD, FA, MD, and eigenvalue ($\lambda 1$, $\lambda 2$, and $\lambda 3$) maps. The average of the second and third eigenvalues of the diffusion tensor was used for the definition of RD. Images were warped to the Montreal Neurological Institute (MNI) 152 template, available as a standard T1 data set in the FSL software package. TBSS was run with FA maps to create the "skeleton," which represents the center of all fiber bundles common to all subjects, and which was used for all other maps. To this purpose, FA images of all subjects ($n = 40$) were aligned to a common target (1 × 1 × 1 mm MNI152 FMRIB58_FA standard space) using nonlinear registration. A mean FA skeleton was then created with threshold of FA > 0.2. Age, gender, and education were considered as covariates. Moreover, the TBSS results were linked to standard anatomic data derived from the International Consortium of Brain Mapping DTI-81 WM label atlas (Johns Hopkins University, Baltimore, MD) [61, 62]. Individual skeleton images were submitted to a general linear model (GLM) analysis with appropriate design matrices and linear contrasts defined for the group comparisons and the correlations between all diffusivity parameters (FA, RD, MD, and AD) and clinical measures of apathy (score on self- and informant-rated AES, including the four factors of AES and *T*-scores of self- and informant-rated versions of the apathy subscale of the FrSBe) and depression (BDI-II scores). The results of voxel-wise correlations were shown on the skeleton map after correction for multiple comparison with the threshold-free cluster enhancement (TFCE) technique [38]. Age, gender, and education were considered as covariates, except for *T*-scores of the apathy subscale of the FrSBe.

3. Results

Demographic (age, gender, and education), clinical (disease duration, UMN scores, ALSFRS-R total score and subscores, and disease progression rate), neuropsychological, and neurobehavioral data of the ALS cohort ($n = 21$) and the HC group ($n = 19$) are reported in Table 1. Patients and HCs did not differ on demographic, cognitive, and behavioral parameters (Table 1). 4.7% of ALS patients ($n = 1$) and 5.2% of healthy subjects ($n = 1$) were above cut-off for apathy on the S-AES. Moreover, the same results were found when apathy was identified by the I-AES.

According to cut-off of BDI-II, 9 ALS patients and 11 healthy controls exhibited minimum depression; 9 ALS patients and 7 healthy controls, mild depression; and 3 ALS patients and 1 healthy control, moderate/severe depression.

3.1. TBSS DTI Analysis. Compared to HCs, ALS patients exhibited a decreased FA ($p < .05$, TFCE corrected) in the WM underneath the precentral gyri, in the body of the corpus callosum (CC) and in the bilateral anterior cingulate bundles (Figure 1), while no significant differences were observed in whole-brain MD, AD, and RD values.

3.2. Correlation between Apathy Scores and MRI Abnormalities. S-AES scores were positively correlated with RD measures (Figure 2) ($p < .05$, TFCE corrected) in the splenium of the CC. Significant inverse correlations were found between the score on the self-rated version of the apathy subscore of FrSBe and FA measures ($p < .05$, TFCE corrected) in the left superior longitudinal fasciculus, in the right and left inferior longitudinal fasciculus, in the left fronto-occipital fasciculus, in the left uncinate fasciculus, in the left anterior cingulum bundle, and in the left thalamus (Figure 2). Moreover, positive correlations were revealed between the score on the self-rated version of the apathy subscore of FrSBe and RD measures ($p < .05$, TFCE corrected) in the splenium of the CC. Score on the informant-rated version of the apathy subscore of FrSBe was found to be inversely correlated with FA ($p < .05$, TFCE corrected) in the WM underneath the left temporal fusiform cortex. Finally, no significant correlation was reported between the BDI-II scores and the DTI measures and between the four factors (i.e.,

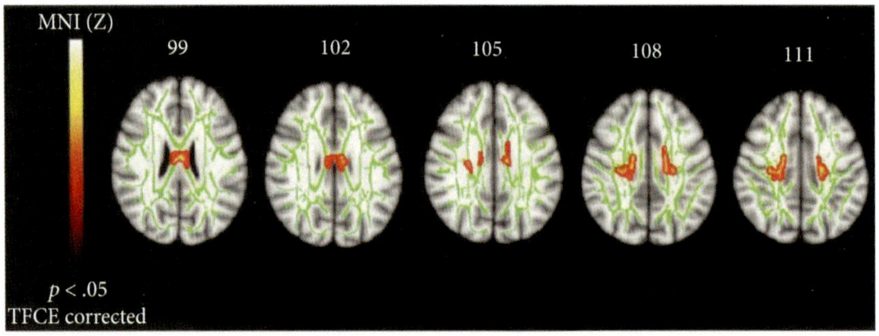

FIGURE 1: Comparison between FA statistic parametric maps of ALS patients versus HCs. FA decrease (red-yellow scale, $p < .05$, TCFE corrected; green: skeleton) is evident bilaterally in the midbody of the corpus callosum and in the anterior cingulum bundles.

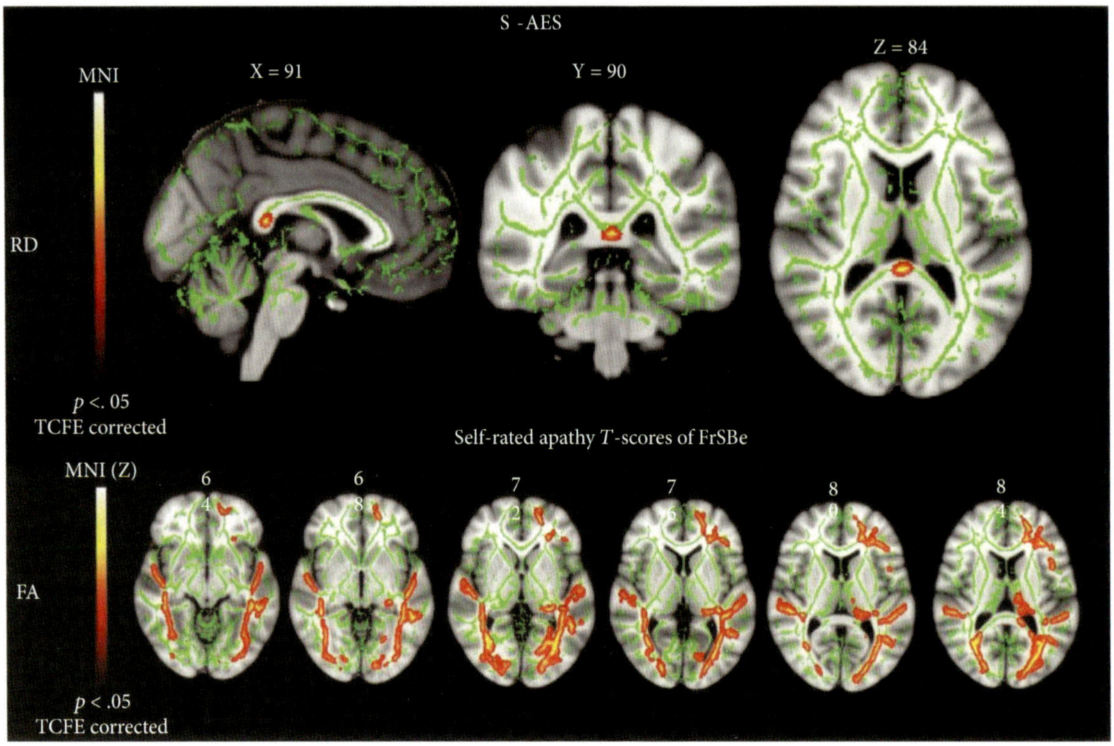

FIGURE 2: Voxel-wise correlation analyses between apathy scores (S-AES scores and self-rated apathy T-scores of FrSBe) and RD/FA in the studied ALS sample. Patterns of positive correlation ($p < .05$, TCFE corrected; red-yellow scale; green: skeleton) between S-AES scores and RD in the splenium of the CC and of negative correlation ($p < .05$, TCFE corrected; red-yellow scale; green: skeleton) between apathy T-scores of FrSBe and FA in several associative WM tracts in the patients' group.

cognitive, behavioral, emotional, and other) of self-rated and informant-rated versions of the AES and the DTI metrics.

4. Discussion

Our findings revealed that ALS patients, in early stages of disease and without cognitive or behavioral impairment, may exhibit microstructural changes in both motor (corticospinal tracts, midbody of CC) and extra-motor (bilateral anterior cingulate bundles) WM tracts. Moreover, in our population, FA and RD changes in several associative fiber tracts in frontal, temporal and parietal lobes were found to be related to severity of apathy when evaluated by self- and informant ratings. Our results thus suggest that subtle WM changes can be associated with mild behavioral symptoms in ALS even in the absence of overt cognitive and behavioral impairment. Besides allowing the confirmation of previous results, the present study expanded previous analyses towards the use of both self- and informant-rated versions of the AES and of the FrSBe to measure the severity of apathy, enabling the investigation of the potential correlations existing between changes in patients' apathy scores and whole-brain DTI measures.

Microstructural alterations in the CC found in our ALS population were similar to those reported in other cohorts of ALS patients [59, 60]. Similar to previous studies, we performed a TBSS analysis of DTI data, a hypothesis-free technique which is capable of detecting structural changes over the whole brain and therefore highlights the structural process of disease spreading across WM fibers known to connect motor areas [59, 60, 63]. Structural neuroimaging evidence of CC damage seems to provide, *in vivo*, the same neuropathological signatures of neurodegeneration widely reported in both animal models [64] and autopsied patients [65]. Interestingly, executive and behavioral dysfunctions have been shown to be associated mainly with a degeneration of the anterior part of CC (e.g., genu) in several cohorts of ALS patients [63, 65] as well as in FTLD phenotypes, in support of the existence of a frontotemporal lobar degeneration continuum [66]. Moreover, among associative WM tracts in the frontal lobe, the anterior cingulum bundle is adjacent to the motor cortex, and its microstructural damage in ALS has been hypothesized to be related to the pattern of corticofugal disease spreading [67, 68]. The functional involvement of the anterior cingulum in a network of multiple frontal brain regions, which are connected to the basal ganglia and limbic system and which substantially regulate goal-directed and socioemotional behaviors [37, 69–71] and inhibitory control [72], may explain the strong association between the alterations in the anterior cingulum bundle and apathy in both FTLD [69] and ALS [6, 26, 27] patients. Moreover, we observed that not only the FA values in the anterior cingulum bundle, together with FA changes in more widespread WM areas, including several long associative WM tracts, were related to severity of apathy when evaluated by the self-rated apathy subscore of FrSBe. This finding suggests an involvement of more distributed cerebral areas in determining apathy, as also revealed in other neurodegenerative diseases, such as Parkinson's [73] and Alzheimer's [74] diseases, and in neuropsychiatric disorders [75]. Taken together, these results substantially expand the microstructural correlates of apathy and may therefore account for the multidomain structure of this behavioral symptom, which has been previously divided into three different subtypes: cognitive, emotional/affective, and initiation apathy [3]. Indeed, although the apathy subscale of FrSBe allows evaluating apathy as a unitary construct, without excluding the potential confounding effects of motor symptoms on the assessment of this behavioral symptom, a neurobiological model of apathy, known as "the ABC model" [27, 76], currently recognizes three aspects of apathy with different clinical manifestations [23]: (i) affective-emotional apathy, affecting the skill of using emotional context to guide behavior and leading to altered social interactions; (ii) behavioral apathy, which may affect spontaneous patterns of motor movement; and (iii) cognitive apathy, which significantly reduces goal-directed behaviors. Moreover, a valuable overcome of this model has been represented by the "Dimensional Apathy Framework," which proposed three types of apathy: "initiation, executive, and emotional" apathy [77]. The three types are measured by the DAS, a reliable scale exploring multidimensional apathy in ALS patients by minimising the effects of motor impairment [20, 77]. In this regard, our findings of the relationship between apathy and changes of DTI metrics in more widespread WM areas, beyond the anterior cingulum bundle, deserve to be further investigated in future studies where apathy should be evaluated by DAS. Conversely, the evidence of no significant differences between the subfactors of the AES between the ALS group and healthy subjects and of no correlation between the subfactors of the AES and DTI parameters within the ALS group may further underline the intrinsic limitation of the AES as a one-dimensional apathy measurement scale, with a unitary outcome score, thereby resulting in not being useful for assessing multidimensional apathy [3]. Importantly, Radakovic et al. [78] revealed that in ALS patients, only "initiation" apathy was significantly associated with verbal fluency deficit, while "emotional" apathy was significantly associated with emotional recognition deficits, suggesting that emotional and initiation apathy may have dissociated neural correlates. However, the implementation of the DAS has been limited by its only recent validation in other languages other than English [79]. In particular, at the time of our data collection, the DAS was still not validated in the Italian language, and therefore, we could not employ it in the present study, prospecting to use this scale in future analyses.

When we assessed apathy by the specific subscale of the FrSBe, our findings revealed significant correlations between apathy *T*-scores and FA measures in several associative WM tracts, resembling the findings by Tsujimoto et al. [36], who reported that the severity of apathy was significantly related to FA decrease within the WM underneath the right medial frontal gyrus. Woolley et al. [37] also revealed a significant correlation between changes of apathy subscores of FrSBe and FA decrease in WM underneath bilateral primary motor areas and in the right anterior cingulum bundle and superior longitudinal fasciculus. However, the diverging results obtained by these studies compared to ours might be related to differences in clinical characteristics of the samples included and to methodological differences.

RD measures in the splenium of the CC were found significantly related to the self-rated AES and FrSBe apathy *T*-scores assessed in our ALS population, as also previously described in some non-ALS cohorts of apathetic patients [80, 81]. In particular, Tu et al. [80] reported that the WM damage of the splenium of the CC in Alzheimer's disease and subcortical ischemic vascular disease patients was correlated with the severity of apathy through the involvement of general cognition and dementia severity. Considering that the WM integrity of the body and splenium of the CC is supposed to be related to general cognition on the basis of their numerous fiber projections [82], the reported association between the severity of apathy and the WM integrity of the splenium adds evidence to the notion that widespread WM disconnection and defective cognition may both significantly affect the mechanisms underlying apathy [80]. In support of the abovementioned suggestion, we also found that the informant-rated apathy subscore of FrSBe was inversely related to FA in the WM underneath the left temporal fusiform cortex, which is in line with recent findings concerning the association between apathy scores and frontotemporal regional cerebral blood flow measures in patients with amnestic mild cognitive impairment (aMCI), especially in those with a high probability of being in the aMCI stage of AD [83].

Major limitations of our study are the use of a non-ALS-specific neuropsychological protocol and the recruitment of a small sample size of ALS patients. Specifically, apathy assessment by the subscale of FrSBe, albeit often adopted for ALS patients [4, 36, 57], may be confounded by the presence of motor and bulbar symptoms. Future investigations using ALS-specific neuropsychological protocols, as well as the DAS, to evaluate the multidimensional nature of apathy, should be performed. Moreover, we did not perform a multimodal neuroimaging analysis to combine (and investigate both) WM and grey matter (GM) correlates of apathy. However, when using available T1 MRI data in a standard voxel-based morphometry (VBM) as described previously [60] (data not shown), we did not detect clusters of significant GM atrophy in ALS patients, likely due to the small sample size. Nonetheless, a voxel-wise meta-analysis of 29 VMB studies involving several cohorts of ALS patients revealed that clusters of GM atrophy were mainly located in the right precentral gyrus, the left rolandic operculum, the left lenticular nucleus, and the right anterior cingulate/ paracingulate gyri [84], confirming the multisystem nature of ALS, involving extra-motor areas besides the motor system. Of note, multimodal structural approaches, combining both DTI and voxel- or surface-based morphometry measures, have been shown to be more sensitive than each modality separately in the individual ALS patient classification [85, 86], thereby overcoming potential limitations related to each technique for diagnostic purposes.

In conclusion, we identified widespread microstructural correlates of apathy in early stages of ALS. These correlates involve the cingulum bundle and further extend over frontotemporal WM areas. The early involvement of nonmotor areas highlights the multisystem nature of ALS already at the early stages of the disease. Thus, more accurate protocols for the multidimensional assessment of apathy should be implemented routinely in the clinical management of ALS patients. This could help to identify early apathy in ALS, to plan tailored therapeutic interventions, and to improve patients' and caregivers' quality of life.

Authors' Contributions

Cinzia Femiano and Francesca Trojsi have equally contributed to this work.

Acknowledgments

The authors are grateful to Dr. Antonella Paccone for her expert technical assistance and to all patients with ALS and control subjects who kindly agreed to take part in this research.

References

[1] R. S. Marin, "Apathy: concept, syndrome, neural mechanisms, and treatment," *Seminars in Clinical Neuropsychiatry*, vol. 1, no. 4, pp. 304–314, 1996.

[2] T. N. Chase, "Apathy in neuropsychiatric disease: diagnosis, pathophysiology and treatment," *Neurotoxicity Research*, vol. 19, no. 2, pp. 266–278, 2011.

[3] R. Radakovic, C. Harley, S. Abrahams, and J. M. Starr, "A systematic review of the validity and reliability of apathy scales in neurodegenerative conditions," *International Psychogeriatrics*, vol. 27, no. 6, pp. 903–923, 2015.

[4] A. B. Grossman, S. Woolley-Levine, W. G. Bradley, and R. G. Miller, "Detecting neurobehavioral changes in amyotrophic lateral sclerosis," *Amyotrophic Lateral Sclerosis*, vol. 8, no. 1, pp. 56–61, 2007.

[5] M. Witgert, A. R. Salamone, A. M. Strutt et al., "Frontal-lobe mediated behavioral dysfunction in amyotrophic lateral sclerosis," *European Journal of Neurology*, vol. 17, no. 1, pp. 103–110, 2010.

[6] P. Lillo, E. Mioshi, M. C. Zoing, M. C. Kiernan, and J. R. Hodges, "How common are behavioural changes in amyotrophic lateral sclerosis?," *Amyotrophic Lateral Sclerosis*, vol. 12, no. 1, pp. 45–51, 2011.

[7] J. R. Burrell, G. M. Halliday, J. J. Kril et al., "The frontotemporal dementia-motor neuron disease continuum," *The Lancet*, vol. 388, no. 10047, pp. 919–931, 2016.

[8] M. J. Strong, S. Abrahams, L. H. Goldstein et al., "Amyotrophic lateral sclerosis - frontotemporal spectrum disorder (ALS-FTSD): revised diagnostic criteria," *Amyotrophic Lateral Sclerosis and Frontotemporal Degeneration*, vol. 18, no. 3-4, pp. 153–174, 2017.

[9] D. Neary, J. S. Snowden, L. Gustafson et al., "Frontotemporal lobar degeneration: a consensus on clinical diagnostic criteria," *Neurology*, vol. 51, no. 6, pp. 1546–1554, 1998.

[10] K. Rascovsky, J. R. Hodges, D. Knopman et al., "Sensitivity of revised diagnostic criteria for the behavioural variant of frontotemporal dementia," *Brain*, vol. 134, no. 9, pp. 2456–2477, 2011.

[11] R. K. Olney, J. Murphy, D. Forshew et al., "The effects of executive and behavioral dysfunction on the course of ALS," *Neurology*, vol. 65, no. 11, pp. 1774–1777, 2005.

[12] Z. Xu, A. R. S. Alruwaili, R. D. Henderson, and P. A. McCombe, "Screening for cognitive and behavioural impairment in amyotrophic lateral sclerosis: frequency of abnormality and effect on survival," *Journal of the Neurological Sciences*, vol. 376, pp. 16–23, 2017.

[13] J. Wolf, A. Safer, J. C. Wöhrle et al., "Variability and prognostic relevance of different phenotypes in amyotrophic lateral sclerosis - data from a population-based registry," *Journal of the Neurological Sciences*, vol. 345, no. 1-2, pp. 164–167, 2014.

[14] W. T. Hu, M. Shelnutt, A. Wilson et al., "Behavior matters – cognitive predictors of survival in amyotrophic lateral sclerosis," *PLoS One*, vol. 8, no. 2, article e57584, 2013.

[15] E. Mioshi, J. Caga, P. Lillo et al., "Neuropsychiatric changes precede classic motor symptoms in ALS and do not affect survival," *Neurology*, vol. 82, no. 2, pp. 149–155, 2014.

[16] J. Caga, M. R. Turner, S. Hsieh et al., "Apathy is associated with poor prognosis in amyotrophic lateral sclerosis," *European Journal of Neurology*, vol. 23, no. 5, pp. 891–897, 2016.

[17] A. Chio, A. Ilardi, S. Cammarosano, C. Moglia, A. Montuschi, and A. Calvo, "Neurobehavioral dysfunction in ALS has a negative effect on outcome and use of PEG and NIV," *Neurology*, vol. 78, no. 14, pp. 1085–1089, 2012.

[18] J. Grace, J. C. Stout, and P. F. Malloy, "Assessing frontal lobe behavioral syndromes with the frontal lobe personality scale," *Assessment*, vol. 6, no. 3, pp. 269–284, 1999.

[19] J. Grace and P. Malloy, *Frontal Systems Behavior Scale (FrSBe): Professional Manual*, Psychological Assessment Resources, Lutz, FL, USA, 2001.

[20] R. Radakovic, L. Stephenson, S. Colville, R. Swingler, S. Chandran, and S. Abrahams, "Multidimensional apathy in ALS: validation of the Dimensional Apathy Scale," *Journal of Neurology, Neurosurgery, and Psychiatry*, vol. 87, no. 6, pp. 663–669, 2016.

[21] R. S. Marin, R. C. Biedrzycki, and S. Firinciogullari, "Reliability and validity of the Apathy Evaluation Scale," *Psychiatry Research*, vol. 38, no. 2, pp. 143–162, 1991.

[22] D. E. Clarke, J. Y. Ko, E. A. Kuhl, R. van Reekum, R. Salvador, and R. S. Marin, "Are the available apathy measures reliable and valid? A review of the psychometric evidence," *Journal of Psychosomatic Research*, vol. 70, no. 1, pp. 73–97, 2011.

[23] R. S. Marin, "Apathy: a neuropsychiatric syndrome," *The Journal of Neuropsychiatry and Clinical Neurosciences*, vol. 3, no. 3, pp. 243–254, 1991.

[24] D. B. Kay, L. Kirsch-Darrow, L. B. Zahodne, M. S. Okun, and D. Bowers, "Dimensions of apathy in Parkinson's disease: exploratory factor analysis of the apathy scale," *Journal of Parkinson's Disease*, vol. 2, no. 2, pp. 161–166, 2012.

[25] G. Santangelo, P. Barone, S. Cuoco et al., "Apathy in untreated, de novo patients with Parkinson's disease: validation study of Apathy Evaluation Scale," *Journal of Neurology*, vol. 261, no. 12, pp. 2319–2328, 2014.

[26] S. L. Meier, A. J. Charleston, and L. J. Tippett, "Cognitive and behavioural deficits associated with the orbitomedial prefrontal cortex in amyotrophic lateral sclerosis," *Brain*, vol. 133, no. 11, pp. 3444–3457, 2010.

[27] R. Levy and B. Dubois, "Apathy and the functional anatomy of the prefrontal cortex–basal ganglia circuits," *Cerebral Cortex*, vol. 16, no. 7, pp. 916–928, 2006.

[28] C. Pierpaoli and P. J. Basser, "Toward a quantitative assessment of diffusion anisotropy," *Magnetic Resonance in Medicine*, vol. 36, no. 6, pp. 893–906, 1996.

[29] D. le Bihan, J.-F. Mangin, C. Poupon et al., "Diffusion tensor imaging: concepts and applications," *Journal of Magnetic Resonance Imaging*, vol. 13, no. 4, pp. 534–546, 2001.

[30] S. J. Teipel, M. Walter, Y. Likitjaroen, P. Schönknecht, and O. Gruber, "Diffusion tensor imaging in Alzheimer's disease and affective disorders," *European Archives of Psychiatry and Clinical Neuroscience*, vol. 264, no. 6, pp. 467–483, 2014.

[31] F. Agosta, M. Weiler, and M. Filippi, "Propagation of pathology through brain networks in neurodegenerative diseases: from molecules to clinical phenotypes," *CNS Neuroscience & Therapeutics*, vol. 21, no. 10, pp. 754–767, 2015.

[32] J. Kassubek and H. P. Müller, "Computer-based magnetic resonance imaging as a tool in clinical diagnosis in neurodegenerative diseases," *Expert Review of Neurotherapeutics*, vol. 16, no. 3, pp. 295–306, 2016.

[33] D. Baldaranov, A. Khomenko, I. Kobor et al., "Longitudinal diffusion tensor imaging-based assessment of tract alterations: an application to amyotrophic lateral sclerosis," *Frontiers in Human Neuroscience*, vol. 11, p. 567, 2017.

[34] E. Kasper, C. Schuster, J. Machts et al., "Microstructural white matter changes underlying cognitive and behavioural impairment in ALS–an *in vivo* study using DTI," *PLoS One*, vol. 9, no. 12, article e114543, 2014.

[35] P. Lillo, S. Savage, E. Mioshi, M. C. Kiernan, and J. R. Hodges, "Amyotrophic lateral sclerosis and frontotemporal dementia: a behavioural and cognitive continuum," *Amyotrophic Lateral Sclerosis*, vol. 13, no. 1, pp. 102–109, 2012.

[36] M. Tsujimoto, J. Senda, T. Ishihara et al., "Behavioral changes in early ALS correlate with voxel-based morphometry and diffusion tensor imaging," *Journal of the Neurological Sciences*, vol. 307, no. 1-2, pp. 34–40, 2011.

[37] S. C. Woolley, Y. Zhang, N. Schuff, M. W. Weiner, and J. S. Katz, "Neuroanatomical correlates of apathy in ALS using 4 Tesla diffusion tensor MRI," *Amyotrophic Lateral Sclerosis*, vol. 12, no. 1, pp. 52–58, 2011.

[38] S. M. Smith, M. Jenkinson, H. Johansen-Berg et al., "Tract-based spatial statistics: voxelwise analysis of multi-subject diffusion data," *NeuroImage*, vol. 31, no. 4, pp. 1487–1505, 2006.

[39] B. R. Brooks, R. G. Miller, M. Swash, T. L. Munsat, and World Federation of Neurology Research Group on Motor Neuron Diseases, "El Escorial revisited: revised criteria for the diagnosis of amyotrophic lateral sclerosis," *Amyotrophic Lateral Sclerosis and Other Motor Neuron Disorders*, vol. 1, no. 5, pp. 293–299, 2009.

[40] A. Chiò, A. Calvo, C. Moglia, L. Mazzini, G. Mora, and PARALS study group, "Phenotypic heterogeneity of amyotrophic lateral sclerosis: a population based study," *Journal of Neurology, Neurosurgery, and Psychiatry*, vol. 82, no. 7, pp. 740–746, 2011.

[41] R. Balendra, A. Jones, N. Jivraj et al., "Use of clinical staging in amyotrophic lateral sclerosis for phase 3 clinical trials," *Journal of Neurology, Neurosurgery, and Psychiatry*, vol. 86, no. 1, pp. 45–49, 2015.

[42] J. M. Cedarbaum, N. Stambler, E. Malta et al., "The ALSFRS-R: a revised ALS functional rating scale that incorporates assessments of respiratory function. BDNF ALS study group (phase III)," *Journal of the Neurological Sciences*, vol. 169, no. 1-2, pp. 13–21, 1999.

[43] M. R. Turner, A. Cagnin, F. E. Turkheimer et al., "Evidence of widespread cerebral microglial activation in amyotrophic lateral sclerosis: an [^{11}C](R)-PK11195 positron emission tomography study," *Neurobiology of Disease*, vol. 15, no. 3, pp. 601–609, 2004.

[44] F. Kimura, C. Fujimura, S. Ishida et al., "Progression rate of ALSFRS-R at time of diagnosis predicts survival time in ALS," *Neurology*, vol. 66, no. 2, pp. 265–267, 2006.

[45] J. Phukan, M. Elamin, P. Bede et al., "The syndrome of cognitive impairment in amyotrophic lateral sclerosis: a population-based study," *Journal of Neurology, Neurosurgery, and Psychiatry*, vol. 83, no. 1, pp. 102–108, 2011.

[46] G. Santangelo, C. Vitale, L. Trojano et al., "Neuropsychological correlates of theory of mind in patients with early Parkinson's disease," *Movement Disorders*, vol. 27, no. 1, pp. 98–105, 2012.

[47] A. Montuschi, B. Iazzolino, A. Calvo et al., "Cognitive correlates in amyotrophic lateral sclerosis: a population-based study in Italy," *Journal of Neurology, Neurosurgery, and Psychiatry*, vol. 86, no. 2, pp. 168–173, 2015.

[48] T. Burke, M. Elamin, P. Bede et al., "Discordant performance on the 'Reading the Mind in the Eyes' test, based on disease onset in amyotrophic lateral sclerosis," *Amyotrophic Lateral Sclerosis and Frontotemporal Degeneration*, vol. 17, no. 7-8, pp. 467–472, 2016.

[49] S. M. Kim, K. M. Lee, Y. H. Hong et al., "Relation between cognitive dysfunction and reduced vital capacity in amyotrophic lateral sclerosis," *Journal of Neurology, Neurosurgery, and Psychiatry*, vol. 78, no. 12, pp. 1387–1389, 2007.

[50] T. J. Braley, A. L. Kratz, N. Kaplish, and R. D. Chervin, "Sleep and cognitive function in multiple sclerosis," *Sleep*, vol. 39, no. 8, pp. 1525–1533, 2016.

[51] P. Y. Gülhan, E. Bulcun, M. Gülhan, D. Çimen, A. Ekici, and M. Ekici, "Low cognitive ability in subjects with bronchiectasis," *Respiratory Care*, vol. 60, no. 11, pp. 1610–1615, 2015.

[52] P. Caffarra, G. Vezzadini, F. Dieci, F. Zonato, and A. Venneri, "A short version of the Stroop test: normative data in an Italian population sample," *Nuova Rivista di Neurologia*, vol. 12, pp. 111–115, 2002.

[53] M. Monaco, A. Costa, C. Caltagirone, and G. A. Carlesimo, "Erratum to: forward and backward span for verbal and visuo-spatial data: standardization and normative data from an Italian adult population," *Neurological Sciences*, vol. 36, no. 2, pp. 345–347, 2015.

[54] H. Spinnler and G. Tognoni, "Standardizzazione e taratura italiana di test neuropsicologici," *Italian Journal of Neurological Sciences*, vol. 8, no. 6, Supplement, pp. 21–120, 1987.

[55] G. Novelli, C. Papagno, E. Capitani, M. Laiacona, S. F. Cappa, and G. Vallar, "Three clinical tests for the assessment of verbal long-term memory function. Norms from 320 normal subjects," *Archivio di Psicologia, Neurologia e Psichiatria*, vol. 47, no. 2, pp. 278–296, 1986.

[56] G. A. Carlesimo, C. Caltagirone, G. Gainotti et al., "The Mental Deterioration Battery: normative data, diagnostic reliability and qualitative analyses of cognitive impairment," *European Neurology*, vol. 36, no. 6, pp. 378–384, 1.

[57] A. Chiò, A. Vignola, E. Mastro et al., "Neurobehavioral symptoms in ALS are negatively related to caregivers' burden and quality of life," *European Journal of Neurology*, vol. 17, no. 10, pp. 1298–1303, 2010.

[58] A. T. Beck, R. A. Steer, and G. K. Brown, *Manual for the Beck Depression Inventory-II*, Psychological Corporation, San Antionio, TX, USA, 1996.

[59] M. Cirillo, F. Esposito, G. Tedeschi et al., "Widespread microstructural white matter involvement in amyotrophic lateral sclerosis: a whole-brain DTI study," *AJNR American Journal of Neuroradiology*, vol. 33, no. 6, pp. 1102–1108, 2012.

[60] F. Trojsi, G. Caiazzo, D. Corbo et al., "Microstructural changes across different clinical milestones of disease in amyotrophic lateral sclerosis," *PLoS One*, vol. 10, no. 3, article e0119045, 2015.

[61] K. Hua, J. Zhang, S. Wakana et al., "Tract probability maps in stereotaxic spaces: analyses of white matter anatomy and tract-specific quantification," *NeuroImage*, vol. 39, no. 1, pp. 336–347, 2008.

[62] S. Wakana, A. Caprihan, M. M. Panzenboeck et al., "Reproducibility of quantitative tractography methods applied to cerebral white matter," *NeuroImage*, vol. 36, no. 3, pp. 630–644, 2007.

[63] M. R. Turner and R. A. L. Menke, "The tough body at the epicentre of amyotrophic lateral sclerosis," *Journal of Neurology, Neurosurgery, and Psychiatry*, vol. 88, no. 5, pp. 369.2–36370, 2017.

[64] G. M. Thomsen, A. M. Ma, A. Ko et al., "A model of recurrent concussion that leads to long-term motor deficits, CTE-like tauopathy and exacerbation of an ALS phenotype," *Journal of Trauma and Acute Care Surgery*, vol. 81, no. 6, pp. 1070–1079, 2016.

[65] A. M. Cardenas, J. E. Sarlls, J. Y. Kwan et al., "Pathology of callosal damage in ALS: an *ex-vivo*, 7 T diffusion tensor MRI study," *NeuroImage: Clinical*, vol. 15, pp. 200–208, 2017.

[66] F. Agosta, S. Galantucci, G. Magnani et al., "MRI signatures of the frontotemporal lobar degeneration continuum," *Human Brain Mapping*, vol. 36, no. 7, pp. 2602–2614, 2015.

[67] A. Eisen, H. Braak, K. del Tredici, R. Lemon, A. C. Ludolph, and M. C. Kiernan, "Cortical influences drive amyotrophic lateral sclerosis," *Journal of Neurology, Neurosurgery, and Psychiatry*, vol. 88, no. 11, pp. 917–924, 2017.

[68] H. Braak, J. Brettschneider, A. C. Ludolph, V. M. Lee, J. Q. Trojanowski, and K. D. Tredici, "Amyotrophic lateral sclerosis–a model of corticofugal axonal spread," *Nature Reviews Neurology*, vol. 9, no. 12, pp. 708–714, 2013.

[69] L. Massimo, J. P. Powers, L. K. Evans et al., "Apathy in frontotemporal degeneration: neuroanatomical evidence of impaired goal-directed behavior," *Frontiers in Human Neuroscience*, vol. 9, p. 611, 2015.

[70] T. Ohtani, S. Bouix, T. Hosokawa et al., "Abnormalities in white matter connections between orbitofrontal cortex and anterior cingulate cortex and their associations with negative symptoms in schizophrenia: a DTI study," *Schizophrenia Research*, vol. 157, no. 1–3, pp. 190–197, 2014.

[71] T. Molesworth, L. K. Sheu, S. Cohen, P. J. Gianaros, and T. D. Verstynen, "Social network diversity and white matter microstructural integrity in humans," *Social Cognitive and Affective Neuroscience*, vol. 10, no. 9, pp. 1169–1176, 2015.

[72] A. F. Santillo, K. Lundblad, M. Nilsson et al., "Grey and white matter clinico-anatomical correlates of disinhibition in neurodegenerative disease," *PLoS One*, vol. 11, no. 10, article e0164122, 2016.

[73] Y. Zhang, J. Wu, W. Wu et al., "Reduction of white matter integrity correlates with apathy in Parkinson's disease," *The International Journal of Neuroscience*, vol. 128, no. 1, pp. 25–31, 2018.

[74] S. K. Tighe, K. Oishi, S. Mori et al., "Diffusion tensor imaging of neuropsychiatric symptoms in mild cognitive impairment and Alzheimer's dementia," *The Journal of Neuropsychiatry and Clinical Neurosciences*, vol. 24, no. 4, pp. 484–488, 2012.

[75] A. Amodio, M. Quarantelli, A. Mucci et al., "Avolition-apathy and white matter connectivity in schizophrenia: reduced fractional anisotropy between amygdala and insular cortex," *Clinical EEG and Neuroscience*, vol. 49, no. 1, pp. 55–65, 2018.

[76] D. T. Stuss, R. Van Reekum, and K. J. Murphy, "Differentiation of states and causes of apathy," in *Series in Affective Science. The Neuropsychology of Emotion*, J. C. Borod, Ed., pp. 340–363, Oxford University Press, New York, NY, USA, 2000.

[77] R. Radakovic and S. Abrahams, "Multidimensional apathy: evidence from neurodegenerative disease," *Current Opinion in Behavioral Sciences*, vol. 22, pp. 42–49, 2018.

[78] R. Radakovic, L. Stephenson, J. Newton et al., "Multidimensional apathy and executive dysfunction in amyotrophic lateral sclerosis," *Cortex*, vol. 94, pp. 142–151, 2017.

[79] G. Santangelo, S. Raimo, M. Siciliano et al., "Assessment of apathy independent of physical disability: validation of the Dimensional Apathy Scale in Italian healthy sample," *Neurological Sciences*, vol. 38, no. 2, pp. 303–309, 2017.

[80] M. C. Tu, W. H. Huang, Y. H. Hsu, C. P. Lo, J. F. Deng, and C. F. Huang, "Comparison of neuropsychiatric symptoms and diffusion tensor imaging correlates among patients with subcortical ischemic vascular disease and Alzheimer's disease," *BioMed Central neurology*, vol. 17, no. 1, p. 144, 2017.

[81] C. Hahn, H. K. Lim, W. Y. Won, K. J. Ahn, W. S. Jung, and C. U. Lee, "Apathy and white matter integrity in Alzheimer's disease: a whole brain analysis with tract-based spatial statistics," *PLoS One*, vol. 8, no. 1, article e53493, 2013.

[82] M. Di Paola, G. Spalletta, and C. Caltagirone, "In vivo structural neuroanatomy of corpus callosum in Alzheimer's disease and mild cognitive impairment using different MRI techniques: a review," *Journal of Alzheimer's Disease*, vol. 20, no. 1, pp. 67–95, 2010.

[83] H. Kazui, R. Takahashi, Y. Yamamoto et al., "Neural basis of apathy in patients with amnestic mild cognitive impairment," *Journal of Alzheimer's Disease*, vol. 55, no. 4, pp. 1403–1416, 2017.

[84] D. Shen, L. Cui, J. Fang, B. Cui, D. Li, and H. Tai, "Voxel-wise meta-analysis of gray matter changes in amyotrophic lateral sclerosis," *Frontiers in Aging Neuroscience*, vol. 8, p. 64, 2016.

[85] F. Agosta, P. M. Ferraro, N. Riva et al., "Structural brain correlates of cognitive and behavioral impairment in MND," *Human Brain Mapping*, vol. 37, no. 4, pp. 1614–1626, 2016.

[86] P. M. Ferraro, F. Agosta, N. Riva et al., "Multimodal structural MRI in the diagnosis of motor neuron diseases," *NeuroImage Clinical*, vol. 16, pp. 240–247, 2017.

17

Gait and Conditioned Fear Impairments in a Mouse Model of Comorbid TBI and PTSD

Peyton Teutsch,[1] Carolyn E. Jones,[1,2] Mara E. Kaiser,[1] Natasha Avalon Gardner,[1,3] and Miranda M. Lim[1,2,4]

[1]*VA Portland Health Care System, Portland, OR, USA*
[2]*Department of Behavioral Neuroscience, Oregon Health & Science University, Portland, OR, USA*
[3]*Portland State University, Portland, OR, USA*
[4]*Department of Neurology, Department of Medicine, Division of Pulmonary and Critical Care Medicine, Oregon Institute of Occupational Health Sciences, Oregon Health & Science University, Portland, OR, USA*

Correspondence should be addressed to Miranda M. Lim; lmir@ohsu.edu

Academic Editor: Laura Piccardi

Study Objectives. Traumatic brain injury (TBI) and posttraumatic stress disorder (PTSD) commonly cooccur. Approaches to research and treatment of these disorders have been segregated, despite overlapping symptomology. We and others have hypothesized that comorbid TBI + PTSD generates worse symptoms than either condition alone. We present a mouse model of comorbid TBI + PTSD to further explore this condition. *Methods.* A mouse model of TBI + PTSD was generated using the single prolonged stress (SPS) protocol in combination with the controlled cortical impact (CCI) protocol. This resulted in four experimental groups: control, TBI, PTSD, and TBI + PTSD. Behavioral phenotyping included gait analysis, contextual fear conditioning, acoustic startle response, and prepulse inhibition. *Results.* Mice in the TBI + PTSD group showed a significantly impaired gait compared to their counterparts with TBI alone as well as control mice. Mice in the TBI + PTSD group showed significantly impaired contextual fear recall compared to controls. Prepulse inhibition testing revealed intact acoustic startle and auditory sensory gating. *Conclusions.* These results indicate that SPS paired with CCI in mice produces unique behavioral impairments in gait and fear recall that are not present in either condition alone. Further studies are underway to examine additional behavioral, physiological, and pathological phenotypes in this combined model of TBI + PTSD.

1. Introduction

Traumatic brain injury (TBI) is a change in neural functioning caused by an external force to the head, resulting in mild to severe injury [1]. TBI results in persistent symptoms including changes in cognition (e.g., difficulty concentrating or remembering), problems with balance, and increased anxiety. TBI is highly prevalent, resulting in approximately 2.5 million yearly diagnoses [2], with an alarming occurrence in the Veteran community of nearly 20% of Veterans reporting a diagnosed TBI [3].

Posttraumatic stress disorder (PTSD) can develop after a traumatizing event and frequently results in behavioral changes that overlap in symptomatology with TBI, including cognitive dysfunction, heightened anxiety, and exaggerated startle response [4]. Compared to the average population, rates and symptom severity of PTSD are reported to be significantly higher in Veterans [5]. Both TBI and PTSD are associated with lower quality of life and increased risk for psychological and medical disorders compared to healthy individuals [6]. Furthermore, Veterans with TBI in particular are at a higher risk for developing PTSD [6].

The comorbidity of TBI and PTSD in the same individual may present a unique symptomology; the extent of which has yet to be fully explored and may depend on the severity of either condition. Conventional approaches to research and treatment of these disorders in the human population have been segregated, despite overlapping symptomology. Thus, the aim of this study was to characterize behavioral outcomes in a mouse model of TBI + PTSD to

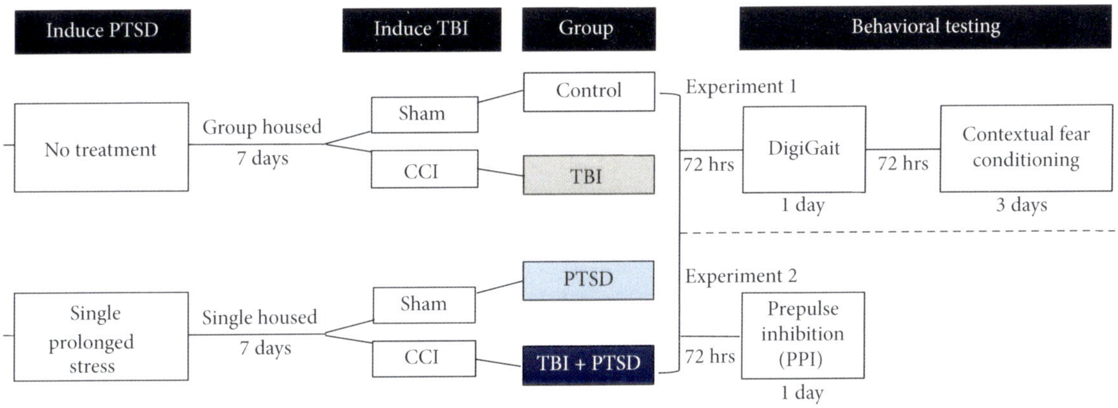

FIGURE 1: Experimental design and timeline. Subjects were randomized to SPS or no treatment. Mice were then further randomized to receive either a CCI or sham surgery to result in our four studied groups: control, TBI, PTSD, and TBI + PTSD. Behavioral testing in experiment 1 began 72 hours after surgeries with one day of gait testing, then 72 hours later began three days of contextual fear conditioning. Experiment 2 consisted of 1 day of PPI testing 72 hours after surgeries.

add to the development and characterization of this emerging field of research [7–10]. We hypothesized that the combination of these two conditions would harbor its own distinct phenotype compared to controls or either condition alone. We used the well-established models of single prolonged stress (SPS) [11] to create a mouse model of PTSD and controlled cortical impact (CCI) [12] as a model of TBI, in order to examine the combined TBI + PTSD behavioral phenotype. Behavior testing reported here includes digital gait analysis, contextual fear conditioning, acoustic startle, and auditory prepulse inhibition.

2. Materials and Methods

2.1. Animals. Male, C57Bl/6J wild-type mice (The Jackson Laboratory), 8-9 weeks in age and weighing 23–30 g, were used for this study. Mice were housed in groups of four and were allowed to acclimate to the colony after shipment for one week prior to beginning the study. Housing was in a 12 : 12 h light : dark cycle (lights on at 0700 h) with ad libitum access to food (LabDiet® PicoLab® Laboratory Rodent Diet, 5L0D) and water. Temperature (21.6°C) and humidity (24%) were monitored and maintained at a constant level throughout the experiment. All protocols and housing were approved by the Institutional Animal Care and Use Committee at the Portland VA and adhered to guidelines set forth by the National Institutes of Health Guide for Care and Use of Laboratory Animals.

2.2. Experimental Design. Mice were randomized into one of four groups (control, TBI, PTSD, and TBI + PTSD; see Figure 1 for design). TBI was generated using the controlled cortical impact (CCI) model, and PTSD was generated using the single prolonged stress (SPS) protocol. Owing to the methodological complexity of SPS, the SPS protocol was performed first, followed by CCI. Two experiments were conducted: in experiment 1, mice underwent gait testing and contextual fear conditioning and in experiment 2, a separate cohort of mice underwent acoustic startle and prepulse inhibition testing (Figure 1).

2.3. Single Prolonged Stress (SPS). Since its initial development in rats [11], SPS has successfully been applied to other rodent models, including mice [13–16]. Briefly, SPS consists of a sequential series of stressors: tube restraint, forced swim, ether anesthesia, and finally social isolation for one week [11]. Half of the mice in all experiments were randomized to receive the SPS protocol. For tube restraint stress, mice were placed into ventilated 50 mL conical vials, which were then placed in a clean cage with bedding, for two hours. After tube restraint, groups of four mice were immediately placed together into a single plastic tub (8.5 × 9.0 × 12.0 in) filled with room temperature water (26°C) deep enough to prevent tails from touching the bottom (three-quarters full). Group forced swim lasted a duration of 20 minutes, during which time the mice and water temperature were closely monitored. Following the group forced swim, mice were towel dried and placed into individual bell jars containing a cotton ball soaked with 1.0 mL of diethyl ether. Mice were carefully monitored and immediately removed from the jar once they lost consciousness. Subsequently, mice were placed in a standard home cage to be individually housed for seven days of social isolation. Each SPS cohort began at 0800 h and ended with individual housing at 1300 h. Mice that were not randomized to SPS remained group housed for the duration of seven days that their counterparts underwent social isolation. Social isolation is a key component of SPS, and it has been shown to be a necessary incubation period for this trauma model [14, 17].

2.4. Controlled Cortical Impact (CCI). Experimental mice were randomized to either a CCI or a sham surgery condition. In combination with SPS above, this resulted in four groups in total (control, TBI, PTSD, and TBI + PTSD). For CCI, mice were weighed, anesthetized using isoflurane (3% to induce, 1% to maintain), and secured to a stereotaxic frame (Stoelting Company). Mice had their heads shaved and sterilized using alcohol and iodine, before topical lidocaine was applied to the shaved head. An incision was made on the right side of the prepared skin to expose the skull landmarks bregma and lambda, and 30% hydrogen peroxide was used on a cotton applicator to remove the membranes covering the skull. Using a hand drill (Fine Science Tools), a 3 mm craniotomy was made to the right of the midline, between bregma and lambda. An impactor arm (Kopf Instruments) was then used to deliver an impact at a depth of 3.0 mm and velocity of 0.5 m/s, with a dwell time of 0.1 s to the cortical surface. The scalp incision was sutured, and triple antibiotic ointment was applied to the incision site. Mice were given a 1.0 mL subcutaneous injection of saline and returned to a standard home cage on a circulating warming pad with access to food, water, nestlets, DietGel® 76A (ClearH_2O®), and 1.0 mL children's cherry flavored acetaminophen (Q-Pap) in 15 mL of water. Mice in the sham surgery condition underwent anesthesia and scalp incision, followed by application of hydrogen peroxide to the skull and immediate closure of the incision with sutures. All mice were housed individually following surgery for the remainder of the study to ensure recovery from surgery.

2.5. Gait Testing. Mice were tested for differences in gait using the DigiGait™ imaging system (Mouse Specifics). The DigiGait system consisted of a transparent treadmill belt surrounded by a Plexiglas compartment (17.4 cm × 5.1 cm × 13.3 cm) that was illuminated and filmed from below by a high-speed imaging video camera shot at 150 frames/s. Mice were given one minute to acclimate to the treadmill testing chamber, then were run for ~5 s at a belt speed of 25 cm/s. Mice were excluded for failure to walk on the treadmill ($n = 2$), failure to walk at least six consecutive strides ($n = 2$), and for technical difficulties of dim lighting affecting usable video acquisition ($n = 4$ per group). Mice were then removed from the treadmill chamber and returned to their home cage. All testing occurred between 0830 and 1000 h. Gait was analyzed using DigiGait imaging software (version 14) according to manufacturer's instructions by a scorer blinded to the group to interpret metrics involving stance and other indices of gait. For the purpose of this study, we focused on measures of stance (e.g., stance duration—time the paw spent in contact with the treadmill belt) and stability (stance width and paw placement positioning) since TBI has been found to affect stance and stature in humans [18]. DigiGait metrics were provided for both fore and hind paws on both sides. Individual values for a priori determined stance and paw placement metrics were analyzed for each paw. A schematic of gait metrics is shown in Figure 2(a).

2.6. Contextual Fear Conditioning. Contextual fear conditioning and recall was conducted over three days in the first four hours of the light cycle (0830 h–1100 h). Behavior was recorded with digital cameras (GoPro Hero Session) that were watched by a trained observer blind to the experimental group and scored manually for freezing upon completion of the experiment. Freezing was defined as the cessation of movement with the exception of respiration. In test sessions, total time freezing over a two-minute period was scored with a stopwatch program (Stopwatch+, Georgia State University) and expressed as a percentage of total time spent freezing. This time period was chosen to examine contextual fear memory recall only, while avoiding engaging fear extinction mechanisms. Scoring of freezing behavior began 20 s after placement into the chamber.

2.6.1. Fear Conditioning Day 1: Contextual Fear Acquisition (Context A). Two identical testing chambers (40.8 cm × 14 cm × 18.4 cm, Omnitech Electronics) were used for fear conditioning. One animal was excluded from fear conditioning due to equipment failure with the shock delivery system. Fear conditioning chambers consisted of four clear acrylic walls and a clear top for overhead video recording. Each chamber had a metal floor that consisted of 45 stainless steel rods spaced 5 mm apart (context A). The unconditional stimulus (US) was a 1.0 mA scrambled footshock (duration = 1 s). Fear conditioning and testing occurred in acoustic isolation boxes configured with a light and fan that provided ambient noise at 65 dB. Mice were placed in the chamber and after three minutes received 5 US deliveries with a fixed intertrial interval (ITI) of 60 s. Mice were removed immediately after the termination of the last shock; as such, there was no freezing measure collected after delivery of the final US.

2.6.2. Fear Conditioning Day 2: Context Generalization (Context B). In order to test contextual discrimination and generalization of fear memories, mice were returned to the fear conditioning boxes the following day with changes in contextual cues from the prior acquisition day. Walls were lined with black and white checkered paper on three of the four walls; a smooth black floor insert covered the shock bars, and a lemon-scented cleaning wipe was used on the pull-out waste tray (context B). Additionally, mice were placed in a different chamber location than the first day of fear conditioning. Mice remained in this new context for two minutes. During this time, no US was delivered.

2.6.3. Fear Conditioning Day 3: Fear Recall Test (Context A). The testing chambers were reverted to context A; the same context was used for fear acquisition—clear walls, floor comprised of parallel metal rods, and no additional scent. A fear recall test was performed by placing mice in the feared context and scoring freezing behavior for two minutes. No US was delivered during this time. A schematic of the contextual fear conditioning protocol is shown in Figure 3(a).

2.7. Acoustic Startle and Prepulse Inhibition (PPI). In experiment 2, the same design of TBI and PTSD was examined for acoustic startle reflex and PPI. Following SPS and/or a CCI depth of 2.5 mm, mice were placed in isolation boxes inside a clear acrylic tube affixed over a piezoelectric accelerometer (San Diego Instruments) that captured animal movement in response to precisely calibrated white noises of varying intensity emitted from a loudspeaker. For each trial, a testing box was left empty, acting as an ambient sensor to capture any background noise that may offer interference to the collected readings. At no point did the ambient sensor register movement higher than that

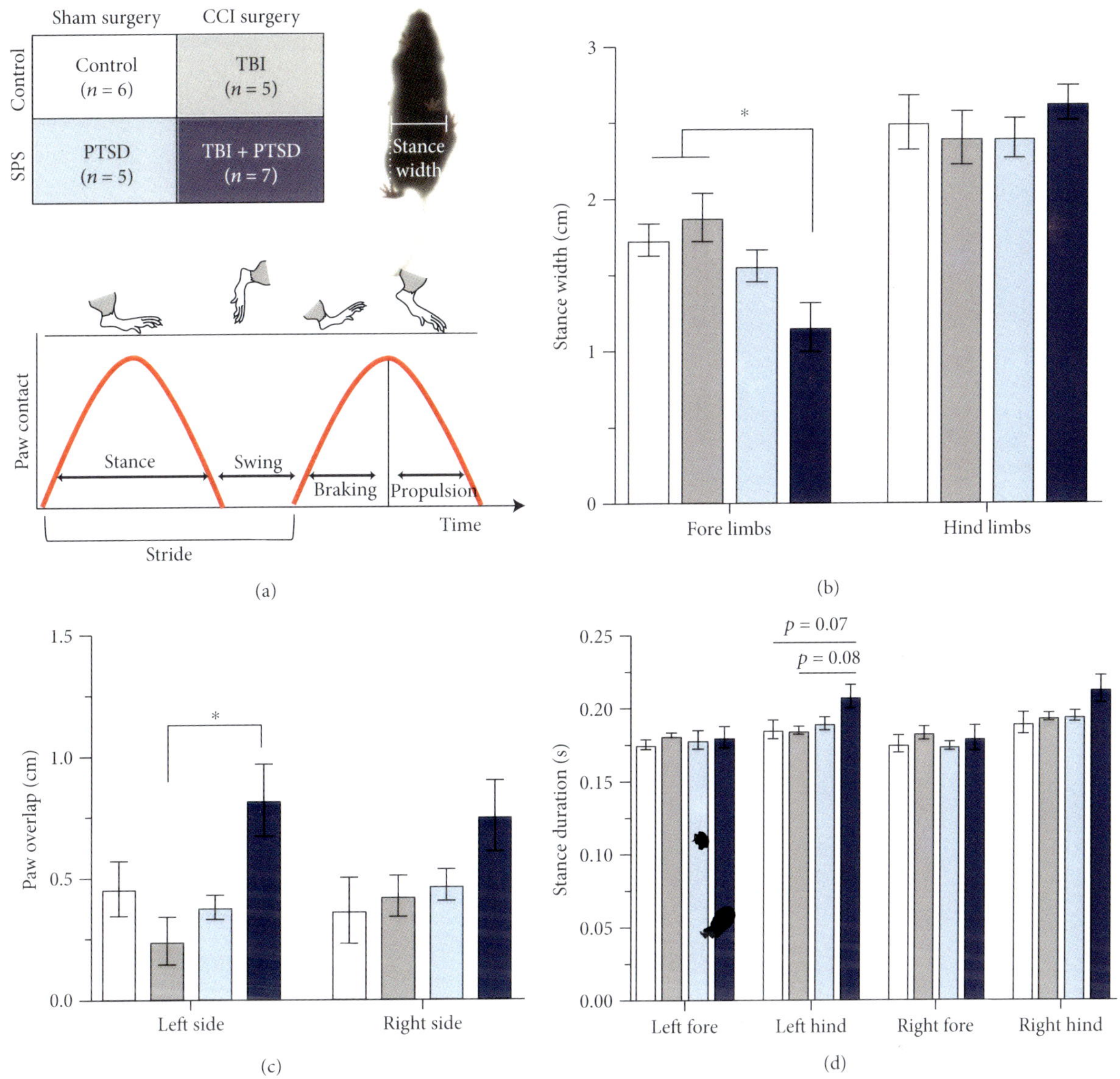

Figure 2: Gait metrics after TBI + PTSD. (a) Experimental design and diagram of the mouse gait representing a step cycle and stance width measures. (b) Stance width in fore and hind limbs. Forelimb stance width was decreased in TBI + PTSD mice compared to TBI alone ($p = 0.008$) and controls ($p = 0.029$). (c) Paw overlap in left and right sides. Paw placement in the left side of TBI + PTSD mice was significantly increased compared to TBI alone mice ($p = 0.018$). (d) Stance duration in each paw. Stance duration in the left hind limbs was significant in the omnibus ANOVA ($p = 0.046$), and post hoc testing was trending in TBI + PTSD relative to control and TBI alone mice. Error bars ± SEM, $^{*}p < 0.05$.

of a box containing an animal. Testing began 5 minutes after mice were placed in the chambers. The test consisted of 66 trials divided into 11 blocks. Each block consisted of null trials with background 65 dB noise only, startle only trials consisting of the pulse (120 dB) alone, and prepulse trials of 72, 80, or 84 dB preceding a 120 dB pulse (fixed interstimulus interval (ISI) = 100 ms). Trial order within each block was pseudorandomized so that no trial type occurred consecutively, and trials were separated by a variable 15 s ITI (maximum ITI = 20 s, minimum ITI = 10 s). All testing occurred between 0900 and 1100 h. A schematic of acoustic startle and PPI apparatus is shown in Figure 4(a).

2.8. Data Analysis. Statistical analyses were performed using one-way analysis of variance (ANOVA) with the treatment group (control, TBI, PTSD, and TBI + PTSD) as the between-subject factor. Significant main effects were explored with Tukey HSD post hoc tests. If measures were taken from animals at repeated time points (PPI testing and contextual fear acquisition), a repeated measures ANOVA was used. When data was not normally distributed, the Kruskal-Wallis nonparametric test was conducted and post hoc comparisons were performed using Dunn's test to follow up significant main effects. Analyses were conducted in IBM SPSS (version 24.0) with figures produced in GraphPad Prism (version 7.0). Results were

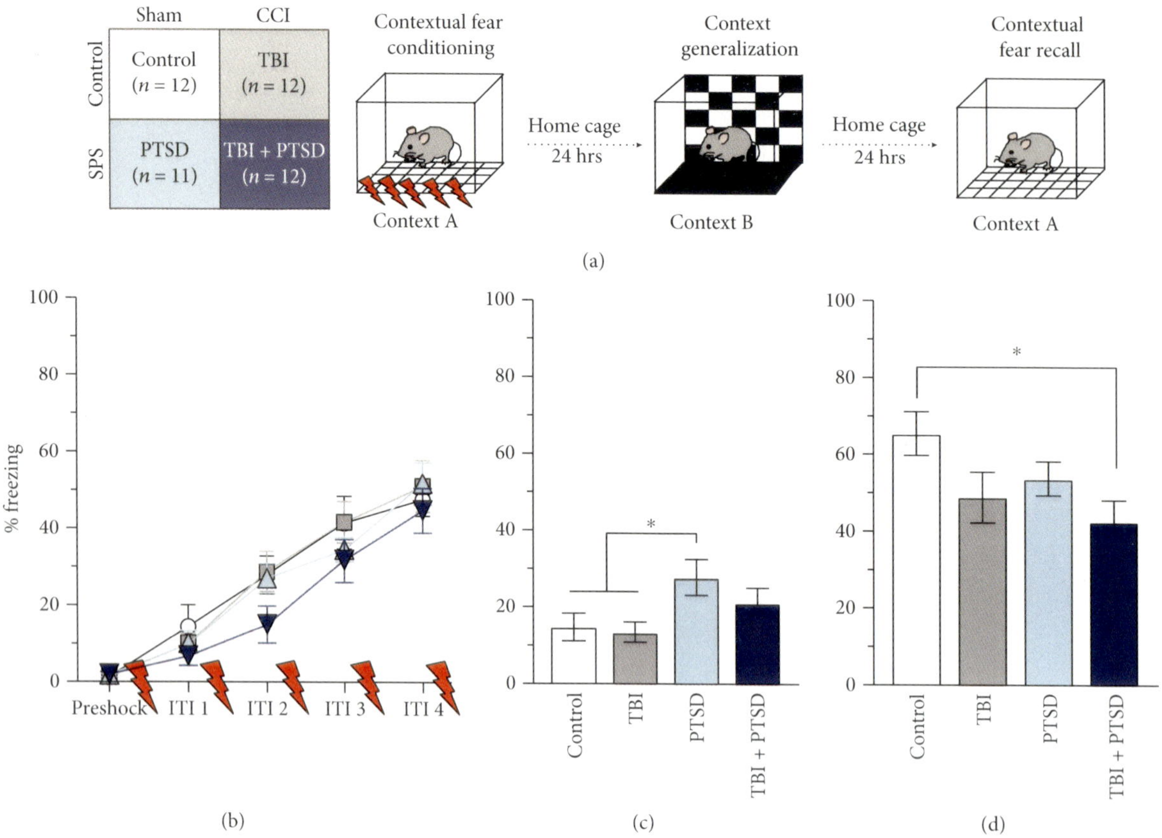

Figure 3: Impaired fear recall in TBI + PTSD mice following contextual fear conditioning. (a) Experimental design and fear conditioning procedure. (b) Contextual fear acquisition. There were no group differences in fear learning. (c) Context generalization. PTSD mice froze significantly more in context B compared to both control ($p = 0.012$) and TBI only mice ($p = 0.010$). (d) Contextual fear recall. TBI + PTSD mice showed deficits in contextual fear recall relative to controls ($p = 0.033$). Error bars ± SEM, $^*p < 0.05$. ITI = intertrial interval.

considered significant at an alpha value of 0.05. All data are represented as means ± standard error of the mean (SEM).

3. Results

3.1. Gait Testing. In the forelimbs, stance width was altered (one-way ANOVA, $F(3,21) = 5.38$, $p = 0.007$), such that the TBI + PTSD mice showed significantly decreased stance width compared to both the TBI group ($p = 0.008$) and the control group ($p = 0.029$), with all other p values > 0.207 (Figure 2(b)). Paw placement positioning was altered in the left side (Kruskal-Wallis, $p = 0.028$), with differences emerging between the TBI + PTSD group and the TBI group ($p = 0.018$) (Figure 2(c)). There was also a significant main effect of the group on stance duration in the left hind paw (one-way ANOVA, $F(3,19) = 3.209$, $p = 0.046$), with a trend towards increased stance duration in TBI + PTSD mice relative to controls ($p = 0.072$) and TBI mice ($p = 0.084$), with all other p values > 0.214 (Figure 2(d)). Between groups, mice did not differ in weight at the time of gait testing (one-way ANOVA; $F(3,26) = 0.303$, $p = 0.828$) (Table 1).

3.2. Contextual Fear Conditioning. All groups acquired contextual fear as evidenced by increased freezing across the acquisition session (repeated measures ANOVA, within subjects: $F(3,111) = 66.843$, $p < 0.0001$), and there were no differences between groups (repeated measures ANOVA, between subjects $F(3,37) = 0.946$, $p = 0.428$) as well as no interaction (repeated measures ANOVA, trial × group interaction, $F(9,111) = 0.425$, $p = 0.919$) (Figure 3(b)). Two animals were excluded from analysis during acquisition because of video camera malfunction. Mice did not display a fear response when first placed in a fear conditioning context (freezing prior to shock onset was less than 2% for all groups, Figure 3(b)).

Generalization of fearful memories was determined by altering the contextual cues associated with the fear conditioning chamber and measuring freezing for a two-minute period. There was a significant main effect of the group on freezing in the new context (Kruskal-Wallis, $p = 0.029$), where PTSD mice froze significantly more than both TBI alone ($p = 0.015$) and controls ($p = 0.017$) (Figure 3(c)).

Fear recall was tested by returning the mice to the fear conditioning context for two minutes and measuring freezing. There was a significant main effect of the group on fear recall as measured by freezing to the fear conditioned context (one-way ANOVA, $F(3,43) = 2.965$, $p = 0.042$). TBI + PTSD mice froze significantly less than controls ($p = 0.033$) during the contextual fear recall test (Figure 3(d)).

3.3. Acoustic Startle and Prepulse Inhibition. Baseline startle to a 120 dB pulse is shown in Figure 4(b). There were no

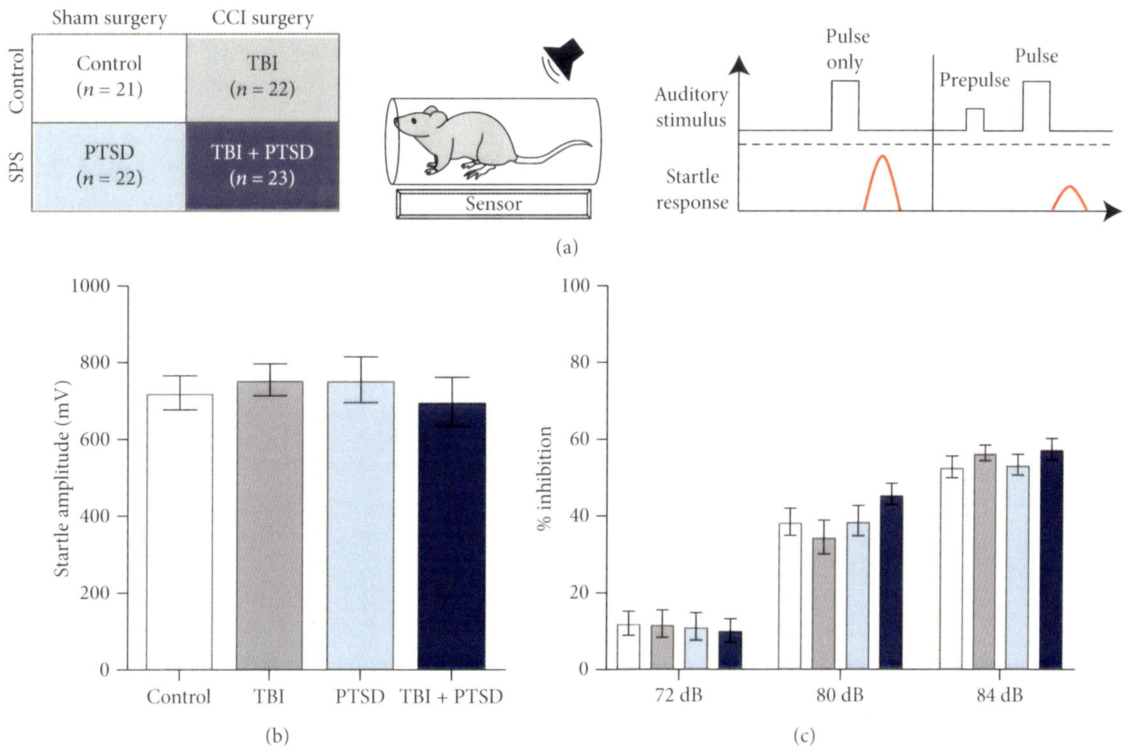

FIGURE 4: Comorbid TBI + PTSD does not affect acoustic startle response or prepulse inhibition. (a) Schematic of experimental design, acoustic testing chamber, and startle protocol. (b) Acoustic startle response. There were no changes in acoustic startle response across groups when the 120 dB pulse was played without a prepulse. (c) Prepulse inhibition. There was a significant interaction between prepulse level and treatment group on inhibition of the startle response to the pulse; however, there were no group differences in overall PPI. Background noise was constantly generated at 65 dB. Error bars ± SEM. dB = decibel.

group differences in average startle response to the 120 dB pulse alone (one-way ANOVA, $F(3,84) = 0.273$, $p = 0.845$).

Prepulse inhibition was determined by comparing percent startle inhibition between groups and prepulse decibel levels. Percent startle inhibition was calculated by dividing the average startle value across each prepulse amplitude by the average startle across trials that were not preceded by a prepulse (pulse alone trials). The following formula was used to calculate percent inhibition at each decibel level: [(1 − (average prepulse startle/average pulse alone startle)) × 100]. Repeated measures ANOVA with the dB level of prepulse (70 dB, 80 dB, and 84 dB) as the within-subject factor and treatment group as the between-subject factor revealed, as expected, a significant within-subject effect of the PPI level with increasing amplitudes of prepulses leading to increased inhibition of the startle response to the subsequent pulse (repeated measures ANOVA, within subjects: $F(2, 168) = 491.153$, $p < 0.0001$). There was a prepulse level × group interaction ($F(6,168) = 2.411$, $p = 0.029$) but no between-group effect ($F(3,84) = 0.366$, $p = 0.778$) (Figure 4(c)).

4. Discussion

We found that mice in the TBI + PTSD group showed a significantly impaired gait compared to mice with TBI alone and controls. Mice in the TBI + PTSD group also showed significantly impaired fear recall compared to controls. Prepulse inhibition testing revealed no overall effect of TBI, PTSD, or combined TBI + PTSD on baseline acoustic startle and sensory gating ability. Taken together, these results indicate that SPS paired with CCI in mice produces unique behavioral impairments in gait and fear recall that are not present in either condition alone.

TABLE 1: Mouse weights at DigiGait testing. There were no weight differences between groups at the time that DigiGait testing was conducted ($p = 0.823$).

Group	Weight (g)	SD	N
Control	28.19	1.55	8
TBI	27.91	2.51	7
PTSD	28.47	2.5	8
TBI + PTSD	28.89	1.09	7

4.1. TBI + PTSD Impairs Gait. Gait is frequently examined in animal models of TBI, likely owing to damage to the motor circuits that control gait caused by CCI and other common TBI protocols. As of now, there are no standardized parameters for TBI induced by CCI and research has shown that variations in speed and/or depth of impact can influence both cognitive and motor outcomes differentially [19]. In our model of TBI, the injury was administered to the right hemisphere of the brain and our results showed predominantly contralateral effects on gait.

In this model of TBI + PTSD, we found that stance width in the forelimbs was dramatically decreased and paw placement position, a measure that indicates the amount of ipsilateral overlap between fore and hind paws, was preferentially increased on the left side in the TBI + PTSD mice. Paw overlap may reflect the ability of mice to balance and may contribute to the instability seen in the decreased forelimb stance width in the TBI + PTSD mice. In humans, narrower stance widths tend to be unstable [20], suggesting that gait alterations in TBI + PTSD mice contribute to unstable walking patterns. Human subjects with TBI have been found to have an increased stance time [18] and often complain of balance problems and difficulty walking, especially when multitasking [21, 22]. The clinical observation that TBI patients have trouble multitasking may provide insight to our results. In our data, we observed distinctive gait impairments only in mice in the TBI + PTSD group. This is consistent with the noted phenomenon in which deficits in TBI in human patients are brought out or worsened with stress or increased cognitive load [21, 23]; the addition of PTSD as a form of chronic or ongoing stress induces gait deficits in TBI mice that are otherwise masked with TBI alone.

TBI alone was not sufficient to induce gait changes, in contrast to what others have found in other CCI mouse models of TBI [24, 25]. In these models, gait changes seem to only emerge after repeated exposure to the treadmill, which we did not incorporate into our protocol [24, 25]. One possibility is that a single test on the DigiGait apparatus may not be complex enough to elicit changes in the TBI only group, whereby postinjury gait impairments may only emerge in subjects with the cognitive burden of PTSD.

Other studies using TBI alone found effects on stance duration that ranged from being present in all paws [24] to only being seen in the contralateral forelimb [25]. In keeping with our findings in the TBI alone group, other studies where mice were also only given one chance to use the treadmill, Luo and colleagues [26] did not observe significant changes in a repetitive, closed-head induced TBI [26]. It is possible that repeated gait testing is more sensitive to detecting gait deficits associated with TBI in rodents. Initially, we chose not to perform gait training and repeated testing due to the injury model of CCI and the timing of its pairing with SPS, as the prolonged length of time required to run SPS would also prolong the length of time elapsed since TBI.

To be able to definitively understand what factors are influencing gait, future studies will look at gait testing in larger cohorts of animals and with altered parameters, such as treadmill training. This will help determine if injury from the TBI is responsible for the effect or if other conditions are driving our results.

4.2. TBI + PTSD Impairs Contextual Fear Recall. In addition to changes in gait, we sought to investigate the pathological fear and startle response characteristic of PTSD within this combined TBI + PTSD mouse model. Overgeneralization of fear responses is common in patients with PTSD, presumably owing to their inability to differentiate between dangerous and neutral contexts [27, 28]. Patients with PTSD may also not be able to use environmental cues to modulate fear expression in the appropriate context [29]. Using contextual fear conditioning, where a previously neutral context is paired with an aversive event (e.g., footshock) such that later exposure to the context elicits a fear response (e.g., freezing), we confirmed that mice that underwent SPS showed increased fear generalization when placed in a new context after associative fear learning, consistent with overgeneralized fear responses present in patients with PTSD [27–29] as well as mouse models of PTSD [30]. Although we hypothesized that mice that had undergone SPS would show increased freezing during fear recall (when returned to context A), we did not observe an increase. One possibility is that the short context B test served as a brief extinction session for the SPS mice potentially reducing the freezing displayed in the following 24 hours.

Additionally, we found that mice with combined TBI + PTSD showed deficits in contextual fear recall 48 hours after contextual fear conditioning as evidenced by decreased freezing when first returned to the feared context. It will be important in future research to determine if this deficit in memory recall is specific to contextual fear learning as well as memory of nonaversive events. We did not find differences during the contextual fear acquisition session, which suggests that fear learning and the expression of freezing are intact in all of our groups. The fear recall deficit is specific to retrieval of the contextual fear memory 48 hours after conditioning and possibly represents impaired memory systems within the combined TBI + PTSD model.

Importantly, our observed contextual fear memory impairment was found only in the combined TBI + PTSD mice and not in mice that received a TBI alone. This suggests that the injury itself is not the cause of the memory impairment. Future research will expand on these results to examine how a contextual fear memory, acquired postinjury, changes over an extended period of time using this model to further explore memory impairments in TBI or TBI + PTSD animals. Sierra-Mercado et al. (2015) also used the CCI method to induce TBI in mice, examined auditory cued fear conditioning, and found no deficits in conditioning, recall, or extinction in CCI mice. Although we used a purely contextual model of fear learning, our TBI results are similar even though our test was conducted only one-week postinjury versus two weeks in the study by Sierra-Mercado et al. Additionally, our results add to data obtained by Ojo et al. [8], who failed to see any differences in spatial learning or memory recall in a TBI group alone but did observe auditory cued fear memory impairments in their model of TBI + PTSD [8]. Our data show that combined TBI + PTSD reduces freezing 48 hours after contextual fear conditioning and suggest that the combined condition impairs contextual fear memory recall. This is consistent with the mixed literature and continues to add to the variable results of fear learning after trauma in animal models.

4.3. Acoustic Startle Response and Prepulse Inhibition Are Intact. We anticipated that mice in the PTSD groups would have an increased baseline acoustic startle response, as has been reported in patients with PTSD [31]. However, we did not observe an increased acoustic startle response in mice in the PTSD groups when pulse trials (120 dB) were presented alone. Our findings are consistent with another study of veterans with PTSD [32], which found no change in acoustic startle response relative to controls. It has been theorized that these inconsistent results in subjects with PTSD may be attributed to differences in symptom severity [33].

Given the phenomenology of human subjects with PTSD, we sought to measure sensory gating in our mouse model of TBI and PTSD using prepulse inhibition testing. Prepulse inhibition tests the phenomenon of sensory gating whereby the occurrence of a low intensity "prepulse" milliseconds before the onset of a high intensity, startle inducing, "pulse," leads to a dampening of the physiological startle response to the pulse. If successful prepulse inhibition has occurred, the recorded startle response would be lower than in the absence of the prepulse. The timing of these trials is on the order of milliseconds and is not consciously detectable to the subject. Importantly, the sensory gating phenomenon and ability to test it with prepulse inhibition testing equipment are conserved across species and altered in some psychiatric conditions.

In human subjects with PTSD, results are mixed regarding the ability to appropriately filter out irrelevant auditory stimuli in tests of prepulse inhibition, with some report finding and others failing to see differences in individuals with PTSD compared to control populations [34]. Here, we add to the growing body of literature investigating sensory gating and the baseline acoustic startle response in PTSD. In our hands, the SPS model of PTSD does not alter startle or prepulse inhibition responses either on its own or in conjunction with a CCI model of TBI, in mice. Taken together, these results suggest that the basic brain circuits underlying both acoustic startle and sensory gating ability remain intact in this population. However, the treatment groups in our study influenced sensory gating changes at different prepulse levels, despite no overall group effects on prepulse inhibition. In our studies, we used a standard 100 ms delay between the prepulse and pulse. TBI work in mice also using the CCI model has found similar interaction effects that become more pronounced at longer delays between the prepulse and pulse (100 ms and 200 ms) [35]. Interestingly, when they shortened the delay to 50 ms, there were no differences in sensory gating ability [35]. This suggests that factors such as the extent of injury and difficulty of a given task are key to consider when interpreting results in animal models of TBI and PTSD [35].

5. Conclusion

Here, we describe a unique model of TBI + PTSD in laboratory mice that recapitulates some of the behavioral impairments found in the patient population with these disease states. By combining single prolonged stress with controlled cortical impact, we have developed a controlled laboratory model of TBI + PTSD. Mice with comorbid TBI + PTSD present with unique impairments in their gait profile and problems with memory recall after contextual fear conditioning without affecting acoustic startle response or their ability to gate sensory stimuli.

Further studies are underway to examine additional behavioral, physiological, and pathological phenotypes in this combined model of TBI + PTSD. As we begin to develop an understanding of how TBI + PTSD symptoms manifest in humans, the use of this animal model to further explore the underlying physiological changes associated with combined TBI + PTSD will be invaluable in both the diagnosis and treatment of this patient population.

Disclosure

The contents do not represent the views of the U.S. Department of Veterans Affairs or the United States Government.

Acknowledgments

The authors would like to express their sincere appreciation and gratitude to Dr. Charles K. Meshul and Madeline L. Churchill for the use of the DigiGait apparatus, Delvin J. Akins for his input early on in establishing the combined TBI + PTSD protocol, Chau Nguyen for the assistance in video scoring, Ryan A. Opel for the surgical training, and the animal care staff in the Portland VA Veterinary Medical Unit. This material is the result of work supported with resources and the use of facilities at the VA Portland Health Care System, VA Career Development Award no. IK2 BX002712, NIH EXITO Institutional Core, no. UL1GM118964, the Oregon Medical Research Foundation New Investigator Award, and the Portland VA Research Foundation to Miranda M. Lim and NIH 5T32AA007468-29 and NIH 5T32HL083808-10 to Carolyn E. Jones.

References

[1] H. S. Wortzel and D. B. Arciniegas, "The DSM-5 approach to the evaluation of traumatic brain injury and its neuropsychiatric sequelae," *NeuroRehabilitation*, vol. 34, no. 4, pp. 613–623, 2014.

[2] C. A. Taylor, J. M. Bell, M. J. Breiding, and X. Likang, "Traumatic brain injury-related emergency department visits, hospitalizations, and deaths — United States, 2007 and 2013," *MMWR Surveillance Summaries*, vol. 66, no. 9, pp. 1–16, 2017.

[3] T. Tanielian, L. H. Jaycox, D. M. Adamson et al., "Invisible wounds of war," in *Psychological and Cognitive Injuries, Their Consequences, and Services to Assist Recovery*, Rand Corporation, 2008.

[4] American Psychiatric Association, *Diagnostic and Statistical Manual of Mental Disorders, 5th Edition (DSM-5)*, Diagnostic and Statistical Manual of Mental Disorders 4th Edition TR, American Psychiatric Association, 2013.

[5] M. A. Gupta, "Review of somatic symptoms in post-traumatic stress disorder," *International Review of Psychiatry*, vol. 25, no. 1, pp. 86–99, 2013.

[6] K. S. Tanev, K. Z. Pentel, M. A. Kredlow, and M. E. Charney, "PTSD and TBI co-morbidity: scope, clinical presentation and treatment options," *Brain Injury*, vol. 28, no. 3, pp. 261–270, 2014.

[7] G. A. Elder, N. P. Dorr, R. de Gasperi et al., "Blast exposure induces post-traumatic stress disorder-related traits in a rat model of mild traumatic brain injury," *Journal of Neurotrauma*, vol. 29, no. 16, pp. 2564–2575, 2012.

[8] J. O. Ojo, M. B. Greenberg, P. Leary et al., "Neurobehavioral, neuropathological and biochemical profiles in a novel mouse model of co-morbid post-traumatic stress disorder and mild traumatic brain injury," *Frontiers in Behavioral Neuroscience*, vol. 8, p. 213, 2014.

[9] G. Perez-Garcia, R. de Gasperi, M. A. Gama Sosa et al., "PTSD-related behavioral traits in a rat model of blast-induced MTBI are reversed by the MGluR2/3 receptor antagonist BCI-838," *ENeuro*, vol. 5, no. 1, 2018.

[10] A. Zuckerman, O. Ram, G. Ifergane et al., "Controlled low-pressure blast-wave exposure causes distinct behavioral and morphological responses modelling mild traumatic brain injury, post-traumatic stress disorder, and comorbid mild traumatic brain injury–post-traumatic stress disorder," *Journal of Neurotrauma*, vol. 34, no. 1, pp. 145–164, 2017.

[11] S. Yamamoto, S. Morinobu, S. Takei et al., "Single prolonged stress: toward an animal model of posttraumatic stress disorder," *Depression and Anxiety*, vol. 26, no. 12, pp. 1110–1117, 2009.

[12] G. B. Fox, L. Fan, R. A. Levasseur, and A. I. Faden, "Sustained sensory/motor and cognitive deficits with neuronal apoptosis following controlled cortical impact brain injury in the mouse," *Journal of Neurotrauma*, vol. 15, no. 8, pp. 599–614, 1998.

[13] A. Arai, Y. Hirota, N. Miyase et al., "A single prolonged stress paradigm produces enduring impairments in social bonding in monogamous prairie voles," *Behavioural Brain Research*, vol. 315, pp. 83–93, 2016.

[14] M. J. Lisieski, A. L. Eagle, A. C. Conti, I. Liberzon, and S. A. Perrine, "Single-prolonged stress: a review of two decades of progress in a rodent model of post-traumatic stress disorder," *Frontiers in Psychiatry*, vol. 9, 2018.

[15] S. A. Perrine, A. L. Eagle, S. A. George et al., "Severe, multimodal stress exposure induces PTSD-like characteristics in a mouse model of single prolonged stress," *Behavioural Brain Research*, vol. 303, pp. 228–237, 2016.

[16] H. Yu, H. Watt, C. Kesavan, and S. Mohan, "The negative impact of single prolonged stress (SPS) on bone development in mice," *Stress*, vol. 16, no. 5, pp. 564–570, 2013.

[17] R. R. Souza, L. J. Noble, and C. K. McIntyre, "Using the single prolonged stress model to examine the pathophysiology of PTSD," *Frontiers in Pharmacology*, vol. 8, 2017.

[18] G. Williams, M. E. Morris, A. Schache, and P. R. McCrory, "Incidence of gait abnormalities after traumatic brain injury," *Archives of Physical Medicine and Rehabilitation*, vol. 90, no. 4, pp. 587–593, 2009.

[19] N. D. Osier, J. R. Korpon, and C. Edward Dixon, "Controlled cortical impact model," in *Brain Neurotrauma: Molecular, Neuropsychological, and Rehabilitation Aspects*, CRC Press/Taylor & Francis, Boca Raton FL USA, 2015.

[20] J. M. Donelan, D. W. Shipman, R. Kram, and A. D. Kuo, "Mechanical and metabolic requirements for active lateral stabilization in human walking," *Journal of Biomechanics*, vol. 37, no. 6, pp. 827–835, 2004.

[21] D. R. Howell, L. R. Osternig, and L. S. Chou, "Dual-task effect on gait balance control in adolescents with concussion," *Archives of Physical Medicine and Rehabilitation*, vol. 94, no. 8, pp. 1513–1520, 2013.

[22] M. Vallée, B. J. McFadyen, B. Swaine, J. Doyon, J. F. Cantin, and D. Dumas, "Effects of environmental demands on locomotion after traumatic brain injury," *Archives of Physical Medicine and Rehabilitation*, vol. 87, no. 6, pp. 806–813, 2006.

[23] T. M. Parker, L. R. Osternig, H.-J. Lee, P. van Donkelaar, and L.-S. Chou, "The effect of divided attention on gait stability following concussion," *Clinical Biomechanics*, vol. 20, no. 4, pp. 389–395, 2005.

[24] M. Neumann, Y. Wang, S. Kim et al., "Assessing gait impairment following experimental traumatic brain injury in mice," *Journal of Neuroscience Methods*, vol. 176, no. 1, pp. 34–44, 2009.

[25] M. Sashindranath, M. Daglas, and R. L. Medcalf, "Evaluation of gait impairment in mice subjected to craniotomy and traumatic brain injury," *Behavioural Brain Research*, vol. 286, pp. 33–38, 2015.

[26] J. Luo, A. Nguyen, S. Villeda et al., "Long-term cognitive impairments and pathological alterations in a mouse model of repetitive mild traumatic brain injury," *Frontiers in Neurology*, vol. 5, 2014.

[27] A. N. Kaczkurkin, P. C. Burton, S. M. Chazin et al., "Neural substrates of overgeneralized conditioned fear in PTSD," *American Journal of Psychiatry*, vol. 174, no. 2, pp. 125–134, 2017.

[28] R. A. Morey, J. E. Dunsmoor, C. C. Haswell et al., "Fear learning circuitry is biased toward generalization of fear associations in posttraumatic stress disorder," *Translational Psychiatry*, vol. 5, no. 12, article e700, 2015.

[29] S. N. Garfinkel, J. L. Abelson, A. P. King et al., "Impaired contextual modulation of memories in PTSD: an FMRI and psychophysiological study of extinction retention and fear renewal," *Journal of Neuroscience*, vol. 34, no. 40, pp. 13435–13443, 2014.

[30] D. E. Aikins, J. A. Strader, R. J. Kohler, N. Bihani, and S. A. Perrine, "Differences in hippocampal serotonergic activity in a mouse single prolonged stress paradigm impact discriminant fear acquisition and retention," *Neuroscience Letters*, vol. 639, pp. 162–166, 2017.

[31] S. P. Orr, L. J. Metzger, and R. K. Pitman, "Psychophysiology of post-traumatic stress disorder," *The Psychiatric Clinics of North America*, vol. 25, no. 2, pp. 271–293, 2002.

[32] C. Grillon, C. A. Morgan, S. M. Southwick, M. Davis, and D. S. Charney, "Baseline startle amplitude and prepulse inhibition in Vietnam veterans with posttraumatic stress disorder," *Psychiatry Research*, vol. 64, no. 3, pp. 169–178, 1996.

[33] R. Yehuda, "Recent advances in the study of biological alterations in post-traumatic stress disorder (PTSD)," *Psychiatric Clinics of North America*, vol. 25, no. 2, pp. xi–xv, 2002.

[34] S. Kohl, K. Heekeren, J. Klosterkötter, and J. Kuhn, "Prepulse inhibition in psychiatric disorders—apart from schizophrenia," *Journal of Psychiatric Research*, vol. 47, no. 4, pp. 445–452, 2013.

18

Quality of Life in Patients with Dementia with Lewy Bodies

Chuo-Yu Lee,[1,2,3] Shih-Jung Cheng,[1,3,4] Hui-Chi Lin,[1] Yu-Lu Liao,[5] and Pei-Hao Chen[1,3,6]

[1]*Department of Neurology, Mackay Memorial Hospital, Taipei, Taiwan*
[2]*Graduate Institute of Chemistry, Tamkang University, New Taipei City, Taiwan*
[3]*Department of Medicine, Mackay Medical College, New Taipei City, Taiwan*
[4]*Department of Physical Therapy and Assistive Technology, National Yang-Ming University, Taipei, Taiwan*
[5]*Department of Accounting Information, Takming University of Science and Technology, Taipei, Taiwan*
[6]*Graduate Institute of Mechanical and Electrical Engineering, National Taipei University of Technology, Taipei, Taiwan*

Correspondence should be addressed to Pei-Hao Chen; a7662888@gmail.com

Academic Editor: Ying-Jui Ho

Dementia with Lewy bodies (DLB) is a complex, multisymptom disorder. When making decisions regarding the treatment of DLB, the patient's quality of life (QoL) should always be the main consideration. To our knowledge, this is the first review article focusing on the QoL in DLB patients. We searched the PubMed database using the keywords "quality of life" and "dementia with Lewy bodies." Previously, no specific instrument had been developed for assessing the QoL in DLB patients. Patients with DLB have a decreased QoL compared to patients with Alzheimer's disease, which is reportedly caused by several factors including level of independence in instrumental activities of daily living, whether the patient is living with the caregiver, apathy, delusion, and dysautonomia. The direct effect of visual hallucination, sleep, and movement disorders on the QoL in DLB patients has not been previously studied. The role of cognitive function on the QoL is still controversial. In a randomized controlled study, memantine may improve the QoL in PDD or DLB patients. We concluded that it is important to develop a specific instrument to assess the QoL in DLB patients. Furthermore, there is an urgent need for large clinical trials to identify factors associated with the QoL and how they can be managed.

1. Introduction

Dementia with Lewy bodies (DLB) is the second most common neurodegenerative dementia after Alzheimer's disease (AD) in people over 65 years of age. A recent published population-based cohort study from the Taiwan National Health Insurance Research Database showed the incidence of DLB was 7.10 per 100,000 person-years [1]. DLB differs from AD as early cognitive symptoms include deficits in visuospatial and executive function, rather than memory. DLB is characterized by parkinsonism, fluctuations in mental status, visual hallucination, and hypersensitivity to neuroleptics. Therefore, it is difficult to discriminate between DLB and Parkinson's disease with dementia (PDD). Both diseases also share a similar pathologic finding, Lewy bodies. Generally, if cognitive impairments appear within a year of parkinsonism, DLB is diagnosed, while patients with parkinsonism for at least a year prior to cognitive impairment are classified as PDD. Early amyloid deposition in DLB relative to PDD may explain the difference in the timing of dementia and parkinsonism [2].

The quality of life (QoL) is a key outcome measure of health and social service interventions. Currently, patient-reported outcome measures are increasingly used in evaluating health and social care. Definitions of health-related QoL include physical, mental, social, and role functioning and health perceptions [3]. Because aging is a global issue, it is critical to identify QoL determinants in the elderly who suffer from chronic disease. A recent study from Southern Taiwan showed Alzheimer disease-8, a screening tool, had the strongest association with the total QoL score in 115 old-age adults suffering from chronic disease. It is important for geriatric health care providers to realize that cognitive impairment among old age adults with chronic disease is a critical determining factor of poor QoL [4].

Assessing the QoL in people with dementia is crucial for evaluating their outcomes; however, it is challenging to interview patients who have a limited ability to express themselves and may lack insight. Meanwhile, there are questions concerning the validity of generic measures of QoL, which are not specific to dementia. Currently, evaluations of QoL largely focus on general dementia or AD. A systematic review [5] regarding the QoL in dementia strongly suggests that depression is consistently related to a decreased QoL. Surprisingly, there is no convincing evidence indicating that lower cognitive ability or greater limitations in the activity are associated with a lower QoL.

Evidence concerning the QoL in DLB patients is limited [6]. In a comparison study, the QoL was measured using the *Alzheimer Disease-Related Quality of Life* (ADRQL) evaluation, a proxy-rated, dementia-specific instrument. The authors concluded that DLB patients have a poorer QoL than AD patients [7]. Figari et al. compared the QoL in 46 AD, 23 DLB, and 39 Huntington's disease (HD) patients, all of whom had dementia for at least two years. Patients with DLB scored significantly lower on the SF-12 Physical and Mental Health Summary than patients with HD and AD. The authors concluded that, when adjusted for age, cognition, comorbidity, and depression, patients with DLB had the poorest QoL [8].

There is only one study whose primary aim was to compare the QoL in patients with DLB and AD [9]. 34 DLB patients and 34 cognitive-matched AD patients were evaluated using two QoL instruments: EQ-5D and QoL-AD. The results showed both patient-rated QoL and proxy-rated QoL were poorer in patients with DLB than those with AD. Due to many differences in clinical symptoms, it is reasonable to predict differences in the QOL between diseases. Herein, we elaborate on studies related to the QoL in DLB patients.

2. Methods

Studies were selected from the PubMed database using keywords "quality of life" and "dementia with Lewy bodies." All languages (with an English abstract) were included. Articles spanned the period between June 1986 and December 2017. Searches yielded 102 citations of which 21 were included as relevant. Other data were collected through references from selected articles and searching relevant journals offline.

2.1. Dementia-Specific QoL Measurement Scales. Unfortunately, there are no instruments available to specifically evaluate the QoL in DLB patients. Therefore, we herein discuss QOL measurement scales for dementia.

There is some debate regarding whether to use the patient's or caregiver's reported QoL as the measurement. Typically, the QoL is rated higher by patients than by caregiver proxy measures. The differences are associated with increased levels of caregiver burden and caregiver depression, rather than lower levels of patients' cognitive performance [10]. Therefore, it is reasonable to directly assess subjective QoL in patients with mild to moderate dementia. Interestingly, Karlawish et al. proposed a method to minimize the discrepancy between patient's and caregiver's QoL scores: caregivers should rate using substituted judgment as if they were the patients [11]. Issues regarding the exclusion of patients with severe dementia from self-reported questionnaires and weak reliability of proxy versions remain unresolved.

There is limited knowledge regarding the standard instruments used to evaluate the QoL in dementia patients. In a recently published review [12], the most frequently used dementia-specific instrument was the Quality of Life in Alzheimer's Disease (QOL-AD) and Dementia Quality of Life questionnaire (DEMQOL). As for generic measures, EuroQol 5-dimension (EQ-5D) and Short Form surveys (SF-36 or SF-12) were widely used. The authors recommended dementia-specific DEMQOL, generic SF-12, and health utility EQ-5D-5L, based on both self- and proxy-report [12]. In the following paragraphs, we will briefly introduce each widely-used measurement scale.

2.2. Quality of Life in Alzheimer's Disease (QOL-AD). The QOL-AD [13] is an instrument specifically developed for mild to severe dementia. It includes 13 items, including physical health, energy, mood, living situation, memory, family, marriage, friends, self, ability to do chores, ability to do things for fun, money, and life as a whole. Each domain is rated from 1 (poor) to 4 (excellent). As for the caregiver version, which contains 15 items, marriage and money are removed, while people who work here, ability to take care of oneself, ability to live with others, and ability to make choices in one's life are added.

2.3. Dementia Quality of Life Questionnaire (DEMQOL). The DEMQOL [14] aims to assess QoL in mild to moderate dementia. It includes 5 domains including daily activities and looking after self, health and well-being, cognitive functioning, social relationships, self-concept, and a total of 28 items. Each item is scored from 1 to 4. A proxy version has been developed for caregivers, DEMQOL-Proxy, which contains 31 items.

2.4. EuroQol 5-Dimension (EQ-5D-5L). The EQ-5D-5L [15] is a generic instrument. Respondents are asked to rate their current health status on 5 dimensions: mobility, hygiene, usual activities, pain/discomfort, and anxiety/depression. For each dimension, the respondent gives 1 of 5 possible ratings according to symptom severity. The questionnaire also includes a visual analog scale (VAS) as a secondary part, ranging from 0 (death) to 100 (perfect health). Thus, two QoL values are acquired with this instrument.

2.5. Short Form-36 and Short Form-12 (SF-36 and SF-12). The SF-36 [16] is a generic measurement containing 36 questions across 8 dimensions of health status: vitality, physical functioning, bodily pain, general health perceptions, physical role functioning, emotional role functioning, social role functioning, and mental health. A shorter version, SF-12, was

TABLE 1: Characteristics of QoL measurement scales for dementia.

Instrument	Patient report	Proxy report	Domains	Items	Measurement	Brief summary
Quality of Life in Alzheimer's Disease (QOL-AD)	Yes	Yes	Physical health Mental health Social and functional domains	13 (15 for proxy version)	Four-point scale score Range 13–52 for patient report and range 15–60 for proxy report Higher scores equal to higher QoL	The best researched of all the dementia measurement scales Relatively brief Suitable for mild to severe dementia
Dementia Quality of Life questionnaire (DEMQOL)	Yes	Yes	Daily activities and looking after self Health and well-being Cognitive functioning Social relationships Self-concept	28 (31 for proxy version)	Four-point scale score Range 28–112 for patient report and range 31–124 for proxy report Higher scores equal to higher QoL	The conceptual framework is based on health-related QoL, with less social relevance The proxy version performed well in psychometric tests Suitable for mild to moderate dementia
EuroQol 5-dimension (EQ-5D-5L)	Yes	No	1st part: Mobility Hygiene Usual activities Pain/discomfort Anxiety/depression 2nd part: Visual analogue scale (VAS)	No	1st part: having no problems for 1, having slight problems for 2, having moderate problems for 3, having severe problems for 4, and being unable to do/having extreme problems for 5 2nd part: 0 for worst; 100 for best health status	A generic, preference-based instrument for health related QoL The 5-digit number for 5 domains can be converted into a single weighted index score Appropriate in people with mild to moderate dementia
Short Form-36 (SF-36)	Yes	No	Vitality Physical functioning Bodily pain General health perceptions Physical role functioning Emotional role functioning Social role functioning Mental health	36	One score in each domain, calculated by special software, representing weighted sums of the questions (0 equivalent to maximum disability; 100 equivalent to no disability)	A generic health status measure A shorter version, SF-12, was developed to minimize respondent burden if only physical and mental health summary scores are of interest

developed to minimize respondent burden if only physical and mental health summary scores are of interest.

A summary of the four widely-used scales is provided in Table 1.

2.6. Reported Symptoms That May Affect QoL in DLB Patients. One study compared the QoL in patients with DLB and AD as its primary aim and demonstrated that the following are important determinants of the QoL in DLB patients: their Neuropsychiatric Inventory score and level of independency in instrumental activities of daily living (ADL), whether the patient lives with the caregiver, apathy, and delusion [9]. Similar to most findings in overall dementia, cognitive function has no strong relation to the QoL in this study.

Caregivers play an important role in affecting a patient's QoL. In a cross-sectional study [17] of 161 patients with dementia (including 13 DLB patients), the QoL was measured using the ADRQL. The results indicated that some predictors of a reduced QoL include behavioral and depressive symptoms, dependency in basic ADL, poorer cognitive function, use of antipsychotic medication, caregiver burden, and caregiver not being an adult child. The role of cognitive function on the QoL is still controversial. Here, we will discuss some reported causative factors for a poorer QoL in DLB patients.

2.7. Visual Hallucinations. Visual hallucinations occur in 60 to 70% of DLB patients, usually beginning in the first 2 or 3 years of the disease [18]. The presentation of visual hallucinations in the first 4 years following the onset of dementia has a positive and negative predictive value for DLB of 81% and 79%, respectively [19]. The most common visual hallucinations are fully formed persons (84%), animals or bugs (37%), and objects (39%) [20]. Early misperceptions and misidentification of family members are usually reported in

DLB. Capgras syndrome, a delusion where a person has been substituted by an imposter with a similar outward, is also common in DLB and is associated with higher rates of visual hallucinations and anxiety [21]. A recently published post-mortem study [22] showed DLB cases had reduced neuronal density in the intermediate gray layer of the superior colliculus tissue, a structure important for directing attention toward visual targets. This finding may provide pathologic evidence for visual hallucinations in DLB.

A cross-sectional and retrospective study of 1025 patients with dementia in Spain found that delusion and hallucinations were more prevalent in DLB patients than those with AD and PDD [23]. In a recent comparative study of 207 delusional and nondelusional patients with DLB, the authors concluded that the delusional patients had poorer cognitive function and more severe neuropsychiatric symptoms [24]. In a cross-sectional study, 21 DLB and 35 PDD patients with recurrent visual hallucinations were evaluated. Most patients had complex hallucinations daily, usually lasting minutes. The study showed that neuropsychiatric symptoms that coexist with hallucinations are apathy, sleep disturbance, and anxiety [25]. The direct effect of visual hallucination on the QoL in DLB patients has not been previously studied.

Treatment of psychosis is challenging in DLB, since many patients are hypersensitive to neuroleptic drugs; therefore, nonpharmacologic treatment approaches should be considered first. Typical antipsychotic agents should be avoided, while the evidence for atypical antipsychotics is controversial. At present, quetiapine and clozapine are usually prescribed. Pimavanserin, a selective serotonin 5-HT2A inverse agonist, has beneficial effects on treating psychosis in PDD [26], while similar results are expected in DLB patients.

2.8. Depression and Apathy. The presence of depression and other behavioral and psychological symptoms of dementia (BPSD) may worsen the QoL of dementia patients and their caregivers [27]. The BPSD can be classified into four clusters: depression, aggressive behaviors, psychosis, and euphoria. In AD and DLB patients, a cross-sectional analysis determined that depressive symptom in patients may be the most important BPSD symptom as it was the only one shown to cause depression in caregivers [28].

A previous literature revealed that DLB is associated with higher scores on the Geriatric Depression Scale compared to AD, and a higher rate of depression is found in the early stages of the disorder [29]. Kurisu et al. compared the QoL of 279 degenerative dementia patients with different subtypes by using the *QOL Questionnaire for Dementia* (QOL-D) as an evaluation scale. The QOL-D comprises six domains: positive affect, negative affect and actions, communication, restlessness, attachment to others, and spontaneity. Results showed that apathy in frontotemporal dementia (FTD) and DLB patients and depression in DLB patients might cause the reduced positive affect in FTD and DLB patients compared to AD patients [30]. Apathy also plays an important role in evaluating the QoL in DLB patients. In a DLB and AD comparison study, DLB patients are less able to complete the QoL questionnaire [6].

In DLB, the presence of Lewy bodies in limbic, paralimbic, and neocortical regions may account for the appearance of depressive symptoms [27]. Early detection of depression in DLB patients is important as these symptoms are treatable. In a recently published review, the authors concluded that neuropsychiatric symptoms, especially psychosis and depression, are priority targets for intervention to improve the outcome of patients with DLB [6].

2.9. Sleep Disorders. Sleep disorders are common in DLB patients, with both rapid eye movement sleep behavior disorder (RBD) and fluctuating cognition being part of the clinical diagnostic criteria. In a contemporary review in sleep medicine, the authors concluded that appropriate management of sleep-related symptoms can improve the QoL in patients with neurodegenerative disorders [31]. Orexins (also known as hypocretins) are secreted in neurons in the lateral hypothalamus that are related to sleep regulation and attention [32]. Lower levels of orexin-1 were detected in the cerebrospinal fluid of DLB patients compared to AD patients and control subjects [33].

76% of DLB patients had RBD [34], which is characterized by acting out dreams, resulting in vocalizations and even violent behavior. Other nocturnal symptoms such as anxiety, periodic leg movements, urinary dysfunction, and difficulty turning over in bed can contribute to sleep problems [31]. In a retrospective study of 78 patients with DLB and sleep disorders who underwent polysomnography, approximately three quarters experienced many arousals not accounted for by a movement or breathing disturbance. Among patients who did not show evidence of significantly disordered breathing, 62% of arousals were arousals for no apparent reason [35]. The direct effect of sleep disorders on the QoL in DLB patients has not been previously studied.

2.10. Dysautonomia. In a study [36] of the prevalence of autonomic symptoms in dementia, the authors concluded that total autonomic symptom scores [37], urinary symptoms, constipation, and postural dizziness were significantly higher in DLB patients than in AD patients. By using the SF-36 [38] as a measurement, higher autonomic symptom scores were related to a lower QoL. The authors proposed that the effect of autonomic symptoms upon the QoL may be due to the limitations in ADL.

A systematic review of autonomic dysfunction in α-synucleinopathies revealed that cardiovascular autonomic failure has a significant impact on daily activities and QoL. Cerebral white matter changes in image and cognitive decline may be related to altered cerebral perfusion, vascular pressure stress, and associated disruption of the blood-brain barrier [39]. In α-synucleinopathies, autonomic dysfunction is more severe in DLB than in PD patients [40].

Both preganglionic and postganglionic dysfunctions may be present in DLB patients [41]. In a retrospective examination of DLB patients, urinary incontinence and constipation were the most commonly presented autonomic symptoms, occurring in 97 and 83% of patients, respectively, while syncope occurred in 28% of patients [42]. Orthostatic hypotension (OH) has been reported in around 50% of DLB patients [43]. OH is defined as the reduction in systolic blood pressure of at least 20 mmHg or diastolic blood pressure of 10 mmHg within 3 minutes of standing from the lying position [44]. Patients may not present with classic postural dizziness, but instead nonspecific malaise or lethargy, which can markedly increase the risk of falls or syncope. Management may include salt supplementation, compression stockings, or oral medication such as midodrine or fludrocortisone [45]. Furthermore, a higher prevalence of carotid sinus syndrome, an altered arterial sinus response to baroceptive stimulation resulting in syncope, was found in 32% of DLB patients compared to 11.1% of AD patients [46].

2.11. Reported Management That May Improve QoL in DLB Patients. It can be helpful to divide the symptoms of DLB into five categories: cognitive, neuropsychiatric, movement, autonomic, and sleep. It is important to take a detailed history and form a comprehensive treatment strategy to improve a patient's QoL [47]. There is little published data regarding the effect of the management of symptoms on the QoL in DLB patients.

2.12. Armodafinil. Because armodafinil has a longer half-life than modafinil, we may predict its better effect at treating patients with excessive daytime sleepiness [48]. In a 12-week pilot trial of oral armodafinil therapy (120–250 mg daily), DLB patients with hypersomnia showed improved scores on the Epworth Sleepiness Scale, Maintenance of Wakefulness Test, and Clinical Global Impression of Change. Moreover, caregivers' overall QoL improved at week 12 [49]. It should be noted that the effect of armodafinil on patients' QoL was not analyzed in this trial.

2.13. Memantine. Memantine, an NMDA receptor antagonist, has been widely used in treating moderate to severe AD. A randomized controlled study was conducted on 70 patients with PDD or DLB over 24 weeks using caregiver-rated QOL-AD as a measurement. A secondary analysis of this study showed that memantine improved the total QoL, body function, physical health, energy, mood, and memory when compared to the placebo group [50]. Large-scale trials are required to confirm these preliminary findings. On the other hand, although cholinesterase inhibitors are widely prescribed for patients with DLB, we found no reported effect of cholinesterase inhibitors on the QoL in DLB patients.

2.14. Exercise. Exercise may improve functional outcomes in PD and AD patients. The multisymptom nature of the DLB (parkinsonism, cognitive, and psychiatric) results in these patients often being excluded from clinical trials to avoid confounding results. A recent systematic review confirms a scarcity of research investigating exercise as a potential therapy in DLB patients [51]. The authors concluded that the effect of exercise on cognitive, psychiatric, QoL, and physiological outcomes remains unclear in DLB patients. Further clinical trials in larger cohorts are necessary.

3. Conclusions

This is, to our knowledge, the first review article focusing on the QoL in patients with dementia with Lewy bodies. Our review may not be fully comprehensive due to the limited literature available regarding this topic. Physicians should keep the patient's QoL in the forefront when managing their symptoms. The following are reported factors leading to poorer QoL in DLB patients: independence in instrumental ADL, whether the patient is living with the caregiver, the presence of depression, apathy, delusion, and dysautonomia.

First, we concluded that it is important to develop a specific instrument to assess the QoL in DLB patients. Apathy is more common in DLB patients, causing them less able to complete the questionnaire [6]. Therefore, it is reasonable to design a scale with proxy version. Since DLB is a complex, multisymptom disorder, we recommend the following domains should be taken into account: health and well-being, daily activities, cognitive functioning, positive and negative affect, restless behavior, social interaction, and satisfaction (i.e., restful sleep). Second, we hope that with the advent of more diagnostic criteria and advances in biomarkers, there will be well-defined DLB cohorts for clinical trials. Further studies may be facilitated by international or multicenter cooperation. For example, a large longitudinal cohort of 5624 DLB patients has been developed recently in 135 dementia centers in Italy (the DLB-SINdem study group) [52]. There is an urgent need for large, cross-sectional, and longitudinal trials to determine other factors associated with the QoL, such as cognition, visual hallucination, sleep, and movement disorders. Finally, because of the poor prognosis and high socioeconomic burden of DBL, we should consider the health-related QoL as one of the outcome measurements when developing new drugs for DLB.

References

[1] S.-K. Yang, W. Chen, C.-H. Su, and C.-H. Liu, "Incidence and comorbidity of dementia with Lewy bodies: a population-based cohort study," *Behavioural Neurology*, vol. 2018, Article ID 7631951, 6 pages, 2018.

[2] D. H. Hepp, D. L. E. Vergoossen, E. Huisman et al., "Distribution and load of amyloid-β pathology in Parkinson disease and dementia with Lewy bodies," *Journal of Neuropathology & Experimental Neurology*, vol. 75, no. 10, pp. 936–945, 2016.

[3] J. E. Ware Jr and C. D. Sherbourne, "The MOS 36-item short-form health survey (SF-36): I. Conceptual framework and item selection," *Medical Care*, vol. 30, no. 6, pp. 473–483, 1992.

[4] H.-M. Chen and C.-M. Chen, "Factors associated with quality of life among older adults with chronic disease in Taiwan," *International Journal of Gerontology*, vol. 11, no. 1, pp. 12–15, 2017.

[5] S. Banerjee, K. Samsi, C. D. Petrie et al., "What do we know about quality of life in dementia? A review of the emerging evidence on the predictive and explanatory value of disease specific measures of health related quality of life in people with dementia," *International Journal of Geriatric Psychiatry*, vol. 24, no. 1, pp. 15–24, 2009.

[6] C. Mueller, C. Ballard, A. Corbett, and D. Aarsland, "The prognosis of dementia with Lewy bodies," *Lancet Neurology*, vol. 16, no. 5, pp. 390–398, 2017.

[7] P. Thomas, F. Lalloué, P. M. Preux et al., "Dementia patients caregivers quality of life: the PIXEL study," *International Journal of Geriatric Psychiatry*, vol. 21, no. 1, pp. 50–56, 2006.

[8] R. Figari-Jordan, K. Anderson, A. Gruber-Baldini et al., "Comparison of quality of life and disability in three different dementias (P07.180)," *Neurology*, vol. 78, no. Meeting Abstracts 1, article P07.180, 2012.

[9] F. Boström, L. Jönsson, L. Minthon, and E. Londos, "Patients with dementia with lewy bodies have more impaired quality of life than patients with Alzheimer disease," *Alzheimer Disease & Associated Disorders*, vol. 21, no. 2, pp. 150–154, 2007.

[10] L. P. Sands, P. Ferreira, A. L. Stewart, M. Brod, and K. Yaffe, "What explains differences between dementia patients' and their caregivers' ratings of patients' quality of life?," *The American Journal of Geriatric Psychiatry*, vol. 12, no. 3, pp. 272–280, 2004.

[11] J. H. T. Karlawish, D. Casarett, J. Klocinski, and C. M. Clark, "The relationship between caregivers' global ratings of Alzheimer's disease patients' quality of life, disease severity, and the caregiving experience," *Journal of the American Geriatrics Society*, vol. 49, no. 8, pp. 1066–1070, 2001.

[12] F. Yang, P. Dawes, I. Leroi, and B. Gannon, "Measurement tools of resource use and quality of life in clinical trials for dementia or cognitive impairment interventions: a systematically conducted narrative review," *International Journal of Geriatric Psychiatry*, vol. 33, no. 2, pp. e166–e176, 2018.

[13] R. G. Logsdon, L. E. Gibbons, S. M. McCurry, and L. Teri, "Quality of life in Alzheimer's disease: patient and caregiver reports," *Journal of Mental health and Aging*, vol. 5, pp. 21–32, 1999.

[14] S. Smith, D. Lamping, S. Banerjee et al., "Measurement of health-related quality of life for people with dementia: development of a new instrument (DEMQOL) and an evaluation of current methodology," *Health Technology Assessment*, vol. 9, no. 10, 2005.

[15] The EuroQol Group, "EuroQol - a new facility for the measurement of health-related quality of life," *Health Policy*, vol. 16, no. 3, pp. 199–208, 1990.

[16] C. Jenkinson, R. Layte, D. Jenkinson et al., "A shorter form health survey: can the SF-12 replicate results from the SF-36 in longitudinal studies?," *Journal of Public Health*, vol. 19, no. 2, pp. 179–186, 1997.

[17] A. A. Mougias, A. Politis, C. G. Lyketsos, and V. G. Mavreas, "Quality of life in dementia patients in Athens, Greece: predictive factors and the role of caregiver-related factors," *International Psychogeriatrics*, vol. 23, no. 3, pp. 395–403, 2011.

[18] C. Ballard, C. Holmes, I. McKeith et al., "Psychiatric morbidity in dementia with Lewy bodies: a prospective clinical and neuropathological comparative study with Alzheimer's disease," *American Journal of Psychiatry*, vol. 156, no. 7, pp. 1039–1045, 1999.

[19] T. J. Ferman, G. E. Smith, B. F. Boeve et al., "Neuropsychological differentiation of dementia with Lewy bodies from normal aging and Alzheimer's disease," *The Clinical Neuropsychologist*, vol. 20, no. 4, pp. 623–636, 2006.

[20] T. J. Ferman, Z. Arvanitakis, H. Fujishiro et al., "Pathology and temporal onset of visual hallucinations, misperceptions and family misidentification distinguishes dementia with Lewy bodies from Alzheimer's disease," *Parkinsonism & Related Disorders*, vol. 19, no. 2, pp. 227–231, 2013.

[21] P. Thaipisuttikul, I. Lobach, Y. Zweig, A. Gurnani, and J. E. Galvin, "Capgras syndrome in dementia with Lewy bodies," *International Psychogeriatrics*, vol. 25, no. 5, pp. 843–849, 2013.

[22] D. Erskine, A. J. Thomas, J. P. Taylor et al., "Neuronal loss and A-synuclein pathology in the superior colliculus and its relationship to visual hallucinations in dementia with Lewy bodies," *The American Journal of Geriatric Psychiatry*, vol. 25, no. 6, pp. 595–604, 2017.

[23] S. López-Pousa, J. Vilalta-Franch, J. Garre-Olmo, S. Pons, and M. G. Cucurella, "Characterisation and prevalence of the psychological and behavioural symptoms in patients with dementia," *Revista de Neurologia*, vol. 45, no. 11, pp. 683–688, 2007.

[24] R.-C. Tzeng, C.-F. Tsai, C.-T. Wang, T.-Y. Wang, and P.-Y. Chiu, "Delusions in patients with dementia with Lewy bodies and the associated factors," *Behavioural Neurology*, vol. 2018, Article ID 6707291, 8 pages, 2018.

[25] U. P. Mosimann, E. N. Rowan, C. E. Partington et al., "Characteristics of visual hallucinations in Parkinson disease dementia and dementia with Lewy bodies," *The American Journal of Geriatric Psychiatry*, vol. 14, no. 2, pp. 153–160, 2006.

[26] J. Cummings, S. Isaacson, R. Mills et al., "Pimavanserin for patients with Parkinson's disease psychosis: a randomised, placebo-controlled phase 3 trial," *The Lancet*, vol. 383, no. 9916, pp. 533–540, 2014.

[27] M. Baquero and N. Martin, "Depressive symptoms in neurodegenerative diseases," *World Journal of Clinical Cases*, vol. 3, no. 8, pp. 682–693, 2015.

[28] K. Ornstein, J. E. Gaugler, D. P. Devanand, N. Scarmeas, C. Zhu, and Y. Stern, "The differential impact of unique behavioral and psychological symptoms for the dementia caregiver: how and why do patients' individual symptom clusters impact caregiver depressive symptoms?," *The American Journal of Geriatric Psychiatry*, vol. 21, no. 12, pp. 1277–1286, 2013.

[29] Y. Yamane, K. Sakai, and K. Maeda, "Dementia with Lewy bodies is associated with higher scores on the Geriatric Depression Scale than is Alzheimer's disease," *Psychogeriatrics*, vol. 11, no. 3, pp. 157–165, 2011.

[30] K. Kurisu, S. Terada, E. Oshima et al., "Comparison of QOL between patients with different degenerative dementias, focusing especially on positive and negative affect," *International Psychogeriatrics*, vol. 28, no. 8, pp. 1355–1361, 2016.

[31] J. A. Pillai and J. B. Leverenz, "Sleep and neurodegeneration: a critical appraisal," *Chest*, vol. 151, no. 6, pp. 1375–1386, 2017.

[32] C. Peyron, D. K. Tighe, A. N. van den Pol et al., "Neurons containing hypocretin (orexin) project to multiple neuronal systems," *Journal of Neuroscience*, vol. 18, no. 23, pp. 9996–10015, 1998.

[33] M. Wennström, E. Londos, L. Minthon, and H. M. Nielsen, "Altered CSF orexin and α-synuclein levels in dementia patients," *Journal of Alzheimer's Disease*, vol. 29, no. 1, pp. 125–132, 2012.

[34] T. J. Ferman, B. F. Boeve, G. E. Smith et al., "Inclusion of RBD improves the diagnostic classification of dementia with Lewy bodies," *Neurology*, vol. 77, no. 9, pp. 875–882, 2011.

[35] W. C. Pao, B. F. Boeve, T. J. Ferman et al., "Polysomnographic findings in dementia with Lewy bodies," *The Neurologist*, vol. 19, no. 1, pp. 1–6, 2013.

[36] L. Allan, I. McKeith, C. Ballard, and R. A. Kenny, "The prevalence of autonomic symptoms in dementia and their association with physical activity, activities of daily living and quality of life," *Dementia and Geriatric Cognitive Disorders*, vol. 22, no. 3, pp. 230–237, 2006.

[37] G. E. Berrios, C. Campbell, and B. E. Politynska, "Autonomic failure, depression and anxiety in Parkinson's disease," *British Journal of Psychiatry*, vol. 166, no. 6, pp. 789–792, 1995.

[38] C. O. L. L. E. E. N. A. MCHORNEY, W. JOHNE JR., and R. ANASTASIAE, "The MOS 36-Item Short-Form Health Survey (SF-36): II. Psychometric and clinical tests of validity in measuring physical and mental health constructs," *Medical Care*, vol. 31, no. 3, pp. 247–263, 1993.

[39] A. Fanciulli, S. Strano, C. Colosimo, C. Caltagirone, G. Spalletta, and F. E. Pontieri, "The potential prognostic role of cardiovascular autonomic failure in α-synucleinopathies," *European Journal of Neurology*, vol. 20, no. 2, pp. 231–235, 2013.

[40] H. Oka, M. Morita, K. Onouchi, M. Yoshioka, S. Mochio, and K. Inoue, "Cardiovascular autonomic dysfunction in dementia with Lewy bodies and Parkinson's disease," *Journal of the Neurological Sciences*, vol. 254, no. 1-2, pp. 72–77, 2007.

[41] H. Oka, M. Yoshioka, M. Morita et al., "Reduced cardiac 123I-MIBG uptake reflects cardiac sympathetic dysfunction in Lewy body disease," *Neurology*, vol. 69, no. 14, pp. 1460–1465, 2007.

[42] Y. Horimoto, M. Matsumoto, H. Akatsu et al., "Autonomic dysfunctions in dementia with Lewy bodies," *Journal of Neurology*, vol. 250, no. 5, pp. 530–533, 2003.

[43] P. Thaisetthawatkul, B. F. Boeve, E. E. Benarroch et al., "Autonomic dysfunction in dementia with Lewy bodies," *Neurology*, vol. 62, no. 10, pp. 1804–1809, 2004.

[44] R. Freeman, W. Wieling, F. B. Axelrod et al., "Consensus statement on the definition of orthostatic hypotension, neurally mediated syncope and the postural tachycardia syndrome," *Autonomic Neuroscience*, vol. 161, no. 1-2, pp. 46–48, 2011.

[45] B. P. Boot, "Comprehensive treatment of dementia with Lewy bodies," *Alzheimer's Research & Therapy*, vol. 7, no. 1, p. 45, 2015.

[46] R. Kenny, F. E. Shaw, J. T. O'Brien, P. H. Scheltens, R. Kalaria, and C. Ballard, "Carotid sinus syndrome is common in dementia with Lewy bodies and correlates with deep white matter lesions," *Journal of Neurology, Neurosurgery & Psychiatry*, vol. 75, no. 7, pp. 966–971, 2004.

[47] K. Stubendorff, O. Hansson, L. Minthon, and E. Londos, "Differences in survival between patients with dementia with Lewy bodies and patients with Alzheimer's disease - measured from a fixed cognitive level," *Dementia and Geriatric Cognitive Disorders*, vol. 32, no. 6, pp. 408–416, 2012.

[48] M. Darwish, M. Kirby, E. T. Hellriegel, and P. Robertson Jr, "Armodafinil and modafinil have substantially different pharmacokinetic profiles despite having the same terminal half-lives," *Clinical Drug Investigation*, vol. 29, no. 9, pp. 613–623, 2009.

[49] M. I. Lapid, K. M. Kuntz, S. S. Mason et al., "Efficacy, safety, and tolerability of armodafinil therapy for hypersomnia associated with dementia with Lewy bodies: a pilot study," *Dementia and Geriatric Cognitive Disorders*, vol. 43, no. 5-6, pp. 269–280, 2017.

[50] V. Larsson, K. Engedal, D. Aarsland, C. Wattmo, L. Minthon, and E. Londos, "Quality of life and the effect of memantine in dementia with Lewy bodies and Parkinson's disease dementia," *Dementia and Geriatric Cognitive Disorders*, vol. 32, no. 4, pp. 227–234, 2011.

[51] M. Inskip, Y. Mavros, P. S. Sachdev, and M. A. Fiatarone Singh, "Exercise for individuals with Lewy body dementia: a systematic review," *PLoS One*, vol. 11, no. 6, article e0156520, 2016.

[52] L. Bonanni, A. Cagnin, F. Agosta et al., "The Italian dementia with Lewy bodies study group (DLB-SINdem): toward a standardization of clinical procedures and multicenter cohort studies design," *Neurological Sciences*, vol. 38, no. 1, pp. 83–91, 2017.

19

Association between Body Mass Index and Migraine

Qingqing Huang, Xiping Liang, Shiqiang Wang, and Xiaosong Mu

Chongqing University Cancer Hospital & Chongqing Cancer Institute & Chongqing Cancer Hospital, Chongqing, China

Correspondence should be addressed to Xiping Liang; liangxiping2006@163.com

Academic Editor: Hailiang Tang

Both migraine and obesity are prevalent disorders in the general population, which are characterized by disability and impaired quality of life. Although so many researches had studied the association between migraine and obesity, there are still no full knowledge of the relationship between body mass index (BMI) and migraine, especially chronic migraine (CM). In this study, we analyzed a previous epidemiological survey data of primary headache patients in Chongqing, which surveyed consecutive neurological outpatients through face-to-face interview with physicians using a headache questionnaire. 166 episodic migraine (EM) patients and 134 chronic migraine (CM) patients were included in the study out of 1327 primary headache patients. And 200 healthy adults from the physical examination center were included as a control group. Finally, we found that the patients with migraine (EM and CM) were more likely to be overweight, obese, or morbidly obese compared to those in the healthy group. Significant difference was found between BMI and frequency of migraine attacks but not severity or duration of headache onset. And no significant difference was found in severity and duration of headache onset between episodic and chronic migraine among different BMI classifications. Such may update our knowledge about the clinical features of migraine and BMI, revealing that the frequency of attacks may be associated with being overweight, obese, or morbidly obese in patients with migraine and that the extent of being overweight, obese, or morbidly obese in CM patients was lower than that in EM patients.

1. Introduction

Migraine is one of the most frequent consultation syndromes at headache clinics with various neurological, gastrointestinal, and autonomic changes and has a worldwide prevalence which ranges from 5 to 35% in females and from 3 to 20% in males [1]. Based on the International Classification of Headache Disorders (ICHD-II) guidelines, migraine is classified as EM and CM, with CM defined as having 15 or more headache days per month, in which at least 8 days meet the criteria for migraine and lasting for at least three months [2].

Obesity is comorbid with a number of chronic pain syndromes. The relationship between obesity and migraine has been the focus of clinical research in recent years. Previous studies had revealed that obesity was related with migraine patients with high frequency, greater severity, and some increased associated symptoms: higher disability grades, aura and an increased frequency of photophobia and phonophobia [3–5]. Individuals with episodic headache and obesity developed chronic daily headache (CDH) 5 times more than normal-weight individuals [6]. A cross-sectional population study also confirmed the relationship between obesity and CDH and suggested that obesity was a risk factor for transforming from EM to CM [5]. What is more is that the risk of transforming from EM to CM was increased in patients with obesity [7]. Taken together, obesity is not only associated with severity and frequency of migraine attacks but also associated with the chronicity of migraine. But there is little knowledge of the association between other BMI classifications and migraine, especially CM, and why obesity was more apt to CM.

Therefore, we played a second analysis of a previous data, which predicted that different BMI classifications might be associated with EM and CM. We focused on the following questions: (1) the relationship between different BMI and migraine (EM and CM); (2) separately exploring the

TABLE 1: Demographic characteristics of the samples.

Characteristics	Control		EM		CM		Total sample	
	n	(%)	n	(%)	n	(%)	n	(%)
Gender								
Male	47	23.5	38	22.89	30	22.38	115	23
Female	153	76.5	128	77.11	104	77.61	385	77
Mean age (year) (mean ± SD)	42.81 ± 0.55		40.42 ± 2.38		43.36 ± 2.93			
Range (year)	18–65		18–65		18–65			18–65
Educational level								
Illiterate	17	8.5	14	8.43	10	7.46	41	8.2
Primary school	38	19	32	19.28	26	15.66	96	19.2
Secondary school	45	22.5	43	25.9	33	24.62	121	24.2
High school	53	26.5	47	28.31	37	27.61	137	27.4
College and above	47	23.5	30	18.07	28	20.9	105	21
Marital status								
Unmarried	35	17.5	29	17.46	14	10.45	78/500	15.6
Married	138	69	109	65.67	93	69.4	340	68
Divorced	17	7	18	10.84	19	14.18	54	10.8
Widowed	10	5	10	6.02	8	5.97	28	5.6

relationship of BMI and the frequency, severity, and duration of headache onset and their influence on migraineurs; and (3) the link between BMI and chronicity of migraine.

2. Methods

This is a second analysis of previous large clinic-based study survey data, which was completed in 2011, conducted at the Neurological Outpatient Department of the First Affiliated Hospital of Chongqing Medical University, China. The target population for this analysis are adults aged 18–65. Younger and older people, as well as pregnant women, were excluded because of their changing weight. The study protocol was reviewed and approved by the Ethics Committee of the First Affiliated Hospital of Chongqing Medical University. Patients were informed of the purpose of the study and provided consent prior to participating.

All patients with a chief complaint of headache were included if they fulfilled "EM" and "CM" criteria according to the ICHD-II criteria. "Frequent" headache was defined as occurring on 10–14 days/month. Each participant was given a questionnaire to record the demographic characteristics, clinical features of the headache (frequency, duration, and intensity), and other information. Electroencephalography (EEG), radiography, transcranial Doppler ultrasound (TCD), and computed tomography (CT) of the brain were carried out if necessary in order to exclude second headache or other diseases.

Pain intensity was assessed on the 11-point pain scale (no pain: 0, mild: 1–3, moderate: 4–6, severe: 7–10). Both body height and weight were measured on subjects with light clothing and without shoes. BMI was calculated as the following formula: BMI = weight (kg)/height $(m)^2$. Using WHO guidelines, we defined five categories based on BMI: underweight (<18.5), normal weight (18.5 to 24.9), overweight (25 to 29.9), obese (30 to 34.9), and morbidly obese (35). We combined the data of obese and morbidly obese patients as one group due to the small number of morbidly obese.

3. Statistical Analysis

Analysis was performed using SPSS version 17.0 program. Data were summarized using frequency counts and descriptive statistics. Measurement data variables were expressed as means ± SEM. One-way ANOVA tests and t-tests were used for comparison when appropriate. A value of $P < 0.05$ was considered statistically significant.

4. Results

4.1. Demographic Characteristics of the Sample. During the study period (July 20, 2011 to December 30, 2011), 10,315 consecutive patients visited the neurological outpatient of the First Affiliated Hospital of Chongqing Medical University. 1327 patients (12.9%) cited headache as their chief complaint, 166 of these headache patients were diagnosed as having EM (128 women and 38 men; mean age ± SD: 40.42 ± 2.38 years), and 134 were diagnosed as having CM (104 women and 30 men; mean age ± SD: 43.36 ± 2.93 years). At enrollment, the distribution of demographic variables was shown in Table 1.

4.2. Proportion of BMI Classifications in Migraine. The proportion of BMI classifications in three groups were shown in Table 2. The normal-weight subjects were more common than the other classifications in the three groups (67.5% for control versus 72.3% for EM versus 69.4% for CM), but no significant difference was found between them. And the underweight subjects showed no difference in the three groups ($P > 0.05$). Compared to the healthy group, both

TABLE 2: Proportion and BMI categories.

Body mass index (BMI)	Control		EM		CM		P
	n	(%)	n	(%)	n	(%)	
Underweight (<18.5)	15	7.5	16	9.6	13	9.7	0.9343
Normal weight (18.5–24.9)	135	67.5	120	72.3	93	69.4	0.094
Overweight (25–29.9)	39	19.5	25	15.1	23	17.2	0.0193
Obese/morbidly obese (>30)	11	5.5	5	3	5	3.7	0.0008

TABLE 3: No correlation between the severity of headache and BMI was found in EM.

Weight category	Mild		Moderate		Severe		P
	n	(%)	n	(%)	n	(%)	
Underweight ($n = 16$)	0	0	9	56.2	7	43.8	0.254
Normal ($n = 120$)	2	1.7	55	45.8	63	52.5	0.259
Overweight ($n = 25$)	1	4	9	36	15	60	0.261
Obese/morbidly obese ($n = 5$)	0	0	4	66.7	1	33.3	0.653

TABLE 4: No correlation between the severity of headache and BMI was found in CM.

Weight category	Mild		Moderate		Severe		P
	n	(%)	n	(%)	n	(%)	
Underweight ($n = 13$)	0	0	5	38.5	8	61.5	0.487
Normal ($n = 93$)	3	3.61	43	44.6	50	53.8	0.251
Overweight ($n = 23$)	0	0	12	52.2	11	47.8	0.651
Obese/morbidly obese ($n = 5$)	0	0	2	40	3	60	0.534

TABLE 5: There was no association between the duration of headache attacks and BMI in EM.

Weight category	<4 h		4–72 h		>72 h		P
	n	(%)	n	(%)	n	(%)	
Underweight ($n = 16$)	6	37.5	7	43.8	3	18.8	0.2415
Normal ($n = 120$)	25	20.8	84	70	11	9.2	0.8176
Overweight ($n = 25$)	6	24	14	56	5	20	0.0529
Obese/morbidly obese ($n = 5$)	0	0	3	60	2	40	0.2076

EM and CM patients had a similar trend; they were less likely to be overweight, obese, and morbidly obese; while when compared with that in EM patients, the proportion of overweight, obese, and morbidly obese in CM patients was significantly higher ($P < 0.05$). In other words, CM patients were more likely to be overweight, obese, or morbidly obese than EM patients.

4.3. Pain Intensity and BMI. We further divided all migraineurs into three groups according to pain severity: mild (1–3), moderate (4–6), and severe (7–10). The results showed that the proportion of four different BMI were not significantly different in three pain severity groups neither in EM nor in CM patients ($P > 0.05$) (Tables 3 and 4). So, maybe we can conclude that pain severity had no correlation with BMI and will not influence the BMI level.

4.4. Duration of Headache Onset and BMI. Most migraine patients had gastrointestinal symptoms, such as nausea and vomiting, which would influence their appetite. As a result, we analyzed whether the duration of headache onset had an effect on the BMI level. Migraineurs were well distributed into three groups (<4 h, 4–72 h, and >72 h) according to the duration of headache onset. The data showed that the proportion of four BMI classifications had no difference between different durations of headache onset in the groups ($P > 0.05$). Both in EM and in CM, the duration of headache onset had no effect on the BMI level. The results were shown in Table 5 for EM and Table 6 for CM.

4.5. Frequency and BMI. Our study had revealed that CM patients were more apt to be overweight, obese, or morbidly obese than EM. We further compared the relationship of

TABLE 6: There was no association between the duration of headache attacks and BMI in CM.

Weight category	<4 h n	(%)	4–72 h n	(%)	>72 h n	(%)	P
Underweight ($n = 13$)	4		5		4		0.2415
Normal ($n = 93$)	21		60		12		0.1025
Overweight ($n = 23$)	8		12		3		0.0529
Obese/morbidly obese ($n = 5$)	1		2		2		0.2076

TABLE 7: Frequency headache was significant associated with BMI.

Weight category	<10 days/ months n	(%)	10–14 days/ months n	(%)	P
Underweight ($n = 16$)	16	100	0	0	0
Normal ($n = 120$)	108	90	12	10	<0.0001
Overweight ($n = 25$)	18	72	7	28	0.0006
Obese/morbidly obese ($n = 5$)	3	60	2	40	0.2392

BMI level and frequency of migraine. We first compared the frequency of migraine attacks in episodic migraine. The result was shown in Table 7. There were 12.7% (21/166) EM patients who had 10–14 headache days per month which was defined as frequent migraine. In the EM group, frequent migraine patients had a less proportion in four BMI classifications than low-frequency migraines (<10 days/month). But we also found that with the increase of BMI level, the proportion of frequency migraine began to increase; meanwhile, the low-frequency migraine presented a negative trend. Maybe, it revealed that the frequency of headache had a positive trend with the increase of BMI. In other words, the more the frequency, the heavier the weight.

4.6. Extent of Overweight, Obese, or Morbidly Obese in EM and CM. Finally, we compared four BMI values in the severity and the duration of headache onset and frequency between EM and CM. In the severity and the duration of headache onset, four BMI classifications had showed no significant difference between EM and CM. Whereas, when we compared CM (>15 days/month) with frequent migraine (10–14 days/month, including EM according to ICHD-II), the results showed that CM had a more BMI score in classification of normal weight but less score in overweight and obese/morbidly obese, but only normal weight and overweight had a significance (Table 8, $P < 0.05$).

Considering the result of Table 2, the proportion of overweight, obese, or morbidly obese was significantly lower in migraineurs compared with healthy controls. In migraineurs, CM patients were more apt to be overweight, obese, or morbidly obese than EM patients, but the extent of being overweight, obese, or morbidly obese was lower than EM patients. Further analysis shows that the frequency of attacks of migraine is associated to the higher proportion of being overweight, obese, or morbidly obese in frequent migraineurs.

5. Discussion

The relationship between obese and migraine in general has been studied in clinical research in recent years [8]. The main findings of our study are the following: compared with the healthy control group, both EM and CM patients were less likely to be overweight, obese, or morbidly obese; while compared to the EM group, the proportion of being overweight, obese, or morbidly obese was higher in the CM group.

The relationship between obesity and migraine was still controversial. Previous studies had reported that obesity was comorbid with migraine in the severity and frequency of migraine attacks [4, 8, 9]. Obesity has also been found to be associated with CM but not chronic tension-type headache [5, 10]. The study of Bond et al. further revealed that the decrease in BMI is associated with the reduction of migraine and migraine outcomes [11]. The association between BMI and migraine was still confined. Some studies found no significant relationship between migraine and BMI [12–14]. A Swedish cross-sectional study showed that there was no relation between obesity and the distribution of frequency, intensity, duration, or severity of attacks compared to nonobese women with migraine [3].

In our case series, we found that overweight and obese/morbidly obese patients had a higher likelihood of having CM than EM. Consistent with a previous study, we found no significant connection between BMI and the severity and the duration of headache onset but a connection with the frequency of migraine attacks was found [3, 14]. It is worth noting that frequent migraine attacks turn to be easily overweight than low-frequency migraine attacks (<10 days/months) in EM patients.

To further study the relationship of migraine and BMI, we tested four different weight classifications in two migraine groups. The significance between migraine and BMI was related neither with severity nor with the duration of headache onset, but was related with the frequency of migraine attacks. CM patients were more likely to have a higher BMI score in the classification of normal weight, but less BMI score in overweight classification comparing with EM patients. It revealed that the frequency of migraine attacks may be associated to the higher proportion of overweight, obesity, or morbidly obese in chronic migraineurs, but the increase extent of BMI was lower than EM.

A similar result was shown in the study of Mamontov et al. [10]. These refined our knowledge on the clinical feature of episodic or chronic migraine. Maybe, further investigation is necessary to better understand the reason and the mechanisms.

Several mechanisms supported that there may exist a possible link between BMI and headaches. Concentrations of calcitonin gene-related peptide (CGRP) levels, which are elevated in obese individuals [15], are a very important mediator of migraine/chronic migraine, and CGRP inhibitors are effective in the treatment of migraine. Additionally, inflammation has been proposed as a possible contributing mechanism for migraine attacks and obesity itself is proinflammatory by the increase in the concentrations of circulating cytokines [16–18]. Furthermore, migraines, like obesity,

Table 8: Frequency of headache was significant among different BMI categories between CM and EM.

Weight classification	Severe			Time of headache onset (>72 h)			Frequency (>10 days/months)		
	EM	CM	P	EM	CM	P	FM	CM	P
Underweight	16.71 ± 0.5884	17.14 ± 0.3642	0.3807	17.82 ± 0.1337	17.77 ± 0.1249	0.4315	0	17.16 ± 0.3904	0
Normal	21.34 ± 0.2356	21.58 ± 0.2831	0.5275	21.44 ± 0.5397	22.22 ± 0.4548	0.2296	21.40 ± 0.3313	21.83 ± 0.2063	<0.0001
Overweight	27.52 ± 0.3692	27.16 ± 0.3680	0.5031	26.17 ± 0.6147	26.34 ± 0.5946	0.1057	27.43 ± 0.3776	27.28 ± 0.2644	0.0001
Obese/morbidly obese	34.22 ± 2.919	34.06 ± 2.729	0.9853	31.35 ± 0.2431	30.85 ± 0.7500	0.3991	38.07 ± 4.157	34.38 ± 0.8696	0.1696

have been reported as a risk factor for cardiovascular disorders, as well as for stroke [6, 7, 19]. Finally, migraine prevention medications, which were used in the preventive treatment of migraine, may also be a possible contributing reason for the change of BMI [20, 21].

Our study evaluated the relationship between BMI and CM and the difference between epidemic and chronic migraine among different weight classifications in a clinic-based study. Diagnosis was made by physician interviewers using a questionnaire based on the ICHD-II criteria. All measurements were recorded by interviewers to confirm the right information of body height and weight. However, there are also some limitations that should be addressed here. It was a hospital-based study, and the results may be inappropriate to the general population. Besides, the study sample was limited. Therefore, further studies should be conducted in bigger population in the future.

In conclusion, overweight, obesity, or morbidly obese was associated with the frequency of migraine attacks but not the severity and duration of headache onset. The frequency of headache is connected with BMI changing. The more frequency, the heavier the weight when the headache was not chronic. Once the patient is transforming from EM to CM, the increasing trend of BMI was decreased. But more researches are needed in this field.

Abbreviations

BMI: Body mass index
CM: Chronic migraine
EM: Episodic migraine
ICHD-II: The International Classification of Headache Disorders
FM: Frequency migraine.

Authors' Contributions

Qingqing Huang carried out all processes of the manuscript. Xiping Liang instructed the statistical analysis; Shiqiang Wang and Xiaosong Mu participated in its revision. And thanks to Jiying Zhou, who allowed us to use the data. All authors read and approved the final manuscript. Qingqing Huang is the first author.

Acknowledgments

Appreciation is expressed to the members of the neurological clinic of The First Affiliated Hospital of Chongqing Medical University for their assistance in screening for eligible participants. The authors heartily thank the participants.

References

[1] K. R. Merikangas, "Contributions of epidemiology to our understanding of migraine," *Headache*, vol. 53, no. 2, pp. 230–246, 2013.

[2] Headache Classification Committee of the International Headache Society (IHS), "The International Classification of Headache Disorders, 3rd edition (beta version)," *Cephalalgia*, vol. 33, no. 9, pp. 629–808, 2013.

[3] A. C. Winter, K. Berger, J. E. Buring, and T. Kurth, "Body mass index, migraine, migraine frequency and migraine features in women," *Cephalalgia*, vol. 29, no. 2, pp. 269–278, 2009.

[4] M. E. Bigal, J. N. Liberman, and R. B. Lipton, "Obesity and migraine a population study," *Neurology*, vol. 66, no. 4, pp. 545–550, 2006.

[5] M. E. Bigal and R. B. Lipton, "Obesity is a risk factor for transformed migraine but not chronic tension-type headache," *Neurology*, vol. 67, no. 2, pp. 252–257, 2006.

[6] T. Kurth, J. M. Gaziano, N. R. Cook, G. Logroscino, H. C. Diener, and J. E. Buring, "Migraine and risk of cardiovascular disease in women," *JAMA*, vol. 296, no. 3, pp. 283–291, 2006.

[7] A. Recober and B. Lee Peterlin, "Migraine and obesity: moving beyond BMI," *Future Neurology*, vol. 9, no. 1, pp. 37–40, 2014.

[8] J. Lillis, J. Graham Thomas, E. K. Seng et al., "Importance of pain acceptance in relation to headache disability and pain interference in women with migraine and overweight/obesity," *Headache*, vol. 57, no. 5, pp. 709–718, 2017.

[9] M. E. Bigal, A. Tsang, E. Loder, D. Serrano, M. L. Reed, and R. B. Lipton, "Body mass index and episodic headaches: a population based study," *Archives of Internal Medicine*, vol. 167, no. 18, pp. 1964–1970, 2007.

[10] O. V. Mamontov, L. Babayan, A. V. Amelin, R. Giniatullin, and A. A. Kamshilin, "Autonomous control of cardiovascular reactivity in patients with episodic and chronic forms of migraine," *The Journal of Headache and Pain*, vol. 17, no. 1, p. 52, 2016.

[11] D. S. Bond, K. C. O'Leary, J. Graham Thomas et al., "Can weight loss improve migraine headaches in obese women? Rationale and design of the WHAM randomized controlled trial," *Contemporary Clinical Trials*, vol. 35, no. 1, pp. 133–144, 2013.

[12] S. Yu, R. Liu, X. Yang et al., "Body mass index and migraine: a survey of the Chinese adult population," *The Journal of Headache and Pain*, vol. 13, no. 7, pp. 531–536, 2012.

[13] L. P. Queiroz, M. F. Peres, E. J. Piovesan et al., "A nationwide population-based study of migraine in Brazil," *Cephalalgia*, vol. 29, no. 6, pp. 642–649, 2009.

[14] R. Ornello, P. Ripa, F. Pistoia et al., "Migraine and body mass index categories: a systematic review and meta-analysis of observational studies," *The Journal of Headache and Pain*, vol. 16, no. 1, p. 27, 2015.

[15] Z. Bic, G. G. Blix, H. P. Hopp, and F. M. Leslie, "In search of the ideal treatment for migraine headache," *Medical Hypotheses*, vol. 50, no. 1, pp. 1–7, 1998.

[16] C. Power, S. K. Miller, and P. T. Alpert, "Promising new causal explanations for obesity and obesity-related diseases," *Biological Research for Nursing*, vol. 8, no. 3, pp. 223–233, 2007.

[17] P. Martelletti, G. Stirparo, and M. Giacovazzo, "Proinflammatory cytokines in cervicogenic headache," *Functional Neurology*, vol. 14, no. 3, pp. 159–162, 1999.

[18] X. Liang, S. Wang, G. Qin et al., "Tyrosine phosphorylation of NR2B contributes to chronic migraines via increased expression of CGRP in rats," *BioMed Research International*, vol. 2017, Article ID 7203458, 8 pages, 2017.

[19] V. Mohamed-Ali, J. H. Pinkney, and S. W. Coppack, "Adipose tissue as an endocrine and paracrine organ," *International Journal of Obesity and Related Metabolic Disorders*, vol. 22, no. 12, pp. 1145–1158, 1998.

[20] A. Sachdev and M. J. Marmura, "Metabolic syndrome and migraine," *Frontiers in Neurology*, vol. 3, p. 161, 2012.

[21] W. B. Young and T. D. Rozen, "Preventive treatment of migraine: effect on weight," *Cephalalgia*, vol. 25, no. 1, pp. 1–11, 2005.

20

Sentence Context and Word-Picture Cued-Recall Paired-Associate Learning Procedure Boosts Recall in Normal and Mild Alzheimer's Disease Patients

Rosario Iodice,[1,2] **Juan José García Meilán**,[2,3] **Juan Carro Ramos**,[2,3] **and Jeff A. Small**[4]

[1]*Catholic University of Pereira, Risaralda, Colombia*
[2]*Institute of Neurosciences of Castilla y León, University of Salamanca, Salamanca, Spain*
[3]*Department of Psychology, University of Salamanca, Salamanca, Spain*
[4]*School of Audiology and Speech Sciences, The University of British Columbia, Vancouver, BC, Canada*

Correspondence should be addressed to Rosario Iodice; rosarioiodice@usal.es

Academic Editor: Raffaella Migliaccio

Introduction. The aim of this study was to employ the word-picture paradigm to examine the effectiveness of combined pictorial illustrations and sentences as strong contextual cues. The experiment details the performance of word recall in healthy older adults (HOA) and mild Alzheimer's disease (AD). The researchers enhanced the words' recall with word-picture condition and when the pair was associated with a sentence contextualizing the two items. *Method.* The sample was composed of 18 HOA and 18 people with mild AD. Participants memorized 15 pairs of words under word-word and word-picture conditions, with and without a sentence context. In the paired-associate test, the first item of the pair was read aloud by participants and used to elicit retrieval of the associated item. *Results.* The findings suggest that both HOA and mild-AD pictures improved item recall compared to word condition such as sentences which further enabled item recall. Additionally, the HOA group performs better than the mild-AD group in all conditions. *Conclusions.* Word-picture and sentence context strengthen the encoding in the explicit memory task, both in HOA and mild AD. These results open a potential window to improve the memory for verbalized instructions and restore sequential abilities in everyday life, such as brushing one's teeth, fastening one's pants, or drying one's hands.

1. Introduction

Alzheimer's disease (AD) is a progressive neurodegenerative disorder that includes deterioration across many cognitive domains. The most commonly reported problem in the early stages of AD is progressive memory loss, in particular episodic recent memory impairment that produces serious difficulty to encode and consolidate new information, resulting from medial temporal lobe (MTL) neural degeneration [1].

Despite the loss of episodic memory in the context of MTL degeneration, there is a relative preservation of semantic knowledge in the AD patients [2, 3] which could represent an opportunity to improve episodic memory, because there exists a relation between semantic and episodic memory. A proof of this is paired associated learning (PAL) in which the encoding of a new episodic memory is affected by the degree of association between the two words (semantic memory) [4]. Generally, the verbal PAL task has been used as an instrument for assessing explicit episodic memory performance in healthy older people, with mild cognitive impairment (MCI) and with early AD [5–8]. In this study, we used PAL task in a new way, not as an assessment instrument but like strategic memory control processes to investigate together the strategic component of episodic memory (organization and manipulation of information during encoding, storage, or retrieval) [9] and the types of mediators (pairs of words, the word followed by an image, and sentence-generation strategies) that determine individuals' encoding performance. The mediator is an aid or strategy that is used to link together the items to be remembered [10]. In these terms, the encoding operation constitutes a control process that can promote the increased levels of recall performance [11].

One possible mediator that has shown improvements in memory performance in healthy young [12] and older adults [13] and has promoted the modality congruency effect (this refers to the congruency between the modality of presentation and the modality of recall) is the interactive imagery strategy. Decades of research (over 50 years) have found that pictures are retained in memory better than words are (picture superiority effect). There exists a wide range of cognitive psychology studies that have shown that pictures enhance recollection compared with words in healthy young and older adults [14]. Consistent empirical finding shows that when a word can evoke an image or have a semantic relation with a pictorial representation, verbal and image codes are stored in interconnected symbolic system memory [15, 16]. The effectiveness of a pictorial representation can improve memory for words, because semantic elaboration enhances the pictorial superiority effect [17, 18]. One theory that explains the picture superiority effect proposes that the pictures allow a deeper and more elaborate conceptual processing than solely words do (semantic processing account) [19, 20]. Several authors have found that individuals with amnesic mild cognitive impairment (aMCI) and mild AD can enhance memory by extracting the conceptual meaning from pictures [21] because they enhance conceptual fluency [22, 23]. Furthermore, the picture enhances perceptual fluency and improves the sense of familiarity [24], which in turn improves accuracy and reduces false recognition [25] compared with words.

Despite that, the widespread limitation found in the experimental designs in which the purpose has been to demonstrate the effectiveness of pictorial representation to improve the memory for words in aMCI or mild AD is that the majority of experimental tasks are based on recognition memory [26].

In this work, we want to propose a sentence's linguistic structure combined with pictorial representation, as a possible mediator to improve the process of encoding new items in mild-AD patients and promote explicit memory retrieval for words. We consider that the linguistic structure of a sentence can be thought as an autopoietic system that receives feedback from itself (in terms of linguistic structure) strengthening the unity between the elements (words). The phrase is inserted in a network that allows it to be activated in different ways (lexical, semantic, and visual). The diversification of activation supports the duration of the memory and therefore access to it [27–29]. There is little research that has directly examined the possibility to use sentence as a mediator in mild AD; generally, the sentence has been used to assess the problem in verbal comprehension in mild AD, as we extensively found in literature [30–33]. We consider that it not is the only form to use the linguistic property of the sentence, because it can be converted into an adequate strategy (mediator) that could improve the process of encoding new items in mild-AD patients, because the sentence favors a sufficient semantic richness which allows it to improve the retrieval of the information preview learned [34]. Sentence processing is a natural task, and it can take advantage of sentence cues when processing the meaning, especially when the sentence context primes certain aspects of a target word's meaning. Retrieval of words in the sentences is facilitated when there is a unique cue-target association that reduces the interference and reliable access to the information. Moreover, a sentential context provides a semantic structure for integration of the meaning across the words and allows the formation of a comprehensive mental image [35, 36].

According to these purposes, it is important to take into account that sentence contexts activate both semantic and lexical hierarchical networks in which stimulation of a concept's representation activates other concept nodes associated with the original concept [37, 38], priming the target words included in a phrase [39] and improving the encoding and retrieval of information [40]. Several authors attributed the advantages of sentence context to an activation of automatic processes, especially when a word is thought to prime other semantically related concepts and boost the processing of a target word [41, 42]. Furthermore, the semantic content of a sentence can provide a semantic structure for the integration of meaning across the words and thus allows the formation of a comprehensive mental image [41].

To further enhance encoding, some authors suggest combining verbal and pictorial stimuli to activate a presemantic level of information that interacts with the episodic and semantic systems. Paivio et al. [43] have shown that the ability to generate interactive visual images facilitates verbal PAL performance, independently from the effect of stimulus relatedness. That is, the interconnectivity of words and images facilitates access to a common conceptual memory storage area [18, 44]. Cherry et al. [45] carried out a study with younger and older adults, where the encoding stimuli consisted of sets of 16 sentences with pictorial illustrations (e.g., The dusty man held the rope), and the retrieval stimuli consisted of "what" question sentences (e.g., "What did the dusty man do?"). They found that the combination of verbal and visual supports allowed retrieval of the main point of the sentences and improved recall performance.

Although these strategies are based on known cognitive paradigms and have a long path of experimentation when they are combined with pictorial and verbal material, the greatest limitation found in previous research is that mild AD is able to extract only the gist from pictorial information, but they can remember the information in verbatim form. The mnemonic strategy is not easy to learn because they are often complex and have a high level of artificiality that generates difficulties using them in daily life. Furthermore, when the therapists interact with mild-AD patients, they found serious difficulties to promote the memorization of complex information such as sentences; generally, the mnemonic method is limited to a simple and short piece of information (face nouns, date, and single words) (see [46] for limitations of mnemonics in clinical applications). In this work, we propose the use of the combinations of two known strategies according to which the sentence context enriched by pictorial illustration represents a form of environmental support where the activation of a sentential semantic network more robustly connects to a visual representation [14, 15, 39, 47]. We consider it important to investigate the relationship between semantic/conceptual (sentences) and visual perception conditions (pictures) during both encoding and retrieval in mild-AD patients, because understanding this relationship would generate new reflections and suggest new forms to use and combine mnemonic strategies that favor the codification of new information.

Taking into account that it is possible to use sentences as contextual cue combined with pictorial representation, we consider that it is also possible in mild AD, because the older adults have a greater experience with sentence processing during their lives because they reprocess the verbal information every day, and they depend more heavily on a set of rich sentential context cues for recalling the information [47]. However, this may have several implications in a clinical context: on the one hand, the linguistic structure of sentences makes mnemonic techniques more natural and familiar, allowing easy use of them in everyday life and promoting the retrieval in explicit memory task.

Despite advances in our understanding of the effects of sentence context as contextual cue, there is little research and timid attempts that have directly examined the importance of the relationship between semantic/conceptual and visual perception conditions during both encoding and retrieval of items embedded in short sentences for healthy older adults (HOA) and persons with mild AD. Understanding these mechanisms would open up new directions for cognitive interventions in older adults with cognitive impairment. Therefore, the specific aim of this work, based on the theoretical models and empirical research described above, was to assess the effectiveness of encoding sentence context as a strong contextual cue (cue-target association) and different types of stimuli in HOA and persons with mild AD. In this study, we used the word-word (WW) and word-picture (WP) conditions as target items [15], comparing the encoding and retrieval of the target item (second item of the pair) in the presence or absence of a sentence contextual cue. Our first hypothesis was that the WP condition would yield a higher recall rate of second pair items compared to the WW condition. Our second hypothesis was that sentence context would improve the recall of the second pair items, in both WW and WP conditions relative to the null sentence context condition. Our third prediction was that the first and second hypotheses would be confirmed for both HOA and mild-AD participants.

2. Method

2.1. Participants. Thirty-six elderly Spanish people were included in the study, forming two groups. The first group was made up of 18 patients at the State Reference Center for people with Alzheimer's disease of Spain (Salamanca). As inclusion criteria, participants had been previously diagnosed with AD (not mixed dementia) for the Spanish National Health System following the criteria of NINCDS-ADRDA [48] and whose diagnosis as AD was later confirmed according to GDS stages 2 and 3 by the center's medical and neurological service (very mild–mild cognitive decline) [49]. The mean age was 83.9 years (SD = 13.573; range 65–90), with a Mini Mental State Examination (MMSE) mean of 20.3, (SD = 2.20; range 18–24) [50]. The families of these patients provided informed consent for their participation in the study. In accordance with the Ethics Committee at the center, a form was sent out to the patients' immediate family or guardian for them to sign and return. The second group was made up of 18 people living in nursing homes who did not have a neurodegenerative pathology and who were classified as cognitively healthy older adults by a physician at the home. The mean age of the group was 80.1 (SD = 7.415; range 63–91) with a MMSE mean of 27.3 (SD = 2.024; range 24–30) [50]. The healthy older adults provided informed consent to participate in the study. We found significant differences between the two experimental groups in terms of their scores on the MMSE, $t\,(32) = 6.2$, $p < .001$ [5]. We confirmed that there were no significant differences between the two groups in terms of educational level, years of schooling, age, or gender distribution (see Table 1). The study excluded those participants with any depressive symptoms, measured by the Beck Depression Inventory (value > 10) [51], as well as those participants with medical backgrounds involving problems in their communication system (auditory or visual) or in their ability to read.

Table 1: Demographic data.

	Groups			
	18 Mild AD		18 healthy older adults	
	Means	SD	Means	SD
Years of education	7.1	3.10	7.0	2.80
Age	83.94	2.62	80.12	1.46
MMSE	20.30	4.10	27.30	2.10
Men	22%		17%	
Women	78%		83%	

MMSE: Mini Mental State Examination.

2.2. Materials. We employed a database of 60 pairs of Spanish words from which we randomly created 4 lists of 15 pairs (e.g., owl-woods, umbrella-winter). We selected and matched all pairs of stimuli based on the factors' "frequency of use" and "proportion" from the normative study by Fernandez et al. [52]. Each list of stimuli contained one of the following four combinations: WW and WP each embedded in a sentence context and WW and WP each not embedded in a sentence context. The pictures for the WP condition were obtained by associating the words with corresponding Snodgrass drawings [53]. The presentation order of these stimuli was counterbalanced across the Paired Associate Learning (PAL) form and, in the embedded context condition, was embedded in a short sentence (sentence context cue), favoring the encoding and retrieval of the second (right) item of the pair. All stimuli were presented using the experimental program E-Prime® V1.1, presented on a 15″ screen with a resolution of 1024 × 768, and placed at a distance of 48″ from participants. The words were displayed in black against a white background, and the images were 3 cm in size (width 45% × height 45% in E-Prime) in the form of line drawings (see Figure 1).

OWL-

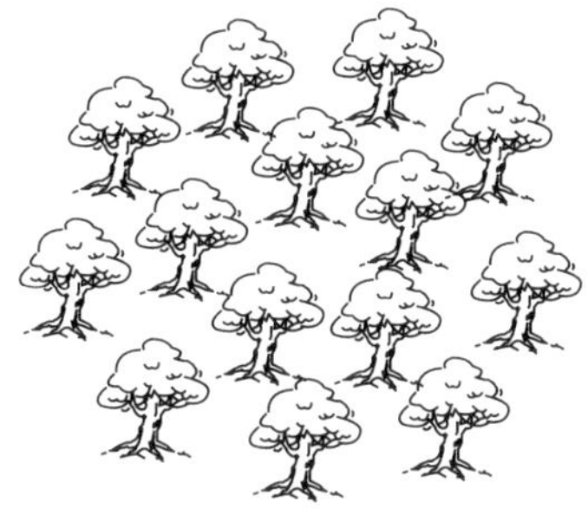

FIGURE 1: Word-picture pair (*owl-woods*) embedded in sentence context *"The owl lives in the woods."*

2.3. Procedure. Each participant was tested individually and completed four 30-minute sessions, each one corresponding to one of the four list types. The order of conditions was counterbalanced across participants, and sessions were held one week apart. The individual sessions were divided into two phases, a study phase and a retrieval phase. In the study phase, 15 pairs of stimuli were presented one at a time on the computer screen for ten seconds. In the null sentence context condition, the stimuli were presented in a PAL task as two words (WW) or as a word followed by picture (WP), and the participants only read the words and named the pictures aloud. In the embedded sentence context condition, the stimuli were again presented in a PAL task (WW or WP), but, in addition, the experimenter read a corresponding sentence (e.g., after presenting the "owl-woods" pair, the experimenter read the embedded sentence: "The *owl* lives in the *woods*"; see Figure 1). In between trials, a fixation point was displayed in the center of the screen for 1 second. After the study phase (approximately 150 seconds), the participants were informed, through instructions presented on the computer screen, that the learning task had been completed and that the retrieval task was to begin immediately. During the retrieval task, the first item in the pair was presented on the screen, and the participants were asked to recall the associated second items. The participant was instructed to say "I do not remember" when he/she thought he/she was not able to recover the information. In these circumstances, the omission of the information was considered as absence of an error instead of a fault; the experimenter provided a phonological cue according to the method of "errorless learning" [54], to corroborate the presence or absence of the encoding process. For example, with the pair "umbrella (word)-winter (image)," to facilitate the recovery of the second element of the pair according to the technique of errorless learning, a phonological cue constituted by the first significant syllables of the word was provided orally, in this case "win-" (for the word winter). With this cue, the participant was invited to complete the word. If the experimenter realized that there was no clarity from the participant about the type of sounds pronounced, the letters were written on a sheet, showed to the person, and pronounced aloud again. The stimulus presentation in the recall phase was not subject to a time limit [15]. The time elapsed in this phase was managed through the recovery process described previously (inviting the participant to remember the associated pair in order to provide a phonetic cue in the absence of the memory and to finalize the recovery phase if the participant had given a correct or incorrect response). The retrieval process took no more than 5 minutes. One point was assigned for each correct retrieval, 0.5 for each retrieval by means of a phonetic cue using "errorless learning" (e.g., "wo" for "woods"), and 0 for each incorrect retrieval or persistent omission of the information. The persistent omission was considered as an omission after it provided four times the phonetic cue [55].

2.3.1. Statistical Analysis. A $2 \times 2 \times 2$ repeated-measures mixed-design analysis of variance model was performed with two within-subject variables: encoding type (WW and WP) and the presence or absence of sentence context (Presence and Absence), and one between-subject variable: participant group (mild-AD and healthy older adults). The dependent variable was the recall accuracy of the second item of each learning pair. The significance level was set at $p < 0.05$. Descriptive data for recall is shown in Table 2.

3. Results

A significant effect of the group factor was also observed, $F(1, 34) = 28.645$, $p < .001$, eta $= .46$, indicating that, as expected, the HOA had 24% greater recall success overall (mean = 12,035) than the mild-AD group had (mean = 8389, $p < .001$). Of the two manipulated variables, we found that there was a significant main effect in the type of encoding, $F(1, 34) = 158.43$, $p < .001$, eta $= .82$). We confirmed the superiority rate recall of WP (mean = 11,528) compared to WW as a contextual cue (mean = 8896, $p < .001$). In this case, we found a significant interaction effect between the type of encoding and group, $F(1, 34) = 6.539$, $p < .05$, eta $= .16$. Pairwise comparisons of the interaction confirmed that there were significant differences between the HOA (mean = 10.87) and mild-AD groups (mean = 6.81; $p < 0.01$) in the WW condition ($p < .001$, eta $= .51$) and in the WP condition (mean = 13.10 for HOA and mean = 9.97 for mild AD; $p < .001$, eta $= .35$) (see Figure 2). We also found differences between WW and WP conditions in both HOA (mean differences = 2097; $p < 0.01$, eta $= .60$) and mild AD (mean differences = 3167; $p < 0.01$, eta $= .77$). There was also a significant main effect of sentence context ($F(1, 34) = 66.768$, $p < .001$, eta $= .66$), in which recall was better when the items were embedded in sentences (mean = 11,556) compared to the null sentence context condition (mean = 8868, $p < .001$). There were no interactions between the use of sentences and the groups, the use of WP and sentences, and the use of WP, sentences, and groups.

4. Discussion

The purpose of this study was to investigate the mechanisms to improve encoding of words in the explicit memory task under WW versus WP, and sentence context versus null sentence conditions, in both HOA and persons with mild AD. The WP and sentence context improved retrieval performance in both groups. The word associated with an image (WP) improves the recall rates (17.54%) with respect to

Table 2: Recall rates of the second element of the pair with and without sentence context.

Variables	18 mild AD: Without sentence Means	SD	18 mild AD: With sentence Means	SD	18 healthy older adults: Without sentence Means	SD	18 healthy older adults: With sentence Means	SD	Means: Means	SD
Word/word	5.50	2.56	8.11*	2.85	9.30	2.39	12.66*	1.63	8.89	2.35
Word/picture	8.94*	2.61	11.00*	3.19	11.72*	2.49	14.44*	1.09	11.52	2.34
Means	7.22	2.58	9.55	3.02	10.51	2.44	13.55	1.36		

ANOVA $2 \times 2 \times 2$ was performed; variables encoding type word-word, word-picture, and the presence or absence of sentence context. *The significance level was set at $p < .05$. A significant main effect in word-picture compared with word-word, and in sentences compared to the null sentence context condition, in both groups was found.

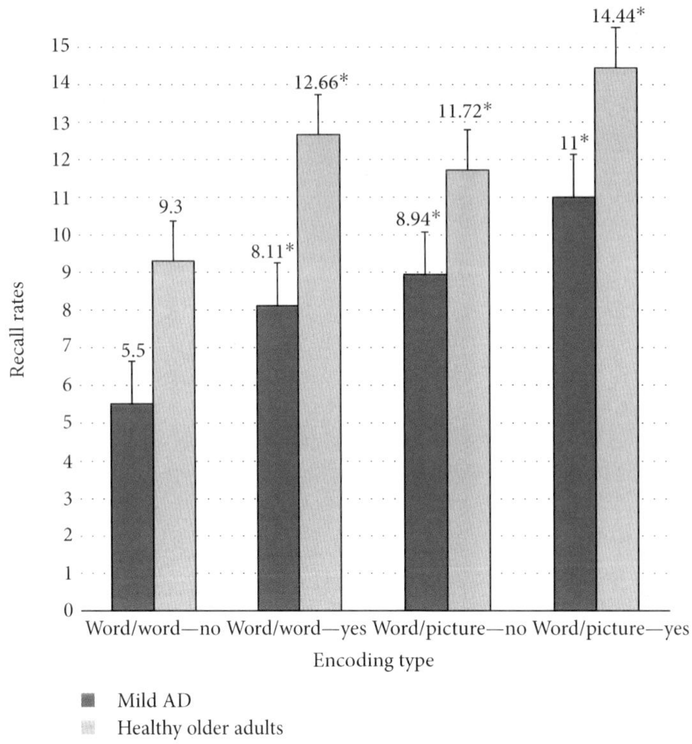

Figure 2: Recall rates of the second element of the pair with (yes) and without (no) sentence context, in healthy older adults and mild AD. ANOVA $2 \times 2 \times 2$ was performed. *The significance level was set at $p < .05$. A significant main effect in word-picture compared with word-word, and in sentences compared to the null sentence context condition, in both groups was found.

WW, with more effectiveness in people with mild AD than in HOA. Similarly, the sentence context condition improves the recall rates (17.91%) compared to the null sentence condition. We found a significant interaction effect between the type of encoding and group. This result can be in agreement with previous studies which show that the magnitude of the picture superiority effect is greater in patients than in HOA [26]. The improvement in recall rates is similar in both coding conditions. Nevertheless, the results do not show an interaction between the variables. Both types of intervention seem to act independently and therefore can be used as a way to improve memory in the elderly. There are several possible reasons for why such an interaction did not emerge. One possibility is that there was such a strong benefit of each cue by itself that any further gains by combining cues were minimal. Another reason could be related to the extra task demands associated with processing stimuli from multiple modalities (word and image) in conjunction with sentential semantic processing. Previous research has shown that processing stimuli under more complex cue conditions can actually create extra attentional demands, leading to declines in performance [56]. Despite the lack of interaction between WP and sentence context, the strong independent effects of each suggest possible intervention approaches capitalizing on the strengths of each cue type, as described below. To understand this possible application in clinical context, we take into account that there is extensive literature which highlights the difficulty of implementing mnemonic strategies for older people, especially for people with mild AD [57, 58]. One of the main criticisms about mnemonic strategies is that they are difficult to learn because they are often complex and have a high level of artificiality that generates difficulties using them in daily life. Our results indicate that, despite the memory deficit based on MTL neural degeneration that causes deficit both in episodic and in semantic memory, the HOA and mild-AD persons are able to extract the gist from pictorial information and learn with less interference because they focus on the conceptual aspect [59, 60]. The HOA individuals process the information with more amplitude as well as depth. The mild-AD persons showed that they were able to benefit from the way material was encoded at acquisition, generating a cued assistance, and that it is related to assistance provided at retrieval, enhancing recall. The results obtained in this study, although they refer to a specific section of a much wider problem (memory problem in the AD), are consistent with cross-sectional studies, where it is reported that the episodic memory impairment of mild-AD patients is characterized by encoding deficit and low retrieval performance compared to HOA [40]. At the same time, the results also show that despite the fact that mild-AD persons were unable to encode and process all the semantic properties, all participants in the present study were able to extract the gist from pictorial information and they were able to learn with less interference because they focus on the conceptual aspect of information. The results of the present study extend past research, in which it was demonstrated that mild-AD persons receive cue benefits when they are provided with instructions to encode the "to be remembered" (TBR). While in this work the patients were able to utilize cues without instructions to encode, they simply received a particular information structure (image and sentence) that generates deep encoding and provides support at retrieval [15, 61].

The results also show that sentences not only serve to assess the problem in verbal comprehension in AD patients [30–33, 62]. The sentences can be used as contextual cue, because the syntactic properties of the sentence (subject, verb, complement (SVC)) create an organized structure where the words are stringed into chunks that improve their recall performance. Several studies have shown that mild-AD patients remained structurally rich with similar syntactic structure as the HOA controls, and mild-AD patients are not impaired to determine aspects of sentence meaning, despite working memory deficits. This means that they can perform relatively normally on some semantic tasks when they are not required to search for, or intentionally manipulate, semantic information [63, 64]. The sentences can be thought as a linguistic structure that strengthens the unity between the elements (words). The simultaneous engagement of the images and words produces an overlap of codes allowing the access to a common conceptual memory storage area [41]. According to some authors, this is because the information has been drawn to a presemantic level and has interacted with episodic and semantic systems [65]. The results from the present study therefore suggest that mnemonic training, based on the WP and sentence context processing, may enhance encoding and recall by persons with mild AD. Moreover, because the WP paradigm targets lexical level processing, it would perhaps be most useful in addressing semantic memory "access" problems in mild-AD persons, whereas the deeper encoding primed by a sentence context may help persons with mild AD encode and recall a higher level of propositional information. Future research is needed to address these possibilities and to explore how mnemonics based on WP and sentence context can be effectively implemented in real-world contexts.

This study indicates that older individuals, with and without dementia, are sensitive to the semantic constraints provided by a sentence context or picture. Thus, it appears that syntactic properties of the sentence can facilitate the abilities of HOA and those with mild AD to carry out operations such as those involved in retrieval of target information [66]. There is data which indicates that patients with mild AD retain their knowledge of semantic features, but they have difficulty voluntarily accessing it because the information is disorganized [67]. The results of the present study suggest that, first of all, these individuals' performance is improved in encoding because the sentence context and picture generate sets of feature restrictions that serve to organize and integrate the words and allow the formation of a comprehensive mental image [15]. Secondly, the sentence and visual representation of the target words creates a context in which there is an accumulation of presemantic activations. This condition enables the person to better process higher-level representations of the meaning of a sentence and a picture, including relevant attributes that are necessary for promoting a deeper encoding of information [68]. Thirdly, reading a sentence requires deeper processing of its constituent words than does reading a pair of nouns [69]. Thus, our two interventions establish a meaningful relationship among its constituent words, thereby reducing the arbitrariness of a pairwise association. The sentence context can be thought of as a mnemonic strategy, whereby the whole promotes greater depth of encoding than the sum of the parts [14].

As a consequence of the discussion and conclusion of this study, we propose a speculative question: if it is possible to increase memory for words when they are embedded in sentence context, can the same pair of target words activate a semantic network that allows to retrieve a sentence in verbatim form? It helps patients to improve memory for sentences in verbatim form, providing a potential window for nonpharmacological therapies. The sentences can be thought as an autopoietic structure. In other words, as it is possible to improve the memorization of words through a sentence by using syntactic and semantic structures which activate semantic networks, in the same way, a pair of words which would have a certain semantic relationship could activate the same networks in order to favor the integral recovery of the sentence. The phrase is inserted in a network that allows it to be activated in different ways (lexical, semantic, and visual). The diversification of activation supports the duration of the memory and therefore access to explicit memory [27–29]. This potential projection represents a premise for future research where it will be studied how to improve the memory for verbalized instructions formulated by simple sentences and when it is needed to restore sequential abilities in everyday life, such as brushing teeth, fastening the pants waist, and drying hands [70].

Authors' Contributions

Rosario Iodice conceived and designed the study, collected the data, and wrote the paper. Juan José Garcia Meilán conceived and designed the study, supervised the data collection, and wrote the paper. Juan Avelino Carro Ramos conducted the statistical analysis. Jeff Small supervised the design and wrote the paper.

Acknowledgments

This work was supported by the Spanish Ministry of Science and Innovation (MICINN, no. BFU2010-17754). The authors acknowledge the contract for research collaboration between the Institute of Neurosciences of Castilla y León, University of Salamanca, Salamanca, Spain, and the National Reference Centre of Alzheimer Disease (CRE Alzheimer, IMSERSO, Salamanca, Government of Spain).

References

[1] E. Tsantali, D. Economidis, and M. Tsolaki, "Could language deficits really differentiate Mild Cognitive Impairment (MCI) from mild Alzheimer's disease?," *Archives of Gerontology and Geriatrics*, vol. 57, no. 3, pp. 263–270, 2013.

[2] M. Irish and O. Piguet, "The pivotal role of semantic memory in remembering the past and imagining the future," *Frontiers in Behavioral Neuroscience*, vol. 7, 2013.

[3] L. J. Tippett, S. McAuliffe, and M. J. Farah, "Preservation of categorical knowledge in Alzheimer's disease: a computational account," *Memory*, vol. 3, no. 3-4, pp. 519–533, 1995.

[4] E. Tulving, "Episodic and semantic memory," in *Organization of memory*, pp. 381–403, New York, Academic Press, 1972.

[5] G. J. Lowndes, M. M. Saling, D. Ames, E. Chiu, L. M. Gonzalez, and G. R. Savage, "Recall and recognition of verbal paired associates in early Alzheimer's disease," *Journal of the International Neuropsychological Society*, vol. 14, no. 4, pp. 591–600, 2008.

[6] J. M. Duchek, M. Cheney, F. R. Ferraro, and M. Storandt, "Paired associate learning in senile dementia of the Alzheimer type," *Archives of Neurology*, vol. 48, no. 10, pp. 1038–1040, 1991.

[7] P. E. J. Spaan, "Episodic and semantic memory impairments in (very) early Alzheimer's disease: the diagnostic accuracy of paired-associate learning formats," *Cogent Psychology*, vol. 3, no. 1, 2016.

[8] R. E. Curiel, E. Crocco, M. Rosado et al., "A brief computerized paired associate test for the detection of mild cognitive impairment in community-dwelling older adults," *Journal of Alzheimer's Disease*, vol. 54, no. 2, pp. 793–799, 2016.

[9] Y. L. Shing, M. Werkle-Bergner, S.-C. Li, and U. Lindenberger, "Associative and strategic components of episodic memory: a life-span dissociation," *Journal of Experimental Psychology: General*, vol. 137, no. 3, pp. 495–513, 2008.

[10] J. T. E. Richardson, "The availability and effectiveness of reported mediators in associative learning: a historical review and an experimental investigation," *Psychonomic Bulletin & Review*, vol. 5, no. 4, pp. 597–614, 1998.

[11] B. B. Murdock, "Context and mediators in a theory of distributed associative memory (TODAM2)," *Psychological Review*, vol. 104, no. 4, pp. 839–862, 1997.

[12] J. T. E. Richardson, *Mental Imagery and Human Memory*, Macmillan Education UK, London, 1980.

[13] P. Verhaeghen, A. Marcoen, and L. Goossens, "Facts and fiction about memory aging: a quantitative integration of research findings," *Journal of Gerontology*, vol. 48, no. 4, pp. P157–P171, 1993.

[14] T. Curran and J. Doyle, "Picture superiority doubly dissociates the ERP correlates of recollection and familiarity," *Journal of Cognitive Neuroscience*, vol. 23, no. 5, pp. 1247–1262, 2011.

[15] R. Iodice, J. J. G. Meilán, and J. Carro, "Improvement of encoding and retrieval in normal and pathological aging with word-picture paradigm," *Aging & Mental Health*, vol. 19, no. 10, pp. 940–946, 2014.

[16] A. Paivio, *Mind and Its Evolution: A Dual Coding Theoretical Approach*, Psychology Press, New York, 2014.

[17] K. E. Cherry, J. Silva Brown, E. Jackson Walker et al., "Semantic encoding enhances the pictorial superiority effect in the oldest-old," *Aging, Neuropsychology, and Cognition*, vol. 19, no. 1-2, pp. 319–337, 2012.

[18] J. A. Small and N. Sandhu, "Episodic and semantic memory influences on picture naming in Alzheimer's disease," *Brain and Language*, vol. 104, no. 1, pp. 1–9, 2008.

[19] M. S. Weldon and H. L. Roediger, "Altering retrieval demands reverses the picture superiority effect," *Memory & Cognition*, vol. 15, no. 4, pp. 269–280, 1987.

[20] M. S. Weldon, H. L. Roediger, and B. H. Challis, "The properties of retrieval cues constrain the picture superiority effect," *Memory & Cognition*, vol. 17, no. 1, pp. 95–105, 1989.

[21] R. G. Deason, E. P. Hussey, S. Flannery, and B. A. Ally, "Preserved conceptual implicit memory for pictures in patients with Alzheimer's disease," *Brain and Cognition*, vol. 99, pp. 112–117, 2015.

[22] A. P. Yonelinas, "The nature of recollection and familiarity: a review of 30 years of research," *Journal of Memory & Language*, vol. 46, no. 3, pp. 441–517, 2002.

[23] C. A. R. Martins and T. J. Lloyd-Jones, "Preserved conceptual priming in Alzheimer's disease," *Cortex*, vol. 42, no. 7, pp. 995–1004, 2006.

[24] C. E. Westerberg, K. A. Paller, S. Weintraub et al., "When memory does not fail: familiarity-based recognition in mild cognitive impairment and Alzheimer's disease," *Neuropsychology*, vol. 20, no. 2, pp. 193–205, 2006.

[25] A. E. Budson, D. A. Wolk, H. Chong, and J. D. Waring, "Episodic memory in Alzheimer's disease: separating response bias from discrimination," *Neuropsychologia*, vol. 44, no. 12, pp. 2222–2232, 2006.

[26] B. A. Ally, "Using pictures and words to understand recognition memory deterioration in amnestic mild cognitive impairment and Alzheimer's disease: a review," *Current Neurology and Neuroscience Reports*, vol. 12, no. 6, pp. 687–694, 2012.

[27] R. K. Moore, "Introducing a pictographic language for envisioning a rich variety of enactive systems with different degrees

of complexity," *International Journal of Advanced Robotic Systems*, vol. 13, no. 2, p. 74, 2017.

[28] A. Kravchenko, *Biology of cognition and linguistic analysis*, Peter Lang, Frankfurt, 2008.

[29] W. Teubert, "Writing, hermeneutics, and corpus linguistics," *Revista Signos*, vol. 40, no. 64, pp. 431–453, 2007.

[30] M. Radanovic and L. Mansur, *Language Disturbances in Adulthood: New Advances from the Neurolinguistics Perspective Language Disturbances in Adulthood*, Bentham Science Publishers Ltd., Sao Paulo, Brazil, 2012.

[31] R. López-Higes, P. Montejo, J. M. Prados, M. Montenegro, and M. Lozano, "¿Hay un déficit de comprensión gramatical multidominio en el Deterioro Cognitivo Leve?," *Universitas Psychologica*, vol. 13, no. 4, 2015.

[32] L. L. Mansur, "Language alterations in alzheimer's disease and other dementias," in *Language Disturbances in Adulthood: New Advances from the Neurolinguistics Perspective*, L. L. Mansur, Ed., pp. 59–70, Bentham Science Publishers, 2011.

[33] J. Marková, L. Horváthová, M. Králová, and Z. Cséfalvay, "Sentence comprehension in Slovak-speaking patients with Alzheimer's disease," *International Journal of Language & Communication Disorders*, vol. 52, no. 4, pp. 456–468, 2017.

[34] M. Sarazin, C. Berr, J. De Rotrou et al., "Amnestic syndrome of the medial temporal type identifies prodromal AD: a longitudinal study," *Neurology*, vol. 69, no. 19, pp. 1859–1867, 2007.

[35] A. Prior and S. Bentin, "Incidental formation of episodic associations: the importance of sentential context," *Memory & Cognition*, vol. 31, no. 2, pp. 306–316, 2003.

[36] A. Prior and S. Bentin, "Word associations are formed incidentally during sentential semantic integration," *Acta Psychologica*, vol. 127, no. 1, pp. 57–71, 2008.

[37] E. M. Arroyo-Anlló, M. Beauchamps, P. Ingrand, J. P. Neau, and R. Gil, "Lexical priming in Alzheimer's disease and aphasia," *European Neurology*, vol. 69, no. 6, pp. 360–365, 2013.

[38] K. Segaert, G. Kempen, K. M. Petersson, and P. Hagoort, "Syntactic priming and the lexical boost effect during sentence production and sentence comprehension: an fMRI study," *Brain and Language*, vol. 124, no. 2, pp. 174–183, 2013.

[39] R. Zeelenberg, D. Pecher, R. M. Shiffrin, and J. G. W. Raaijmakers, "Semantic context effects and priming in word association," *Psychonomic Bulletin & Review*, vol. 10, no. 3, pp. 653–660, 2003.

[40] F. Clément, S. Belleville, and S. Mellah, "Functional neuroanatomy of the encoding and retrieval processes of verbal episodic memory in MCI," *Cortex*, vol. 46, no. 8, pp. 1005–1015, 2010.

[41] R. D. Nebes, D. C. Martin, and L. C. Horn, "Sparing of semantic memory in Alzheimer's disease," *Journal of Abnormal Psychology*, vol. 93, no. 3, pp. 321–330, 1984.

[42] R. D. Nebes and C. B. Brady, "The effect of contextual constraint on semantic judgments by Alzheimer patients," *Cortex*, vol. 27, no. 2, pp. 237–246, 1991.

[43] A. Paivio, M. Khan, and I. Begg, "Concreteness and relational effects on recall of adjective-noun pairs," *Canadian Journal of Experimental Psychology/Revue canadienne de psychologie expérimentale*, vol. 54, no. 3, pp. 149–160, 2000.

[44] V. A. Kazmerski and D. Friedman, "Old/new differences in direct and indirect memory tests using pictures and words in within- and cross-form conditions: event-related potential and behavioral measures," *Cognitive Brain Research*, vol. 5, no. 4, pp. 255–272, 1997.

[45] K. E. Cherry, D. K. Dokey, C. M. Reese, and S. Brigman, "Pictorial illustrations enhance memory for sentences in younger and older adults," *Experimental Aging Research*, vol. 29, no. 3, pp. 353–370, 2003.

[46] B. A. Wilson, *Memory Rehabilitation: Integrating Theory and Practice*, The Guilford Press, New York, 2009.

[47] L. E. Matzen and A. S. Benjamin, "Older and wiser: older adults' episodic word memory benefits from sentence study contexts," *Psychology and Aging*, vol. 28, no. 3, pp. 754–767, 2013.

[48] G. McKhann, D. Drachman, M. Folstein, R. Katzman, D. Price, and E. M. Stadlan, "Clinical diagnosis of Alzheimer's disease: report of the NINCDS-ADRDA Work Group under the auspices of Department of Health and Human Services Task Force on Alzheimer's Disease," *Neurology*, vol. 34, no. 7, pp. 939–944, 1984.

[49] B. Reisberg, S. H. Ferris, M. J. de Leon, and T. Crook, "The Global Deterioration Scale for assessment of primary degenerative dementia," *American Journal of Psychiatry*, vol. 139, no. 9, pp. 1136–1139, 1982.

[50] M. F. Folstein, S. E. Folstein, and P. R. McHugh, "Mini-mental state: a practical method for grading the cognitive state of patients for the clinician," *Journal of Psychiatric Research*, vol. 12, no. 3, pp. 189–198, 1975.

[51] A. T. Beck, R. A. Steer, and G. K. Brown, "BDI-II. Beck Depression Inventory-II," The Psychological Corporation, San Antonio, TX, 1996.

[52] A. Fernandez, E. Diez, M. A. Alonso, and M. S. Beato, "Free-association norms for the Spanish names of the Snodgrass and Vanderwart pictures," *Behavior Research Methods, Instruments, & Computers*, vol. 36, no. 3, pp. 577–583, 2004.

[53] J. G. Snodgrass and M. Vanderwart, "A standardized set of 260 pictures: norms for name agreement, image agreement, familiarity, and visual complexity," *Journal of Experimental Psychology: Human Learning and Memory*, vol. 6, no. 2, pp. 174–215, 1980.

[54] T. Hopper, M. Bourgeois, J. Pimentel et al., "An evidence-based systematic review on cognitive interventions for individuals with dementia," *American Journal of Speech-Language Pathology*, vol. 22, no. 1, pp. 126–145, 2013.

[55] A. Baddeley and B. A. Wilson, "When implicit learning fails: amnesia and the problem of error elimination," *Neuropsychologia*, vol. 32, no. 1, pp. 53–68, 1994.

[56] C. Jacquemot, E. Dupoux, O. Decouche, and A.-C. Bachoud-Levi, "Misperception in sentences but not in words: speech perception and the phonological buffer," *Cognitive Neuropsychology*, vol. 23, no. 6, pp. 949–971, 2006.

[57] J. O. Brooks, L. Friedman, and J. A. Yesavage, "A study of the problems older adults encounter when using a mnemonic technique," *International Psychogeriatrics*, vol. 5, no. 1, pp. 57–65, 1999.

[58] A. L. Gross, J. Brandt, K. Bandeen-Roche et al., "Do older adults use the method of loci? Results from the ACTIVE study," *Experimental Aging Research*, vol. 40, no. 2, pp. 140–163, 2014.

[59] D. Bunce, "Cognitive support at encoding attenuates age differences in recollective experience among adults of lower frontal lobe function," *Neuropsychology*, vol. 17, no. 3, pp. 353–361, 2003.

[60] J. R. Quamme, A. P. Yonelinas, K. F. Widaman, N. E. A. Kroll, and M. J. Sauvé, "Recall and recognition in mild

hypoxia: using covariance structural modeling to test competing theories of explicit memory," *Neuropsychologia*, vol. 42, no. 5, pp. 672–691, 2004.

[61] F. I. M. Craik and R. S. Lockhart, "Levels of processing: a framework for memory research," *Journal of Verbal Learning and Verbal Behavior*, vol. 11, no. 6, pp. 671–684, 1972.

[62] R. López-Higes, J. M. Prados, S. Rubio, P. Montejo, and D. Del Río, "Executive functions and linguistic performance in SCD older adults and healthy controls," *Aging, Neuropsychology, and Cognition*, vol. 24, no. 6, pp. 717–734, 2016.

[63] Y.-h. Lai, H.-h. Pai, and Y.-t. Lin, "To be semantically-impaired or to be syntactically-impaired: Linguistic patterns in Chinese-speaking persons with or without dementia," *Journal of Neurolinguistics*, vol. 22, no. 5, pp. 465–475, 2009.

[64] G. Waters and D. Caplan, "Working memory and online syntactic processing in Alzheimer's disease: studies with auditory moving window presentation," *The Journals of Gerontology Series B: Psychological Sciences and Social Sciences*, vol. 57, no. 4, pp. P298–P311, 2002.

[65] P. Garrard, M. Lambonralph, K. Patterson, K. Pratt, and J. Hodges, "Semantic feature knowledge and picture naming in dementia of Alzheimer's type: a new approach," *Brain and Language*, vol. 93, no. 1, pp. 79–94, 2005.

[66] E. M. Arroyo-Anlló, S. Bellouard, P. Ingrand, and R. Gil, "Effects of automatic/controlled access processes on semantic memory in Alzheimer's disease," *Journal of Alzheimer's Disease*, vol. 25, no. 3, pp. 525–533, 2011.

[67] L. R. Duarte, A. Syssau, M. Jiménez, M. Launay, and P. Terrier, "Deficit of access or storage: semantic memory processing in Alzheimer disease," *Canadian Journal on Aging*, vol. 26, no. 03, pp. 227–239, 2007.

[68] D. Caplan and G. Waters, "Memory mechanisms supporting syntactic comprehension," *Psychonomic Bulletin & Review*, vol. 20, no. 2, pp. 243–268, 2013.

[69] E. W. Wlotko and K. D. Federmeier, "Age-related changes in the impact of contextual strength on multiple aspects of sentence comprehension," *Psychophysiology*, vol. 49, no. 6, pp. 770–785, 2012.

[70] R. Iodice, *Enriquecimiento visual del aprendizaje de palabras*, M. JJG, Ed., Guía Practica de terapias estimulativas en el Alzhéimer, Madrid: Sintesis, 2015.

PPAR-γ Promotes Hematoma Clearance through Haptoglobin-Hemoglobin-CD163 in a Rat Model of Intracerebral Hemorrhage

Gaiqing Wang,[1,2] Tong Li,[1] Shu-na Duan,[1] Liang Dong,[1] Xin-gang Sun,[2] and Fang Xue[2]

[1]*Department of Neurology, Shanxi Medical University, 56 Xinjian S Rd., Yingze, Taiyuan, Shanxi 030001, China*
[2]*Department of Neurology, The Second Hospital, Shanxi Medical University, 382 WuYi St., Taiyuan, Shanxi 030001, China*

Correspondence should be addressed to Gaiqing Wang; wanggq08@163.com

Academic Editor: Hailiang Tang

Background and Purpose. PPAR-γ is a transcriptional factor which is associated with promoting hematoma clearance and reducing neurological dysfunction after intracerebral hemorrhage (ICH). Haptoglobin- (Hp-) hemoglobin- (Hb-) CD163 acts as a main pathway to Hb scavenging after ICH. The effect of PPAR-γ on the Hp-Hb-CD163 signaling pathway has not been reported. We hypothesized that PPAR-γ might protect against ICH-induced neuronal injury via activating the Hp-Hb-CD163 pathway in a rat ICH model. *Methods.* 107 Sprague-Dawley rats were used in this research. They were randomly allocated to 4 groups as follows: sham group, vehicle group, monascin-treated group, and Glivec-treated group. Animals were euthanized at 3 days after the model was established successfully. We observed the effects of PPAR-γ on the brain water content, hemoglobin levels, and the expressions of CD163 and Hp in Western blot and real-ime PCR; meanwhile, we measured hematoma volumes and edema areas by MRI scanning. *Result.* The results showed that PPAR-γ agonist significantly reduced hematoma volume, brain edema, and hemoglobin after ICH. It also enhanced CD163 and Hp expression while PPAR-γ antagonist had the opposite effects. *Conclusions.* PPAR-γ promotes hematoma clearance and plays a protective role through the Hp-Hb-CD163 pathway in a rat collagenase infusion ICH model.

1. Introduction

In Western societies, intracerebral hemorrhage (ICH) takes up for 8–15% of all strokes and 20–30% in the Asian area, and there is no definite effective therapy so far [1, 2]. Understanding the complex pathophysiology of cerebral injury after ICH is crucial to developing new approaches to reduce the harmful impacts on ICH.

The occurrence of ICH begins with a vast release of blood within the brain parenchyma [3, 4]. Erythrocytes, as the major cellular components of the hematoma, dissolves and releases hemoglobin (Hb) which subsequently broke down into heme and iron after ICH within a few days [5]. These cytotoxins mainly cause secondary brain injury following ICH [6]. Haptoglobin-Hb-CD163 as well as hemopexin-heme-LRP1 (low-density lipoprotein receptor-related protein-1) is believed to be the most important endogenous scavenging pathway which participates in hematoma/blood component resolution following ICH [6]. The cell-free Hb can trigger oxidative damages caspase activation, blood-brain barrier disruption, and neuronal death and result in irreversible brain damages [7]. CD163, which is the only hemoglobin clearance receptor expressed in the mononuclear phagocyte system, is formed during the hemolysis of erythrocytes and mediates the endocytosis of the Hb, leading to the degradation of the ligand protein and cytoplasmic heme oxygenase [8]. Haptoglobin (Hp), which is a primary Hb-binding protein, attenuates the destructive effects of Hb in the plasma [6, 9, 10]. Superabundant Hb in the plasma can upregulate the expression of Hp and the Hb-Hp receptor CD163 in neurons [11]. Hp is bound to free Hb and once Hp-Hb complex is endocytosed by CD163 may cause an anti-inflammatory response. The Hp-Hb-

CD163 acts as the main pathway in Hb scavenging and exerts a pivotal protective role [9, 12].

PPAR-γ is a transcription factor which can regulate the expression of catalase and superoxide dismutase which are two important antioxidant genes [13, 14]. It is also associated with promoting hematoma clearance and reducing neurological dysfunction [15]. As a PPAR-γ agonist, monascin is the main component of red yeast rice with a Chinese traditional technique and has been shown to have a protective effect by promoting hematoma clearance and reducing cerebral edema in rats after ICH [13], but the specific mechanism of monascin in ICH has not been clarified so far.

We hypothesize that PPAR-γ will promote hematoma clearance via CD163 and Hp upregulation, therefore reducing brain edema and improving BBB integrity after ICH. So we designed the study to test the effect of PPAR-γ on the Hp-Hb-CD163 pathway through PPAR-γ agonist monascin and its antagonist Glivec which mediates PPAR-γ by declining the phosphorylation level [16] in a collagenase-induced ICH rat model.

2. Materials and Methods

2.1. Animal Preparation. This study used 107 male adult Sprague-Dawley rats, weighing about 250~300 g (from Shanxi Medical University Animal Laboratory). The protocol for using these animals was in accordance with the Animal Utilization and Management Committee which was made by Shanxi Medical University. All rats were available to get fodder and water freely in the research.

2.2. Animal Treatments and Experimental and Control Groups. All rats were randomized to the following groups: sham operation group ($n = 25$), vehicle group ($n = 27$), monascin-treated group (10 mg/kg twice a day, $n = 26$), and Glivec-treated group (100 mg/kg/day, $n = 29$). Dead animals were replaced before final assessment. All gavages were administered by gastric perfusion 6 h after ICH until the endpoint.

2.3. Intracerebral Hemorrhage Model of Rats. The intracerebral hemorrhage model was made by injecting collagenase IV to the corpus striatum under a head stereotaxic apparatus [13]. Briefly, experimental rats were anesthetized by hydrated chloric aldehyde (300–350 mg/kg) in an intraperitoneal injection method. After being anesthetized, rats were positioned in the stereotactic instrument (Jiangwan type 1 C Instrument, Shanghai, China). A 1 mm needle was inserted through a cranial burr hole into the striatum to the following frame of references: 0.5 0mm anterior, 5.8 mm ventral, and 2.3 mm lateral to the bregma. Then, we used a 5 μL flat-headed microsyringe (Hamilton 600, Switzerland) to infuse 0.5 U type IV collagenase (Sigma-Aldrich, USA) which was dissolved in 2.5 μL saline solution. After infusion, the needle needs to be maintained in there for extra 3 minutes and subsequently be pulled out slowly. In the sham group, 2.5 μL saline solution was infused using the same method. After the surgery, the hole in the skull was sealed and the scalp was well sutured. Animals were bred in a specific facility which was pathogen free. Besides, they can get food and water uncontrolled.

2.4. Brain Water Content. The water content of rat brain tissue was performed as earlier described [13]. We used 4% chloral hydrate for intraperitoneal injection to deeply anesthetize the rat, and then the rat was decapitated to measure the cerebral water content. The brain tissue was removed from the skull rapidly and then divided into 4 mm sections in the portion around the puncture point. All brain tissue samples we got from the ipsilateral basal ganglia were instantly weighed by an electric microbalance to know the wet weight (Ww). Then tissues were placed in a 100°C drying oven for 48 hours to desiccation. After that, we can obtain dry weight (Dw). The brain water content was calculated by the following formula: $(\mathrm{Ww} - \mathrm{Dw})/\mathrm{Ww} \times 100\%$.

2.5. Hemoglobin Assay. Quantitation of brain hemoglobin after ICH was measured by hemoglobin assay under the guidance of the manufacturer's instructions. Briefly, successful modeling rats were sacrificed and the brain tissues were quickly removed and put into four glass dishes, respectively. A total of 1000 μL prerefrigerated PBS buffer was added into each glass dish. Brain tissue was smashed by sonication, collected in a centrifuged tube, and centrifuged at 4°C, 12000 rpm for 30 minutes. 25 μL of the supernatant of each group was put into a 96-well plate, and Drabkin's reagent was added to the supernatant in a ratio of 1 : 4. After incubation for 5 minutes at room temperature, OD value was measured by a spectrophotometer in 400 nm. The OD value of each sample was calibrated by a blank group.

2.6. Expression of PPAR-γ, CD163, and Hp in Different Groups by Western Blot. The brain tissue was smashed, and RIPA Lysis Buffer with PMSF was added for extracted total protein in each sample for Western blot analysis. Protein concentration was determined by a bicinchoninic acid (BCA) assay. 50 μg of each sample lysis was loaded on a 10% sodium dodecyl sulfate gel and electrophoresed in 90 volts for 2 hours. Belt was transferred to the polyvinylidene fluoride membrane after an electrophoresis process. Membranes were blocked with 5% BSA blocking buffer at 37°C for 2 hours and incubated with first antibodies: polyclonal anti-PPAR-γ of rabbit (1 : 1000, Bioss), anti-CD163 of rabbit (1 : 500, Bioss), and polyclonal anti-Hp of rabbit (1 : 500, Bioss) at 4°C in a thermostat shaker overnight. Meanwhile, other membranes were probed with β-actin (1 : 3000, Bioworld) as an internal control. After being washed by the TBST buffer, all membranes were incubated with the second antibodies at 37°C for 2 hours. Immunoreactive membranes were processed with an ECL Plus chemiluminescence assay kit. After that, it can be visualized through an imaging system (Bio-Rad, ChemiDoc). Finally, band intensities were normalizing with their internal controls, respectively, and digitizing using ImageJ software.

2.7. Measurements of Volume of Hematoma and Cerebral Edema by MRI. All rats were given brain MRI scan on a 1.5 T clinical scanner (GE Signa HDx, GE healthcare Milwaukee) with a knee coil 3 days post-ICH at the Second Hospital affiliated to Shanxi Medical University. During the

MRI imaging scanning, rats were maintained well anesthetized after the use of 5% chloral hydrate with the prone position. A series of MR sequences were acquired in our study, the protocol included T2-weighted imaging (T2WI) and T2 Flair to assess the edema, and scanning parameters [13] are listed as follows: repetition time (TR)/echo time (TE) = 2400/129 ms, field of view (FOV) = 18 × 18 mm, slice thickness = 2.0 mm, matrix size = 512 × 448, and interval = 0.2 mm. In T2 fluid-attenuated inversion recovery (T2 Flair), TR/TE = 8502/128.6 ms, FOV = 12 × 12 mm, slice thickness = 2.0 mm, matrix size = 512 × 448, and interval = 0.2 mm. T2*-weighted imaging (T2*WI) and susceptibility weighted imaging (SWI) were used to determine the hematoma size; scan parameters are as follows: in T2*WI, TR/TE = 400/15 ms, FOV = 18 × 18 mm, slice thickness = 2.0 mm, matrix size = 448 × 384, interval = 0.2 mm, and flip angle = 15°. In SWI: TR/TE = 49.9/4.5 ms, FOV = 18 × 18 mm, slice thickness = 1.5 mm, flip angle = 15°, and matrix size = 448 × 448. MRI postprocessing was performed on an off-line workstation by two experienced neurologists who were blinded to the group set and scan date. The absolute volume of intracerebral hemorrhage area which contains the outer amount of edema and hematoma was adopted during the measurement process. The total value of the absolute volume was calculated by integrating injured areas of brain hemorrhage slices. All the assessments were repeated three times, respectively. The results were shown as the mean and standard deviation.

2.8. Assay of Haptoglobin and CD163 in Different Groups by Real-Time PCR. The total RNA of different groups was extracted from the brain tissue surrounding hematoma by using TRIzol Reagent (Takara Inc., Japan) complied with the manufacturer's instructions. After completing the extraction process, total RNA was determined by Nano-drop 2000 (Thermo Fisher, USA) with the UV absorbance at 260 nm to ensure purity. Complementary DNA was reverse transcribed by using a one-step PrimeScript™ RT Master Mix kit (Takara Inc., Japan), and a total of 20 μL reaction mixture system which contained 1 μg total RNA was carried out at 37°C for 15 minutes; finally, the complementary DNA was kept at a minus 80°C environment. Real-time PCR analysis was processed in a BIO-RAD iCycler Thermal Cycler for RT-PCR (Bio-rad, USA) with the complementary DNA and SYBR® Premix Ex Taq™ Kit (Takara Inc., Japan). Oligonucleotide PCR-based primers are as follows: haptoglobin: 5′-gaaaggcgctgtaagtcctg-3′ (forward primer) and 5′-tcctcttccagggtgaattg-3′(reverse primer) and CD163: 5′-gacagacccaacggcttaca-3′ (forward primer) and 5′-ggtcacaaaacttcaaccgga-3′(reverse primer). The experiment uses a 25 μL volume total reaction mixture reaction system which contains 2 μL of the diluted complementary DNA product, 12.5 μL of the SYBR Premix Ex Taq Mix (Takara Inc., Japan), 1 μL of forward/reverse primers, respectively, and 8.5 μL of RNase-free water. The condition of real-time PCR reaction was implemented as follows: predenaturation step was processed at 95°C for 1 minute. The extended process sets the denaturation at 95°C for 30 seconds and annealing and elongation at 55°C for 45 seconds, and the extended process was repeated for 40 cycles. Reverse transcription PCR was performed three times for each sample. To standardize the expression of haptoglobin and CD163 mRNA, the levels of the reference gene β actin were determined for each sample parallelly. Expression of final results was ratios of the target gene copy numbers to β-actin transcripts. The expression of the targeted gene was computed by the $2^{-\Delta\Delta Ct}$ method.

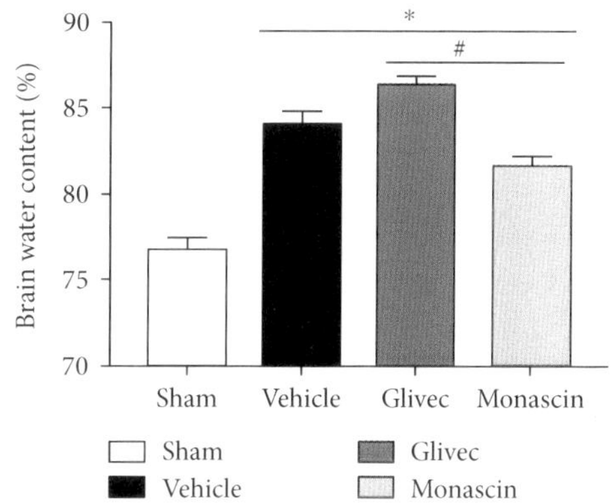

FIGURE 1: Effect of PPAR-γ on brain water content associated with ICH 3 days after surgery ($^*p < 0.05$ versus sham; $^\#p < 0.05$ versus vehicle).

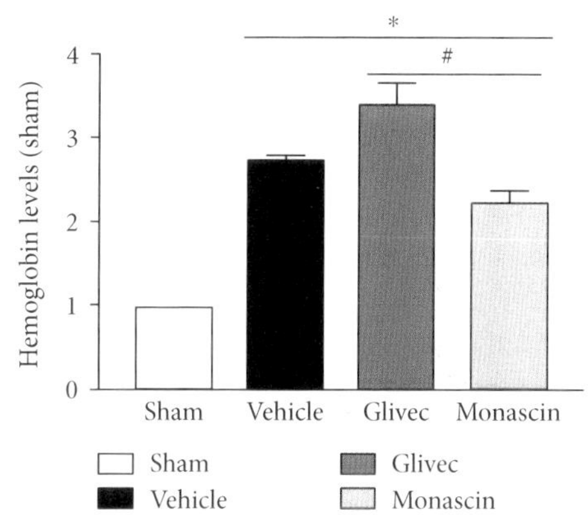

FIGURE 2: Effect of PPAR-γ on hemoglobin levels associated with ICH 3 days after surgery ($^*p < 0.05$ versus sham; $^\#p < 0.05$ versus vehicle).

2.9. Statistical Analysis. Quantitative data were sorted out as the mean ± SD. One-way ANOVA was taken for multiple comparisons. The SNK-q test was adopted for the comparison of the differences between groups of brain water content, hemoglobin levels, and real-time PCR assay, while the differences of MRI parameter and Western blot results were determined by Tukey's post hoc test. $p < 0.05$ was denoted the difference processing statistical significance among all groups.

3. Results

3.1. Mortality. The overall mortality in operative rats was approximately 10.2% ($n = 11$). All the sham group rats

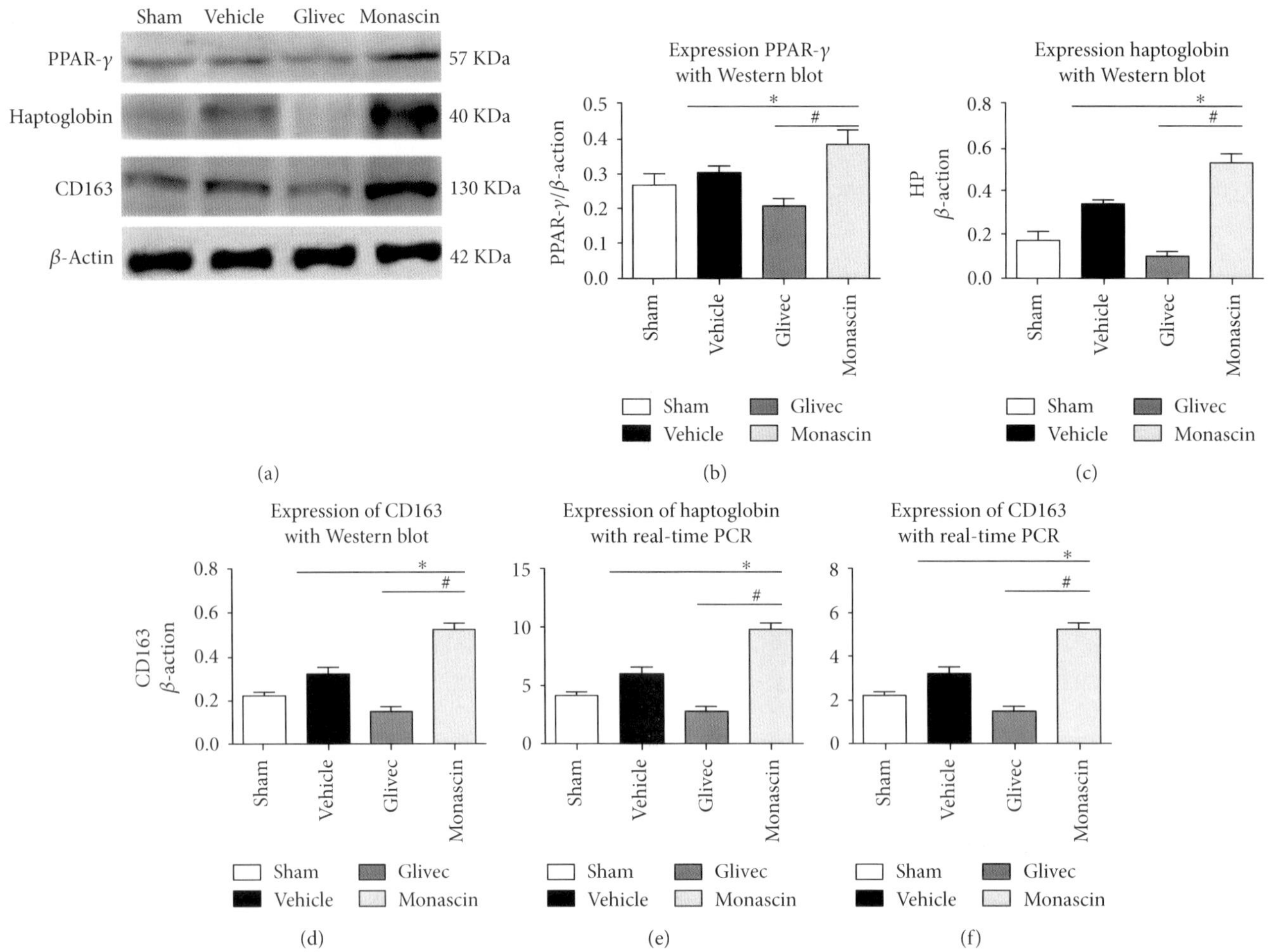

FIGURE 3: Effect of Glivec and monascin on PPAR-γ, haptoglobin, and CD163 associated with ICH 3 days after surgery. Representative images are shown of Western blot assay (a–d) and real-time PCR (e and f) for PPAR-γ, haptoglobin, and CD163 levels within ipsilateral brain tissues. One-way ANOVA followed by Tukey's tests was used. ($^*p < 0.05$ versus sham; $^{\#}p < 0.05$ versus vehicle).

survived, and there was no significant difference in the mortality of each group (data not shown).

3.2. PPAR-γ Agonist Monascin Decreased Brain Water Content. All the operative groups showed a significant increase in brain water content when compared to the sham group ($^*p < 0.05$ versus sham; Figure 1). PPAR-γ agonist monascin significantly lowed the water content of brain tissue around hematoma while PPAR-γ antagonist Glivec acted the opposite way, in comparison with the vehicle group ($^{\#}p < 0.05$; Figure 1).

3.3. PPAR-γ Agonist Monascin Reduced Hemoglobin Level. The hemoglobin level of all the operative groups was obviously higher than that of the sham group ($^*p < 0.05$; Figure 2). Compared to the vehicle group, monascin significantly decreased the level of hemoglobin ($^{\#}p < 0.05$ versus vehicle), while Glivec increased it ($^{\#}p < 0.05$ versus vehicle).

3.4. Effect of Monascin and Glivec on CD163 and Hp Expression following ICH. The results of Western blot and PCR showed a significant increase in PPAR-γ, Hp, and CD163 expression within ipsilateral brain tissues after ICH when compared to sham ($^*p < 0.05$, Figure 3). Compared to vehicle, monascin increased PPAR-γ, Hp, and CD163 expression with Western blot ($^{\#}p < 0.05$, Figures 3(a)–3(d)) and real-time PCR ($^{\#}p < 0.05$, Figures 3(e) and 3(f)). Meanwhile, the administration of Glivec downregulated the expression of PPAR-γ, Hp, and CD163 ($^{\#}p < 0.05$, Figure 3).

3.5. Monascin Decreased the Volume of Hematoma (T2 WI/SWI) and Brain Edema (T2WI/T2 Flair) in the Rat Model after ICH.* The volumes of hematoma and edema of all groups were measured at 3 days after modeling successfully (showed in Figure 4). The volume of hematoma and edema was reduced in the monascin group compared to the vehicle group. While Glivec extended the volume of hematoma and edema 3 days after ICH. The link assay between brain edema and hematoma lesion showed a positive correlation between them ($r = 0.989$, $p = 0.011$).

4. Discussion

In our study, we demonstrated that PPAR-γ is neuroprotective through decreasing hematoma size and hemoglobin

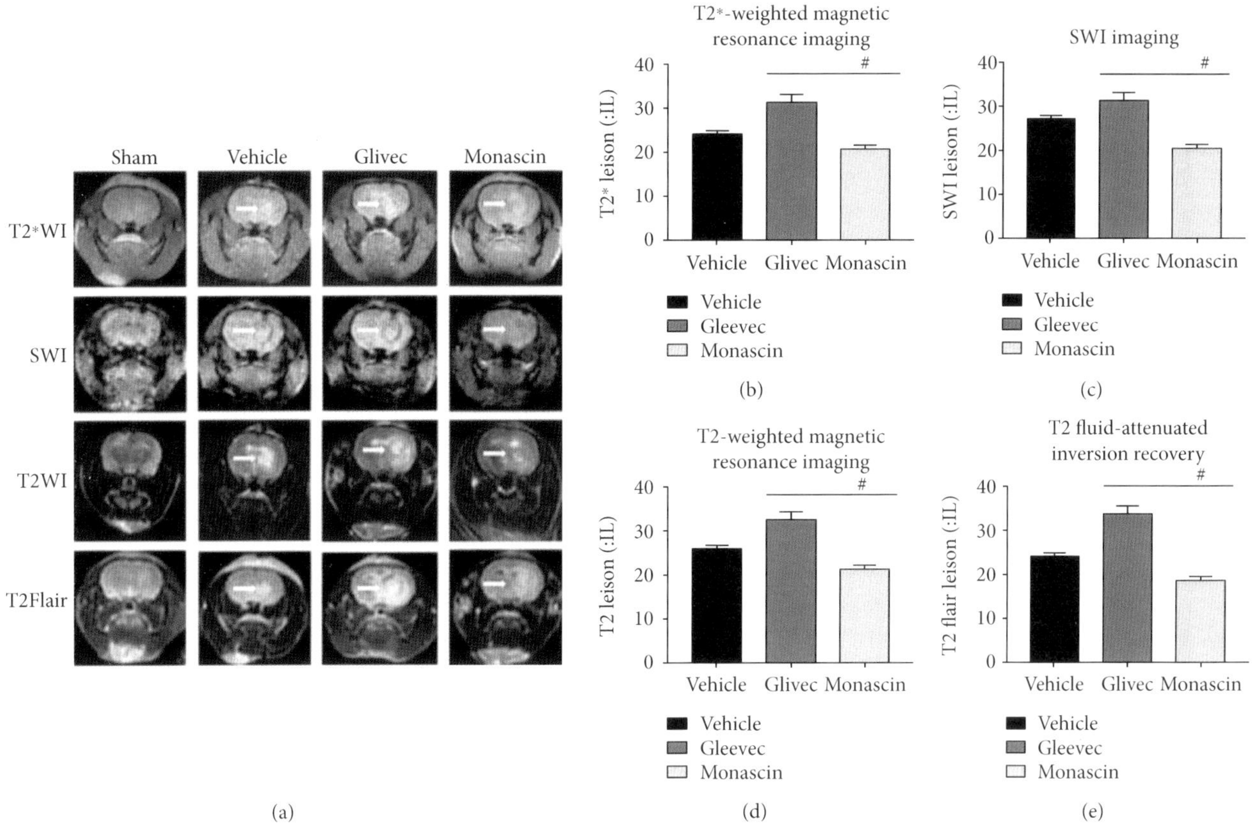

FIGURE 4: Effect of PPAR-γ on hematoma volume (a–c) and brain edema (a, d, and e) associated with ICH 3 days after surgery. Representative images are shown of T2*WI (a and b), SWI (a and c) for hematoma volume, T2WI (a and d), and T2 Flair (a and e) for brain edema within ipsilateral brain tissues. One-way ANOVA followed by Tukey's tests were used ($^{\#}p < 0.05$ versus vehicle).

levels then reduced brain edema. PPAR-γ agonist monascin enhanced haptoglobin and CD163 expression whereas PPAR-γ antagonist Glivec had the opposite effects on a rat ICH model.

Intracerebral hemorrhage is a devastating disease, and there has been no specific therapy to reduce the mortality [17]. It started from the blood's massive release into the brain parenchyma [3, 11, 18]. The red blood cell (RBC) lyses within several days and releases Hb at the same time [6]. The hematoma is the culprit of brain insults after ICH, so how to effectively remove blood products is crucial in ICH-induced brain injury [19].

Hp is a glycoprotein which is abundant in the plasma [20]. It is mainly secreted by hepatocytes, and a mononuclear phagocyte system can also produce it [21]. The levels of Hp in the plasma increases to answer stress response and anti-inflammation, which bond to free Hb after cerebral hemorrhage [14, 19]. The formation of Hp-Hb complex protects Hb from oxidative modifications. Otherwise, oxidative modification can prevent the clearance processing and lead the releasing of free Hb into the circulation of the blood [22]. Besides, the Hp-Hb-CD163 complex has a high-affinity site for CD163 to recognize and promote hemoglobin clearance [8, 9, 14].

CD163 acts as a hemoglobin scavenger receptor. It is only expressed in the monocyte-macrophage system [9] and is a 130 kDa transmembrane glycoprotein which can be combined with a variety of ligands. It also belongs to scavenger receptor superfamily class B [18]. CD163 is the cellular receptor target of Hp after ICH [10]. After recognization by the Hp-Hb complex, the Hp-Hb-CD163 complex system is formed during the hemolysis of erythrocytes and mediates the endocytosis of the hemoglobin, leading to the degradation of the lysosomal ligand protein [8]. The Hp-Hb-CD163 acts as the main pathway in Hb scavenging and exerts a pivotal protective role [9].

PPAR-γ is a transcription factor belonging to the nuclear hormone receptor superfamily. During the past years, the transcription factors of PPAR-γ [19, 23] were validated as important players in regulating phagocyte-mediated cleanup processes and able to promote endogenous hematoma absorption, decrease neuronal damage, and improve functional recovery in a rodent model of ICH [24]. It not only increased microglia-mediated phagocytosis of RBC in rat primary microglia in culture but also reduced the generation of peroxide during the phagocytic process [25]. The specific mechanism of PPAR-γ in ICH has not been completely clarified so far.

In the present study, we found that PPAR-γ agonist monascin is neuroprotective by decreasing the brain water content and the level of hemoglobin. Besides, it also enhanced CD163 and Hp expression in Western blot and real-time PCR results whereas Glivec reduced Hp and CD163 expression.

Magnetic resonance imaging (MRI) is a medical imaging technique and has been extensively used in the study of intracerebral hemorrhage [14]. It has high sensitivity for presenting the temporal and spatial shifts of hematoma and edema after ICH. At 3 days after surgery, we assessed the volume of hematoma and cerebral edema via T2*WI/SWI and T2WI/T2 FLAIR sequences [7]. The results showed PPAR-γ agonist monascin evidently reduced hematoma volume and cerebral edema after ICH, while the Glivec expanded the hematoma and edema areas.

Our results demonstrated that PPAR-γ agonist monascin decreased hematoma volume and brain edema in a collagenase-induced ICH rat model via histology, molecular biology, and MRI imaging methods. Meanwhile, monascin upregulated the expression of CD163 and Hp which belong to the endogenous hemoglobin scavenging system in ICH.

PPAR-γ activation reinforced microglia-induced erythrocyte phagocytosis. Our previous study demonstrated that PPAR-γ agonist improved outcome through reducing hematoma volume and edema formation following ICH [13]. While macrophages play a central role in hematoma clearance, hemoglobin mostly remains encapsulated within erythrocytes until they are phagocytosed and degraded by microglia and infiltrating macrophages [1]. CD163, a hemoglobin scavenger receptor, is mainly expressed on macrophages/microglia, and it plays a major role in scavenging free hemoglobin released during erythrolysis after ICH. CD163 transports hemoglobin into microglia/macrophages and functions as a membrane-bound scavenger receptor for clearing extracellular haptoglobin-hemoglobin (Hp-Hb) complexes [11]. Excessive Hb upregulated the expression of Hp and the Hb/Hp receptor CD163 in vivo and in vitro. Free Hb binds to Hp and once Hp-Hb complex is endocytosed by CD163, which mediated the delivery of Hb to the macrophage, may fuel an anti-inflammatory response because heme metabolites have potent anti-inflammatory effects [6]. So PPAR-γ activation possibly reinforced microglia-induced Hp-Hb complex phagocytosis through enhancing CD163 expression.

In conclusion, PPAR-γ promotes hematoma clearance and plays a protective role possibly through the Hp-Hb-CD163 pathway in a rat collagenase-induced ICH model. Monascin, as a PPAR-γ agonist, will be a potential medical treatment for ICH in the future.

Authors' Contributions

Gaiqing Wang and Tong Li contributed equally to this work.

Acknowledgments

This study was supported by a project from the National Natural Science Foundation of China (Project no. 81771294).

References

[1] R. Liu, S. Cao, Y. Hua, R. F. Keep, Y. Huang, and G. Xi, "CD163 expression in neurons after experimental intracerebral hemorrhage," *Stroke*, vol. 48, no. 5, pp. 1369–1375, 2017.

[2] J. Chen-Roetling and R. F. Regan, "Haptoglobin increases the vulnerability of CD163-expressing neurons to hemoglobin," *Journal of Neurochemistry*, vol. 139, no. 4, pp. 586–595, 2016.

[3] X. Zhao, S. Song, G. Sun et al., "Neuroprotective role of haptoglobin after intracerebral hemorrhage," *The Journal of Neuroscience*, vol. 29, no. 50, pp. 15819–15827, 2009.

[4] S. Cao, M. Zheng, Y. Hua, G. Chen, R. F. Keep, and G. Xi, "Hematoma changes during clot resolution after experimental intracerebral hemorrhage," *Stroke*, vol. 47, no. 6, pp. 1626–1631, 2016.

[5] H. Zhao, X. Zhang, Z. Dai et al., "P2X7 receptor suppression preserves blood-brain barrier through inhibiting RhoA activation after experimental intracerebral hemorrhage in rats," *Scientific Reports*, vol. 6, no. 1, article 23286, 2016.

[6] G. Wang, L. Wang, X. G. Sun, and J. Tang, "Haematoma scavenging in intracerebral haemorrhage: from mechanisms to the clinic," *Journal of Cellular and Molecular Medicine*, vol. 22, no. 2, pp. 768–777, 2017.

[7] X. Zhao, G. Sun, J. Zhang et al., "Transcription factor Nrf2 protects the brain from damage produced by intracerebral hemorrhage," *Stroke*, vol. 38, no. 12, pp. 3280–3286, 2007.

[8] J. H. Thomsen, A. Etzerodt, P. Svendsen, and S. K. Moestrup, "The haptoglobin-CD163-heme oxygenase-1 pathway for hemoglobin scavenging," *Oxidative Medicine and Cellular Longevity*, vol. 2013, Article ID 523652, 11 pages, 2013.

[9] J. Galea, G. Cruickshank, J. L. Teeling et al., "The intrathecal CD163-haptoglobin-hemoglobin scavenging system in subarachnoid hemorrhage," *Journal of Neurochemistry*, vol. 121, no. 5, pp. 785–792, 2012.

[10] J. L. Leclerc, A. S. Lampert, C. Loyola Amador et al., "The absence of the CD163 receptor has distinct temporal influences on intracerebral hemorrhage outcomes," *Journal of Cerebral Blood Flow & Metabolism*, vol. 38, no. 2, pp. 262–273, 2017.

[11] D. J. Schaer, A. I. Alayash, and P. W. Buehler, "Gating the radical hemoglobin to macrophages: the anti-inflammatory role of CD163, a scavenger receptor," *Antioxidants & Redox Signaling*, vol. 9, no. 7, pp. 991–999, 2007.

[12] C. J. Roche, D. Dantsker, A. I. Alayash, and J. M. Friedman, "Enhanced nitrite reductase activity associated with the haptoglobin complexed hemoglobin dimer: functional and antioxidative implications," *Nitric Oxide*, vol. 27, no. 1, pp. 32–39, 2012.

[13] J. Wang, G. Wang, J. Yi et al., "The effect of monascin on hematoma clearance and edema after intracerebral hemorrhage in rats," *Brain Research Bulletin*, vol. 134, pp. 24–29, 2017.

[14] X. Wang, T. Mori, T. Sumii, and E. H. Lo, "Hemoglobin-induced cytotoxicity in rat cerebral cortical neurons: caspase activation and oxidative stress," *Stroke*, vol. 33, no. 7, pp. 1882–1888, 2002.

[15] J. Zhao, N. Kobori, J. Aronowski, and P. K. Dash, "Sulforaphane reduces infarct volume following focal cerebral ischemia in rodents," *Neuroscience Letters*, vol. 393, no. 2-3, pp. 108–112, 2006.

[16] S. S. Choi, E. S. Kim, J. E. Jung et al., "PPARγ antagonist gleevec improves insulin sensitivity and promotes the browning of white adipose tissue," *Diabetes*, vol. 65, no. 4, pp. 829–839, 2016.

[17] H. B. Brouwers and J. N. Goldstein, "Therapeutic strategies in acute intracerebral hemorrhage," *Neurotherapeutics*, vol. 9, no. 1, pp. 87–98, 2012.

[18] M. Roy-O'Reilly, L. Zhu, L. Atadja et al., "Soluble CD163 in intracerebral hemorrhage: biomarker for perihematomal edema," *Annals of Clinical Translational Neurology*, vol. 4, no. 11, pp. 793–800, 2017.

[19] J. Aronowski and X. Zhao, "Molecular pathophysiology of cerebral hemorrhage: secondary brain injury," *Stroke*, vol. 42, no. 6, pp. 1781–6, 2011.

[20] D. H. Ko, H. E. Chang, T. S. Kim et al., "A review of haptoglobin typing methods for disease association study and preventing anaphylactic transfusion reaction," *BioMed Research International*, vol. 2013, Article ID 390630, 6 pages, 2013.

[21] C. Burkard, S. G. Lillico, E. Reid et al., "Precision engineering for PRRSV resistance in pigs: macrophages from genome edited pigs lacking CD163 SRCR5 domain are fully resistant to both PRRSV genotypes while maintaining biological function," *PLoS Pathogens*, vol. 13, no. 2, article e1006206, 2017.

[22] C. A. Gleissner, I. Shaked, C. Erbel, D. Bockler, H. A. Katus, and K. Ley, "CXCL4 downregulates the atheroprotective hemoglobin receptor CD163 in human macrophages," *Circulation Research*, vol. 106, no. 1, pp. 203–211, 2010.

[23] X. Zhao, J. Grotta, N. Gonzales, and J. Aronowski, "Hematoma resolution as a therapeutic target: the role of microglia/macrophages," *Stroke*, vol. 40, no. 3, Supplement 1, pp. S92–S94, 2009.

[24] X. R. Zhao, N. Gonzales, and J. Aronowski, "Pleiotropic role of PPARγ in intracerebral hemorrhage: an intricate system involving Nrf2, RXR, and NF-κB," *CNS Neuroscience & Therapeutics*, vol. 21, no. 4, pp. 357–366, 2015.

[25] F. A. Monsalve, R. D. Pyarasani, F. Delgado-Lopez, and R. Moore-Carrasco, "Peroxisome proliferator-activated receptor targets for the treatment of metabolic diseases," *Mediators of Inflammation*, vol. 2013, Article ID 549627, 18 pages, 2013.

Histone Deacetylase Inhibitor Scriptaid Alleviated Neurological Dysfunction after Experimental Intracerebral Hemorrhage in Mice

Heng Yang, Wei Ni, Hanqiang Jiang, Yu Lei, Jiabin Su, Yuxiang Gu, and Liangfu Zhou

Department of Neurosurgery, Huashan Hospital, Fudan University, Shanghai, China

Correspondence should be addressed to Liangfu Zhou; lfzhouc@126.com

Academic Editor: Hu Qin

Objectives. To investigate the role of Scriptaid in reducing brain injury after intracerebral hemorrhage (ICH) in mice. *Methods.* An ICH model was constructed by injecting autologous blood into the right basal ganglia in mice. The animals were administered 3.5 mg/kg of Scriptaid intraperitoneally after ICH. The hematoma volume and hemoglobin level were measured to examine hematoma resolution. A behavior test and brain edema and white matter injury examinations indicated brain injury after ICH. *Results.* Scriptaid treatment promoted hematoma resolution and reduced the hematoma volume 7 d after ICH compared with the vehicle group ($P < 0.05$). Scriptaid treatment also alleviated the brain water content in the ipsilateral basal ganglia ($P < 0.05$) and cortex ($P < 0.01$) 3 d after ICH. In addition, Scriptaid improved neurological function recovery and alleviated white matter injury 35 d after ICH. *Conclusions.* Scriptaid can protect against brain injury after ICH and may be considered a new medical therapy method for ICH.

1. Introduction

Intracerebral hemorrhage (ICH) is a fatal subtype of stroke with high morbidity and mortality that accounts for 10%–15% of all strokes [1]. The mechanisms of brain injury following ICH have achieved great understanding in past decades, including primary and secondary brain injuries. Primary brain damage is mainly due to the mass effect and mechanical disruption from extravasated blood. Secondary brain injury is much more complicated and is mainly caused by the physiological response to the hematoma and toxic blood components [2–4]. Unfortunately, no effective medical treatment is available to improve functional outcomes in patients with ICH.

Neuroinflammation plays a key role in secondary brain injury after ICH and is associated with both brain damage and recovery from ICH [5]. First, as resident immune cells in the central nervous system (CNS), activated microglia release many inflammatory factors. Then, systemic immune cells infiltrate and produce cytokines, chemokines, extracellular proteases, and reactive oxygen species (ROS) and induce a severe inflammatory reaction [6–9] after ICH. When microglia/macrophages are activated, they switch into two phenotypes (the M1 and M2 phenotypes) through the so-called microglia/macrophage polarization process [10]. Many previous studies have demonstrated that microglia/microphage polarization is dynamic during a central nervous system injury and modulating microglia/macrophage polarization ameliorates inflammatory injuries after traumatic brain injury (TBI) and ischemic and hemorrhagic strokes [11–13]. Recent studies have also demonstrated that activating microglia/macrophages enhances hematoma resolution and improves functional outcomes in a rat model of ICH [14, 15]. In addition, blood-brain barrier (BBB) disruption, which contributes to the development of perihematomal edema, is an important cause of secondary injury after ICH [3, 16].

Histone deacetylases (HDACs) are a class of enzymes that remove acetyl groups ($O = C - CH_3$) from an ε-N-acetyl lysine amino acid on a histone, thereby allowing the histones to wrap the DNA more tightly. Histone deacetylase inhibitors (HDACis) have been widely used for the treatment of

TABLE 1: General physiological information for the different groups.

Group	MABP (mmHg)	pH	PO_2 (mmHg)	PCO_2 (mmHg)	Hct. (%)	Glucose (mg/dl)	Core body temperature
Sham	72.1 ± 7.9	7.42 ± 0.03	98.3 ± 4.1	42.3 ± 4.3	41.3 ± 0.5	91.5 ± 11.2	36.2 ± 0.4
ICH + vehicle	73.5 ± 8.4	7.36 ± 0.02	96.9 ± 2.4	41.5 ± 3.1	41.8 ± 1.1	92.3 ± 8.1	36.5 ± 0.2
ICH + Scriptaid	73.2 ± 9.1	7.38 ± 0.04	97.3 ± 2.8	42.1 ± 2.5	42.1 ± 0.8	94.2 ± 10.5	36.1 ± 0.8

epilepsy, neurodegenerative diseases, and cancer [17–19]. Recently, significant progress has been made in increasing the understanding of the roles of HDACs in regulating inflammation and immunoreactions. Therapeutic application of HDACis for inflammatory and infectious diseases has also been described in many previous reports [20, 21]. In addition, an effort has been made to develop HDACis for the treatment of traumatic brain injury and stroke. For example, HDACis suppress immune activation and alleviate brain injury in TBI and ischemic stroke in animal models [22–25]. Scriptaid is a novel histone deacetylase inhibitor, and recent studies have indicated that Scriptaid modulates microglia/macrophage polarization and protects against traumatic brain injury [25, 26]. However, few studies have investigated the application of Scriptaid in therapy for intracerebral hemorrhage. Therefore, the present study investigated the effect of Scriptaid on the amelioration of brain injury in a mouse ICH model.

2. Materials and Methods

2.1. Animals and ICH Model Construction. C57BL/6 male mice (8–10 weeks, 20–26 g) were purchased from the Chinese Academy of Sciences at Shanghai. All animals were provided free access to food and water, and all experiments were approved by the Animal Ethics Committee of Fudan University. Moreover, all experiments were performed and reported according to the ARRIVE guidelines (http://www.nc3rs.org.uk/arrive). ICH model construction was established previously [27, 28]. Briefly, animals were intraperitoneally anesthetized with 4% chloral hydrate. Blood was obtained from a femoral artery catheter for analysis of pH, PaO_2, $PaCO_2$, and blood glucose. The core body temperature was maintained at 36.0 ± 1.0°C with a feedback-controlled heating pad. The physiological information is shown in Table 1. The mice were positioned in a mouse stereotaxic frame, and 30 μl of nonanticoagulated autologous blood obtained from the femoral artery of the mouse or saline was injected straight into the right basal ganglia (0.2 mm anterior, 3.5 mm ventral, and 2.5 mm lateral to the bregma) at a rate of 2 μl/min with a microinfusion pump. The needle remained in position for an additional 10 minutes after the blood was fully injected and then was removed gently. The burr hole was filled with bone wax, and the skin incision was sutured.

2.2. Experimental Groups. The animals were divided into three groups: sham, ICH + vehicle, and ICH + Scriptaid (3.5 mg/kg). Animal group assignments for the ICH or sham operation, treatment with Scriptaid or vehicle, and neurobehavioral testing or sacrifice for hematoma measurement, brain water content assessment, and immunostaining were performed randomly using a lottery drawing box. All main outcome studies, including neurobehavioral tests, hematoma volume, brain water content, and immunohistochemistry, were performed by investigators blinded to the group assignments and experimental conditions. As described previously [25], the animals were administered 3.5 mg/kg of Scriptaid intraperitoneally at 2, 26, and 50 hours after ICH. The ICH + vehicle group was treated with an equivalent volume and concentration of dimethyl sulfoxide diluted in saline on the same time course. Then, behavioral testing was performed on the animals, and the animals were euthanized at days 1, 3, 7, and 35 after ICH for hematoma measurement, brain water content calculation, and immunohistochemistry assays.

2.3. Hematoma Measurement. As described previously [29], the brains were removed after perfusion and sliced into 1 mm-thick sections. ImageJ (version 1.49, NIH) was used to measure the ICH volumes. Additionally, the hemoglobin levels in the brain tissues were measured to quantify the hematoma size [15]. After ICH, the contralateral hemisphere and ipsilateral cortex were removed and the remaining brain tissue was dissolved in Drabkin's reagent. Then, the supernatant of the homogenate was collected and measured using a spectrophotometer. The hematoma volume (microliters) was calculated using the standard curve.

2.4. Behavior Tests. The behavior tests included the corner turn test and the wire hanging test, which were described previously [25, 26, 30]. Before the behavior tests, all animals underwent behavior training for three days and abnormal animals were excluded. The corner turn test was performed as follows. Mice were allowed to proceed into a corner with a 30° angle. The directions (left or right) of the turns made by the mice were recorded. Every mouse repeated this procedure 20 times. The percentage of right turns was calculated. The wire hanging apparatus was a stainless steel bar (50 cm length, 2 mm diameter) resting on two vertical supports and elevated 37 cm above a flat surface. Mice were placed on the middle of the bar and were observed for 30 seconds in 4 trials. The amount of time spent hanging was recorded and scored according to the following system: 0, fell off; 1, hung onto the bar with two forepaws; 2, hung onto the bar with added attempt to climb onto the bar; 3, hung onto the bar with two forepaws and one or two hind paws; 4, hung onto the bar with all four paws and with tail wrapped around the bar; and 5, escaped to one of the supports. All behavior tests were performed and evaluated by a blinded observer.

2.5. Brain Water Content. The brain water content measurement was performed as previously reported [31]. After euthanization and decapitation, the mouse brains were removed and divided into the following five parts: the ipsilateral cortex, ipsilateral basal ganglia, contralateral cortex, contralateral basal ganglia, and cerebellum. Every brain part was weighed with an electronic balance to obtain the wet weight and then dried in a gravity oven at 100°C for 24 hours to obtain the dry weight. The brain water content was calculated with the following formula: brain water content (%) = (wet weight − dry weight)/wet weight * 100%.

2.6. Immunohistochemistry Staining. Brains were removed after perfusions with saline and 4% paraformaldehyde (Sigma-Aldrich, St. Louis, MO, USA) and gradient dehydrated with 20% and 30% sucrose in PBS. Then, the sample brains were sectioned into 25 μm-thick sections on a freezing microtome and subjected to immunohistochemistry. Immunohistochemistry staining was performed as previously described [12]. The primary antibodies included rabbit anti-MBP (myelin basic protein) (Abcam, 1 : 500 dilution, Cambridge, MA, USA) and mouse antinonphosphorylated neurofilaments (SMI-32, 1 : 500 dilution, Abcam). Alexa Flour conjugated antibodies (Invitrogen, Grand Island, NY, USA, 1 : 1000) were used as the secondary antibodies. The slides were covered with Fluoroshield with DAPI (Sigma-Aldrich, St. Louis, MO, USA). Double labeling was analyzed using an epifluorescence microscope.

2.7. Statistical Analysis. All data in this study are presented as the mean ± standard error of the mean (SEM) and have been analyzed using the SPSS 19.0 software. Student's *t*-test was used to analyze differences between two groups, whereas differences between multiple groups were analyzed with one-way ANOVA. Two-way ANOVA was used to evaluate differences in the behavior tests between groups and between time points. Differences were considered significant when $P < 0.05$.

3. Results

3.1. Scriptaid Improved Hematoma Resolution after Intracerebral Hemorrhage. The hematoma mass effect is an important factor for brain injury after ICH. The hematoma morphology and size at 1, 3, and 7 d post-ICH are demonstrated in Figure 1(a) and show the hematoma absorption process (Figure 1(b)). In addition, the hemoglobin level indirectly demonstrated dynamic changes in the hematoma volume (Figure 1(c)). Compared with the vehicle group, Scriptaid treatment improved hematoma absorption at 7 d post-ICH (Figure 1(d)). Scriptaid treatment reduced the hematoma volume by 44% (3.29 ± 0.41 mm^3 in the vehicle group versus 1.85 ± 0.32 mm^3 in the Scriptaid group; $P < 0.05$) at 7 d post-ICH (Figure 1(e)). The hemoglobin level also decreased by 44.4% (3.73 ± 0.77 μl in the vehicle group versus 2.08 ± 0.68) at 7 d post-ICH, although the difference was not significant (Figure 1(f)).

3.2. Scriptaid Improved Neurological Dysfunction after Intracerebral Hemorrhage. Scriptaid treatment ameliorated both sensorimotor functions after ICH. In the corner turn test, Scriptaid administration reduced the corner turn score significantly at 1 and 3 d post-ICH (Figure 2(a), $P < 0.05$). Additionally, the wire hanging test showed motor deficit improvement in the Scriptaid treatment group at 1 and 3 d post-ICH compared with the vehicle group (Figure 2(b), $P < 0.05$).

3.3. Scriptaid Reduced the Brain Water Content 3 Days after Intracerebral Hemorrhage. Scriptaid treatment reduced brain edema in the ipsilateral basal ganglia (brain water content 81.53 ± 1.68 versus 77.31 ± 2.52 in the vehicle-treated controls, $P < 0.05$) and ipsilateral cortex (brain water content 81.43 ± 1.72 versus 76.74 ± 1.34 in the vehicle-treated controls, $P < 0.01$) at 3 d post-ICH. However, no significant difference was found in the brain water content in the contralateral basal ganglia and cortex between the Scriptaid treatment group and the vehicle group (Figure 3).

3.4. Scriptaid Conferred Long-Term Preservation of White Matter after ICH. White matter injury was evaluated by double immunofluorescent staining for MBP and SMI-32 in the ipsilateral striatum and corpus callosum at 35 d post-ICH (vehicle and Scriptaid groups) or after sham surgery (sham group) (Figures 4(a) and 4(b)). In the sham group, SMI-32 immunoreactivity and high MBP expression were rarely observed in the ipsilateral striatum and corpus callosum, which demonstrated no white matter injury. Scriptaid failed to alleviate MBP expression at 35 d post-ICH in the ipsilateral striatum and corpus callosum compared with those in the vehicle group (Figures 4(c) and 4(e)). However, Scriptaid treatment reduced SMI-32 expression at 35 d post-ICH, which demonstrated alleviation of white matter injury. The relative ratio of the ipsilateral versus contralateral SMI-32 immunostaining intensity was lower in the Scriptaid group than in the vehicle group (1.83 ± 0.14 versus 2.64 ± 0.34 in the striatum, $P < 0.05$; 1.30 ± 0.09 versus 1.62 ± 0.10 in the corpus callosum, $P < 0.01$; Figures 4(d) and 4(f)).

4. Discussion

Although many previous studies have described the mechanism of ICH and have attempted to find a therapy, no effective medical treatment for ICH is available at present. HDACis have been shown to possess neuroprotective effects in animal models of TBI and stroke [22–25]. As a novel histone deacetylase inhibitor, Scriptaid was demonstrated to protect against white matter injury in a mouse TBI model. However, the neuroprotective effects of Scriptaid in ICH remain unknown. In the present study, we found that Scriptaid improved hematoma resolution and alleviated brain edema after ICH. In addition, Scriptaid treatment had an effect on preserving white matter integrity at 35 d post-ICH and promoting neurological behavioral functions, thereby facilitating long-term functional recovery after ICH.

Secondary brain injury due to ICH is mainly caused by direct toxicity and inflammation induced by toxic blood components and hematoma metabolic products. Therefore, hematoma removal is an important target for ICH treatment because this process can relieve mass effects, alleviate

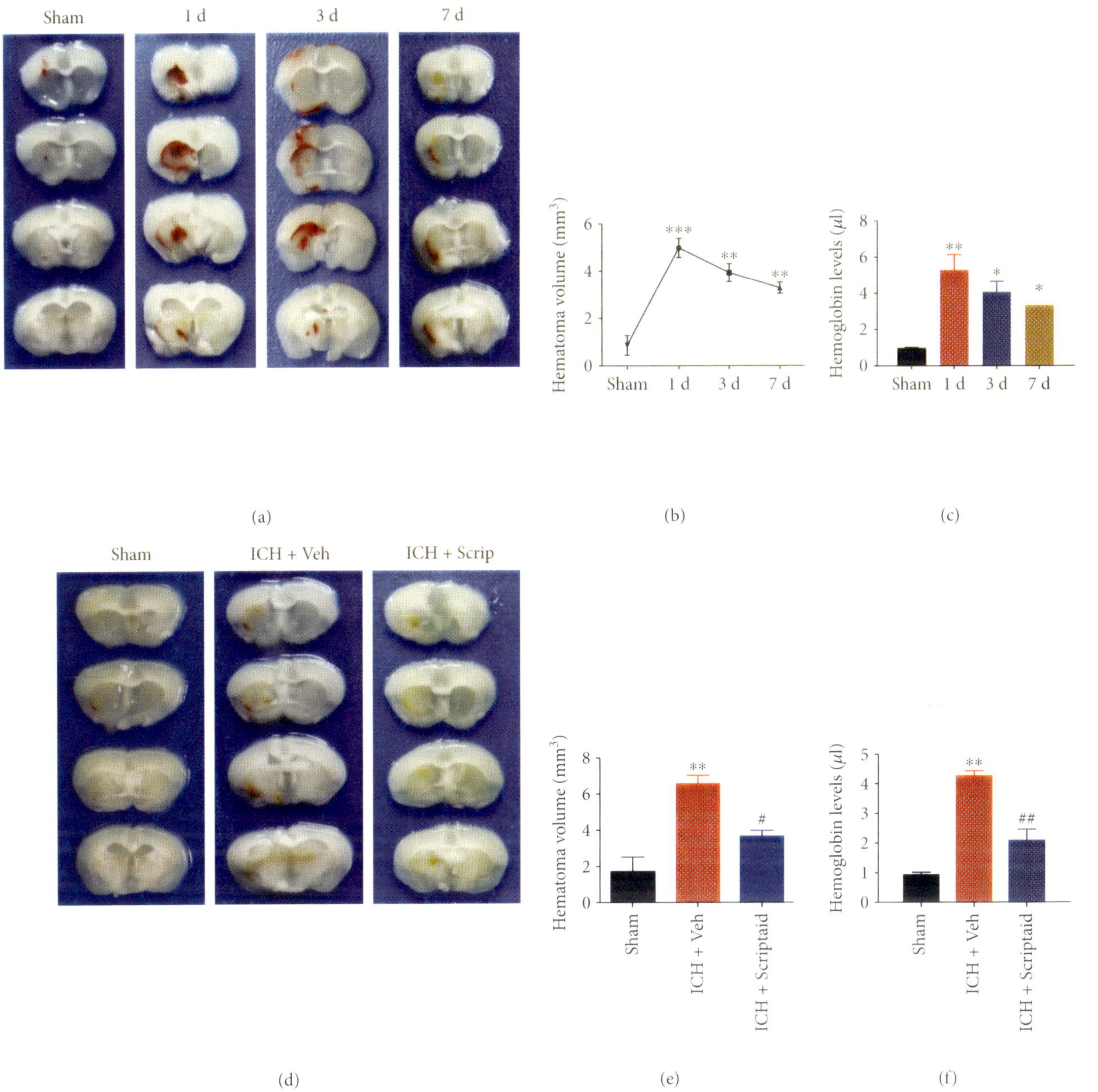

FIGURE 1: Scriptaid promoted hematoma resolution in an experimental intracerebral hemorrhage model. (a) Representative images of hematoma volumes at 1 d, 3 d, and 7 d after ICH. Time course of hematoma volume (b) and hemoglobin level (c) changes after ICH ($^{*}P < 0.05$, $^{**}P < 0.01$, and $^{***}P < 0.001$). (d) Serial coronal sections of mouse brain tissues at 7 d after ICH. The hematoma volumes (e) and hemoglobin levels (f) at 7 d after ICH ($^{**}P < 0.01$ versus the sham group; $^{\#}P < 0.05$ versus the vehicle group).

inflammation, and improve the recovery of neuronal function [14, 15, 29]. In our study, Scriptaid improved hematoma resolution through a mechanism that might be related to modulation of microglia/macrophage polarization. As a novel histone deacetylase inhibitor, Scriptaid can shift microglia/macrophage polarization toward the M2 phenotype and mitigate inflammation [25]. Microglia/macrophages play a significant role in hematoma clearance. Recent studies indicated that activating microglia/macrophages promoted hematoma absorption and neurological outcomes after ICH [14, 15, 28, 32]. However, the specific mechanism by which Scriptaid treatment improves hematoma resolution remains unknown and requires further research. In mouse TBI models, 3.5 mg/kg is the optimal dose of Scriptaid for TBI treatment [26]. Although many differences in the mechanism of brain injury exist between TBI and ICH, both conditions involve hematoma and brain edema. Therefore, we also chose 3.5 mg/kg for the treatment of ICH in our study.

Perihematomal brain edema can occur within hours of ICH and peak at several days [33, 34]. Brain edema after ICH can increase intracranial pressure and induce herniation. Edema formation after ICH has several phases,

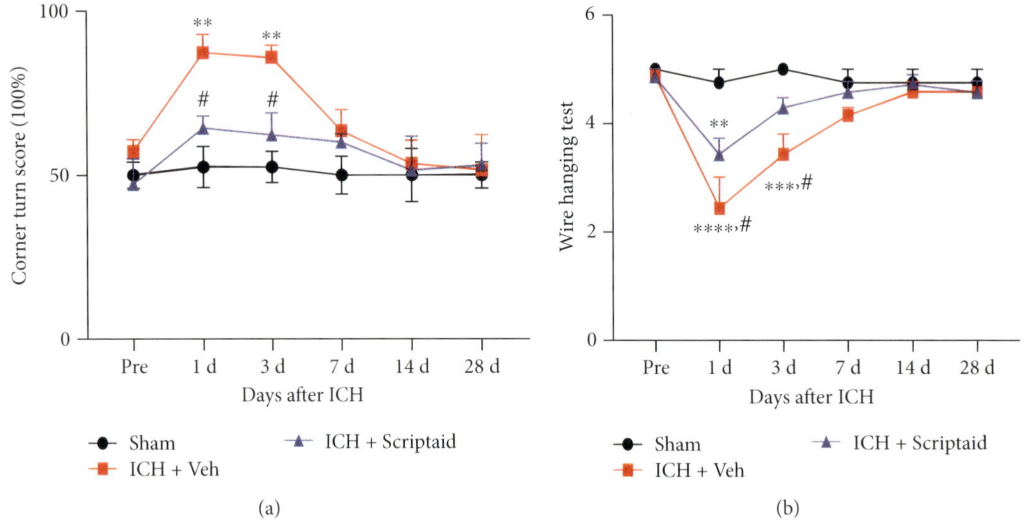

FIGURE 2: Scriptaid improved the neurological function deficit after ICH. (a) Corner turn test: Scriptaid treatment alleviated sensory deficits at 1 d and 3 d after ICH compared with the ICH + vehicle group ($^{**}P < 0.01$ versus the sham group; $^{\#}P < 0.05$ versus the ICH + vehicle group). (b) Wire hanging test: Scriptaid treatment alleviated motor deficits at 1 d and 3 d after ICH compared with the ICH + vehicle group ($^{**}P < 0.01$, $^{***}P < 0.001$, and $^{****}P < 0.001$ versus the sham group; $^{\#}P < 0.05$ versus the ICH + vehicle group).

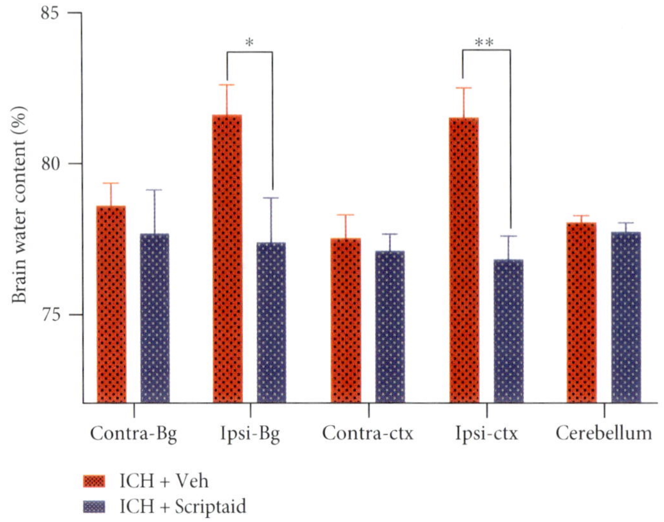

FIGURE 3: Scriptaid reduced the brain water content at 3 d after ICH. Compared with the vehicle group, the Scriptaid treatment group exhibited a significantly reduced brain water content in the ipsilateral basal ganglia and ipsilateral cortex at 3 d after ICH ($^{*}P < 0.05$, $^{**}P < 0.01$ versus the vehicle group). No significant difference in the brain water content in the contralateral basal ganglia and cortex was found between the Scriptaid treatment group and the vehicle group.

including an early phase (involving clot retraction and serum protein accumulation around the hematoma), a second phase (involving thrombin), and a third phase (involving erythrocyte components) [3, 33]. In the present study, Scriptaid treatment reduced perihematomal brain tissue edema at 3 d post-ICH. Thus, Scriptaid can improve hematoma clearance and reduce the mass effect, whereas HDACis can reduce inflammation and then protect the blood-brain barrier from disruption in mouse and rat ICH models [23, 24]. White matter injury is another important reason for poor outcomes of ICH. Recently, significant progress has been made in increasing the understanding of the role of white matter injury after ICH [35, 36]. Consistent with the present finding, Scriptaid has been described to prevent white matter injury in mouse TBI models [25]. Our data also showed that Scriptaid reduced white matter injury in mouse ICH models. Moreover, reducing white matter after ICH could improve neurological behavioral functions, such as sensorimotor function.

Although this study is a novel evaluation focused on the preservation of brain injury in ICH by Scriptaid, there are still several limitations: (1) no information was provided about the anti-inflammatory effect of Scriptaid and (2) no data demonstrated the relationship between

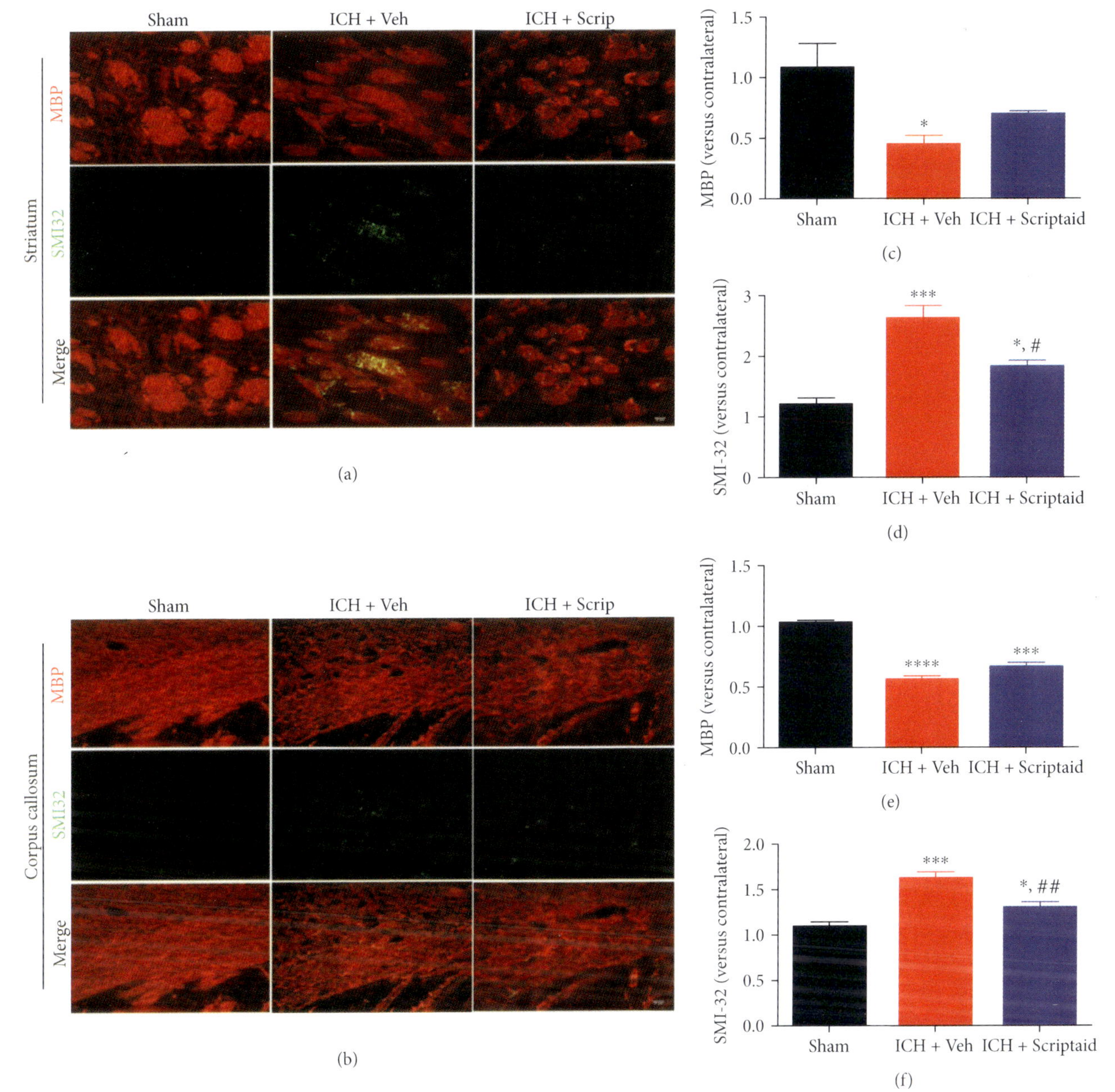

Figure 4: Scriptaid alleviated white matter injury at 35 d after ICH. (a, b) Representative images of myelin basic protein (MBP) (red) and SMI32 (green) immunostaining in the striatum (a) and corpus callosum (b) (scale bar = 25 μm). (c, d) The relative ratio of ipsilateral versus contralateral MBP (c) and SMI32 (d) immunostaining intensity 35 d after ICH in the striatum. (e, f) The relative ratio of ipsilateral versus contralateral MBP (e) and SMI32 (f) immunostaining intensity 35 d after ICH in the corpus callosum ($^{*}P < 0.05$, $^{***}P < 0.001$, and $^{****}P < 0.0001$ versus the sham group; $^{\#}P < 0.05$ and $^{\#\#}P < 0.01$ versus the vehicle group).

microglia/macrophage polarization and hematoma resolution after ICH. Therefore, we will conduct further research on the mechanism by which Scriptaid preserves brain injury in ICH.

In conclusion, our data demonstrate that Scriptaid treatment protects against brain injury by improving hematoma resolution, reducing brain edema, and alleviating white matter injury in a mouse ICH model. Thus, the histone deacetylase inhibitor Scriptaid can be considered a new medical therapy method for ICH.

Acknowledgments

The study was supported by grants from the national 973 Programs (2014CB541604-LFZ), the National Natural Science Foundation of China (NSFC) (81500987 and 81771237), and the Science and Technology Commission of Shanghai Municipality (STCSM) (15140902300).

References

[1] C. J. van Asch, M. J. A. Luitse, G. J. E. Rinkel, I. van der Tweel, A. Algra, and C. J. M. Klijn, "Incidence, case fatality, and functional outcome of intracerebral haemorrhage over time, according to age, sex, and ethnic origin: a systematic review and meta-analysis," *Lancet Neurology*, vol. 9, no. 2, pp. 167–176, 2010.

[2] R. F. Keep, Y. Hua, and G. Xi, "Intracerebral haemorrhage: mechanisms of injury and therapeutic targets," *Lancet Neurology*, vol. 11, no. 8, pp. 720–731, 2012.

[3] G. Xi, R. F. Keep, and J. T. Hoff, "Mechanisms of brain injury after intracerebral haemorrhage," *Lancet Neurology*, vol. 5, no. 1, pp. 53–63, 2006.

[4] Y. Zhou, Y. Wang, J. Wang, R. Anne Stetler, and Q. W. Yang, "Inflammation in intracerebral hemorrhage: from mechanisms to clinical translation," *Progress in Neurobiology*, vol. 115, pp. 25–44, 2014.

[5] J. Wang, "Preclinical and clinical research on inflammation after intracerebral hemorrhage," *Progress in Neurobiology*, vol. 92, no. 4, pp. 463–477, 2010.

[6] W. B. Rolland, T. Lekic, P. R. Krafft et al., "Fingolimod reduces cerebral lymphocyte infiltration in experimental models of rodent intracerebral hemorrhage," *Experimental Neurology*, vol. 241, pp. 45–55, 2013.

[7] J. Wang and S. Dore, "Heme oxygenase-1 exacerbates early brain injury after intracerebral haemorrhage," *Brain*, vol. 130, no. 6, pp. 1643–1652, 2007.

[8] J. Wang and S. Dore, "Inflammation after intracerebral hemorrhage," *Journal of Cerebral Blood Flow and Metabolism*, vol. 27, no. 5, pp. 894–908, 2007.

[9] J. Wang and S. E. Tsirka, "Contribution of extracellular proteolysis and microglia to intracerebral hemorrhage," *Neurocritical Care*, vol. 3, no. 1, pp. 077–085, 2005.

[10] X. Hu, R. K. Leak, Y. Shi et al., "Microglial and macrophage polarization-new prospects for brain repair," *Nature Reviews Neurology*, vol. 11, no. 1, pp. 56–64, 2015.

[11] X. Hu, P. Li, Y. Guo et al., "Microglia/macrophage polarization dynamics reveal novel mechanism of injury expansion after focal cerebral ischemia," *Stroke*, vol. 43, no. 11, pp. 3063–3070, 2012.

[12] G. Wang, J. Zhang, X. Hu et al., "Microglia/macrophage polarization dynamics in white matter after traumatic brain injury," *Journal of Cerebral Blood Flow and Metabolism*, vol. 33, no. 12, pp. 1864–1874, 2013.

[13] H. Zhao, T. Garton, R. F. Keep, Y. Hua, and G. Xi, "Microglia/macrophage polarization after experimental intracerebral hemorrhage," *Translational Stroke Research*, vol. 6, no. 6, pp. 407–409, 2015.

[14] X. Zhao, J. Grotta, N. Gonzales, and J. Aronowski, "Hematoma resolution as a therapeutic target the role of microglia/macrophages," *Stroke*, vol. 40, no. 3, Supplement 1, pp. S92–S94, 2009.

[15] X. Zhao, G. Sun, J. Zhang et al., "Hematoma resolution as a target for intracerebral hemorrhage treatment: role for peroxisome proliferator-activated receptor gamma in microglia/macrophages," *Annals of Neurology*, vol. 61, no. 4, pp. 352–362, 2007.

[16] G. Xi, J. Strahle, Y. Hua, and R. F. Keep, "Progress in translational research on intracerebral hemorrhage: is there an end in sight?," *Progress in Neurobiology*, vol. 115, pp. 45–63, 2014.

[17] J. Hrebackova, J. Hrabeta, and T. Eckschlager, "Valproic acid in the complex therapy of malignant tumors," *Current Drug Targets*, vol. 11, no. 3, pp. 361–379, 2010.

[18] B. Monti, E. Polazzi, and A. Contestabile, "Biochemical, molecular and epigenetic mechanisms of valproic acid neuroprotection," *Current Molecular Pharmacology*, vol. 2, no. 1, pp. 95–109, 2009.

[19] T. Nuutinen, T. Suuronen, A. Kauppinen, and A. Salminen, "Valproic acid stimulates clusterin expression in human astrocytes: implications for Alzheimer's disease," *Neuroscience Letters*, vol. 475, no. 2, pp. 64–68, 2010.

[20] F. Blanchard and C. Chipoy, "Histone deacetylase inhibitors: new drugs for the treatment of inflammatory diseases?," *Drug Discovery Today*, vol. 10, no. 3, pp. 197–204, 2005.

[21] R. Glauben and B. Siegmund, "Molecular basis of histone deacetylase inhibitors as new drugs for the treatment of inflammatory diseases and cancer," *Methods in Molecular Biology*, vol. 512, pp. 365–376, 2009.

[22] R. Patnala, T. V. Arumugam, N. Gupta, and S. T. Dheen, "HDAC inhibitor sodium butyrate-mediated epigenetic regulation enhances neuroprotective function of microglia during ischemic stroke," *Molecular Neurobiology*, vol. 54, no. 8, pp. 6391–6411, 2017.

[23] D. I. Sinn, S. J. Kim, K. Chu et al., "Valproic acid-mediated neuroprotection in intracerebral hemorrhage via histone deacetylase inhibition and transcriptional activation," *Neurobiology of Disease*, vol. 26, no. 2, pp. 464–472, 2007.

[24] S. Sukumari-Ramesh, C. H. Alleyne, and K. M. Dhandapani, "The histone deacetylase inhibitor suberoylanilide hydroxamic acid (SAHA) confers acute neuroprotection after intracerebral hemorrhage in mice," *Translational Stroke Research*, vol. 7, no. 2, pp. 141–148, 2016.

[25] G. Wang, Y. Shi, X. Jiang et al., "HDAC inhibition prevents white matter injury by modulating microglia/macrophage polarization through the GSK3β/PTEN/Akt axis," *Proceedings of the National Academy of Sciences of the United States of America*, vol. 112, no. 9, pp. 2853–2858, 2015.

[26] G. Wang, X. Jiang, H. Pu et al., "Scriptaid, a novel histone deacetylase inhibitor, protects against traumatic brain injury via modulation of PTEN and AKT pathway," *Neurotherapeutics*, vol. 10, no. 1, pp. 124–142, 2013.

[27] T. Nakamura, G. Xi, Y. Hua, T. Schallert, J. T. Hoff, and R. F. Keep, "Intracerebral hemorrhage in mice: model characterization and application for genetically modified mice," *Journal of Cerebral Blood Flow and Metabolism*, vol. 24, no. 5, pp. 487–494, 2016.

[28] W. Ni, S. Mao, G. Xi, R. F. Keep, and Y. Hua, "Role of erythrocyte CD47 in intracerebral hematoma clearance," *Stroke*, vol. 47, no. 2, pp. 505–511, 2016.

[29] H. Fang, J. Chen, S. Lin et al., "CD36-mediated hematoma absorption following intracerebral hemorrhage: negative regulation by TLR4 signaling," *Journal of Immunology*, vol. 192, no. 12, pp. 5984–5992, 2014.

[30] Y. Hua, T. Schallert, R. F. Keep, J. Wu, J. T. Hoff, and G. Xi, "Behavioral tests after intracerebral hemorrhage in the rat," *Stroke*, vol. 33, no. 10, pp. 2478–2484, 2002.

[31] F. P. Huang, G. Xi, R. F. Keep, Y. Hua, A. Nemoianu, and J. T. Hoff, "Brain edema after experimental intracerebral hemorrhage: role of hemoglobin degradation products," *Journal of Neurosurgery*, vol. 96, no. 2, pp. 287–293, 2002.

[32] X. Zhao, G. Sun, S. M. Ting et al., "Cleaning up after ICH: the role of Nrf2 in modulating microglia function and hematoma clearance," *Journal of Neurochemistry*, vol. 133, no. 1, pp. 144–152, 2015.

[33] G. Xi, R. F. Keep, and J. T. Hoff, "Pathophysiology of brain edema formation," *Neurosurgery Clinics of North America*, vol. 13, no. 3, pp. 371–383, 2002.

[34] A. R. Zazulia, M. N. Diringer, C. P. Derdeyn, and W. J. Powers, "Progression of mass effect after intracerebral hemorrhage," *Stroke*, vol. 30, no. 6, pp. 1167–1173, 1999.

[35] W. Ni, M. Okauchi, T. Hatakeyama et al., "Deferoxamine reduces intracerebral hemorrhage-induced white matter damage in aged rats," *Experimental Neurology*, vol. 272, pp. 128–134, 2015.

[36] Q. Xie, Y. Gu, Y. Hua, W. Liu, R. F. Keep, and G. Xi, "Deferoxamine attenuates white matter injury in a piglet intracerebral hemorrhage model," *Stroke*, vol. 45, no. 1, pp. 290–292, 2013.

Prophylactic use of Troxerutin can Delay the Development of Diabetic Cognitive Dysfunction and Improve the Expression of Nrf2 in the Hippocampus on STZ Diabetic Rats

Songyun Zhang, Lingling Yuan, Lihui Zhang, Caige Li, and Jie Li

The Second Hospital of Hebei Medical University, No. 215 Heping Road (West), Shijiazhuang City, Hebei Province, China

Correspondence should be addressed to Lihui Zhang; zhanglihui10510@163.com

Academic Editor: Tauheed Ishrat

Background. With the change in lifestyle and the aging population, the incidence of cognitive dysfunction in diabetes mellitus is rising sharply. Oxidative stress is an important mechanism in the development of diabetic cognitive dysfunction. Nuclear factor E2-related factor 2 (Nrf2) is the core transcription factor of antioxidative stress. Early prevention and treatment of diabetic cognitive dysfunction can reduce the incidence of dementia and improve the quality of life of diabetic patients. *Aim.* This study was aimed at determining effect of troxerutin on the development of cognitive dysfunction and the expression level of Nrf2 in the hippocampus of streptozotocin (STZ) diabetic rats, when used in the early preventive stage. *Methods.* An STZ-induced diabetic rat model was established ($n = 30$), and the animals were randomly divided into 2 groups: diabetic control group (DC, $n = 15$) and diabetic troxerutin intervention group (DT, $n = 15$). Another 10 normoglycemic rats were put into a normal control group (NC, $n = 10$). While the DT group was injected with troxerutin (60 mg/kg), the DC group and the NC group were injected with physiological saline for 12 weeks daily. Learning and memory behaviors were tested using the Morris water maze test. The superoxide dismutase (SOD) activity, malondialdehyde (MDA) content, mRNA level, and protein level of Nrf2 were measured. Data were collected and analyzed by the statistical software package SPSS 19.0, which included one-way analysis of variance with completely randomized design. *Results.* Learning and memory levels were significantly improved in the DT group compared with the DC group. Moreover, in the DT group, the expression level of Nrf2 in the hippocampus was increased, activity of SOD was elevated, and MDA content was decreased. *Conclusion.* Prophylactic use of troxerutin delays the development of diabetic cognitive dysfunction and increases the expression level of Nrf2 in the hippocampus of STZ diabetic rats.

1. Introduction

As diabetes mellitus can cause cognitive dysfunction, it has become an important research domain. However, the exact mechanisms of diabetic encephalopathy are yet to be identified. Nevertheless, increasing evidence indicates that oxidative stress is an important mechanism in the development of diabetic cognitive dysfunction. Malondialdehyde (MDA) content and superoxide dismutase (SOD) activity are classic indicators in assessing the balance between oxidative and antioxidant systems. Nrf2 is considered to be the main transcription factor of antioxidative stress [1, 2]. In addition, Nrf2 is closely related with cognitive dysfunction [3, 4].

Troxerutin is a flavonol (a type of flavonoid) or, more accurately, a hydroxyethylrutoside. Troxerutin has been reported to possess strong antioxidant and anti-inflammatory properties [5–9]. Importantly, early prevention and treatment of diabetic cognitive dysfunction can reduce the incidence of dementia and improve the quality of life of diabetic patients [3–7]. This study aimed to observe the development of cognitive dysfunction and determine the expression levels of Nrf2 in the hippocampus of streptozotocin (STZ) diabetic rats when using troxerutin in the early preventive stage.

2. Results

2.1. Morris Water Maze Test

2.1.1. Basic Swimming Speed. There was no statistical difference in swimming speed between the three groups (Table 1).

2.1.2. Navigation Test. Repeated measures ANOVA was used to compare the data between each group. The effect of time did not result in significant changes among the groups ($P = 0.058$). The escape latency of the DC group was significantly longer when compared with that of the NC group ($P < 0.001$). This indicated that diabetic rats had cognitive dysfunction after having successfully modeled for 12 weeks. The DT group had a shorter escape latency than the DC group ($P < 0.001$). This suggests that treatment with troxerutin for 12 weeks can reduce cognitive dysfunction. There were no significant differences in escape latency among the NC, DC, and DT groups after the first day (day 1, $P = 0.256$). Compared with the NC group, the escape latency of DC rats was longer during the subsequent 4 days (day 2, $P < 0.001$; day 3, $P < 0.001$; day 4, $P < 0.001$; day 5, $P < 0.001$). On day 2, the escape latency of the DC group was not significantly different from that of the DT group ($P = 0.061$). From the third to the fifth day, the escape latency of the DT group was significantly shorter than that of the DC group (day 3–day 5: $P < 0.001$) (Table 2).

2.1.3. Probe Test. When comparing the number of times the rats crossed to the platform in 60s, the number of the NC group was greater than those of the DC group and DT group. Moreover, the number of the DT group was greater than that of the DC group ($F_{2,27} = 185.33$, $P < 0.001$) (Table 3).

2.2. HE Staining. After observing a series of histopathologic alterations in the hippocampal neurons of the DC group, the number of normal neurons significantly decreased. On the contrary, the majority of the CAl neurons in the DT and NC groups maintained normal morphology, showing integrated structures and being lined up in order. Moreover, there was less neuron depletion in the DT and NC groups compared to the DC group (Figure 1).

2.3. Immunohistochemical Staining. The optical density (OD) value of the Nrf2-positive cells in the hippocampus of rats in the NC group was higher than that of rats in the DC group and the DT group. Compared with the DC group, the OD value of the Nrf2-positive hippocampal cells of rats in the DT group was increased ($F_{2,87} = 64.67$, $P < 0.001$) (Figure 2).

2.4. Nrf2 mRNA Expression. When compared with the NC group, mRNA expression of Nrf2 decreased in the DC group and the DT group. Moreover, there was a statistically significant difference between the DC group and the DT group, the Nrf2 mRNA level being higher in the latter ($F_{2,15} = 2815.91$, $P < 0.001$) (Figure 3(a)).

TABLE 1: The basic swimming speed of the rats in different groups (cm/s, $\bar{x} + s$).

Group	n	The swimming speed
NC	10	30.67 ± 2.58
DC	10	$28.32 \pm 1.65^{\triangle}$
DT	10	$30.06 \pm 2.58^{\triangle\blacktriangle}$

Note: compared to NC, $^{\triangle}P > 0.05$; compared to DC, $^{\blacktriangle}P > 0.05$.

2.5. Nrf2 Protein Expression. Total Nrf2 protein: The expression level of total Nrf2 protein in the hippocampus of rats in the DC and the DT groups was lower than that of rats in the NC group. Moreover, the total Nrf2 protein expression of the DT group was significantly higher than that of the DC group ($F_{2,15} = 107.95$, $P < 0.001$) (Figure 3(b)).

Nuclear Nrf2 protein: The expression level of nuclear Nrf2 protein in the hippocampus of rats in groups DC and DT was lower than that of rats in the NC group. Furthermore, the expression level of nuclear Nrf2 protein of rats in the DT group was higher than that of rats in the DC group ($F_{2,15} = 65.73$, $P < 0.001$) (Figure 3(c)).

2.6. SOD Activity and MDA Content. SOD activity: The SOD activity of the NC group was higher than that of the DC group. There was no statistical significance between groups NC and DT. However, the SOD activity of the DT group was increased compared with that of the DC group ($F_{2,15} = 5.873$, $P = 0.013$) (Figure 4(a)).

MDA content: The MDA content of the NC group was lower than that of the DC group. There was no statistical significance between the NC group and the DT group. However, the MDA content of the DT group was decreased compared with that of the DC group ($F_{2,15} = 7.868$, $P = 0.005$) (Figure 4(b)).

3. Discussion

Modeling is crucial during an experiment, because if an animal model fails, the experimental results will not be reliable.

To successfully develop the rat model of type 1 diabetes mellitus, rats with blood glucose level ≥ 16.7 mmol/L at 72 h after an STZ injection (60 mg/kg) were included in the model.

Rats with blood glucose level < 16.7 mmol/L were rejected once a week [10, 11]. According to the test proposed by Wang et al. [12], 72 SD male rats, aged 8 weeks, were used. Type 1 diabetes mellitus rats began to show cognitive dysfunction symptoms after 6 weeks. More importantly, the symptoms became more apparent after 12 weeks. In this study, rat cognitive function was tested via the Morris water maze, and the results demonstrated that type 1 diabetes mellitus rats became cognitively dysfunctional after 12 weeks.

Troxerutin is 3-hydroxy-rutin and soluble in water [13]. Compared to the intragastric administration, intraperitoneal injection has shorter administration time and is easier to operate. A liquid volume equivalent to 3–8% of animal weight can be absorbed in one hour. This is because a larger area of the peritoneum and clouds of blood vessels are

Table 2: The escape latencies of the rats in different groups in place navigation test (s, $\bar{x} + s$).

Group	n	Day 1	Day 2	Day 3	Day 4	Day 5
NC	10	22.08 ± 12.22	11.01 ± 4.19	7.82 ± 3.84	7.52 ± 3.06	5.81 ± 2.33
DC	10	29.22 ± 14.10$^{\triangle}$	32.56 ± 15.66$^{\triangle}$	28.58 ± 12.21$^{\triangle}$	28.72 ± 3.59$^{\triangle}$	24.68 ± 8.02$^{\triangle}$
DT	10	25.94 ± 15.03$^{\triangle\blacktriangle}$	25.38 ± 16.21$^{\triangle\blacktriangle}$	16.00 ± 8.33$^{\triangle\blacktriangle}$	14.72 ± 6.29$^{\triangle\blacktriangle}$	15.04 ± 10.20$^{\triangle\blacktriangle}$

Note: compared to NC, $^{\triangle}P < 0.01$; compared to DC, $^{\blacktriangle}P < 0.01$.

Table 3: The times of crossing platform in 60s in different groups in spatial probe test ($\bar{x} + s$).

Group	n	Times of cross the platform area
NC	10	16.00 ± 1.83
DC	10	3.00 ± 0.91$^{\triangle}$
DT	10	13.00 ± 1.83$^{\triangle\blacktriangle}$

Note: compared to NC, $^{\triangle}P < 0.001$; compared to DC, $^{\blacktriangle}P < 0.001$.

exposed, and the peritoneum has a particularly strong lymphatic absorption capacity for the drug. Clinical trials found that troxerutin has a high safety profile, tolerability, and other advantages, even at high doses [13]. Moreover, a previous study [14] confirmed that 150 mg/kg/d (ig) is the optimal dose for treatment of cognitive dysfunction of diabetic rats.

Furthermore, the dose administered to the rats was equivalent to that previously administered to mice, and the dose administered intraperitoneally was 0.3 to 0.5 times greater than the dose administered intragastrically.

Therefore, in this experiment, rats in the DT group were injected with 60 mg/kg/d (i.e., 150 × 0.4 mg/kg/d) of troxerutin.

In the present study, the Morris water maze test was proven to be a credible test for cognitive dysfunction related to hippocampal synaptic plasticity [15]. The navigation test was used to test the spatial learning ability of rats, whereas the probe test was used to test their spatial memory. The basis of cognitive dysfunction in pathology is the connecting dysfunction of the prefrontal-striatum-thalamus-temporal lobe, which features the hippocampus and plays an important role [16]. The hippocampus is one of the most important nerve centers in learning and memory. Its structure and function are closely linked to diabetic cognitive dysfunction [17]. SOD activity reflects antioxidant levels, and MDA content reflects oxidative levels; thus, these measurements are frequently used to assess oxidative damage [18]. Our results were consistent with those of other recent studies, in that troxerutin has strong antioxidant and anti-inflammatory properties [19]. An important cellular defense mechanism under oxidative stress is the Nrf2-mediated expression of endogenous antioxidants [20].

In this experiment, hippocampus tissues were stained with HE, and CA1 hippocampal nerve cells of rats in the NC group were eumorphic, structurally integral, and ordered; cells in the DC group were disordered, with shrunken cell bodies and red cytoplasm, and the number of nerve cells with normal morphology was significantly reduced; cells in the DT group were arranged in order, structurally integrated. These results suggest that the hippocampal damage in the DC group is morphological, which affects the cognitive function. The degree of hippocampal impairment in the DT group was lower than that in the DC group; thus, the preventive use of troxerutin could alleviate damage to the hippocampus and reduce cognitive impairment, to a certain extent.

In this experiment, the blood glucose level of rats in the DT group was not significantly different from that of rats in the DC group. This illustrates that troxerutin cannot decrease blood glucose level, which agrees with the results of Geetha et al., who tested 36 rats weighing 25~30 g by administrating a high-fat, high-carbohydrate diet. The results suggested that troxerutin reduces body weight, blood pressure, and insulin resistance [21], but does not induce a significant decrease in blood glucose level. In this study, the results of the Morris water maze test proved that the prophylactic use of troxerutin can delay the development of diabetic cognitive dysfunction in STZ diabetic rats. Additionally, the prophylactic use of troxerutin can increase SOD activity in the hippocampus, suggesting that it can improve the antioxidant ability. Both the mRNA and protein expression of Nrf2 were higher in the DT group than in the DC group. This demonstrated that the prophylactic use of troxerutin in rats increases Nrf2 content in the hippocampus. Therefore, troxerutin administered prophylactically delays the development of diabetes-induced cognitive dysfunction in rats by increasing the Nrf2 content in the hippocampus.

4. Methods

4.1. Animals and Drug Administration. All procedures involving animals were in accordance with the *Guide for the Care and Use of Laboratory Animals.* Forty male Sprague-Dawley rats (age 6–8 weeks, from Beijing Vital River Laboratory Animal Technology Co., certificate number 1100195543) were randomly divided into a normal control group (NC group, $n = 10$ rats) and a diabetic group ($n = 30$ rats). The rats fasted overnight. Then, STZ was dissolved in 0.1 mol/L sodium citrate buffer, pH 4.4, and the 30 rats were intraperitoneally injected with STZ citrate buffer (60 mg/kg/d, Sigma Company, USA). At 72 hours after the injection, the blood glucose level of the rats was determined via their tail veins using a blood glucose meter. Fasted rats with a blood glucose level above 16.7 mmol/L were considered to be diabetic and were randomly divided between a diabetic control group (DC group, $n = 15$) and a diabetic troxerutin intervention group (DT group, $n = 15$).

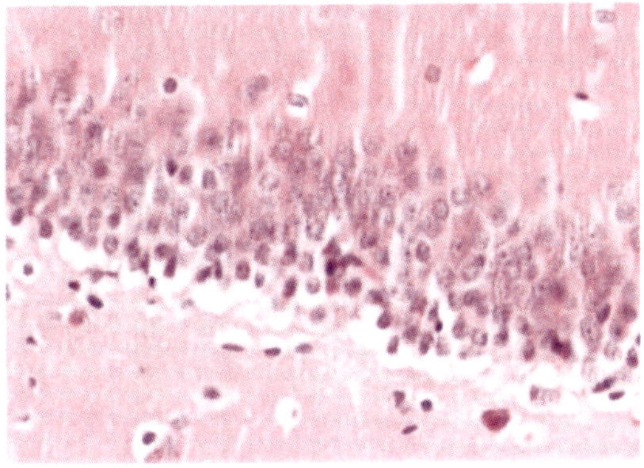

NC

(a)

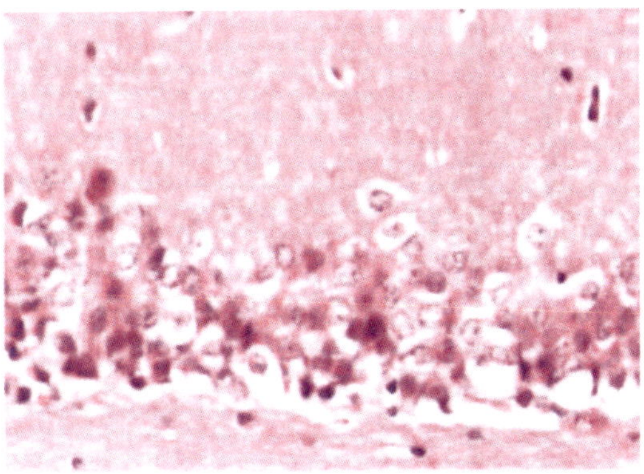

DC

(b)

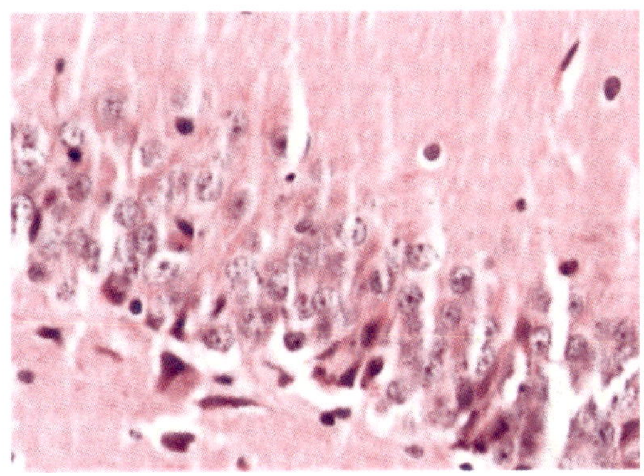

DT

(c)

FIGURE 1: Representative photomicrographs of the hippocampal CA1 area showing the histological changes in different groups (HE, ×200). NC: normal control group; DC: diabetic control group; DT: diabetic troxerutin intervention group.

Rats in the DT group were intraperitoneally injected with troxerutin (60 mg/kg, 1 mL/kg, Jingchun Biochemistry Technology Corporation, Shanghai, China), while those in the DC and NC groups were intraperitoneally injected with physiological saline once daily for 12 weeks. Finally, the blood glucose levels were measured after 12 weeks of troxerutin treatment.

4.2. Morris Water Maze Test. The rats were tested in the Morris water maze at the end of the treatment period (12 weeks). Basic swimming speed of the rats was assessed the day prior to the test. Rats were pretested to determine their treadmill running willingness and those rats which refused to run were excluded from the water maze experiments. The maze consisted of a circular pool (150 cm in diameter and 60 cm in height) that contained a hidden platform. The apparatus was used to assess the learning and memory performance of rats. Rats were trained to locate the hidden platform using only distal extra maze cues.

For the navigation test, the tracks of rats were recorded and analyzed by using a camera connected to a video recorder and the EthoVision tracking system (Zhenghua Bio-instruments Co. Ltd., Huaibei, Anhui). Each rat was allowed to search for the platform for 60 seconds, and rest on the platform for 30 seconds once found. Then, the rats were placed back in their respective cages. Rats that failed to find the platform within 60 seconds were manually guided to the platform and placed on the platform for 30 seconds before being returned to their cages. Each rat received four learning trials in the four quadrants (N, S, E, and W) per day for five consecutive days. The times spent searching for the platform and the mounting latency were calculated.

On the sixth day, the rats were given the probe test, in which the platform was removed from the pool. Rats were randomly placed into a quadrant and were allowed to swim freely for 60 s. The number of times the rats swarm across the platform in 60 s was recorded [15].

4.3. Biochemical Assessment. On the seventh day, the rats were sacrificed, and their left and right hippocampus was removed promptly. The right side of the hippocampus was used for hematoxylin and eosin (HE) staining and immunohistochemistry. The left side of the hippocampus was transferred to a 4°C ice-cold board for dissection and then used to measure SOD activity and MDA content and to detect the mRNA (reverse transcription polymerase chain

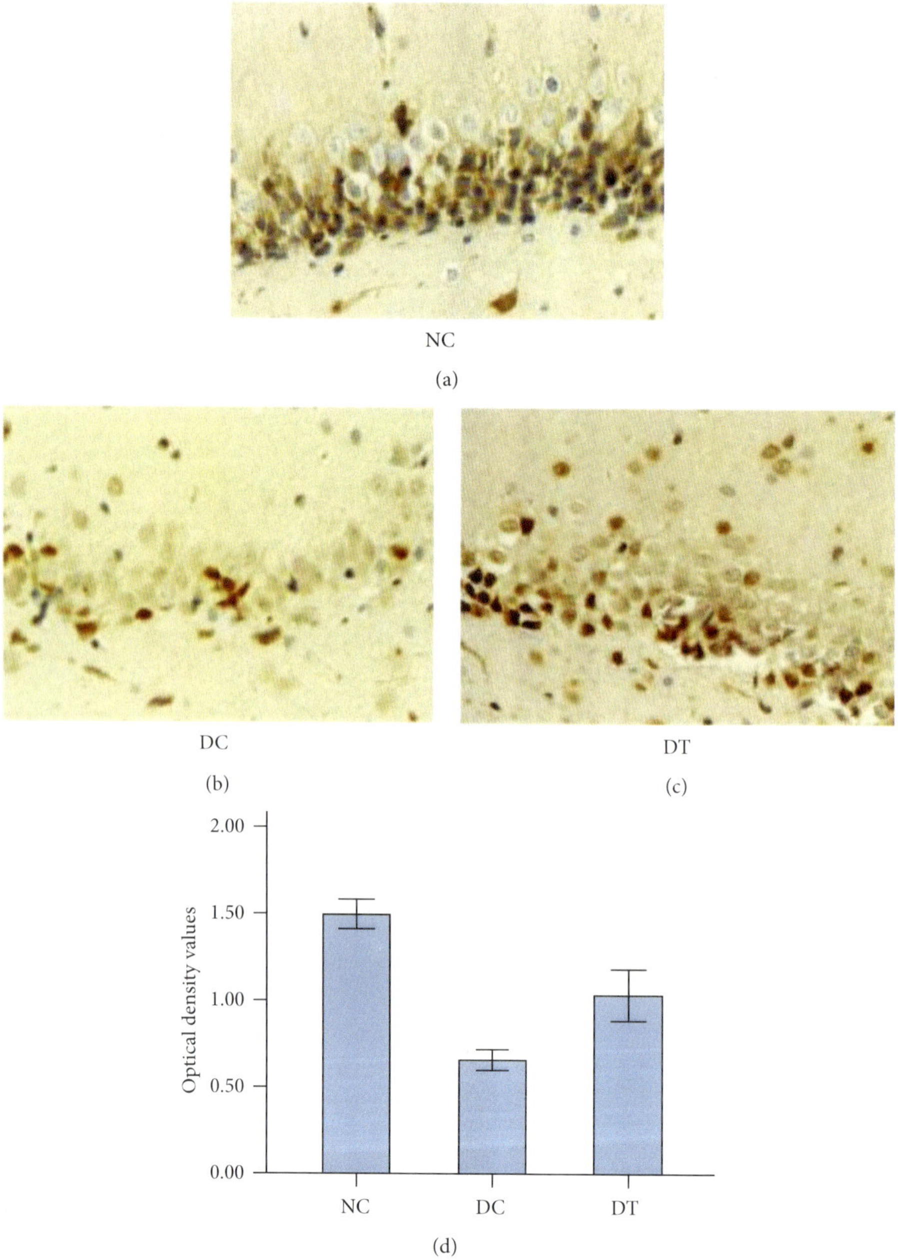

FIGURE 2: The optical density values of Nrf2 in hippocampal CA1 area of each group (IHC, ×200). Results shown are mean ± SD ($n = 6$). $P < 0.001$ DT versus DC.

reaction, RT-PCR) and protein (Western blot analysis) levels of Nrf2 in both cytoplasm and nucleus.

4.3.1. HE Staining. The syringe containing the sample was kept vertically and still for 10 to 20 minutes, with the needle end pointing downward. The glass slides were cleaned, disinfected with 75% ethanol, and then dried. One droplet of test solution was added to the glass slide and dried at room temperature. The sample was then fixed in methanol solution for 30 minutes. The methanol solution was removed, and the sample was hydrated with distilled water and subjected to conventional HE staining.

4.3.2. Immunohistochemistry for Nrf2 Expression. Sections were dehydrated in xylene and graded alcohol series. The sections were then rinsed for 5 minutes with tap water and incubated for 30 minutes in 0.3% H_2O_2 in methanol. After, they were washed for 5 minutes with buffer and incubated for 20 minutes in diluted normal serum from the species in which the secondary antibody was obtained. Excess serum from sections was blotted. Then, the sections were incubated for 30 minutes in primary antiserum diluted with buffer. Slides were subsequently washed for 5 minutes with buffer. Sections were incubated for 30 minutes in diluted biotinylated secondary antibody solution, followed by a 5-minute

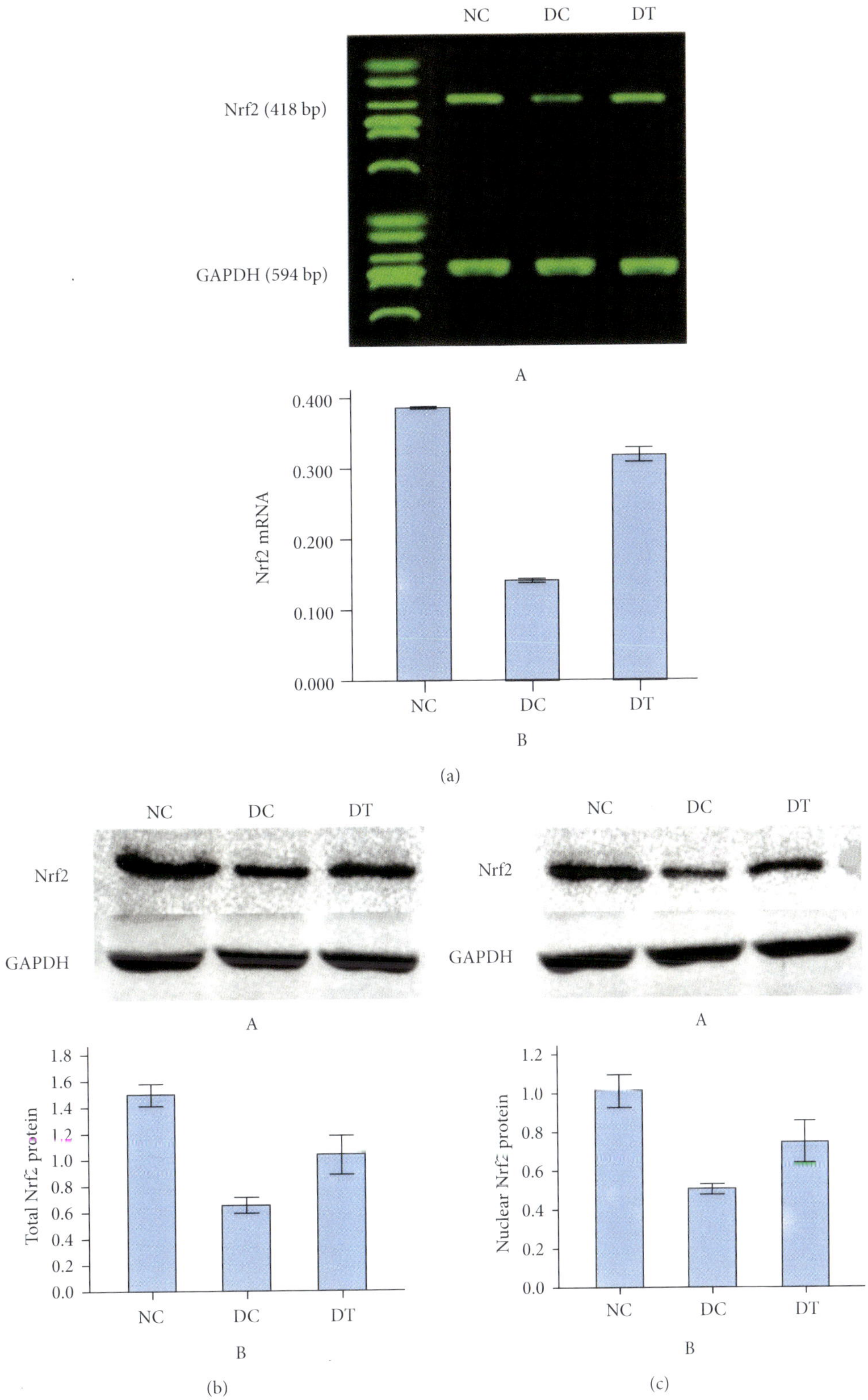

FIGURE 3: (a) The expression of total Nrf2 mRNA in different groups. Results shown are mean ± SD ($n = 6$), $P < 0.001$ DT versus DC. (b) The expression of total Nrf2 protein in different groups. Results shown are mean ± SD ($n = 6$), $P < 0.001$ DT versus DC. (c) The expression of nuclear Nrf2 protein in different groups. Results shown are mean ± SD ($n = 6$), $P < 0.001$ DT versus DC.

washing step in buffer. Sections were then incubated for 30 minutes in VECTASTAIN ABC Reagent and washed for another 5 minutes with buffer. Next, sections were incubated in peroxidase substrate solution until the stain developed to the desired intensity. Lastly, sections were rinsed with tap water, counterstained, cleared, and mounted for observation.

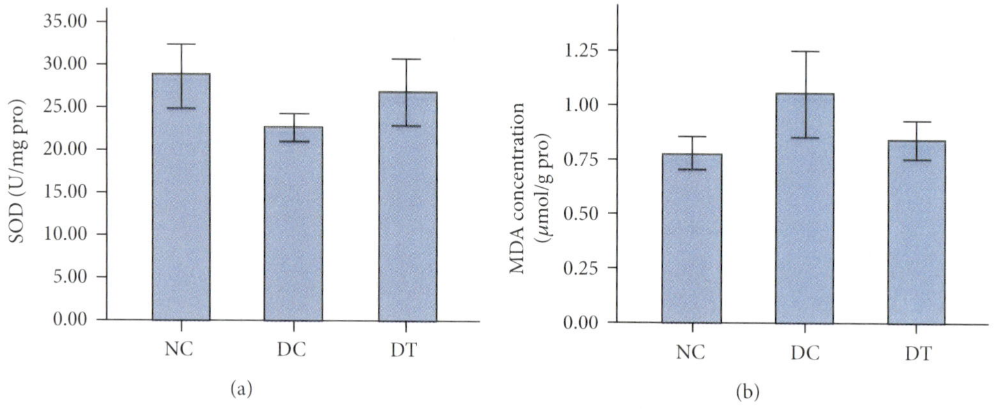

FIGURE 4: (a) The activity of SOD in different groups. Results shown are mean ± SD ($n = 6$), $P < 0.05$ DT versus DC. (b) The MDA concentration in different groups. Results shown are mean ± SD ($n = 6$), $P < 0.01$ DT versus DC.

4.3.3. Quantitative Assessment of Nrf2 mRNA by RT-PCR. Four rats from each group were randomly selected. Total RNA from the hippocampus was isolated using Trizol (Invitrogen Co.), according to the manufacturer's instructions. Reverse transcription was performed using the DEPC (USA Co.). The expression of the housekeeping gene glyceraldehyde-3-phosphate dehydrogenase (GAPDH) mRNA was used as an internal standard. PCR was performed for 30 cycles in an Eppendorf Mastercycler. Denaturing, annealing, and extension reactions were performed at 94°C for 30 minutes, 60°C for 30 seconds, and 72°C for 1 minute, respectively. Then, the PCR products were separated by 1% agarose gel electrophoresis, stained with GoldView, photographed under ultraviolet illumination, compared with a known standard ladder, and quantified by densitometry using the Bio-1D system. The levels of Nrf2 mRNA were expressed as their respective ratios to GAPDH mRNA.

4.3.4. Western Blotting Analysis for Determining the Nrf2 Protein Levels. Approximately 500–600 mg of tissue homogenate were added to 1 mL of extraction solution. The mixture was then centrifuged at 12,000 rpm for 5 minutes, at 4°C, and the supernatant was collected. An equal volume of sample buffer was added to the supernatant on χSDS. The sample was then boiled for 5 min at 100°C. The same amount of total protein was added to each well, to undergo polyacrylamide gel electrophoresis. The proteins were transferred to a membrane by electric water bath blotting. After the membrane was shaken in a petri dish for 2 hours at room temperature, primary antibody (diluted 1:250 in blocking buffer) [Nrf2 (C-20) is an affinity purified rabbit polyclonal antibody raised against a peptide mapping at the C-terminus of Nrf2 of human origin, Santa Cruz Biotechnology] was added and incubated for 2 hours at room temperature. The membrane was subsequently washed with PBS-Tween three times. After washing, labeled horseradish peroxidase (HRP) secondary antibody (diluted 1 : 5000 in blocking buffer) [GAPDH(0411) is a mouse monoclonal antibody raised against recombinant GAPDH of human origin] was added, and the petri dish was shaken for 1 hour at room temperature. After washing the membrane sufficiently with PBS-Tween, the membrane was immersed in DAB color development solution and was let to sit at room temperature for full color development. Then, the membrane was washed with distilled water and immediately transferred to PBS for observation. Lastly, the membrane was photographed and analyzed.

4.3.5. SOD Activity and MDA Content. SOD activity is measured by testing the capacity of pyrogallol to autoxidize. The inhibition of autoxidation of this compound occurs when SOD (Jian Cheng Technology Corporation, China) is present, and the enzymatic activity can be assayed indirectly using a temperature-controlled double-beam spectrophotometer at an absorbance of 420 nm. A 50% inhibition of pyrogallol autoxidation is defined as 1 U SOD. For testing MDA (Jian Cheng Technology Corporation, China) levels, the samples were mixed with 1 mL of 10% trichloroacetic acid and 1 mL of 0.67% thiobarbituric acid and then heated in a boiling water bath for 30 minutes. Malondialdehyde equivalents were detected in both tissue and submitochondrial particles of the rats' brain using a spectrophotometer at an absorbance of 532 nm.

4.4. Statistical Analysis. Data were collected and analyzed by the statistical software package SPSS 19.0, which includes one-factor ANOVA with completely randomized design. Repeated measures ANOVA was used to analyze the results of the Morris water maze test. The method of Bonferroni was used to perform pairwise comparisons of the repeatedly measured data from the different measurement times of each treated group, as previously described [22]. As the data passed the normality test ($P > 0.10$), the results were evaluated as the mean ± standard deviation. Values of $P < 0.05$ were considered statistically significant.

Additional Points

Highlights. (1) This research emphasizes the importance of preventive intervention. (2) The mechanism of diabetic cognitive dysfunction relies on oxidative stress. (3) The prophylactic use of troxerutin can delay the development of diabetic cognitive dysfunction. (4) The prophylactic use of troxerutin can improve the expression of Nrf2 in the hippocampus of STZ diabetic rats.

Ethical Approval

This research states that all animal experiments conformed to institutional standards.

References

[1] K. Itoh, T. Chiba, S. Takahashi et al., "An Nrf2/small Maf heterodimer mediates the induction of phase II detoxifying enzyme genes through antioxidant response elements," *Biochemical and Biophysical Research Communications*, vol. 236, no. 2, pp. 313–322, 1997.

[2] T. H. Rushmore, M. R. Morton, and C. B. Pickett, "The antioxidant responsive element. Activation by oxidative stress and identification of the DNA consensus sequence required for functional activity," *Journal of Biological Chemistry*, vol. 266, no. 18, pp. 11632–11639, 1991.

[3] Z. Wang, C. Ji, L. Wu et al., "Tert-butylhydroquinone alleviates early brain injury and cognitive dysfunction after experimental subarachnoid hemorrhage: role of Keap1/Nrf2/ARE pathway," *PLoS One*, vol. 9, no. 5, article e97685, 2014.

[4] R. Chandran, T. Kim, S. L. Mehta et al., "A combination antioxidant therapy to inhibit NOX2 and activate Nrf2 decreases secondary brain damage and improves functional recovery after traumatic brain injury," *Journal of Cerebral Blood Flow & Metabolism*, pp. 1–9, 2017.

[5] S. H. Fan, Z. F. Zhang, Y. L. Zheng et al., "Troxerutin protects the mouse kidney from D-galactose-caused injury through anti-inflammation and anti-oxidation," *International Immunopharmacology*, vol. 9, no. 1, pp. 91–96, 2009.

[6] C. M. Liu, J. Q. Ma, and Y. Lou, "Chronic administration of troxerutin protects mouse kidney against D-galactose-induced oxidative DNA damage," *Food and Chemical Toxicology*, vol. 48, no. 10, pp. 2809–2817, 2010.

[7] Z. F. Zhang, S. H. Fan, Y. L. Zheng et al., "Troxerutin protects the mouse liver against oxidative stress-mediated injury induced by D-galactose," *Journal of Agricultural and Food Chemistry*, vol. 57, no. 17, pp. 7731–7736, 2009.

[8] J. Lu, D. M. Wu, B. Hu, Y. L. Zheng, Z. F. Zhang, and Y. J. Wang, "NGF-dependent activation of TrkA pathway: a mechanism for the neuroprotective effect of troxerutin in D-galactose-treated mice," *Brain Pathology*, vol. 20, no. 5, pp. 952–965, 2010.

[9] J. Lu, D. M. Wu, Z. H. Zheng, Y. L. Zheng, B. Hu, and Z. F. Zhang, "Troxerutin protects against high cholesterol-induced cognitive deficits in mice," *Brain*, vol. 134, no. 3, pp. 783–797, 2011.

[10] Z. Razga, G. Kovacs, N. Bódi, T. P3, and J. R. Nyengaard, "Heterogeneous downregulation of angiotensin II AT1-A and AT1-B receptors in arterioles in STZ-induced diabetic rat kidneys," *BioMed Research International*, vol. 2014, Article ID 947506, 6 pages, 2014.

[11] T. Baluchnejadmojarad and M. Roghani, "Chronic oral epigallocatechin-gallate alleviates streptozotocin-induced diabetic neuropathic hyperalgesia in rat: involvement of oxidative stress," *Iranian Journal of Pharmaceutical Research*, vol. 11, no. 4, pp. 1243–1253, 2012.

[12] F. Wang, G. Z. Yang, and S. Liu, "Observational research on type 1 diabetes mellitus rats complicated cognitive dysfunction," in *Chinese Medical Association the Seventh Nationwide Young Laboratory Medicine Conference Proceedings*, pp. 548-549, 2012, http://219.140.69.158/D/Conference_8575243.aspx.

[13] Y. Q. Fu, "Troxerutin pharmacological properties and clinical application profiles," *China Pharmaceutical Directory*, vol. 10, no. 7, pp. 59-60, 2012.

[14] D. K. Maurya, S. Balakrishnan, V. P. Salvi, and C. K. Nair, "Protection of cellular DNA from γ-radiation-induced damages and enhancement in DNA repair by troxerutin," *Molecular and Cellular Biochemistry*, vol. 280, no. 1-2, pp. 57–68, 2005.

[15] C. V. Vorhees and M. T. Williams, "Morris water maze: procedures for assessing spatial and related forms of learning and memory," *Nature Protocols*, vol. 1, no. 2, pp. 848–858, 2006.

[16] Q. F. Wei, H. L. Lan, and H. Y. Tan, "Research related to diabetes mellitus and cognitive impairment," *Medical Review*, vol. 16, no. 11, pp. 1696–1699, 2010.

[17] S. H. Wang, X. M. Jia, and H. L. Ke, "Hippocampus and diabetic cognitive dysfunction," *Neuroanatomy*, vol. 20, no. 6, pp. 637–640, 2004.

[18] F. Atig, M. Raffa, H. B. Ali, A. Saad, and M. Ajina, "Altered antioxidant status and increased lipid peroxidation in seminal plasma of Tunisian infertile men," *International Journal of Biological Sciences*, vol. 8, no. 1, pp. 139–149, 2012.

[19] J. Lu, D. M. Wu, Y. L. Zheng et al., "Troxerutin counteracts domoic acid–induced memory deficits in mice by inhibiting CCAAT/enhancer binding protein β–mediated inflammatory response and oxidative stress," *The Journal of Immunology*, vol. 190, no. 7, pp. 3466–3479, 2013.

[20] H. Y. Cho, S. P. Reddy, and S. R. Kleeberger, "Nrf2 defends the lung from oxidative stress," *Antioxidants & Redox Signaling*, vol. 8, no. 1-2, pp. 76–87, 2006.

[21] R. Geetha, B. Yogalakshmi, S. Sreeja, and C. V. Anuradha, "Troxerutin suppresses lipid abnormalities in the heart of high-fat–high-fructose diet-fed mice," *Molecular and Cellular Biochemistry*, vol. 387, no. 1-2, pp. 123–134, 2014.

[22] H. Qiu, G. Q. Jin, R. F. Jin, and W. K. Zhao, "Analysis of variance of repeated data measured by water maze with SPSS," *Journal of Chinese Integrative Medicine*, vol. 5, pp. 101–105, 2007.

24

Incidence and Comorbidity of Dementia with Lewy Bodies: A Population-Based Cohort Study

Sheng-Kung Yang,[1] Weishan Chen,[2,3] Chun-Hsien Su,[4] and Chung-Hsiang Liu[5]

[1] *Department of Neurology, Chang Bing Show Chwan Memorial Hospital, Changhua County, Taiwan*
[2] *Management Office for Health Data, China Medical University Hospital, Taichung, Taiwan*
[3] *College of Medicine, China Medical University, Taichung, Taiwan*
[4] *Department of Exercise and Health Promotion, College of Education, Chinese Culture University, Taipei, Taiwan*
[5] *Department of Neurology, China Medical University Hospital, Taichung, Taiwan*

Correspondence should be addressed to Chung-Hsiang Liu; greengen@gmail.com

Academic Editor: Shinro Matsuo

Background and Aims. Dementia with Lewy bodies (DLB) is the third most common form of dementia. Epidemiological studies of DLB in Taiwan are scarce. In this study, we estimated the incidence of DLB and comorbidity in the population of Taiwan. *Methods.* Data were obtained from the Taiwan National Health Insurance Research Database (NHIRD). DLB patients between 2000 and 2013 were enrolled in assessments of incidence and comorbidity. *Results.* The incidence of DLB was shown to be 7.10 per 100,000 person-years (95% CI = 6.63–7.59), which increased with age. The average age at diagnosis was 76.3, and this was higher for males than for females. The comorbidity rates of hypertension and hyperlipidemia in DLB patients were higher in females than in males. *Conclusions.* Epidemiologic data from large-scale retrospective studies is crucial to the prevention of DLB.

1. Introduction

Dementia is a major health issue around the globe. Affected individuals can have considerable difficulty in their daily functioning, due to an inability to maintain cogent thought processes or keep their memories in order [1]. Dementia with Lewy bodies (DLB) is the third most common form of dementia after Alzheimer's disease and vascular dementia [2]. In America, DLB has been shown to influence 10–25% of cases of dementia, affecting 1%-2% of the population aged over 65 years [3]. The comedian Robin Williams suffered from DLB at the time of his suicide in 2014 [4]. Lewy bodies are abnormal microscopic deposits that consist primarily of alpha-synuclein (a protein found widely in the brain). They were discovered by Frederick H. Lewy, M.D., in the early 1900s [5]. These abnormal aggregations lead to the gradual destruction of certain brain cells over time, resulting in a progressive decline in reasoning capacity and the ability to function independently.

The fact that DLB is a degenerative dementia with alpha-synuclein pathology makes it clinically different from other types of dementia [6]. The distinctive clinical features include visual hallucinations, Parkinsonism, cognitive impairment with fluctuations, autonomic dysfunction, rapid eye movement sleep behavior disorder (RBD), and neuroleptic sensitivity. Parkinson's disease with dementia (PDD) is another major neurocognitive disorder with Lewy bodies. DLB and PDD share many clinical and neuropathological features. It is always a challenge for physicians to differentiate DLB from PDD. Clinically, patients with DLB present with less tremor but more orthostatic hypotension, delusion, attention fluctuation, and visual hallucination. Poor balance and early onset of dementia are more frequent in DLB. However, patients with DLB vary in the severity of these symptoms, and many individuals lack standard signs in the early stages of the disease. Furthermore, because of the morphological heterogeneity of the DLB/PDD group within synucleinopathies, it would be difficult to differentiate DLB from PDD simply from neuropathological findings without sufficient clinical data [7]. This means that no single test or combination of tests can conclusively diagnose DLB in a living patient. As a result, DLB is often misdiagnosed or progresses unrecognized, according to the criteria last revised in 2015 [2, 8, 9]. Palmqvist et al. found that more than 50% of cases with DLB go undiagnosed [10]. This led to the establishment of new criteria at the 2017 International Dementia with Lewy Bodies (DLB) Conference [11]. The new criteria feature sensitivity of 83% and specificity of 95%, based on research confirmed by postmortem autopsy [12]. So far, there is no clear or objective distinction between the two entities established, except the arbitrary timing of the appearance of cognitive impairments and Parkinsonism (1-year rule) [13].

One population-based prospective cohort study estimated the incidence of suspected DLB at 112/100,000 person-years among individuals aged 65 and over [14]. A systemic review revealed that DLB incidence ranges from 50 to 160 per 100,000 person-years [15]. Currently, very few studies focused on comorbidities of DLB. There was one linkage study indicating a worse comorbidity profile in DLB patients, with a higher prevalence of depression, stroke, and migraine, compared with the AD population [16]. Awareness of DLB has increased following the adoption of revised diagnostic criteria and the publishing of new studies reporting primary data; however, epidemiological and comorbidity studies of DLB in Taiwan remain scarce. In this study, we investigated the incidence and comorbidity of DLB in a national retrospective study.

2. Data Source

The Taiwanese government established the National Health Insurance (NHI) in 1995, and more than 99% of the population of Taiwan is currently enrolled [17]. Research institutes under the NHI have released databases to promote research as subsets of the National Health Insurance Research Database (NHIRD). The Longitudinal Health Insurance Database 2000 (LHID2000) includes a random selection of 1 million patients from the NHIRD. From this database, we were able to obtain registration and claim information of patients. To ensure the privacy of patients, personal ID numbers were reencoded prior to the release of information. This study was approved by the International Review Board, China Medical University and Hospital Research Ethics Committee (IRB permit number: CMUH-104-REC2-115).

3. Sampled Participant, Relevant Variables, and Comorbidities

In this study, DLB was defined as having been diagnosed based on ICD-9-CM code 331.82 or following the 1-year rule or having been diagnosed with Parkinson's disease (PD) or Parkinsonism (ICD-9-CM codes 332 and 333, excluding 333.1–333.8) within 1 year before or after the development of dementia (ICD-9-CM codes 290.0, 290.1, 290.2, 290.3, 294.1, and 331.0) [11]. The index date was the date of diagnosis according to ICD-9-CM code 331.82 or diagnosis with dementia. Patients who had been diagnosed with stroke (430–435), head injury (850–854, 959.01), or hydrocephalus (331.3, 331.4, 331.5, 741.0, and 742.3) prior index date were excluded.

The comorbidities discussed for DLB patients were diabetes mellitus (DM) (ICD-9-CM code 250), hypertension (HTN) (ICD-9-CM codes 401–405), hyperlipidemia (ICD-9-CM code 272), coronary artery disease (CAD) (ICD-9-CM codes 410–414), congestive heart failure (CHF) (ICD-9-CM code 428), and chronic kidney disease (CKD) (ICD-9-CM code 585). According to the location of insurance coverage, the patients were classified within Northern, Central, Southern, or Eastern Taiwan.

4. Statistical Analysis

We began by calculating the incidence of DLB between 2000 and 2013 according to the number of patients diagnosed with DLB during that period divided by the number of individuals in the LHID2000 in each year of the study period. We assembled 95% confidence intervals of incidence according to Poisson distribution. We compared the demographics of male and female DLB patients using the chi-squared test for categorical variables and the *t*-test for continuous variables. Data analysis in this study was performed using SAS statistical software (Version 9.4 for Windows; SAS Institute Inc., Cary, NC, USA), with statistical significance set at a p value < 0.05.

5. Results

Between 2000 and 2013, 872 patients were newly diagnosed with DLB, which translated to an incidence rate of 7.10 per 100,000 person-years (95% CI = 6.63–7.59). The incidence rates among males and females were 7.06 and 7.14, respectively, per 100,000 person-years. The incidence rate increased with age regardless of sex. The incidence was higher in Southern and Eastern Taiwan than in other areas.

Then patients were divided into four groups according to the type of DLB with which they had been diagnosed as shown in Figure 1. Patients in Group A were diagnosed with PD within 1 year following diagnosis with dementia, whereas those in Group B were diagnosed with Parkinsonism within 1 year prior to the onset of dementia. Patients in Group C were diagnosed with DLB according to ICD-9-CM code 331.82. Patients in Group D were diagnosed with dementia and PD and/or Parkinsonism on the same day. We identified no patients diagnosed with DLB using ICD-9-CM code 331.82. Most of the patients belonged to Group A or B, regardless of gender, age, area, or the level of hospital. We also identified many patients in Group D. As shown in Table 1, the mean age of patients diagnosed with DLB was 76.3, and the average age was higher for males than for females. The mean age at the time of death was 83.3. Among patients with a history of HTN, 74.9% were diagnosed with DLB. We observed no significant differences between male and female patients with regard to the comorbidities DM, CAD, CHF, or CKD. A higher proportion of female patients presented HTN or hyperlipidemia.

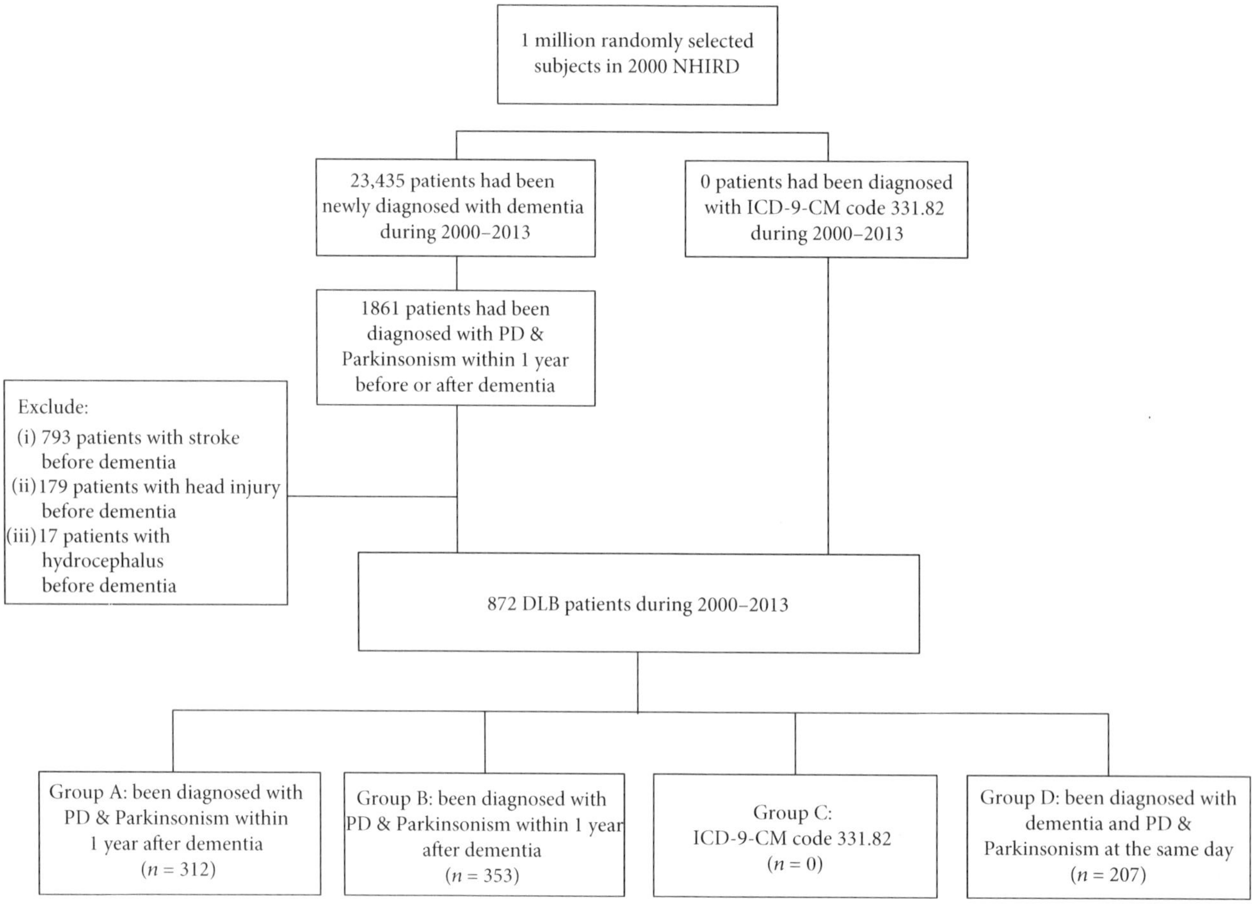

FIGURE 1: Flowchart of DLB patient selection from the National Health Insurance Research Database in Taiwan.

TABLE 1: Characteristics of DLB.

	Total ($n = 872$)	Male ($n = 438$)	Female ($n = 434$)	p value
Age				
<65	89 (10.2)	40 (9.13)	49 (11.3)	0.27
65–74	246 (28.2)	117 (26.7)	129 (29.7)	
75–84	397 (45.5)	202 (46.1)	195 (44.9)	
≥85	140 (16.1)	79 (18.0)	61 (14.1)	
Mean (SD)	76.3 (9.84)	77.1 (9.48)	75.6 (10.1)	0.03
Death	176 (20.2)	95 (21.7)	81 (18.7)	0.27
Mean age at death (SD)	83.3 (6.56)	83.5 (6.24)	83.1 (6.95)	0.70
Comorbidity				
Diabetes mellitus	230 (26.4)	104 (23.7)	126 (29.0)	0.08
Hypertension	653 (74.9)	313 (71.5)	340 (78.3)	0.02
Hyperlipidemia	340 (39.0)	148 (33.8)	192 (44.2)	0.002
CAD	420 (48.2)	201 (45.9)	219 (50.5)	0.18
CHF	148 (17.0)	66 (15.1)	82 (18.9)	0.13
CKD	70 (8.03)	40 (9.13)	30 (6.91)	0.23

CAD: coronary artery disease; CHF: congestive heart failure; CKD: chronic kidney disease.

TABLE 2: Incidence rate of DLB.

	n	Cases	2000–2013 Incidence per 100,000 person-years	(95% CI)
Total	12,284,820	872	7.10	(6.63–7.59)
Sex				
Male	6,202,935	438	7.06	(6.42–7.75)
Female	6,081,806	434	7.14	(6.48–7.84)
Age				
<65	10,968,984	89	0.81	(0.65–1.00)
65–74	760,233	246	32.4	(28.4–36.7)
75–84	440,724	397	90.1	(81.4–99.4)
≥85	114,879	140	122	(103–144)
Area				
Northern	5,602,310	309	5.52	(4.92–6.17)
Central	2,531,483	169	6.68	(5.71–7.76)
Southern	3,140,566	302	9.62	(8.56–10.8)
Eastern & island	1,010,198	92	9.11	(7.34–11.2)

6. Discussion

DLB is the second most common cause of degenerative dementia; however, there has been a dearth of research into the incidence of DLB in Taiwan. Rongve and Aarsland found its incidence at 0.7–1.4 new cases/100,000 person-years [18]. Another geographically defined population in Olmsted County, Minnesota (MN), reported an overall DLB incidence of 3.5 per 100,000 person-years, which increased sharply with age [19]. Table 2 lists the age-, sex-, and area-specific incidence rates (new cases per 100,000 person-years) of DLB in Taiwan. Between 2000 and 2013, the overall incidence of DLB in Taiwan was 7.10 per 100,000 person-years (95% CI = 6.63–7.59), and the incidence was slightly lower among men than among women (7.06 versus 7.14, resp.). The incidence of DLB increased with age, ranging from 0.81 among those <65 years old and peaking at 122 among those >85 years old, with an overall DLB incidence of 244.5 cases per 100,000 person-years among subjects aged 65 and older. The overall incidence of DLB was shown to increase consistently with age. In Southern Taiwan, the overall incidence of DLB was 9.62 per 100,000 person-years (95% CI = 8.56–10.8), which was higher than in other regions of Taiwan. The incidence values in this study may have been influenced by ascertainment bias. Rather than adopting a clinical or pathological diagnosis of DLB, we defined DLB based on ICD-9 and diagnoses of Parkinsonism as well as dementia within 1 year. It is therefore possible that cases of early onset DLB without Parkinsonism or dementia may have been missed. It is also possible that we failed to exclude other non-DLB diseases presenting both Parkinsonism and dementia. Thus, our estimates pertaining to the incidence of DLB must be regarded as imprecise. Nonetheless, these are currently the only large-population estimates in Taiwan. One previous study found that among patients with DLB, the median age at the time of death was 78 years [20]. In the present study, the mean age at death was 83.3 years (Table 2).

DLB is difficult to differentiate from Alzheimer's disease (AD) or PD with dementia due to similarities in cognitive and motor symptoms. Table 3 shows that no patients were diagnosed with DLB using ICD-9-CM code 331.82 in Taiwan. This cannot be attributed to an inability to diagnose patients with DLB. Other explanations are at work. First, ICD-9-CM codes 294.20 (dementia without behavioral disturbance) and 294.21 (dementia with behavioral disturbance) were widely used as an alternative to definite diagnostic codes. Second, cholinesterase inhibitors and memantine are the only medications currently available for patients with dementia. Unfortunately, those medications are not covered by the NHI, even after DLB is clinically diagnosed. It is for this reason that ICD-9-CM code 331.82 is not used for DLB in Taiwan. This left us no alternative but to select Groups A, B, and D in order to form a cohort of DLB patients for subsequent investigations.

HTN is a major risk factor for cerebrovascular disorders; however, it increases the risk of cognitive decline and dementia. A growing body of evidence indicates that chronic HTN is an important factor associated with the microstructural damage of brain white matter and cognitive decline [21]. Control of HTN is a key intervention in the prevention of dementia, and the effects are similar to those obtained from most antihypertensive agents [22, 23]. Nonetheless, a very limited number of studies have investigated the association between HTN and DLB. One nationwide, population-based, cross-sectional study of dementia among individuals aged 65 years and over in Taiwan revealed that 52.94% of patients with dementia presented HTN levels exceeding those in the population with normal cognition [24]. As shown in Table 1, there is a high rate of HTN as a comorbidity of DLB (74.9%), and the proportion of HTN is higher among males versus among females (71.5% versus 78.3%, resp.). These results imply that the proportion of HTN in patients with DLB is higher among females However, there is little evidence concerning the association between DLB and NTN and the underlying mechanisms.

TABLE 3: Classified DLB patients.

	Cases	2000–2013 Group A n (%)	B n (%)	C n (%)	D n (%)
Total	872	312 (35.8)	353 (40.5)	0 (0)	207 (23.7)
Sex					
Male	438	155 (35.4)	179 (40.9)	0 (0)	104 (23.7)
Female	434	157 (36.2)	174 (40.1)	0 (0)	103 (23.7)
Age					
<65	89	41 (46.1)	26 (29.2)	0 (0)	22 (24.7)
65–74	246	98 (39.8)	97 (39.4)	0 (0)	51 (20.7)
75–84	397	132 (33.2)	167 (42.1)	0 (0)	98 (24.7)
≥85	140	41 (29.3)	63 (45.0)	0 (0)	36 (25.7)
Area					
Northern	309	112 (36.2)	112 (36.2)	0 (0)	85 (27.5)
Central	169	51 (30.2)	80 (47.3)	0 (0)	38 (22.5)
Southern	302	115 (38.1)	123 (40.7)	0 (0)	64 (21.2)
Eastern & island	92	34 (37.0)	38 (41.3)	0 (0)	20 (21.7)
Accreditation level of hospital					
Medical center	217	77 (35.5)	83 (38.2)	0 (0)	57 (26.3)
District hospital	343	116 (33.8)	139 (40.5)	0 (0)	88 (25.7)
Local hospital	197	69 (35.0)	87 (44.2)	0 (0)	41 (20.8)
Other	114	50 (43.9)	44 (38.6)	0 (0)	20 (17.5)

Group A: been diagnosed with PD & Parkinsonism within 1 year after dementia. Group B: been diagnosed of PD & Parkinsonism within 1 year before dementia. Group C: ICD-9-CM code 331.82. Group D: been diagnosed with dementia, PD, & Parkinsonism at the same day

Lewy bodies composed of alpha-synuclein fibrils are abundant in the cortical neurons of patients with DLB. Evidence suggests that the interaction between alpha-synuclein and lipids on the cell membrane can trigger alpha-synuclein aggregation [25]. However, the relationship between hyperlipidemia and cognition remains an issue of controversy. One large study of older adults identified a correlation between higher low-density lipoproteins and better cognitive performance [26]. A longitudinal study of 1159 elderly Chinese people found that higher amounts of low-density lipoproteins are associated with accelerated cognitive decline [27]. However, a meta-analysis of four large randomized trials among patients diagnosed with AD revealed that lipid-lowering therapy using statins had no effect on cognition in the treatment or prevention of dementia [28]. One study of dementia among a population aged 65 years and over in Taiwan revealed that the proportions of patients with hyperlipidemia comorbidity are similar among those with dementia and among those with normal cognition (16.79% and 18.71%, resp.). In this study, we found that 39.0% of DLB patients also presented with hyperlipidemia and that the rates were higher among females. Interestingly, no previous studies have focused on the association between hyperlipidemia and DLB.

This study was subject to a number of limitations that warrant consideration. First, diagnosing DLB is difficult, and the definition of DLB in this study inevitably leads to the identification of non-DLB patients and patients in the early stages of DLB. Second, we were unable to obtain information on factors that could affect the results, such as duration of the comorbidity and use of medication.

This is the first large-population retrospective study on the incidence of DLB and cardiovascular comorbidities in Taiwan. Our results showed the incidence of DLB and higher comorbidity HTN and hyperlipidemia in female DLB patients in Taiwan. In the future, more generalizable studies concerning the association between DLB and vascular risk factors and cardiovascular disease are warranted.

Acknowledgments

This work was supported by grants from the Ministry of Health and Welfare, Taiwan (MOHW107-TDU-B-212-123004); China Medical University Hospital, Academia Sinica Stroke Biosignature Project (BM10701010021); MOST Clinical Trial Consortium for Stroke (MOST 106-2321-B-039-005); Tseng-Lien Lin Foundation, Taichung, Taiwan; and Katsuzo and Kiyo Aoshima Memorial Funds, Japan.

References

[1] J. L. Cummings, "Alzheimer's disease," *The New England Journal of Medicine*, vol. 351, no. 1, pp. 56–67, 2004.

[2] I. G. McKeith, D. Galasko, K. Kosaka et al., "Consensus guidelines for the clinical and pathologic diagnosis of dementia with Lewy bodies (DLB): report of the consortium on DLB international workshop," *Neurology*, vol. 47, no. 5, pp. 1113–1124, 1996.

[3] R. H. Perry, D. Irving, and B. E. Tomlinson, "Lewy body prevalence in the aging brain: relationship to neuropsychiatric disorders, Alzheimer-type pathology and catecholaminergic nuclei," *Journal of the Neurological Sciences*, vol. 100, no. 1-2, pp. 223–233, 1990.

[4] S. S. Williams, "The terrorist inside my husband's brain," *Neurology*, vol. 87, no. 13, pp. 1308–1311, 2016.

[5] B. Holdorff, "Friedrich Heinrich Lewy (1885–1950) and his work," *Journal of the History of the Neurosciences*, vol. 11, no. 1, pp. 19–28, 2002.

[6] I. G. McKeith, D. W. Dickson, J. Lowe et al., "Diagnosis and management of dementia with Lewy bodies: third report of the DLB Consortium," *Neurology*, vol. 65, no. 12, pp. 1863–1872, 2005.

[7] G. M. Halliday, J. L. Holton, T. Revesz, and D. W. Dickson, "Neuropathology underlying clinical variability in patients with synucleinopathies," *Acta Neuropathologica*, vol. 122, no. 2, pp. 187–204, 2011.

[8] J. Zaccai, C. McCracken, and C. Brayne, "A systematic review of prevalence and incidence studies of dementia with Lewy bodies," *Age and Ageing*, vol. 34, no. 6, pp. 561–566, 2005.

[9] S. A. Vann Jones and J. T. O'Brien, "The prevalence and incidence of dementia with Lewy bodies: a systematic review of population and clinical studies," *Psychological Medicine*, vol. 44, no. 4, pp. 673–683, 2014.

[10] S. Palmqvist, O. Hansson, L. Minthon, and E. Londos, "Practical suggestions on how to differentiate dementia with Lewy bodies from Alzheimer's disease with common cognitive tests," *International Journal of Geriatric Psychiatry*, vol. 24, no. 12, pp. 1405–1412, 2009.

[11] I. G. McKeith, B. F. Boeve, D. W. Dickson et al., "Diagnosis and management of dementia with Lewy bodies: fourth consensus report of the DLB Consortium," *Neurology*, vol. 89, no. 1, pp. 1–13, 2017.

[12] O. L. Lopez, J. T. Becker, D. I. Kaufer et al., "Research evaluation and prospective diagnosis of dementia with Lewy bodies," *Archives of Neurology*, vol. 59, no. 1, pp. 43–46, 2002.

[13] C. F. Lippa, J. E. Duda, M. Grossman et al., "DLB and PDD boundary issues: diagnosis, treatment, molecular pathology, and biomarkers," *Neurology*, vol. 68, no. 11, pp. 812–819, 2007.

[14] F. Perez, C. Helmer, J. F. Dartigues, S. Auriacombe, and F. Tison, "A 15-year population-based cohort study of the incidence of Parkinson's disease and dementia with Lewy bodies in an elderly French cohort," *Journal of Neurology, Neurosurgery & Psychiatry*, vol. 81, no. 7, pp. 742–746, 2010.

[15] D. B. Hogan, K. M. Fiest, J. I. Roberts et al., "The prevalence and incidence of dementia with Lewy bodies: a systematic review," *Canadian Journal of Neurological Sciences*, vol. 43, no. S1, pp. S83–S95, 2016.

[16] S.-M. Fereshtehnejad, S. Damangir, P. Cermakova, D. Aarsland, M. Eriksdotter, and D. Religa, "Comorbidity profile in dementia with Lewy bodies versus Alzheimer's disease: a linkage study between the Swedish Dementia Registry and the Swedish National Patient Registry," *Alzheimer's Research & Therapy*, vol. 6, no. 5-8, p. 65, 2014.

[17] "Database NHIR," http://nhird.nhri.org.tw/en/index.html.

[18] A. Rongve and D. Aarsland, "Dementia in Parkinson's disease and dementia with Lewy bodies," in *Oxford Textbook of Old Age Psychiatry*, T. Dening and A. Thomas, Eds., pp. 469–478, Oxford University Press, Oxford, 2nd edition, 2013.

[19] R. Savica, B. R. Grossardt, J. H. Bower, B. F. Boeve, J. E. Ahlskog, and W. A. Rocca, "Incidence of dementia with Lewy bodies and Parkinson disease dementia," *JAMA Neurology*, vol. 70, no. 11, pp. 1396–1402, 2013.

[20] M. M. Williams, C. Xiong, J. C. Morris, and J. E. Galvin, "Survival and mortality differences between dementia with Lewy bodies vs Alzheimer disease," *Neurology*, vol. 67, no. 11, pp. 1935–1941, 2006.

[21] R. A. Gons, L. J. van Oudheusden, K. F. de Laat et al., "Hypertension is related to the microstructure of the corpus callosum: the RUN DMC study," *Journal of Alzheimer's Disease*, vol. 32, no. 3, pp. 623–631, 2012.

[22] M. D. Murray, H. C. Hendrie, K. A. Lane et al., "Antihypertensive medication and dementia risk in older adult African Americans with hypertension: a prospective cohort study," *Journal of General Internal Medicine*, vol. 33, no. 4, pp. 455–462, 2018.

[23] M. Stuhec, J. Keuschler, J. Serra-Mestres, and M. Isetta, "Effects of different antihypertensive medication groups on cognitive function in older patients: a systematic review," *European Psychiatry*, vol. 46, pp. 1–15, 2017.

[24] T. B. Chen, S. Y. Yiao, Y. Sun et al., "Comorbidity and dementia: a nationwide survey in Taiwan," *PLoS One*, vol. 12, no. 4, article e0175475, 2017.

[25] A. van Maarschalkerweerd, V. Vetri, and B. Vestergaard, "Cholesterol facilitates interactions between α-synuclein oligomers and charge-neutral membranes," *FEBS Letters*, vol. 589, no. 19, Part B, pp. 2661–2667, 2015.

[26] Y. B. Lv, Z. X. Yin, C. L. Chei et al., "Serum cholesterol levels within the high normal range are associated with better cognitive performance among chinese elderly," *The Journal of Nutrition, Health & Aging*, vol. 20, no. 3, pp. 280–287, 2016.

[27] C. Ma, Z. Yin, P. Zhu, J. Luo, X. Shi, and X. Gao, "Blood cholesterol in late-life and cognitive decline: a longitudinal study of the Chinese elderly," *Molecular Neurodegeneration*, vol. 12, no. 1, p. 24, 2017.

[28] B. McGuinness, D. Craig, R. Bullock, R. Malouf, and P. Passmore, "Statins for the treatment of dementia," *Cochrane Database of Systematic Reviews*, no. 8, article CD007514, 2010.

25

REM Sleep Behavior Disorder (RBD) in Dementia with Lewy Bodies (DLB)

Po-Chi Chan[1] **Hsun-Hua Lee,**[2,3,4,5] **Chien-Tai Hong,**[2,3] **Chaur-Jong Hu,**[2,3,5] **and Dean Wu**[2,3,4]

[1]*Department of Neurology, Show Chwan Memorial Hospital, Changhua, Taiwan*
[2]*Department of Neurology, Taipei Medical University Shuang Ho Hospital, New Taipei City, Taiwan*
[3]*Department of Neurology, School of Medicine, College of Medicine, Taipei Medical University, Taipei, Taiwan*
[4]*Sleep Center, Taipei Medical University Shuang Ho Hospital, New Taipei City, Taiwan*
[5]*Vertigo and Balance Impairment Center, Taipei Medical University Shuang Ho Hospital, New Taipei City, Taiwan*

Correspondence should be addressed to Dean Wu; tingyu02139@gmail.com

Academic Editor: Ying-Jui Ho

Rapid eye movement sleep behavior disorder (RBD) is a parasomnia, with abnormal dream-enacting behavior during the rapid eye movement (REM) sleep. RBD is either idiopathic or secondary to other neurologic disorders and medications. Dementia with Lewy bodies (DLB) is the third most common cause of dementia, and the typical clinical presentation is rapidly progressive cognitive impairment. RBD is one of the core features of DLB and may occur either in advance or simultaneously with the onset of DLB. The association between RBD with DLB is widely studied. Evidences suggest that both DLB and RBD are possibly caused by the shared underlying synucleinopathy. This review article discusses history, clinical manifestations, possible pathophysiologies, and treatment of DLB and RBD and provides the latest updates.

1. Introduction

Lewy body dementia (LBD), including dementia with Lewy bodies (DLB) and Parkinson's disease dementia (PDD), is often discussed simultaneously because of the overlaps in pathological features, such as the presence of Lewy bodies and intracellular inclusions of α-synuclein and ubiquitin in the brain stem, limbic area, forebrain, and neocortex. It is still not clear whether DLB and PDD are distinct disorders or the same disease but at different stages. DLB is the third most common type of dementia in the world [1]. The annual incidence is 0.1% of the general population and 3.2% of all new dementia population [2]. The prevalence of DLB varied from 3.0% to 26.3% of patients who are above 65 years old [3, 4]. On the other hand, rapid eye movement sleep behavior disorder (RBD) is a disorder with abnormal behavior during the rapid eye movement (REM) sleep. RBD is acknowledged as a core clinical feature of DLB because the prevalence is up to 76% [5]. RBD not only precedes or coincides with the onset of DLB but also occurs during the course of the progression [6]. The cooccurrence of RBD, DLB, and Parkinson's disease is an important topic. In this review, we aimed to review the clinical features of DLB and its sleep manifestations. New advances in diagnosis, management, and underlying pathophysiology of DLB and RBD would also be discussed and summarized.

2. Dementia with Lewy Bodies

DLB was first clearly defined in 1996, at the First International Workshop of the Consortium on Dementia with Lewy Bodies [7]. The clinical diagnostic criteria include rapid progressive mental impairment to dementia as the central feature of DLB. Specific core features include fluctuated cognitive function, persistent well-formed visual hallucinations, and spontaneous motor features of parkinsonism. DLB is distinct from PDD, Alzheimer's disease (AD), and other types of dementia in several aspects, including clinical symptoms,

Table 1: Revised [7, 121] criteria for the clinical diagnosis of probable and possible dementia with Lewy bodies (DLB).

Essential for a diagnosis of DLB is dementia, defined as a progressive cognitive decline of sufficient magnitude to interfere with normal social or occupational functions, or with usual daily activities. Prominent or persistent memory impairment may not necessarily occur in the early stages but is usually evident with progression. Deficits on tests of attention, executive function, and visuoperceptual ability may be especially prominent and occur early.
Core clinical features (The first 3 typically occur early and may persist throughout the course.) (i) Fluctuating cognition with pronounced variations in attention and alertness (ii) Recurrent visual hallucinations that are typically well formed and detailed (iii) REM sleep behavior disorder, which may precede cognitive decline (iv) One or more spontaneous cardinal features of parkinsonism: these are bradykinesia (defined as slowness of movement and decrement in amplitude or speed), rest tremor, or rigidity
Supportive clinical features Severe sensitivity to antipsychotic agents; postural instability; repeated falls; syncope or other transient episodes of unresponsiveness; severe autonomic dysfunction, for example, constipation, orthostatic hypotension, urinary incontinence; hypersomnia; hyposmia; hallucinations in other modalities; systematized delusions; apathy, anxiety, and depression
Indicative biomarkers (i) Reduced dopamine transporter uptake in basal ganglia demonstrated by SPECT or PET (ii) Abnormal (low uptake) ^{123}iodine-MIBG myocardial scintigraphy (iii) Polysomnographic confirmation of REM sleep without atonia
Supportive biomarkers (i) Relative preservation of medial temporal lobe structures on CT/MRI scan (ii) Generalized low uptake on SPECT/PET perfusion/metabolism scan with reduced occipital activity 6 the cingulate island sign on FDG-PET imaging (iii) Prominent posterior slow-wave activity on EEG with periodic fluctuations in the prealpha/theta range
Probable DLB can be diagnosed if (a) Two or more core clinical features of DLB are present, with or without the presence of indicative biomarkers, or (b) Only one core clinical feature is present, but with one or more indicative biomarkers.
Probable DLB should not be diagnosed on the basis of biomarkers alone. *Possible DLB* can be diagnosed if (a) Only one core clinical feature of DLB is present, with no indicative biomarker evidence, or (b) One or more indicative biomarkers is present but there are no core clinical features.
DLB is less likely (a) In the presence of any other physical illness or brain disorder including cerebrovascular disease sufficient to account in part or in total for the clinical picture, although these do not exclude a DLB diagnosis and may serve to indicate mixed or multiple pathologies contributing to the clinical presentation, or (b) If parkinsonian features are the only core clinical feature and appear for the first time at a stage of severe dementia.
DLB should be diagnosed when dementia occurs before or concurrently with parkinsonism. The term Parkinson disease dementia (PDD) should be used to describe dementia that occurs in the context of well-established Parkinson disease. In a practice setting, the term that is most appropriate to the clinical situation should be used and generic terms such as Lewy body disease are often helpful. In research studies in which distinction needs to be made between DLB and PDD, the existing 1-year rule between the onset of dementia and parkinsonism continues to be recommended.

(Adapted from Ian G. McKeith et al., Neurology 89 July 4, 2017).

pathological findings, and nuclear imaging studies [8]. The extrapyramidal symptoms of DLB are extremely sensitive to neuroleptic medications [7]. Lower dopamine transporter uptake in the basal ganglia is demonstrated by SPECT or PET imaging. They are also the suggestive features of DLB [9]. The confirmation of DLB is based on pathology which shows Lewy bodies in the brain stem or cerebral cortex [10]. Lewy-related neurites, Alzheimer pathology, and spongiform change may also be presented, but they are not necessary features for diagnosis.

In 2017, the diagnostic criteria have been updated for the fourth time (Table 1) [5]. The revised criteria had made some changes and defined essential diagnosis of dementia in a more detailed way. Dementia, defined by progressive cognitive decline of sufficient magnitude, interferes with normal social or occupational functions, or usual daily activities are still essential for the diagnosis of DLB. Unlike AD, patients are not necessary to have prominent or persistent memory impairment in the early stages, instead of dysfunction of attention, executive function, and visuoperceptual ability [11]. Core clinical features may precede dementia including fluctuating cognition with pronounced variations in attention and alertness, recurrent well-formed and detailed visual hallucinations, and RBD [12]. One or more spontaneous cardinal features of parkinsonism may also present such as bradykinesia, rest tremor, and rigidity. Supportive clinical features include severe sensitivity to antipsychotic agents, postural instability, repeated falls, syncope or other transient episodes of unresponsiveness, severe autonomic dysfunction, hyposmia, hallucinations in other modalities, delusions, apathy, anxiety, and depression and may exist in the early stage [13].

The revised DLB consensus criteria are now distinguished clearly between clinical features and diagnostic biomarkers. If one or more of the indicative biomarkers are identified and are associated with one or more core clinical features, then probable DLB should be diagnosed. Dementia without any core clinical features, but with one or more indicative biomarkers, may be classified as possible DLB. For the supportive biomarkers, these are biomarkers consistent with DLB that help the diagnostic evaluation, but without clear diagnostic specificity.

3. Recommended Management of DLB

With few randomized controlled trials in DLB, recommendations about clinical management are largely based upon expert opinions. Management of DLB is complex, and the approach with a multidisciplinary team is helpful. It is recommended that the combination of pharmacologic and nonpharmacologic approaches might result in an optimal outcome. Among others, exercise [14], cognitive training [15], and caregiver-oriented education and training are promising nonpharmacologic managements for DLB patients [16, 17]. For the pharmacologic therapy, there are four clinical aspects that should be considered:

(1) Cognitive functions

It is well established that the involvement of cholinergic deficits in DLB and cholinesterase inhibitors (ChEIs) is beneficial for better clinical courses by lowering the choline degradation [18]. Either rivastigmine or donepezil may improve cognition, global function, and activities of living [19, 20]. On the other hand, there are evidences of hyperactivity of glutamatergic neurons in both human and animal studies [21, 22]. It is likely that memantine, the N-methyl-D-aspartate receptor antagonist, may be effective by amelioration of glutamatergic neurotransmission for cognitive improvement of DLB patients. However, memantine produced remarkable efficacy on global assessment, but the cognitive function, behavioral symptoms, and activities of daily living are based on current evidence [19].

(2) Psychiatric symptoms

ChEIs may reduce apathy, visual hallucinations, delusion, and associated anxiety and agitation [23]. The use of antipsychotics should be avoided because of the increased risk of mortality [24]. The second generation of antipsychotics, such as quetiapine, may be beneficial and safer based on a previous study [25]. However, efficacy and tolerability are not well established yet. On the other hand, the incidence of depression ranged from 22 to 53 per 100 person-years in atypical PD, including DLB, which is higher as compared to PD [26]. Regarding the management of depression in DLB patients, serotoninergic-targeted therapy would be an option based on individual response. Furthermore, selective serotonin reuptake inhibitor treatment may even be associated with increased hippocampal neurogenesis and preservation of cognition in DLB/PDD patients according to a recent study [27].

(3) Extrapyramidal symptoms

Previous studies mostly revealed no benefits or mild improvement with levodopa treatment in motor symptoms of DLB patients [28, 29]. The use of dopaminergic medications in DLB is often withheld by fears of aggravating psychosis and confusion. However, although the response to dopaminergic treatment in DLB for its motor symptoms is poor, a low dose of levodopa is still an alternative and should be titrated slowly in order to avoid psychiatric side effects [28, 30].

(4) Sleep disturbances

DLB patients frequently have several sleep problems, and they often occur simultaneously. Excessive daytime sleepiness can be managed by improving sleep hygiene. Previous studies regarding central nervous system stimulants such as modafinil and armodafinil revealed inconsistent results [31]. Armodafinil has been associated with increased wakefulness but may exacerbate agitation and hallucinations [32]. It is critical to prevent sleep-related injuries in DLB patients with RBD. Taking clonazepam before bedtime may reduce the RBD and consequent injuries. However, it may worsen the cognitive function and daytime sleepiness.

4. REM Sleep Behavior Disorder (RBD)

The first major classification of sleep disorders, the Diagnostic Classification of Sleep and Arousal Disorders, was published in 1979 [33]. In 2014, the International Classification of Sleep Disorders (ICSD) made the 3rd revised version of the American Academy of Sleep Medicine's manual of sleep disorders nosology [34]. A parasomnia involves undesired events that happen during sleeping. It also involves three different classifications: nonrapid eye movement- (NREM-) related parasomnias, REM-related parasomnias, and other parasomnias. RBD is one of the REM-related parasomnias.

RBD was first described in 1986 by Schenck et al. [35]. In this 2-year study, 5 patients were found to have similar behavioral disturbances during REM sleep. They were associated with loss of chin and limb electromyography atonia [12, 36, 37]. RBD is either idiopathic or secondary [34]. Idiopathic RBD is cryptogenic since Lewy bodies were demonstrated by autopsy in two cases of presumptive idiopathic

RBD [38, 39]. Idiopathic RBD is also found to have α-synuclein accumulation and thought to be the prodromal stage of many neurodegenerative disorders, such as PD and DLB, multiple system atrophy (MSA), and a pure autonomic failure [40]. Secondary RBD is defined to be caused by other diseases, most commonly in neurodegenerative or other neurologic disorders, sleep disorders, medications, and withdrawal states. Known causes of secondary RBD up to date are spinocerebellar ataxia [41], limbic encephalitis [42], brain tumors [42], multiple sclerosis [43], stroke [44], different antidepressants [45–47], alcohol [48], and barbiturate withdrawal [49].

5. Clinical Presentation of RBD

RBD has special clinical dream-enacting behavior symptoms such as repeated episodes of sleep-related vocalization and/or complex motor behaviors during REM sleep, correlating with dreams [50]. Patients with RBD act out their dreams and commonly have violent or injurious behavior during sleep [35, 51, 52]. The behavior includes purposeful movements of short duration and can be really violent thrashing, punching, kicking, and even falling out of the bed [53]. The patients also have loud vocalizations, screaming, and talking. Under normal conditions, the skeletal muscles lose muscle tone physiologically when dreaming [54]. In RBD, a loss of atonia causes self-injury and injury to their bed partners. Diagnosing RBD needs a careful and detailed history taking [55]. Males are much more than females in RBD patient groups. The median age at diagnosis is between 60 and 70 years [56]. The symptoms progress gradually; they can occur daily or once per year [57]. Dream contents of RBD patients are different from the normal population. Their dreams are mostly unpleasant and more violent. Patients do not usually consider this a problem, until themselves or their bed partners get hurt [58].

6. Clinical Implications of RBD and Its Relationship to DLB

RBD can be either idiopathic and a marker of prodromal neurodegeneration or secondary to neurodegeneration [59]. Longitudinal studies of idiopathic RBD had shown evidence of a strong association with eventual phenoconversion to a neurodegenerative disease. Phenoconversion risk between two and five years is about 15% to 35%, and the risk may increase to 41% to 90.9% if extending the follow-up period up to 12 to 25 years. When patients have RBD, compared to those without RBD, the accompanied neurodegenerative disease tends to be worse, such as more severe parkinsonian symptoms, autonomic dysfunction, and cognitive impairment [37].

Overall, idiopathic RBD patients convert to PD eventually and accomplish with 5 years. Those PD patients converted from RBD were faster motor progression, less response to levodopa therapy, and more severe postural instability [60, 61]. RBD appears to be associated with the α-synucleinopathies [62]. Previous studies showed that 38%–65% of RBD patients have developed α-synucleinopathy from 10 to 20 years after RBD presentation; it could be most likely PD, DLB, or multiple system atrophy [63, 64]. Other cohort studies have provided evidence that patients with idiopathic RBD will eventually develop a synucleinopathy, such as PD, DLB, or MSA [37, 40, 65–68].

Prevalence of RBD in the general population is between 0.38 and 0.5%, but RBD has been found in 70% of patients with MSA, 40% of patients with DLB, and between 15% and 33% of patients with PD [69–71]. Another study even showed that 74% of the DLB population had RBD [72, 73]. By using diffusion magnetic resonance imaging (MRI), PD patients with RBD showed microstructural white matter changes in the bilateral cingulum, inferior front occipital fasciculus, bilateral corticospinal tracts, and middle cerebellar peduncles. However, PD patients without RBD do not have such signal changes [74]. A series of autopsies of RBD patients shows underlying synucleinopathy up to 94% of patients [65, 75–77]. Furthermore, peripheral tissues such as submandibular glands and the enteric nervous system from living patients with idiopathic RBD also show abnormal α-synuclein immunoreactivity [78, 79]. The implication from these evidences aforementioned is that RBD onset in older adults is associated with underlying synucleinopathy in pathology.

7. Diagnoses and Treatment of RBD

The diagnosis of RBD is based on clinical features and polysomnography (PSG) findings. Firstly, the patients must have repeated episodes of complex motor behaviors or vocalization during REM sleep, and they can be documented by PSG or reports of dream enactment. Secondly, it must have evidence of REM sleep without atonia on PSG, namely, REM sleep without atonia (RSWA). Other clinical findings are strongly suggested by the diagnosis of RBD, but RSWA is not observed, yet the diagnosis can still be given. RBD can be secondary to several medications, most of which are antidepressants [80, 81]. When RBD is believed as a secondary cause of medication use, a diagnosis of RBD is still applicable.

The management of RBD should be applied carefully because around 33% to 65% RBD patients have sleep-related injuries that are caused by the patients themselves [82]. Sleep disruption usually happens because of abnormal or disruptive, or even violent, behavior during REM sleep [83]. So, modifying the sleep environment is necessary for RBD patients to prevent from getting sleep-related injuries. Under certain circumstances, separating bedrooms may be necessary to prevent bed partners from getting injuries. Pharmacologic therapy includes clonazepam and melatonin [82, 84]. Both are modestly effective in preventing sleep-related injuries. Clonazepam is a long-acting benzodiazepine with increased risks of falls and cognitive impairment. It should be used with caution in RBD patients with dementia, gait disorders, or concomitant obstructive sleep apnea. Melatonin is a hormone releasing from the pineal gland with favorable safety and tolerability. Thus, RBD patients not suitable for clonazepam should consider melatonin as their first-line treatment [85]. Other dopaminergic medications, such as pramipexole, paroxetine, or levodopa, show no therapeutic effect, sometimes even worsen RBD [86]. Only few studies have discussed about the drug effect of ChEIs [87]. They are considered to treat RBD patients with a concomitant synucleinopathy. Other medications are used for RBD treatment, with less evidence, such as zopiclone, benzodiazepines, desipramine, clozapine, carbamazepine, and sodium oxybate [88–91].

8. Pathophysiology of RBD

Sleep is a physiological state, which is defined by consciousness loss, reduced responsiveness to the environment, and decreased body movement [66]. Two different states with different biochemical, neuronal, and metabolic properties are involved in sleep: non-REM sleep and REM sleep. REM sleep was named because of its most obvious behavior—rapid eye movements during sleep [92, 93]. Besides rapid eye movement, one of the features of REM is muscle atonia, which means the muscle activity is inhibited, except middle ear muscle activity and eye movement. A recent study has proved that the modulation of dorsal medulla GABAergic neurons control the REM phenomenon in rodents [94]. The atonia is believed to be controlled by nuclei in the lower pons and medulla, particularly the perilocus ceruleus area. This area directly innervates the spinal interneurons and induces REM atonia via a flip-flop switch [32]. During REM sleep, excitatory sublateral dorsal/subcoeruleus nucleus glutamatergic neurons activate spinal cord inhibitory interneurons to hyperpolarize and thereby inhibit the spinal motoneuron pool and cause REM sleep atonia. It is proposed that hypocretin neurons, located in the posterior hypothalamus, may further stabilize the REM-active and REM-inactive centers [95].

The key structure for modulating REM sleep is the brain stem, particularly the pons and adjacent portions of the midbrain. During REM sleep, cholinergic neurons in the pontine tegmentum of the reticular formation are active. GABAergic neurons and orexin/hypocretin neurons also regulate REM sleep [96]. REM sleep has special EEG characteristics with low-amplitude desynchronized theta activity with the presence of saw-tooth waves, the presence of pontine–geniculate–occipital (PGO) waves, and hippocampal theta activity. PGO waves occur during the transition from non-REM sleep to REM sleep or during REM sleep itself. REM sleep is the sleep state with the highest physiological arousal.

Currently, the loss of REM sleep atonia control is well accepted in RBD patients. However, the underlying mechanisms for RBD or RSWA are far from clear. Motor circuits involve afferent, integrative, and efferent systems in the spinal cord, the brain stem, the basal ganglia, the cerebellum, and the limbic/cerebral cortex. Abnormal activation and disinhibition of these motor circuits may explain this sleep-related motor manifestation. During REM sleep, there are physiologic intermittent muscle twitches that could be originated from the red nucleus, pedunculopontine nucleus, and lateral dorsal tegmental nucleus. Dysfunction of sublateral dorsal/subcoeruleus nucleus from brain lesions in the dorsal pons was proved to cause RSWA and may cause clinical RBD [97, 98]. It is proposed that the accumulation of Lewy bodies in the pontine and medullary structures, which is in advance to the degeneration of the substantia nigra according to the Braak stage [99], will result in RSWA and RBD. With the ascending of Lewy bodies to the substantia nigra and cortex, the motor symptoms and dementia evolved [100]. On the other hand, regarding DLB, before the development of parkinsonism and other features, RBD typically begins many years before cognitive dysfunction. It can be explained that the nigrostriatal system is later or less involved in DLB as compared to PD and PDD, and the neocortex is involved in an earlier phase.

Animal experiments can help understand the biological mechanism, pathogenesis, and treatment of RBD. In 1965, Jouvet and Delorme first reported a cat model of loss of REM atonia, which was induced by bilateral, symmetrical, and mediodorsal pontine tegmental electrolytic injury [101]. These 35 pontine-impaired cats have de novo "hallucinatory-type" behavior during REM sleep. During non-REM sleep, the hallmark phasic REM sleep PGO waves were frequently seen [102]. Jouvet's group then discovered that bilateral lesions of the caudal and ventral pons were descending pathways for REM atonia [103]. Morrison's group designed an idiopathic RBD cat and dog animal model and discovered clonazepam as an effective therapeutic medication [35, 104]. Valenica Garcia et al. developed the RBD rat model for pharmacotherapies of clonazepam and melatonin [82]. Also, the rat model can be used for studying other medication effects, such as antidepressants [105]. Currently, Lyon's group developed a novel rat model of RBD with precision techniques that deepen the understanding of the human RBD basic and clinical research [106].

The specific neuronal networks and neuropathology involved in human RBD pathogenesis have not been identified with certainty; more work is needed for determination. RBD shares similar pathological changes with PD and DLB in sleep-related brainstem nuclei, specifically those in the rostral pontine tegmentum. In PD and DLB, α-synuclein immunoreactive Lewy-related pathology and neuronal loss are discovered in the same area [107–109]. But DLB with or without RBD differs clinically or pathologically. DLB without RBD has early involvement of corticolimbic areas and later extension to brainstem nuclei. DLB with RBD has early brainstem involvement then extends to forebrain structures [110–112]. AD-type neuropathology is frequent in DLB. Some of the DLB and PD patients, especially those with PD with later developing dementia, can have β-amyloid plaques and tau-positive neurofibrillary degeneration, which belongs to AD. RBD is uncommon in AD, but when RBD occurred, α-synuclein deposition is discovered [113]. Another study showed that probable RBD is associated with DLB and less severe AD-related pathology in the medial temporal lobes. If the absence of probable RBD, AD-like atrophy patterns on MRI and increased phospho-tau burden are noted [114, 115]. The cholinergic mechanism is an important modulatory role of RBD. Cholinergic depletion is also known to be severe in DLB, even in the early beginning of the dementia [116]. Loss of neurons in the locus coeruleus and substantia nigra in DLB with subsequent dysregulation of cholinergic neurons in the pedunculopontine nucleus increased REM sleep drive and RBD [116, 117]. The pedunculopontine/laterodorsal tegmental nuclei (PPN/LDT) are active during REM sleep which contain cholinergic neurons. In an animal study, damage in PPN/LDT leads to RBD-like behavior. Cholinergic neurons decrease, and α-synuclein accumulation in the PPN/LDT is seen in DLB with and without RBD, also in PD and AD. But different from AD, significant neuronal loss was only detected in these nuclei in DLB [69, 77, 118–120]. With the help of these innovative research methodologies and materials, further insight of mechanisms of pathogenesis can be expected in the near future.

9. Conclusions

Compelling evidence has suggested that both DLB and RBD are possibly caused by underlying synucleinopathy, and RBD often precedes DLB. Currently, the mainstay of pharmacological treatment of RBD is clonazepam and melatonin, which may reduce the possibility of sleep-related injuries. As a sentinel of possible DLB and other synucleinopathy, RBD may be the beginning of degenerative diseases and provide opportunities for preemptive treatment for earlier disease-modifying therapy, targeting α-synuclein or its regulatory pathways. Further studies need to address factors that will determine its phenoconversion to different types of synucleinopathy. Early interventional strategies should be developed to prevent or at least delay the consequences of devastating dementia, parkinsonism, and autonomic failures.

Authors' Contributions

Po-Chi Chan and Hsun-Hua Lee contributed equally to this study.

Acknowledgments

This work was supported by Taipei Medical University Research Fund, Grant no. TMU103-AE1-B33.

References

[1] J. L. Heidebrink, "Is dementia with Lewy bodies the second most common cause of dementia?," *Journal of Geriatric Psychiatry and Neurology*, vol. 15, no. 4, pp. 182–187, 2002.

[2] J. Zaccai, C. McCracken, and C. Brayne, "A systematic review of prevalence and incidence studies of dementia with Lewy bodies," *Age and Ageing*, vol. 34, no. 6, pp. 561–566, 2005.

[3] S. S. M. Chan, H. F. K. Chiu, L. C. W. Lam, and V. P. Y. Leung, "Prevalence of dementia with Lewy bodies in an inpatient psychogeriatric population in Hong Kong Chinese," *International Journal of Geriatric Psychiatry*, vol. 17, no. 9, pp. 847–850, 2002.

[4] S. Shergill, E. Mullan, P. D'ath, and C. Katona, "What is the clinical prevalence of Lewy body dementia?," *International Journal of Geriatric Psychiatry*, vol. 9, no. 11, pp. 907–912, 1994.

[5] I. G. McKeith, B. F. Boeve, D. W. Dickson et al., "Diagnosis and management of dementia with Lewy bodies: fourth consensus report of the DLB Consortium," *Neurology*, vol. 89, no. 1, pp. 88–100, 2017.

[6] M. Onofrj, A. Thomas, G. D'Andreamatteo et al., "Incidence of RBD and hallucination in patients affected by Parkinson's disease: 8-year follow-up," *Neurological Sciences*, vol. 23, no. 0, pp. s91–s94, 2002.

[7] I. G. McKeith, D. Galasko, K. Kosaka et al., "Consensus guidelines for the clinical and pathologic diagnosis of dementia with Lewy bodies (DLB) report of the consortium on DLB international workshop," *Neurology*, vol. 47, no. 5, pp. 1113–1124, 1996.

[8] R. B. Postuma and C. Trenkwalder, "Neurodegeneration in REM sleep behavior disorder stratification keeps improving," *Neurology*, vol. 88, no. 16, pp. 1486-1487, 2017.

[9] J. Heller, N. Brcina, I. Dogan et al., "Brain imaging findings in idiopathic REM sleep behavior disorder (RBD) – a systematic review on potential biomarkers for neurodegeneration," *Sleep Medicine Reviews*, vol. 34, pp. 23–33, 2017.

[10] A. Iranzo, H. Stockner, M. Serradell et al., "Five-year follow-up of substantia nigra echogenicity in idiopathic REM sleep behavior disorder," *Movement Disorders*, vol. 29, no. 14, pp. 1774–1780, 2014.

[11] J. M. Hamilton, K. M. Landy, D. P. Salmon, L. A. Hansen, E. Masliah, and D. Galasko, "Early visuospatial deficits predict the occurrence of visual hallucinations in autopsy-confirmed dementia with Lewy bodies," *The American Journal of Geriatric Psychiatry*, vol. 20, no. 9, pp. 773–781, 2012.

[12] A. Iranzo, A. Fernández-Arcos, E. Tolosa et al., "Neurodegenerative disorder risk in idiopathic REM sleep behavior disorder: study in 174 patients," *PLoS One*, vol. 9, no. 2, article e89741, 2014.

[13] K. Li, S. H. Li, W. Su, and H. B. Chen, "Diagnostic accuracy of REM sleep behaviour disorder screening questionnaire: a meta-analysis," *Neurological Sciences*, vol. 38, no. 6, pp. 1039–1046, 2017.

[14] E. Y. Uc, K. C. Doerschug, V. Magnotta et al., "Phase I/II randomized trial of aerobic exercise in Parkinson disease in a community setting," *Neurology*, vol. 83, no. 5, pp. 413–425, 2014.

[15] I. H. K. Leung, C. C. Walton, H. Hallock, S. J. G. Lewis, M. Valenzuela, and A. Lampit, "Cognitive training in Parkinson disease: a systematic review and meta-analysis," *Neurology*, vol. 85, no. 21, pp. 1843–1851, 2015.

[16] T. J. Huh, P. A. Areán, H. Bornfeld, and A. Elite-Marcandonatou, "The effectiveness of an environmental and behavioral approach to treat behavior problems in a patient with dementia with Lewy bodies: a case study," *The Annals of Long-Term Care*, vol. 16, no. 11, pp. 17–21, 2008.

[17] L. N. Gitlin, L. Winter, M. P. Dennis, N. Hodgson, and W. W. Hauck, "A biobehavioral home-based intervention and the well-being of patients with dementia and their caregivers: the COPE randomized trial," *JAMA*, vol. 304, no. 9, pp. 983–991, 2010.

[18] P. Tiraboschi, L. A. Hansen, M. Alford et al., "Cholinergic dysfunction in diseases with Lewy bodies," *Neurology*, vol. 54, no. 2, pp. 407–411, 2000.

[19] H. F. Wang, J. T. Yu, S. W. Tang et al., "Efficacy and safety of cholinesterase inhibitors and memantine in cognitive impairment in Parkinson's disease, Parkinson's disease dementia, and dementia with Lewy bodies: systematic review with meta-analysis and trial sequential analysis," *Journal of Neurology, Neurosurgery & Psychiatry*, vol. 86, no. 2, pp. 135–143, 2015.

[20] C. Stinton, I. McKeith, J. P. Taylor et al., "Pharmacological management of Lewy body dementia: a systematic review and meta-analysis," *The American Journal of Psychiatry*, vol. 172, no. 8, pp. 731–742, 2015.

[21] E. Dalfó, J. L. Albasanz, M. Martin, and I. Ferrer, "Abnormal metabotropic glutamate receptor expression and signaling in the cerebral cortex in diffuse Lewy body disease is associated with irregular α-synuclein/phospholipase C (PLCβ_1) interactions," *Brain Pathology*, vol. 14, no. 4, pp. 388–398, 2004.

[22] M. S. Starr, "Glutamate/dopamine D_1/D_2 balance in the basal ganglia and its relevance to Parkinson' disease," *Synapse*, vol. 19, no. 4, pp. 264–293, 1995.

[23] I. McKeith, T. del Ser, P. F. Spano et al., "Efficacy of rivastigmine in dementia with Lewy bodies: a randomised, double-blind, placebo-controlled international study," *The Lancet*, vol. 356, no. 9247, pp. 2031–2036, 2000.

[24] I. McKeith, A. Fairbairn, R. Perry, P. Thompson, and E. Perry, "Neuroleptic sensitivity in patients with senile dementia of Lewy body type," *BMJ*, vol. 305, no. 6855, pp. 673–678, 1992.

[25] D. T. Maust, H. M. Kim, L. S. Seyfried et al., "Antipsychotics, other psychotropics, and the risk of death in patients with dementia: number needed to harm," *JAMA Psychiatry*, vol. 72, no. 5, pp. 438–445, 2015.

[26] L. Almeida, B. Ahmed, R. Walz et al., "Depressive symptoms are frequent in atypical parkinsonian disorders," *Movement Disorders Clinical Practice*, vol. 4, no. 2, pp. 191–197, 2017.

[27] A. Gatt, A. Ekonomou, A. Somani et al., "Importance of proactive treatment of depression in Lewy body dementias: the impact on hippocampal neurogenesis and cognition in a post-mortem study," *Dementia and Geriatric Cognitive Disorders*, vol. 44, no. 5-6, pp. 283–293, 2018.

[28] S. Molloy, I. McKeith, J. T. O'Brien, and D. J. Burn, "The role of levodopa in the management of dementia with Lewy bodies," *Journal of Neurology, Neurosurgery & Psychiatry*, vol. 76, no. 9, pp. 1200–1203, 2005.

[29] S. B. Bonelli, G. Ransmayr, M. Steffelbauer, T. Lukas, C. Lampl, and M. Deibl, "L-dopa responsiveness in dementia with Lewy bodies, Parkinson disease with and without dementia," *Neurology*, vol. 63, no. 2, pp. 376–378, 2004.

[30] J. G. Goldman, C. G. Goetz, M. Brandabur, M. Sanfilippo, and G. T. Stebbins, "Effects of dopaminergic medications on psychosis and motor function in dementia with Lewy bodies," *Movement Disorders*, vol. 23, no. 15, pp. 2248–2250, 2008.

[31] E. Prado, P. Paholpak, M. Ngo et al., "Agitation and psychosis associated with dementia with Lewy bodies exacerbated by modafinil use," *American Journal of Alzheimer's Disease & Other Dementias*, vol. 27, no. 7, pp. 468–473, 2012.

[32] M. I. Lapid, K. M. Kuntz, S. S. Mason et al., "Efficacy, safety, and tolerability of armodafinil therapy for hypersomnia associated with dementia with Lewy bodies: a pilot study," *Dementia and Geriatric Cognitive Disorders*, vol. 43, no. 5-6, pp. 269–280, 2017.

[33] P. R. Howard, "Sleep Disorders Classification Committee, Association of Sleep Disorders Centers," *Sleep*, vol. 2, no. 1, pp. 1–137, 1979.

[34] M. J. Sateia, "International Classification of Sleep Disorders-Third Edition," *Chest Journal*, vol. 146, no. 5, pp. 1387–1394, 2014.

[35] C. H. Schenck, S. R. Bundlie, M. G. Ettinger, and M. W. Mahowald, "Chronic behavioral disorders of human REM sleep: a new category of parasomnia," *Sleep*, vol. 9, no. 2, pp. 293–308, 1986.

[36] T. J. Ferman, B. F. Boeve, G. E. Smith et al., "Inclusion of RBD improves the diagnostic classification of dementia with Lewy bodies," *Neurology*, vol. 77, no. 9, pp. 875–882, 2011.

[37] R. B. Postuma, J. F. Gagnon, M. Vendette, M. L. Fantini, J. Massicotte-Marquez, and J. Montplaisir, "Quantifying the risk of neurodegenerative disease in idiopathic REM sleep behavior disorder," *Neurology*, vol. 72, no. 15, pp. 1296–1300, 2009.

[38] M. Uchiyama, K. Tanaka, K. Isse, and M. Okawa, "Lewy body disease in a patient with REM sleep disorder," *Neurology*, vol. 46, no. 5, p. 1493, 1996.

[39] B. F. Boeve, M. H. Silber, C. B. Saper et al., "Pathophysiology of REM sleep behaviour disorder and relevance to neurodegenerative disease," *Brain*, vol. 130, no. 11, pp. 2770–2788, 2007.

[40] C. H. Schenck, B. F. Boeve, and M. W. Mahowald, "Delayed emergence of a parkinsonian disorder or dementia in 81% of older men initially diagnosed with idiopathic rapid eye movement sleep behavior disorder: a 16-year update on a previously reported series," *Sleep Medicine*, vol. 14, no. 8, pp. 744–748, 2013.

[41] S. M. Boesch, B. Frauscher, E. Brandauer, G. K. Wenning, B. Högl, and W. Poewe, "Disturbance of rapid eye movement sleep in spinocerebellar ataxia type 2," *Movement Disorders*, vol. 21, no. 10, pp. 1751–1754, 2006.

[42] A. Iranzo, J. Santamaria, and E. Tolosa, "The clinical and pathophysiological relevance of REM sleep behavior disorder in neurodegenerative diseases," *Sleep Medicine Reviews*, vol. 13, no. 6, pp. 385–401, 2009.

[43] M. J. Gómez-Choco, A. Iranzo, Y. Blanco, F. Graus, J. Santamaria, and A. Saiz, "Prevalence of restless legs syndrome and REM sleep behavior disorder in multiple sclerosis," *Multiple Sclerosis Journal*, vol. 13, no. 6, pp. 805–808, 2007.

[44] Z. Xi and W. Luning, "REM sleep behavior disorder in a patient with pontine stroke," *Sleep Medicine*, vol. 10, no. 1, pp. 143–146, 2009.

[45] J. M. Parish, "Violent dreaming and antidepressant drugs: or how paroxetine made me dream that I was fighting Saddam Hussein," *Journal of Clinical Sleep Medicine*, vol. 3, no. 5, pp. 529–531, 2007.

[46] C. H. Schenck, M. W. Mahowald, S. W. Kim, K. A. O'Connor, and T. D. Hurwitz, "Prominent eye movements during NREM sleep and REM sleep behavior disorder associated with fluoxetine treatment of depression and obsessive-compulsive disorder," *Sleep*, vol. 15, no. 3, pp. 226–235, 1992.

[47] S. Schutte, "REM sleep behavior disorder seen with venlafaxine (Effexor)," *Sleep Research*, vol. 25, p. 364, 1996.

[48] A. Iranzo and J. Santamaria, "Bisoprolol-induced rapid eye movement sleep behavior disorder," *The American Journal of Medicine*, vol. 107, no. 4, pp. 390–392, 1999.

[49] M. Silber, "REM sleep behavior disorder associated with barbiturate withdrawal," *Sleep Research*, vol. 25, p. 371, 1996.

[50] R. B. Postuma, "REM sleep behavior disorder," in *Oxford Textbook of Sleep Disorders*, p. 375, Oxford University Press, 2017.

[51] C. H. Schenck and M. W. Mahowald, "REM sleep behavior disorder: clinical, developmental, and neuroscience perspectives 16 years after its formal identification in *SLEEP*," *Sleep*, vol. 25, no. 2, pp. 120–138, 2002.

[52] C. H. Schenck, S. R. Bundlie, A. L. Patterson, and M. W. Mahowald, "Rapid eye movement sleep behavior disorder: a treatable parasomnia affecting older adults," *JAMA*, vol. 257, no. 13, pp. 1786–1789, 1987.

[53] A. D'Agostino, R. Manni, I. Limosani, M. Terzaghi, S. Cavallotti, and S. Scarone, "Challenging the myth of REM sleep behavior disorder: no evidence of heightened aggressiveness in dreams," *Sleep Medicine*, vol. 13, no. 6, pp. 714–719, 2012.

[54] T. Sasai, Y. Inoue, and M. Matsuura, "Do patients with rapid eye movement sleep behavior disorder have a disease-specific personality?," *Parkinsonism & Related Disorders*, vol. 18, no. 5, pp. 616–618, 2012.

[55] C. H. Schenck, T. D. Hurwitz, and M. W. Mahowald, "REM sleep behaviour disorder: an update on a series of 96 patients and a review of the world literature," *Journal of Sleep Research*, vol. 2, no. 4, pp. 224-231, 1993.

[56] E. J. Olson, B. F. Boeve, and M. H. Silber, "Rapid eye movement sleep behaviour disorder: demographic, clinical and laboratory findings in 93 cases," *Brain*, vol. 123, no. 2, pp. 331–339, 2000.

[57] E. Sforza, J. Krieger, and C. Petiau, "REM sleep behavior disorder: clinical and physiopathological findings," *Sleep Medicine Reviews*, vol. 1, no. 1, pp. 57–69, 1997.

[58] Y. K. Wing, S. P. Lam, S. X. Li et al., "REM sleep behaviour disorder in Hong Kong Chinese: clinical outcome and gender comparison," *Journal of Neurology, Neurosurgery & Psychiatry*, vol. 79, no. 12, pp. 1415-1416, 2008.

[59] S. M. Fereshtehnejad, J. Y. Montplaisir, A. Pelletier, J. F. Gagnon, D. Berg, and R. B. Postuma, "Validation of the MDS research criteria for prodromal Parkinson's disease: longitudinal assessment in a REM sleep behavior disorder (RBD) cohort," *Movement Disorders*, vol. 32, no. 6, pp. 865–873, 2017.

[60] R. B. Postuma, A. Iranzo, B. Hogl et al., "Risk factors for neurodegeneration in idiopathic rapid eye movement sleep behavior disorder: a multicenter study," *Annals of Neurology*, vol. 77, no. 5, pp. 830–839, 2015.

[61] E. J. Slow, R. B. Postuma, and A. E. Lang, "Implications of nocturnal symptoms towards the early diagnosis of Parkinson's disease," *Journal of Neural Transmission*, vol. 121, Supplement 1, pp. 49–57, 2014.

[62] M. W. Mahowald, C. H. Schenck, and M. A. Cramer Bornemann, "Pathophysiologic mechanisms in REM sleep behavior disorder," *Current Neurology and Neuroscience Reports*, vol. 7, no. 2, pp. 167–172, 2007.

[63] C. H. Schenck, S. R. Bundlie, and M. W. Mahowald, "Delayed emergence of a parkinsonian disorder in 38% of 29 older men initially diagnosed with idiopathic rapid eye movement sleep behavior disorder," *Neurology*, vol. 46, no. 2, pp. 388–393, 1996.

[64] C. Schenck, "REM behavior disorder (RBD) : delayed emergence of parkinsonism and/or dementia in 65% of older men initially diagnosed with idiopathic RBD, and an analysis of the minimum & maximum tonic and/or phasic electromyographic abnormalities found during REM sleep," *Sleep*, vol. 26, article A316, 2003.

[65] A. Iranzo, E. Tolosa, E. Gelpi et al., "Neurodegenerative disease status and post-mortem pathology in idiopathic rapid-eye-movement sleep behaviour disorder: an observational cohort study," *The Lancet Neurology*, vol. 12, no. 5, pp. 443–453, 2013.

[66] A. Iranzo, J. Santamaria, and E. Tolosa, "Idiopathic rapid eye movement sleep behaviour disorder: diagnosis, management, and the need for neuroprotective interventions," *The Lancet Neurology*, vol. 15, no. 4, pp. 405–419, 2016.

[67] Y. K. Wing, S. X. Li, V. Mok et al., "Prospective outcome of rapid eye movement sleep behaviour disorder: psychiatric disorders as a potential early marker of Parkinson's disease," *Journal of Neurology, Neurosurgery, and Psychiatry*, vol. 83, no. 4, pp. 470–472, 2012.

[68] B. P. Boot, B. F. Boeve, R. O. Roberts et al., "Probable rapid eye movement sleep behavior disorder increases risk for mild cognitive impairment and Parkinson disease: a population-based study," *Annals of Neurology*, vol. 71, no. 1, pp. 49–56, 2012.

[69] B. F. Boeve, M. H. Silber, T. J. Ferman, J. A. Lucas, and J. E. Parisi, "Association of REM sleep behavior disorder and neurodegenerative disease may reflect an underlying synucleinopathy," *Movement Disorders*, vol. 16, no. 4, pp. 622–630, 2001.

[70] M. D. Gjerstad, B. Boeve, T. Wentzel-Larsen, D. Aarsland, and J. P. Larsen, "Occurrence and clinical correlates of REM sleep behaviour disorder in patients with Parkinson's disease over time," *Journal of Neurology, Neurosurgery & Psychiatry*, vol. 79, no. 4, pp. 387–391, 2008.

[71] J.-F. Gagnon, M. A. Bedard, M. L. Fantini et al., "REM sleep behavior disorder and REM sleep without atonia in Parkinson's disease," *Neurology*, vol. 59, no. 4, pp. 585–589, 2002.

[72] H. Chiu, Y. K. Wing, L. C. Lam et al., "Sleep-related injury in the elderly—an epidemiological study in Hong Kong," *Sleep*, vol. 23, no. 4, pp. 513–517, 2000.

[73] C. Idzikowski, "An essay on sleep-related sexual behaviours and offences related to sexual behaviours," in *Sleep and Its Disorders Affect Society*, pp. 51–76, InTech, 2014.

[74] M. Ansari, F. Rahmani, M. Dolatshahi, A. Pooyan, and M. H. Aarabi, "Brain pathway differences between Parkinson's disease patients with and without REM sleep behavior disorder," *Sleep and Breathing*, vol. 21, no. 1, pp. 155–161, 2017.

[75] B. F. Boeve, M. H. Silber, T. J. Ferman et al., "Clinicopathologic correlations in 172 cases of rapid eye movement sleep behavior disorder with or without a coexisting neurologic disorder," *Sleep Medicine*, vol. 14, no. 8, pp. 754–762, 2013.

[76] M. Uchiyama, K. Isse, K. Tanaka et al., "Incidental Lewy body disease in a patient with REM sleep behavior disorder," *Neurology*, vol. 45, no. 4, pp. 709–712, 1995.

[77] B. F. Boeve, D. W. Dickson, E. J. Olson et al., "Insights into REM sleep behavior disorder pathophysiology in brainstem-predominant Lewy body disease," *Sleep Medicine*, vol. 8, no. 1, pp. 60–64, 2007.

[78] D. Vilas, et al.A. Iranzo, E. Tolosa et al., "Assessment of α-synuclein in submandibular glands of patients with idiopathic rapid-eye-movement sleep behaviour disorder: a case-control study," *The Lancet Neurology*, vol. 15, no. 7, pp. 708–718, 2016.

[79] F. S. Sprenger, N. Stefanova, E. Gelpi et al., "Enteric nervous system α-synuclein immunoreactivity in idiopathic REM sleep behavior disorder," *Neurology*, vol. 85, no. 20, pp. 1761–1768, 2015.

[80] Y. Dauvilliers, P. Jennum, and G. Plazzi, "Rapid eye movement sleep behavior disorder and rapid eye movement sleep without atonia in narcolepsy," *Sleep Medicine*, vol. 14, no. 8, pp. 775–781, 2013.

[81] J. W. Winkelman and L. James, "Serotonergic antidepressants are associated with REM sleep without atonia," *Sleep*, vol. 27, no. 2, pp. 317–321, 2004.

[82] R. N. Aurora, R. S. Zak, R. K. Maganti et al., "Best practice guide for the treatment of REM sleep behavior disorder (RBD)," *Journal of Clinical Sleep Medicine*, vol. 6, no. 1, pp. 85–95, 2010.

[83] C. L. Comella, T. M. Nardine, N. J. Diederich, and G. T. Stebbins, "Sleep-related violence, injury, and REM sleep behavior disorder in Parkinson's disease," *Neurology*, vol. 51, no. 2, pp. 526–529, 1998.

[84] H. Shinno, M. Kamei, Y. Inami, J. Horiguchi, and Y. Nakamura, "Successful treatment with *Yi-Gan San* for rapid eye movement sleep behavior disorder," *Progress in Neuro-Psychopharmacology and Biological Psychiatry*, vol. 32, no. 7, pp. 1749–1751, 2008.

[85] C. H. Schenck, J. Y. Montplaisir, B. Frauscher et al., "Rapid eye movement sleep behavior disorder: devising controlled active treatment studies for symptomatic and neuroprotective therapy—a consensus statement from the International Rapid Eye Movement Sleep Behavior Disorder Study Group," *Sleep Medicine*, vol. 14, no. 8, pp. 795–806, 2013.

[86] M. L. Fantini, J. F. Gagnon, D. Filipini, and J. Montplaisir, "The effects of pramipexole in REM sleep behavior disorder," *Neurology*, vol. 61, no. 10, pp. 1418–1420, 2003.

[87] J. M. Ringman and J. H. Simmons, "Treatment of REM sleep behavior disorder with donepezil: a report of three cases," *Neurology*, vol. 55, no. 6, pp. 870-871, 2000.

[88] A. Bonakis, R. S. Howard, I. O. Ebrahim, S. Merritt, and A. Williams, "REM sleep behaviour disorder (RBD) and its associations in young patients," *Sleep Medicine*, vol. 10, no. 6, pp. 641–645, 2009.

[89] K. N. Anderson and J. M. Shneerson, "Drug treatment of REM sleep behavior disorder: the use of drug therapies other than clonazepam," *Journal of Clinical Sleep Medicine*, vol. 5, no. 3, pp. 235–239, 2009.

[90] M. J. Howell, P. A. Arneson, and C. H. Schenck, "A novel therapy for REM sleep behavior disorder (RBD)," *Journal of Clinical Sleep Medicine*, vol. 7, no. 6, pp. 639–644A, 2011.

[91] J. M. Shneerson, "Successful treatment of REM sleep behavior disorder with sodium oxybate," *Clinical Neuropharmacology*, vol. 32, no. 3, pp. 158-159, 2009.

[92] B. Y. Mileykovskiy, L. I. Kiyashchenko, and J. M. Siegel, "Behavioral correlates of activity in identified hypocretin/orexin neurons," *Neuron*, vol. 46, no. 5, pp. 787–798, 2005.

[93] J. M. Siegel, "Clues to the functions of mammalian sleep," *Nature*, vol. 437, no. 7063, pp. 1264–1271, 2005.

[94] F. Weber, S. Chung, K. T. Beier, M. Xu, L. Luo, and Y. Dan, "Control of REM sleep by ventral medulla GABAergic neurons," *Nature*, vol. 526, no. 7573, pp. 435–438, 2015.

[95] S. Knudsen, S. Gammeltoft, and P. J. Jennum, "Rapid eye movement sleep behaviour disorder in patients with narcolepsy is associated with hypocretin-1 deficiency," *Brain*, vol. 133, no. 2, pp. 568–579, 2010.

[96] H. Zepelin, J. M. Siegel, and I. Tobler, "Mammalian sleep," *Principles and Practice of Sleep Medicine*, vol. 4, pp. 91–100, 2005.

[97] E. K. St. Louis, S. J. McCarter, B. F. Boeve et al., "Lesional REM sleep behavior disorder localizes to the dorsomedial pons," *Neurology*, vol. 83, no. 20, pp. 1871–1873, 2014.

[98] S. J. McCarter, M. Tippmann-Peikert, D. J. Sandness et al., "Neuroimaging-evident lesional pathology associated with REM sleep behavior disorder," *Sleep Medicine*, vol. 16, no. 12, pp. 1502–1510, 2015.

[99] H. Braak and K. Del Tredici, "Invited article: nervous system pathology in sporadic Parkinson disease," *Neurology*, vol. 70, no. 20, pp. 1916–1925, 2008.

[100] H. Braak, E. Ghebremedhin, U. Rüb, H. Bratzke, and K. del Tredici, "Stages in the development of Parkinson's disease-related pathology," *Cell and Tissue Research*, vol. 318, no. 1, pp. 121–134, 2004.

[101] M. Jouvet and F. Delorme, "Locus coeruleus et sommeil paradoxal," *Comptes Rendus des Seances de la Societe de Biologie et de ses Filiales*, vol. 159, no. 4, p. 895, 1965.

[102] P. J.-P. Sastre and M. Jouvet, "Le comportement onirique du chat," *Physiology & Behavior*, vol. 22, no. 5, pp. 979–989, 1979.

[103] T. Harada, A. Tanoue, and H. Takeuchi, "Epidemiological studies on dreams, sleep habits and mental symptoms in students aged 18–25 years and the 24 hour a day commercialization of Japanese society (1)," *Sleep and Biological Rhythms*, vol. 4, no. 3, pp. 274–281, 2006.

[104] J. Hendricks, A. Lager, D. O'Brien, and A. R. Morrison, "Movement disorders during sleep in cats and dogs," *Journal of the American Veterinary Medical Association*, vol. 194, no. 5, pp. 686–689, 1989.

[105] R. B. Postuma, J. F. Gagnon, M. Tuineaig et al., "Antidepressants and REM sleep behavior disorder: isolated side effect or neurodegenerative signal?," *Sleep*, vol. 36, no. 11, pp. 1579–1585, 2013.

[106] S. Valencia Garcia, et al.P.-A. Libourel, M. Lazarus, D. Grassi, P.-H. Luppi, and P. Fort, "Genetic inactivation of glutamate neurons in the rat sublaterodorsal tegmental nucleus recapitulates REM sleep behaviour disorder," *Brain*, vol. 140, no. 2, pp. 414–428, 2017.

[107] L. T. Grinberg, U. Rueb, A. T. L. Alho, and H. Heinsen, "Brainstem pathology and non-motor symptoms in PD," *Journal of the Neurological Sciences*, vol. 289, no. 1-2, pp. 81–88, 2010.

[108] H. Braak, K. D. Tredici, U. Rüb, R. A. I. de Vos, E. N. H. Jansen Steur, and E. Braak, "Staging of brain pathology related to sporadic Parkinson's disease," *Neurobiology of Aging*, vol. 24, no. 2, pp. 197–211, 2003.

[109] A. M. Schmeichel, L. C. Buchhalter, P. A. Low et al., "Mesopontine cholinergic neuron involvement in Lewy body

dementia and multiple system atrophy," *Neurology*, vol. 70, no. 5, pp. 368–373, 2008.

[110] G. Thomas, C. H. Adler, L. F. Lue et al., "Unified staging system for Lewy body disorders: correlation with nigrostriatal degeneration, cognitive impairment and motor dysfunction," *Acta Neuropathologica*, vol. 117, no. 6, pp. 613–634, 2009.

[111] R. Frigerio, H. Fujishiro, T. B. Ahn et al., "Incidental Lewy body disease: do some cases represent a preclinical stage of dementia with Lewy bodies?," *Neurobiology of Aging*, vol. 32, no. 5, pp. 857–863, 2011.

[112] B. N. Dugger, B. F. Boeve, M. E. Murray et al., "Rapid eye movement sleep behavior disorder and subtypes in autopsy-confirmed dementia with Lewy bodies," *Movement Disorders*, vol. 27, no. 1, pp. 72–78, 2012.

[113] C. H. Schenck, E. Garcia-Rill, R. D. Skinner, M. L. Anderson, and M. W. Mahowald, "A case of REM sleep behavior disorder with autopsy-confirmed Alzheimer's disease: postmortem brain stem histochemical analyses," *Biological Psychiatry*, vol. 40, no. 5, pp. 422–5, 1996.

[114] Y. Chiba, E. Iseki, H. Fujishiro et al., "Primary visual cortical metabolism and rapid eye movement sleep behavior disorder in dementia with Lewy bodies," *Psychiatry and Clinical Neurosciences*, vol. 68, no. 2, pp. 137–144, 2014.

[115] M. E. Murray, T. J. Ferman, B. F. Boeve et al., "MRI and pathology of REM sleep behavior disorder in dementia with Lewy bodies," *Neurology*, vol. 81, no. 19, pp. 1681–1689, 2013.

[116] K. Kasanuki, T. J. Ferman, M. E. Murray et al., "Daytime sleepiness in dementia with Lewy bodies is associated with neuronal depletion of the nucleus basalis of Meynert," *Parkinsonism & Related Disorders*, vol. 50, pp. 99–103, 2018.

[117] R. S. Turner, C. J. D'Amato, R. D. Chervin, and M. Blaivas, "The pathology of REM sleep behavior disorder with comorbid Lewy body dementia," *Neurology*, vol. 55, no. 11, pp. 1730–1732, 2000.

[118] Y. Y. Lai, K. C. Hsieh, D. Nguyen, J. Peever, and J. M. Siegel, "Neurotoxic lesions at the ventral mesopontine junction change sleep time and muscle activity during sleep: an animal model of motor disorders in sleep," *Neuroscience*, vol. 154, no. 2, pp. 431–443, 2008.

[119] M. Emre, D. Aarsland, R. Brown et al., "Clinical diagnostic criteria for dementia associated with Parkinson's disease," *Movement Disorders*, vol. 22, no. 12, pp. 1689–1707, 2007.

[120] B. N. Dugger, M. E. Murray, B. F. Boeve et al., "Neuropathological analysis of brainstem cholinergic and catecholaminergic nuclei in relation to rapid eye movement (REM) sleep behaviour disorder," *Neuropathology and Applied Neurobiology*, vol. 38, no. 2, pp. 142–152, 2012.

[121] I. G. McKeith, D. W. Dickson, J. Lowe et al., "Diagnosis and management of dementia with Lewy bodies: third report of the DLB consortium," *Neurology*, vol. 65, no. 12, pp. 1863–1872, 2005.

The Pathogenesis of Necroptosis-Dependent Signaling Pathway in Cerebral Ischemic Disease

Yang Xu,[1,2] Ji Zhang,[1] Lingsong Ma,[1] Shoucai Zhao,[1] Shizun Li,[1] Tingting Huang,[1] and Zhaohu Chu[1]

[1]*Department of Neurology, First Affiliated Hospital of Wannan Medical College, No. 2, ZheShanXi Road, Wuhu 241001, China*
[2]*Non-Coding RNA of Major Diseases Research Center, Central Laboratory, First Affiliated Hospital of Wannan Medical College, No. 2, ZheShanXi Road, Wuhu 241001, China*

Correspondence should be addressed to Shizun Li; lishizun1212@163.com, Tingting Huang; 1006551570@qq.com, and Zhaohu Chu; chuzhaohu0991@163.com

Academic Editor: Hu Qin

Necroptosis is the best-described form of regulated necrosis at present, which is widely recognized as a component of caspase-independent cell death mediated by the concerted action of receptor-interacting protein kinase 1 (RIPK1) and receptor-interacting protein kinase 3 (RIPK3). Mixed-lineage kinase domain-like (MLKL) was phosphorylated by RIPK3 at the threonine 357 and serine 358 residues and then formed tetramers and translocated onto the plasma membrane, which destabilizes plasma membrane integrity leading to cell swelling and membrane rupture. Necroptosis is downstream of the tumor necrosis factor (TNF) receptor family, and also interaction with NOD-like receptor pyrin 3 (NLRP3) induced inflammasome activation. Multiple inhibitors of RIPK1 and MLKL have been developed to block the cascade of signal pathways for procedural necrosis and represent potential leads for drug development. In this review, we highlight recent progress in the study of roles for necroptosis in cerebral ischemic disease and discuss how these modifications delicately control necroptosis.

1. Introduction

For a long time, necrosis was classified as nonprogrammed cell death as a response to extreme stress. The integrity of the plasma membrane was attacked by uncontrolled and accidental necrosis causing the collapse of the cell, though the nuclei keep substantially intact on the way [1]. However, in recent years, there is strong evidence confirming that part of necrosis also contained program control, therefore proposing the new concept as programmed necrosis or necroptosis. Apoptosis, autophagy, and necroptosis are all classified as programmed cell death (PCD) based on morphological and biochemical features [2, 3]. These phenomena have been observed in the ischemic stroke model [4–6]. Due to technical limitations, many studies considered necroptosis equated with apoptosis. Necroptosis is not induced by the caspase activation which is a typical requirement of the apoptotic pathway [7]. Wang et al. systematically exposed the classic signal pathway of necroptosis to further understand this form of cell death [8]. It was found that necroptotic cell death participates in a variety of cerebrovascular diseases. These mechanisms are reviewed in this paper, since they could be targets of new therapeutic approaches for these diseases.

2. Research Progress of the Signal Pathway of Programmed Necrosis

In the 1990s, researchers observed that caspase inhibition cannot fully block tumor necrosis factor- (TNF-) induced cell death but rather switches the cell fate to the necrotic death signal pathway similar to apoptosis [9, 10]. This is the first time that procedural necroptosis has been observed. In the activation of downstream necroptosis of the pathway, caspase-8 plays a critical regulatory role in the switch. Caspase-8 acts as an endogenous inhibitor of the necroptosis signal. It not only cleaves but also activates and initiates the execution phase of apoptosis. When FADD-caspase-8-FLIP complex functions are inhibited, the pathway of cell death switches from apoptosis to typical necroptosis features [11–14]. On the other side, when RIP3 kinase activity is inhibited, necroptosis may also lead to the activation of the FADD-RIPK1-RIPK3-caspase-8 complex to induce apoptosis [15]. TNF-α is the major trigger of necroptosis, which is capable of initiating RIPK1 kinase-dependent necroptosis as well as caspase-8-dependent apoptosis [16].

So what is the most classic feature of procedural necroptosis? TNF-α-induced necroptosis is mostly intensively investigated. TNF receptor 1 (TNFR1) ligation recruits complex I which contains TRADD, TRAF2, and cIAP1/2 [17]. Complex I transits into the cytosol activating death-inducing TNFR1 complex II via cylindromatosis (CYLD) [18]. In the necrotic signal pathway, receptor-interacting kinase 1 (RIPK1 or RIP1) was the first molecule recognized as the central components of the necroptotic machinery [19]. When FADD or caspase-8 is inactivated or absent, RIPK1 and TRIF include a RIP homotypic interaction motif (RHIM) domain that permits RIPK3 activation via RHIM-mediated interactions. RIPK3 kinase activity and RIPK3 RHIM domain are the requirement of necroptosis induction [20, 21]. RIPK1 and RIPK3 were phosphorylated, then formed a necrosome through their RHIM domains, and activate their kinase activities [22]. This RIPK1-RIPK3 interacts with mixed-lineage kinase domain-like (MLKL) phosphorylation [23], which consists of an N-terminal 4-helical-bundle domain (4HBD) linked by a brace region to a C-terminal pseudokinase domain [24]. MLKL was phosphorylated by RIP3 at the serine 358 and threonine 357 residues, which induces a conformational change into its active state [25], and then formed tetramers and translocated onto the plasma membrane, which injures cellular membrane integrity resulting in cell swelling and membrane rupture [26]. Downstream of the necrosome are two splice variants of phosphoglycerate mutase family member 5 (PGAM5), PGAM5S and PGAM5L. It was first reported to be a key substrate associated with the RIP1-RIP3-MLKL complex in necroptosis. PGAM5S and PGAM5L are both requirements of intrinsic necroptosis. The presence of the necrosis inhibitor necrosulfonamide (NSA) does not affect PGAM5L bound to the necrosome. However, the binding of PGAM5S is blocked by NSA. PGAM5S is normally located on the mitochondria and becomes related to the upstream necrosis-inducing complex probably through interactions with RIP3 resulting in the activation of PGAM5S by phosphorylation [27]. Furthermore, mitochondrial fragmentation caused by the mitochondrial phosphatase PGAM5S which recruited the mitochondrial fission factor dynamin-related protein 1 (Drp1) may upregulate ROS generation [27].

RIP3 is a nucleocytoplasmic shuttling protein whose nuclear distribution is temperature-sensitive. RIP3 possesses two classical unconventional nuclear localization signals (NLS, aa 442–472) and two classical nuclear export signals (NES) [28]. The above two localization signals and amino acid residue 452 within NLS participated in the necroptosis signal pathway [29]. Therefore, some studies began to explore the existence of the RIP3 nuclear pathway in addition to the classic mitochondrial pathway. Recent literature suggests that RIP3 binds to the apoptosis-inducing factor (AIF) nuclear pathway which is also involved in the process of procedural necrosis [14]. AIF is discharged from mitochondria and combines with RIP3 to form RIP3-AIF complexes. The new RIP3-AIF complex translocates into the nucleus leading to DNA degradation, and then the neurons are induced to suffer the necroptosis signal pathway (Figure 1).

3. Necroptosis in Cerebral Ischemia Disease

In the field of cerebral ischemia, the recognition of procedural necrosis can be traced back to 2005; Degterev et al. found that cerebral ischemia in mice in the absence of apoptotic signaling is contributing to the nonapoptotic death pathway like necroptosis. Necroptosis delayed mouse ischemic brain injury distinct from that of apoptosis [30]. Vieira et al. established oxygen-glucose deprivation (OGD) models in vitro and explored the mechanism underlying OGD-induced necroptosis in hippocampal neurons, and they found that although ischemic insults induced caspase-8 mRNA downregulation, they also induced RIP3 mRNA and protein level upregulation. The changes in RIP3 protein level were positively related to hippocampal neuronal death. Similar to RIP3, RIP1 protein levels were positively related to the activation of neuronal death. Both RIP1 and RIP3 contribute to necrotic cell death in hippocampal neurons challenged with OGD insult. Consistent with the classical procedural necroptosis cellular pathways, upregulation of RIP1-RIP3 expression and negative change of caspase-8 can afterwards be used to activate necroptotic signaling [31].

Global brain ischemia and reperfusion (I/R) injury acts as another manifestation of brain cell injury, in which the hippocampal CA1 layer is especially vulnerable [32, 33]. Yin et al. built rat 20 min global cerebral ischemia model to explore intracellular changes [5]. As a marker of necroptosis, RIP3 upregulated and transferred into the nucleus after cerebral ischemia and reperfusion injury. The RIP1-RIP3 complex plays crucial roles for TNF-induced necroptosis in the cell cytosol. ATP depletion is one of the results of the mitochondrial permeability transition pore (mPTP) leading to mitochondrial swelling. Fakharnia et al. presented additional arguments in the classical mitochondrial pathway. As a gatekeeper of mPTP, CypD, which mediated mPTP opening, may contribute to not only apoptosis but also necroptotic cell death in cerebral I/R injury and alleviated the levels of RIP1 and RIP3 [34]. However, the RIP3 function in the nucleus is not completely dependent on the RIP3-RIP1 complex. It needs future studies to examine other nuclear proteins that interacted with RIP3 [5]. Xu et al. continued to explore the role of RIP3 mechanisms in the nucleus. The interaction between activated RIP3 and AIF occurs in the cytoplasm after I/R injury. AIF and RIP3 translocation into the nucleus is critical to neuronal necroptosis, and AIF translocation into the nucleus may be RIP3-dependent [14]. As a key mediator, AIF links caspase-independent PCD with the necroptotic pathway.

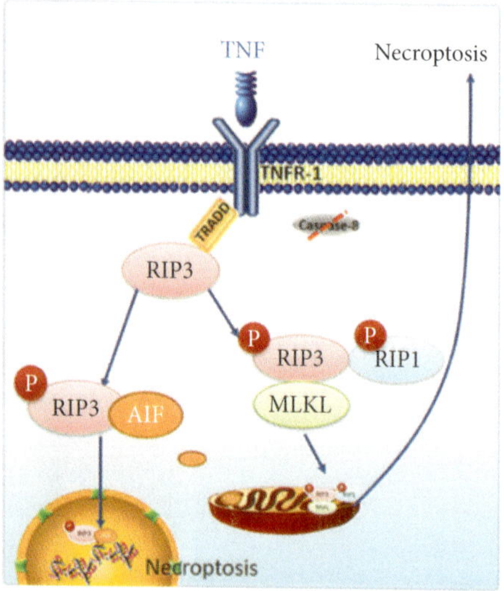

Figure 1: Two classic pathways of necroptosis. One of the classic pathways is RIP3 binding to RIP1 to form procedural necrosis complex II, which in turn binds to MLKL and mediates necroptosis of the mitochondrial pathway. The other is RIP1 binding to AIF, which translocated into the nucleus and mediates necroptosis of the nuclear pathway.

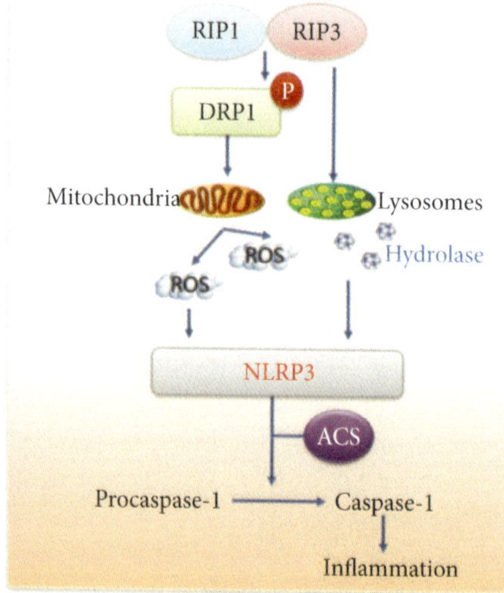

Figure 2: The activation of the NLRP3 inflammasome through the RIP1-RIP3 signaling pathway. The activation of RIP1-RIP3 damages the mitochondria by activating the DRP1. This results in excessive production of ROS and subsequent trigger activation of the NLRP3 inflammasome. RIP3 also destructs lysosomal membrane stability, leading to hydrolase release (such as cathepsin-B) and activation of NLRP3-mediated inflammatory factors.

Nerve cell necrosis was observed following the focal middle carotid artery occlusion/reperfusion (MCAO/R) ischemic stroke model. TNFR1 and RIP3 were positively expressed and significantly increased following the volume of cerebral infarction postreperfusion. Caspase inhibitor z-VAD-FMK (z-VAD) treatment markedly increased RIP3 expression during ischemia injury [35]. Compared with the classic procedural necrosis pathway, Lu et al. put forward the opposite view on the MCAO model, which is mainly concentrated in the downstream of RIP1-RIP3-MLKL. They found the mitochondria-enriched RIP1/RIP3 complex in necroptosis; nevertheless, PGAM5 had hardly any effect on RIP1-RIP3 recruitment. PGAM5 gene knockout in mice exacerbated necroptosis rather than reduced necroptosis. It causes abnormal mitochondrial accumulation and increases ROS generation [36].

In addition to phosphorylation modification, Miao et al. tested RIP3 S-nitrosylation in I/R paralleled with elevated phosphorylation. It means that phosphorylation and activation of RIP3 could be modulated by its S-nitrosylation triggered by NMDAR-dependent nNOS activation [37].

4. The Activation of the NLRP3 Inflammasome by a Mechanism Involving the RIP1-RIP3 Signaling Pathway

Neuroinflammation is still the primary cause of morbidity and mortality in cerebral ischemia [38–40]. The NOD-like receptor pyrin 3 (NLRP3) inflammasome is considered an effective therapeutic target. The abnormalities of structure and expression of the NLRP3 inflammasome could affect the development or progression of ischemic stroke. After OGD, MCAO, or global cerebral ischemia injury, NLRP3 inflammasome and other proinflammatory cytokines were activated [41]. These cytokines could be the mediating molecules during postischemic inflammation and immune responses. Following the detection of cellular stress, NLRP3 was exposed to interact with the adaptor apoptosis-associated speck-like protein containing a CARD (ASC). After binding with NLRP3, ASC recruits procaspase-1 clustering which permits autocleavage and formation of the active caspase-1, which mediates the release of the mature, biologically active cytokines to engage in immune defense [42]. The downstream of NLRP3 was explored relatively and clearly in neuronal cell experiments, primarily associated with inflammatory factors. Caspase-1 and both IL-6 and IL-1β are involved in mouse primary cortical neurons' ischemic conditions [43, 44]. In particular, caspase-1 inhibitor treatment protected neurons in experimental stroke models through suppression of NLRP3 inflammasome activity [45]. These mechanisms have been confirmed in the cerebral ischemic disease model. However, we know very little about its upstream studies. So far, the mechanism that activates NLRP3 inflammasome in ischemia injury generalizations in two main models, lysosomal damage or ROS release, is mutually connected and associated with NLRP3 in ischemia injury (Figure 2). Although there are many pathways of ROS production after ischemia [46, 47], necroptosis is one of the ways.

As mentioned before, caspase-8 is a regulatory molecule. Kang found certain cells deficient in caspase-8 prompting which is mediated by RIP1 and RIP3. Caspase-8 deficiency dendritic cells (DCs) expressed to accentuated activation of the inflammasome through the functions of RIP1, RIP3, and MLKL [7]. And Gurung et al. considered caspase-8 an apical mediator of NLRP3 inflammasome priming [48]. MLKL, a key component downstream of necrosome components, is considered an executor of necroptosis. In MLKL-knockout mice, NLRP3 activation was inhibited, which means that the potential function of MLKL is the regulation of inflammasome activation [17]. Beyond their core role in necrosis, the necrosome components RIP1 and RIP3 have been proposed to be hyperresponsive to the induction of assembly, which were applied to the NLRP3 inflammasome. When inhibitory factors of necrosomes are blocked, RIP1-RIP3 could promote inflammasome activation spontaneously. Wang et al. discovered that the RIP1-RIP3 complex participates in RNA virus-induced NLRP3 activation through the GTPase DRP1 pathway. This promoted the mitochondrial damage leading to the production of ROS and stimulus NLRP3 [49].

The relationship between the procedural necrosis and inflammation is likely clearer, but this may not be the only signaling pathways that intersect. At least downstream studies, including the relationship between necroptosis and inflammation in cerebral infarction, indicate the direction of the study.

5. The Regulation of Necroptosis in the Cerebral Ischemic Model

Many studies focus on how to block the cascade of signal pathways for procedural necrosis. The most classic inhibitor is the small-molecule compound necrosulfonamide (NSA). NSA did not block interactions between necrosis-induced RIP1 and RIP3, but it blocks necroptosis downstream of RIP3 activation. NSA targets the N-terminal Cys86 residue MLKL which has a drawback that is specifically inhibiting necroptosis in multiple human cell lines. In human glioblastoma cells, NSA switches from necrosis to apoptosis in edelfosine-treated cells [50]. In a HeLa cell line in which caspase-8 was knocked down and RIP3 was expressed, necrosis induced by TNF-α plus Smac mimetic (no need for z-VAD) was efficiently blocked by NSA, while necrosis induced by either TNF-α or z-VAD was insensitive to NSA in a 3T3 cell line expressing mouse RIP3 [23]. NSA also significantly reduces BV6/MS275-induced cell death in acute myeloid leukemia (AML) cell lines [51].

In the field of cerebral ischemia, some of the inhibitors of programmed necrosis have been demonstrated in animal models. Degterev et al. reported that as an identified small-molecule inhibitor of necroptosis, necrostatin-1 (NEC-1) has been shown to ameliorate tissue damage in ischemic brain injury animal models [30]. NEC-1 has a selective primary cellular target responsible for the death domain receptor-associated adaptor kinase RIP1 activity [52, 53]. The crystal structures of the RIP1 kinase domain bound to NEC-1 and are caged in a hydrophobic pocket between the N- and C-lobes of the kinase domain. This structure stabilizes RIP1 in an inactive conformation. DAXX is a novel substrate of RIP3 in global cerebral ischemia and ischemia of the retinal cell animal model and is translocated from the nucleus to the cytoplasm in response to stress. Pretreatment with Nec-1 can block DAXX translocation from the nucleus to the cytoplasm, which resulted in the inactivation of DAXX [54–56]. NEC-1 not only inhibited the expression of RIP1 and prevented the upregulation and nuclear translocation of RIP3 but also decreased cathepsin-B release in the globe cerebral ischemic model. This suggests that there may be a signal transduction between programmed necrosis and autophagy [5]. The recent literature highlights the intricate interplay between necroptosis and autophagy. CA074-me and 3-methyladenine (3-MA), as autophagy inhibitors [46], were used to determine what is beneficial for global cerebral ischemia in the process of necroptosis signal pathways. CA074-me and 3-MA pretreatment greatly inhibited rat mortality rates and neuronal death. The mechanism of 3-MA is the inhibition of the nuclear translocation and colocalization of RIP3 and AIF, as it is significant for ischemic neuronal DNA degradation and necroptosis for the nuclear translocation of the RIP3-AIF complex [14]. In the stabilization of the lysosomal membrane, CA074-me has an indirect effect by maintaining energy balance and inhibiting RIP3 expression and nuclear translocation [57]. Besides this, CA074-me almost completely hampered the loss of mitochondrial membrane depolarization, phosphatidylserine (PS) translocation, and plasma membrane rupture [58].

Multitargeted kinase inhibitors, such as dabrafenib, vemurafenib, sorafenib, pazopanib, and ponatinib, are currently used for the treatment of cancer, which have later emerged as having antinecroptotic activity [59–61]. Among them, dabrafenib may block TNF-α-induced necroptosis as an effective high-affinity inhibitor of RIP3. Dabrafenib administered intraperitoneally after mouse cerebral ischemic injury markedly reduced infarct lesion size along with significantly attenuated upregulation of TNF-α [59].

6. Future Research about Necroptosis

Previous studies suggested that PGAM5 promotes necroptosis by associating with necrosome. However, the role of PGAM5 intrinsically is still controversial [62]. In response to multiple necroptotic stimuli, PGAM5 deficiency aggravated rather than mitigated necroptosis in brain ischemic reperfusion injury [36]. The loss of PGAM caused abnormal mitochondrial accumulation and increased ROS generation. In oxidative damage and necroptosis-dependent stroke, PGAM5 could drive pathology, and thus targeting PGAM5 may be of benefit.

The core of procedural necrosis is RIP1 RIP3 and its downstream signaling pathways. In addition to the above-mentioned inhibitors, the drugs used in the experiments and the clinical use of drugs have been developed. This is because the understanding of this pathway is still relatively limited. After the classic pathway was proposed, there are many studies that questioned the effect of RIP3 on the necrosis of the bypass signals, such as dynamin-related protein 1 and proteasome beta-4 subunit (PSMB4) [63, 64]. These need to be systematically assessed. Furthermore, the most critical problem is that for a long time, both necrotic and apoptotic cells dominated the theory of neuronal death in the penumbra zone. The clarification of the relationship between procedural necroptosis and necrosis and autophagy still needs a lot of work to do. This cross-channel signal path may be complexity over imagination.

Acknowledgments

This work was supported by the National Natural Science Foundation of China (Grant nos. 81701161 and 81371295).

References

[1] D. V. Krysko, T. vanden Berghe, K. D'Herde, and P. Vandenabeele, "Apoptosis and necrosis: detection, discrimination and phagocytosis," *Methods*, vol. 44, no. 3, pp. 205–221, 2008.

[2] Y. Fuchs and H. Steller, "Programmed cell death in animal development and disease," *Cell*, vol. 147, no. 4, pp. 742–758, 2011.

[3] Y. Fuchs and H. Steller, "Live to die another way: modes of programmed cell death and the signals emanating from dying cells," *Nature Reviews Molecular Cell Biology*, vol. 16, no. 6, pp. 329–344, 2015.

[4] B. Pourheydar, S. Soleimani Asl, M. Azimzadeh, A. Rezaei Moghadam, A. Marzban, and M. Mehdizadeh, "Neuroprotective effects of bone marrow mesenchymal stem cells on bilateral common carotid arteries occlusion model of cerebral ischemia in rat," *Behavioural Neurology*, vol. 2016, Article ID 2964712, 10 pages, 2016.

[5] B. Yin, Y. Xu, R. L. Wei, F. He, B. Y. Luo, and J. Y. Wang, "Inhibition of receptor-interacting protein 3 upregulation and nuclear translocation involved in necrostatin-1 protection against hippocampal neuronal programmed necrosis induced by ischemia/reperfusion injury," *Brain Research*, vol. 1609, pp. 63–71, 2015.

[6] H. Wei, Y. Li, S. Han et al., "cPKCγ-modulated autophagy in neurons alleviates ischemic injury in brain of mice with ischemic stroke through Akt-mTOR pathway," *Translational Stroke Research*, vol. 7, no. 6, pp. 497–511, 2016.

[7] A. Kaczmarek, P. Vandenabeele, and D. V. Krysko, "Necroptosis: the release of damage-associated molecular patterns and its physiological relevance," *Immunity*, vol. 38, no. 2, pp. 209–223, 2013.

[8] S. He, L. Wang, L. Miao et al., "Receptor interacting protein kinase-3 determines cellular necrotic response to TNF-alpha," *Cell*, vol. 137, no. 6, pp. 1100–1111, 2009.

[9] A. Kawahara, Y. Ohsawa, H. Matsumura, Y. Uchiyama, and S. Nagata, "Caspase-independent cell killing by Fas-associated protein with death domain," *The Journal of Cell Biology*, vol. 143, no. 5, pp. 1353–1360, 1998.

[10] D. Vercammen, R. Beyaert, G. Denecker et al., "Inhibition of caspases increases the sensitivity of L929 cells to necrosis mediated by tumor necrosis factor," *The Journal of Experimental Medicine*, vol. 187, no. 9, pp. 1477–1485, 1998.

[11] C. Günther, E. Martini, N. Wittkopf et al., "Caspase-8 regulates TNF-α-induced epithelial necroptosis and terminal ileitis," *Nature*, vol. 477, no. 7364, pp. 335–339, 2011.

[12] W. J. Kaiser, J. W. Upton, A. B. Long et al., "RIP3 mediates the embryonic lethality of caspase-8-deficient mice," *Nature*, vol. 471, no. 7338, pp. 368–372, 2011.

[13] A. Oberst, C. P. Dillon, R. Weinlich et al., "Catalytic activity of the caspase-8-FLIP(L) complex inhibits RIPK3-dependent necrosis," *Nature*, vol. 471, no. 7338, pp. 363–367, 2011.

[14] Y. Xu, J. Wang, X. Song et al., "RIP3 induces ischemic neuronal DNA degradation and programmed necrosis in rat via AIF," *Scientific Reports*, vol. 6, no. 1, p. 29362, 2016.

[15] I. Shlomovitz, S. Zargrian, and M. Gerlic, "Mechanisms of RIPK3-induced inflammation," *Immunology and Cell Biology*, vol. 95, no. 2, pp. 166–172, 2017.

[16] P. Vandenabeele, L. Galluzzi, T. vanden Berghe, and G. Kroemer, "Molecular mechanisms of necroptosis: an ordered cellular explosion," *Nature Reviews Molecular Cell Biology*, vol. 11, no. 10, pp. 700–714, 2010.

[17] X. Zhang, C. Fan, H. Zhang et al., "MLKL and FADD are critical for suppressing progressive lymphoproliferative disease and activating the NLRP3 inflammasome," *Cell Reports*, vol. 16, no. 12, pp. 3247–3259, 2016.

[18] J. Hitomi, D. E. Christofferson, A. Ng et al., "Identification of a molecular signaling network that regulates a cellular necrotic cell death pathway," *Cell*, vol. 135, no. 7, pp. 1311–1323, 2008.

[19] N. Holler, R. Zaru, O. Micheau et al., "Fas triggers an alternative, caspase-8-independent cell death pathway using the kinase RIP as effector molecule," *Nature Immunology*, vol. 1, no. 6, pp. 489–495, 2000.

[20] Y. S. Cho, S. Challa, D. Moquin et al., "Phosphorylation-driven assembly of the RIP1-RIP3 complex regulates programmed necrosis and virus-induced inflammation," *Cell*, vol. 137, no. 6, pp. 1112–1123, 2009.

[21] J. W. Upton, W. J. Kaiser, and E. S. Mocarski, "Virus inhibition of RIP3-dependent necrosis," *Cell Host & Microbe*, vol. 7, no. 4, pp. 302–313, 2010.

[22] J. Li, T. McQuade, A. B. Siemer et al., "The RIP1/RIP3 necrosome forms a functional amyloid signaling complex required for programmed necrosis," *Cell*, vol. 150, no. 2, pp. 339–350, 2012.

[23] L. Sun, H. Wang, Z. Wang et al., "Mixed lineage kinase domain-like protein mediates necrosis signaling downstream of RIP3 kinase," *Cell*, vol. 148, no. 1-2, pp. 213–227, 2012.

[24] J. M. Murphy, P. E. Czabotar, J. M. Hildebrand et al., "The pseudokinase MLKL mediates necroptosis via a molecular switch mechanism," *Immunity*, vol. 39, no. 3, pp. 443–453, 2013.

[25] D. A. Rodriguez, R. Weinlich, S. Brown et al., "Characterization of RIPK3-mediated phosphorylation of the activation loop of MLKL during necroptosis," *Cell Death and Differentiation*, vol. 23, no. 1, pp. 76–88, 2016.

[26] Z. Cai, S. Jitkaew, J. Zhao et al., "Plasma membrane translocation of trimerized MLKL protein is required for TNF-induced necroptosis," *Nature Cell Biology*, vol. 16, no. 1, pp. 55–65, 2014.

[27] Z. Wang, H. Jiang, S. Chen, F. du, and X. Wang, "The mitochondrial phosphatase PGAM5 functions at the convergence point of multiple necrotic death pathways," *Cell*, vol. 148, no. 1-2, pp. 228–243, 2012.

[28] Y. Yang, J. Ma, Y. Chen, and M. Wu, "Nucleocytoplasmic shuttling of receptor-interacting protein 3 (RIP3): identification of novel nuclear export and import signals in RIP3," *The Journal of Biological Chemistry*, vol. 279, no. 37, pp. 38820–38829, 2004.

[29] M. Li, S. Feng, and M. Wu, "Multiple roles for nuclear localization signal (NLS, aa 442-472) of receptor interacting protein 3 (RIP3)," *Biochemical and Biophysical Research Communications*, vol. 372, no. 4, pp. 850–855, 2008.

[30] A. Degterev, Z. Huang, M. Boyce et al., "Chemical inhibitor of nonapoptotic cell death with therapeutic potential for ischemic brain injury," *Nature Chemical Biology*, vol. 1, no. 2, pp. 112–119, 2005.

[31] M. Vieira, J. Fernandes, L. Carreto et al., "Ischemic insults induce necroptotic cell death in hippocampal neurons through the up-regulation of endogenous RIP3," *Neurobiology of Disease*, vol. 68, pp. 26–36, 2014.

[32] K. R. Dave, D. Della-Morte, I. Saul, R. Prado, and M. A. Perez-Pinzon, "Ventricular fibrillation-induced cardiac arrest in the rat as a model of global cerebral ischemia," *Translational Stroke Research*, vol. 4, no. 5, pp. 571–578, 2013.

[33] J. J. Szymanski, H. Wang, J. T. Jamison, and D. J. DeGracia, "HuR function and translational state analysis following global brain ischemia and reperfusion," *Translational Stroke Research*, vol. 4, no. 6, pp. 589–603, 2013.

[34] F. Fakharnia, F. Khodagholi, L. Dargahi, and A. Ahmadiani, "Prevention of cyclophilin D-mediated mPTP opening using cyclosporine-a alleviates the elevation of necroptosis, autophagy and apoptosis-related markers following global cerebral ischemia-reperfusion," *Journal of Molecular Neuroscience*, vol. 61, no. 1, pp. 52–60, 2017.

[35] Y. Dong, C. Bao, J. Yu, and X. Liu, "Receptor-interacting protein kinase 3-mediated programmed cell necrosis in rats subjected to focal cerebral ischemia-reperfusion injury," *Molecular Medicine Reports*, vol. 14, no. 1, pp. 728–736, 2016.

[36] W. Lu, J. Sun, J. S. Yoon et al., "Mitochondrial protein PGAM5 regulates mitophagic protection against cell necroptosis," *PLoS One*, vol. 11, no. 1, article e0147792, 2016.

[37] W. Miao, Z. Qu, K. Shi et al., "RIP3 S-nitrosylation contributes to cerebral ischemic neuronal injury," *Brain Research*, vol. 1627, pp. 165–176, 2015.

[38] M. Ahmad and S. H. Graham, "Inflammation after stroke: mechanisms and therapeutic approaches," *Translational Stroke Research*, vol. 1, no. 2, pp. 74–84, 2010.

[39] J. Montaner, D. Salat, T. García-Berrocoso et al., "Reperfusion therapy for acute stroke improves outcome by decreasing neuroinflammation," *Translational Stroke Research*, vol. 1, no. 4, pp. 261–267, 2010.

[40] J. C. Pena-Philippides, Y. Yang, O. Bragina, S. Hagberg, E. Nemoto, and T. Roitbak, "Effect of pulsed electromagnetic field (PEMF) on infarct size and inflammation after cerebral ischemia in mice," *Translational Stroke Research*, vol. 5, no. 4, pp. 491–500, 2014.

[41] S. K. McCann, F. Cramond, M. R. Macleod, and E. S. Sena, "Systematic review and meta-analysis of the efficacy of interleukin-1 receptor antagonist in animal models of stroke: an update," *Translational Stroke Research*, vol. 7, no. 5, pp. 395–406, 2016.

[42] W. L. Lu, D. Z. Song, J. L. Yue et al., "NLRP3 inflammasome may regulate inflammatory response of human periodontal ligament fibroblasts in an apoptosis-associated speck-like protein containing a CARD (ASC)-dependent manner," *International Endodontic Journal*, vol. 50, no. 10, pp. 967–975, 2017.

[43] J. A. Switzer, A. Sikora, A. Ergul, J. L. Waller, D. C. Hess, and S. C. Fagan, "Minocycline prevents IL-6 increase after acute ischemic stroke," *Translational Stroke Research*, vol. 3, no. 3, pp. 363–368, 2012.

[44] C. P. Wang, L. Z. Zhang, G. C. Li et al., "Mulberroside A protects against ischemic impairment in primary culture of rat cortical neurons after oxygen-glucose deprivation followed by reperfusion," *Journal of Neuroscience Research*, vol. 92, no. 7, pp. 944–954, 2014.

[45] J. Qiu, M. Wang, J. Zhang et al., "The neuroprotection of sinomenine against ischemic stroke in mice by suppressing NLRP3 inflammasome via AMPK signaling," *International Immunopharmacology*, vol. 40, pp. 492–500, 2016.

[46] H. Li, A. Gao, D. Feng et al., "Evaluation of the protective potential of brain microvascular endothelial cell autophagy on blood-brain barrier integrity during experimental cerebral ischemia-reperfusion injury," *Translational Stroke Research*, vol. 5, no. 5, pp. 618–626, 2014.

[47] L. J. Wu, "Microglial voltage-gated proton channel Hv1 in ischemic stroke," *Translational Stroke Research*, vol. 5, no. 1, pp. 99–108, 2014.

[48] P. Gurung, P. K. Anand, R. K. S. Malireddi et al., "FADD and caspase-8 mediate priming and activation of the canonical and noncanonical Nlrp3 inflammasomes," *The Journal of Immunology*, vol. 192, no. 4, pp. 1835–1846, 2014.

[49] X. Wang, W. Jiang, Y. Yan et al., "RNA viruses promote activation of the NLRP3 inflammasome through a RIP1-RIP3-DRP1 signaling pathway," *Nature Immunology*, vol. 15, no. 12, pp. 1126–1133, 2014.

[50] S. Melo-Lima, M. C. Lopes, and F. Mollinedo, "Necroptosis is associated with low procaspase-8 and active RIPK1 and -3 in human glioma cells," *Oncoscience*, vol. 1, no. 10, pp. 649–664, 2014.

[51] S. Steinwascher, A. L. Nugues, H. Schoeneberger, and S. Fulda, "Identification of a novel synergistic induction of cell death by Smac mimetic and HDAC inhibitors in acute myeloid leukemia cells," *Cancer Letters*, vol. 366, no. 1, pp. 32–43, 2015.

[52] A. Degterev, J. Hitomi, M. Germscheid et al., "Identification of RIP1 kinase as a specific cellular target of necrostatins," *Nature Chemical Biology*, vol. 4, no. 5, pp. 313–321, 2008.

[53] P. Vandenabeele, W. Declercq, and T. V. Berghe, "Necrotic cell death and 'necrostatins': now we can control cellular explosion," *Trends in Biochemical Sciences*, vol. 33, no. 8, pp. 352–355, 2008.

[54] T. Xie, W. Peng, Y. Liu et al., "Structural basis of RIP1 inhibition by necrostatins," *Structure*, vol. 21, no. 3, pp. 493–499, 2013.

[55] R. Yang, K. Hu, J. Chen et al., "Necrostatin-1 protects hippocampal neurons against ischemia/reperfusion injury via the RIP3/DAXX signaling pathway in rats," *Neuroscience Letters*, vol. 651, pp. 207–215, 2017.

[56] Y. S. Lee, Y. Dayma, M. Y. Park, K. I. Kim, S. E. Yoo, and E. Kim, "Daxx is a key downstream component of receptor interacting protein kinase 3 mediating retinal ischemic cell death," *FEBS Letters*, vol. 587, no. 3, pp. 266–271, 2013.

[57] Y. Xu, J. Wang, X. Song et al., "Protective mechanisms of CA074-me (other than cathepsin-B inhibition) against programmed necrosis induced by global cerebral ischemia/reperfusion injury in rats," *Brain Research Bulletin*, vol. 120, pp. 97–105, 2016.

[58] Z. A. Dunai, G. Imre, G. Barna et al., "Staurosporine induces necroptotic cell death under caspase-compromised conditions in U937 cells," *PLoS One*, vol. 7, no. 7, article e41945, 2012.

[59] S. A. Cruz, Z. Qin, A. F. R. Stewart, and H. H. Chen, "Dabrafenib, an inhibitor of RIP3 kinase-dependent necroptosis, reduces ischemic brain injury," *Neural Regeneration Research*, vol. 13, no. 2, pp. 252–256, 2018.

[60] P. Geserick, J. Wang, R. Schilling et al., "Absence of RIPK3 predicts necroptosis resistance in malignant melanoma," *Cell Death & Disease*, vol. 6, no. 9, p. e1884, 2015.

[61] F. Feldmann, B. Schenk, S. Martens, P. Vandenabeele, and S. Fulda, "Sorafenib inhibits therapeutic induction of necroptosis in acute leukemia cells," *Oncotarget*, vol. 8, no. 40, pp. 68208–68220, 2017.

[62] W. Xu, L. Jing, Q. Wang et al., "Bax-PGAM5L-Drp1 complex is required for intrinsic apoptosis execution," *Oncotarget*, vol. 6, no. 30, pp. 30017–30034, 2015.

[63] C. Wu, J. Chen, Y. Liu et al., "Upregulation of PSMB4 is associated with the necroptosis after spinal cord injury," *Neurochemical Research*, vol. 41, no. 11, pp. 3103–3112, 2016.

[64] T. Yamada, Y. Adachi, M. Fukaya, M. Iijima, and H. Sesaki, "Dynamin-related protein 1 deficiency leads to receptor-interacting protein kinase 3-mediated necroptotic neurodegeneration," *The American Journal of Pathology*, vol. 186, no. 11, pp. 2798–2802, 2016.

27

MST1 Suppression Reduces Early Brain Injury by Inhibiting the NF-κB/MMP-9 Pathway after Subarachnoid Hemorrhage in Mice

Jie Qu, Hengli Zhao, Qiang Li, Pengyu Pan, Kang Ma, Xin Liu, Hua Feng, and Yujie Chen

Department of Neurosurgery, Southwest Hospital, Third Military Medical University, Chongqing, China

Correspondence should be addressed to Hua Feng; fenghua8888@vip.163.com and Yujie Chen; yujiechen6886@foxmail.com

Academic Editor: Hailiang Tang

Background. Mammalian sterile 20-like kinase 1 (MST1), the key component of the Hippo-YAP pathway, exhibits an important role in the pathophysiological process of various neurological disorders, including ischemic stroke and spinal cord injury. However, during subarachnoid hemorrhage, the involvement of MST1 in the pathophysiology of early brain injury remains unknown. *Methods.* We employed intravascular filament perforation to establish the subarachnoid hemorrhage (SAH) mouse model. The MST1 inhibitor XMU-MP-1 was intraperitoneally injected at 1 h after SAH, followed by daily injections. MST1 in vivo knockdown was performed 3 weeks prior to SAH via intracerebroventricular injection of adeno-associated virus (AAV) packaged with MST1 shRNA. The SAH grade, behavioral deficits, TUNEL staining, Evans blue dye extravasation and fluorescence, brain water content, protein and cytokine expressions by Western blotting, immunofluorescence, and proteome cytokine array were evaluated. *Results.* Following SAH, the phosphorylation level of MST1 was upregulated at 12 h, with a peak at 72 h after SAH. It was colocalized with the microglial marker Iba1. Both XMU-MP-1 and MST1 shRNA alleviated the neurological deficits, blood-brain barrier (BBB) disruption, brain edema, neuroinflammation, and white matter injury, which were induced by SAH in association with nuclear factor- (NF-) κB p65 and matrix metallopeptidase-9 (MMP-9) activation and downregulated endothelial junction protein expression. *Conclusions.* The current findings indicate that MST1 participates in SAH-induced BBB disruption and white matter fiber damage via the downstream NF-κB-MMP-9 signaling pathway. Therefore, MST1 antagonists may serve as a novel therapeutic target to prevent early brain injury in SAH patients.

1. Introduction

Subarachnoid hemorrhage (SAH) is identified as a subtype of hemorrhage stroke; it is mainly caused by a ruptured aneurysm, with high mortality and morbidity worldwide [1]. Recent studies have indicated the pivotal role of the vascular neural network in the pathophysiological process of early brain injury after SAH [2]. The blood-brain barrier (BBB), identified as a component of this vascular neural network, is critical for brain homeostasis. After SAH, BBB disruption is an important pathological change, which contributes to brain edema, thus leading to poor outcomes [3]. Therefore, targeting BBB disruption may represent a prospective strategy to prevent early brain injury after SAH.

Mammalian sterile 20-like kinase 1 (MST1), a core component of the Hippo pathway, regulates multiple biological effects, including the response to oxidative stress, apoptosis, cell growth, and tumor suppression [4, 5]. In the central nervous system, many studies have demonstrated that oxidative stress-induced neuronal and neuroglia death is associated with MST1 activation [6–8]. In addition, MST1 exhibits fundamental functions in various central nervous system diseases, including vascular dementia, Alzheimer's disease, amyotrophic lateral sclerosis, and cerebral cavernous malformation [9–12]. Furthermore, genetic deletion of MST1 provides neuroprotection against ischemic stroke and spinal cord injury by attenuating neuronal apoptosis and the inflammatory response [13, 14].

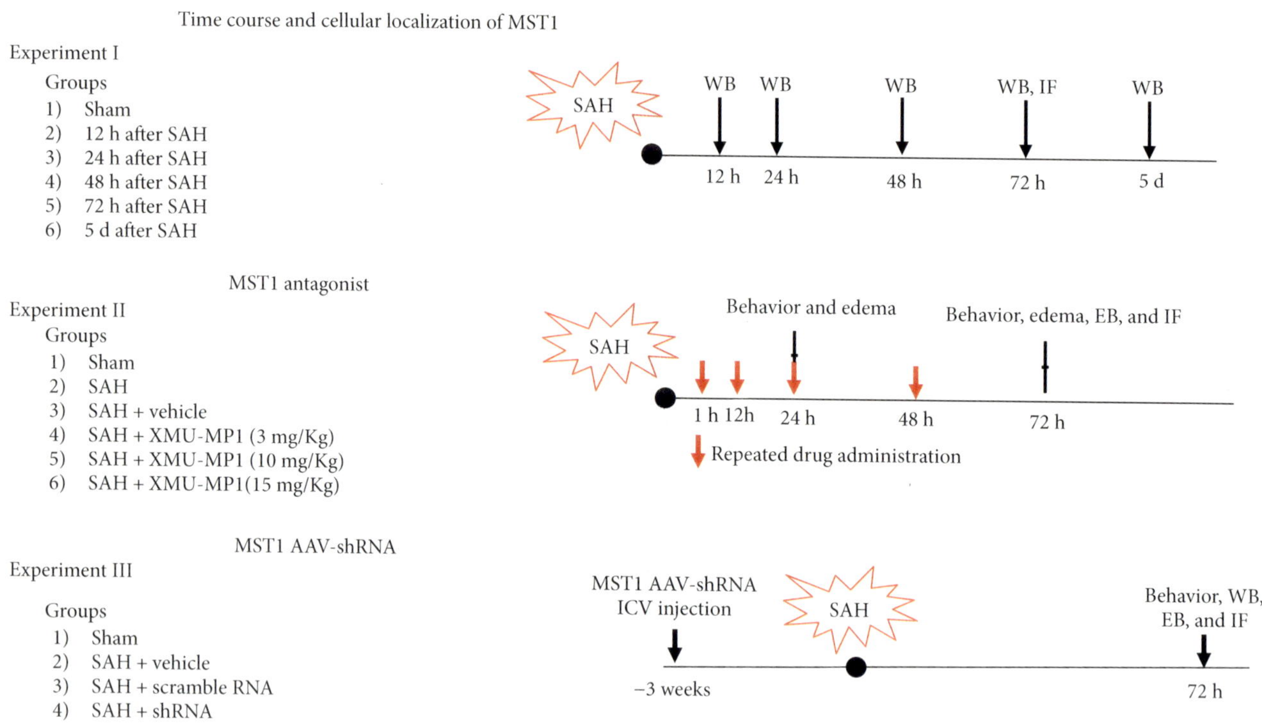

FIGURE 1: Brief illustration of the experimental design. WB: Western blot; EB: Evans blue extravasation; IF: immunofluorescence; ICV: intracerebroventricular.

MST1 has been shown to be upstream of nuclear factor-(NF-) κB, a well-established conserved factor, for regulating neuroinflammation in many neurological diseases. However, the specific role of MST1 in the pathophysiological process of early brain injury remains elusive. Therefore, we aim to investigate the potential role of MST1 in a mouse model of SAH to determine its effects on early brain injury.

2. Materials and Methods

2.1. Experimental Animals. Two hundred and sixty-one (261) male C57B6J mice, 23 g to 28 g in weight, were raised and housed by the Experimental Animal Center of Third Military Medical University (Chongqing, China). All animal experimental procedures were evaluated and approved by the Ethics Committee of Southwest Hospital, Third Military Medical University; the procedures were performed in accordance with the National Institutes of Health (NIH) Guide for the Care and Use of Laboratory Animals and are reported in accordance with the ARRIVE guideline. The mice were randomly allocated to different experimental groups as shown in Figure 1.

2.2. SAH Model. The mice underwent intravascular perforation procedures to mimic SAH as previously described [15]. Briefly, sodium pentobarbital (intraperitoneal injection, 40 mg/kg) was used to anesthetize the animals. The external carotid artery (ECA) was isolated and cut distally into a 2 mm stump. A 5-0 filament suture was subsequently threaded through the ECA to the inner carotid artery (ICA). The sharpened suture was pushed 2 mm further during resistance to penetrate the bifurcation of the anterior cerebral artery (ACA) and middle cerebral artery (MCA). The ICA reperfused after filament suture was subsequently withdrawn. Sham-operated mice underwent the same procedure, without perforating the cerebral artery.

Following euthanasia, the severity of the SAH grade was blindly evaluated as previously reported [16]. In general, the scores from 6 segments of the SAH were summed. Mice that exhibited a score < 8 with no obvious neurological deficits were excluded from the following experiments.

2.3. Adeno-Associated Virus (AAV) Vector Administration. Sodium pentobarbital (40 mg/kg, ip) was used to anaesthetize the mice. Three microliters of AAV (Vigene Biosciences Inc., Shandong, China) or AAV empty were intraventricularly administered into the lateral ventricles (0.33 μl/min) using specific coordinates (0.5 mm posterior to bregma, 3 mm ventral to the skull, and 1 mm lateral to the sagittal line) and a stereotaxic frame. The SAH model was performed 3 weeks after AAV infusion. To improve the knockdown efficiency, four different shRNA duplexes were designed and mixed in the present study. Their sequences are provided in their $5' \rightarrow 3'$ orientation:

shRNA1:
GCGGACCTGCATTATGGACAATCTCGAGATTGT
CCATAATGCAGGTCCGTTTTT
shRNA2:
GCCAGGAATGTAACACGAAGTACTCGAGTACTT
CGTGTTACATTCCTGGTTTTT

shRNA3:
GCCCGAATGTTGAGCGAGAATTCTCGAGAATTC
TCGCTCAACATTCGGGTTTTT
shRNA4:
GCGTGAGAATTTCTGCCGGAATCTCGAGATTCC
GGCAGAAATTCTCACGTTTTT

2.4. Neurological Scoring. The modified Garcia scale was employed to evaluate the neurological function at 24 and 72 h after SAH and included six measurements as follows: spontaneous activity, forepaw outstretching, symmetry of limb climbing, responses to body proprioception, and vibrissae touch [17]. For the Beam Balance Score text, the mice were placed on the center of a wooden beam to assess the walking distance within 1 min and were subsequently assigned 0–4 points in total. The neurologic scores determined by the two blinded observers were used to determine the grade.

2.5. Brain Edema. The brain edema of the mice was evaluated using a previously described method [15]. Under deep anesthesia, brain tissues were rapidly dissected and separated into two cerebral hemispheres and cerebellum on tin foil paper, and the wet weights of the specimens were determined. The brain specimens were subsequently incubated in a 75°C oven for 72 h, and the dry weights were recorded. The brain edema/brain water content was calculated as (wet weight − dry weight)/wet weight × 100%.

2.6. Evans Blue Dye Extravasation and Autofluorescence. As previously reported, the BBB permeability was evaluated by Evans blue dye extravasation and autofluorescence. Under deep anesthesia, Evans blue dye (2%, 5 ml/kg) was administered into the caudal vein. After 2 h, the mice were intracardially perfused with phosphate-buffered solution (PBS), and brain specimens were collected and rapidly weighed. Two milliliters of 50% trichloroacetic acid was added to the ipsilateral/right hemisphere, tightly homogenized, and subsequently centrifuged at 10,000 ×g for 30 min. The homogenates were then incubated overnight at 4°C. Supernatants that contained the Evans blue dye were collected following a subsequent centrifugation at 10,000 ×g for 30 min, and a spectrophotometer was used to measure the absorbance of the supernatant at 615 nm.

2.7. Immunofluorescence Staining. Immunofluorescence staining was performed at 72 h after the operation. Briefly, the mice were anesthetized and perfused with 4% paraformaldehyde. Brain specimens were rapidly collected and postfixed in 4% paraformaldehyde for 1 day and a 30% sucrose solution for the following 3 days. Fifteen μm thick coronal sections were cut and treated with 0.3% Triton for 30 min. The brain sections were subsequently treated with 5% donkey serum for 1 h for antigen block and incubated with the primary antibodies overnight in a 4°C freezer, including anti-zonula occludens-1 (1 : 100, Invitrogen, Grand Island, NY), anti-von Willebrand factor (1 : 100 Abcam), anti-Iba1 (1 : 100, Abcam), and anti-MST1 (1 : 100, Invitrogen, Grand Island, NY), followed by FITC-conjugated secondary antibody (1 : 200, Beyotime Biotechnology, Shanghai, China) and cy3-conjugated secondary antibodies (1 : 200, Beyotime Biotechnology, Shanghai, China) for 1.5 h at room temperature. A confocal laser scanning microscope (Zeiss, Oberkochen, Germany) was used to detect the expression of fluorescent dyes.

2.8. Terminal Deoxynucleotidyl Transferase-Mediated dUTP Nick-End Labeling (TUNEL) Staining. The In Situ Cell Apoptosis Detection Kit I (Boster Biological Technology, Wuhan, China) was used to detect DNA fragmentation in the cell nuclei of brain specimen sections by following the operating manual. Sections were illustrated with DAB solution, and the apoptotic nuclei were identified by the presence dark-brown staining. TUNEL-positive cells were counted by two researchers in a blinded manner.

2.9. Western Blotting. The ipsilateral/right cortex was isolated and homogenized for Western blotting as previously described [15] with the following primary antibodies: anti-MST1 (1 : 1000, Cell Signaling Technology, Danvers, MA, USA), anti-phosphorylated MST1 (1 : 1000, Cell Signaling Technology, Danvers, MA, USA), anti-ZO-1 (1 : 500 Invitrogen, Grand Island, NY, USA), anti-occludin (1 : 1000 Abcam, Shanghai, China), anti-claudin-5 (1 : 1000, Abcam, Shanghai, China), anti-NF-κB (1 : 1000, Cell Signaling Technology, Danvers, MA, USA), and anti-matrix metallopeptidase-(MMP-) 9 (1 : 1000, Cell Signaling Technology, Danvers, MA, USA). GAPDH (1 : 10,000, Proteintech, Rosemont, IL, USA) was used as an internal loading control. The relative density of the Western blots was normalized to the sham group.

2.10. Proteome Profiler Mouse Cytokine Array. Protein expression analysis of the sham group, MST1 shRNA group, and negative control group (sh-NC) was performed 72 h after SAH using the Proteome Profiler Antibody Arrays—Mouse Cytokine Antibody Array, Panel A (Catalog Number ARY006, R&D Systems, Minneapolis, MN, USA) according to the manufacturer's instructions as previously reported.

2.11. Statistical Analysis. All data are presented as the me an + standard deviation (mean ± SD) and were analyzed using GraphPad Prism 6 (GraphPad Software, San Diego, CA). One-way ANOVA and Tukey's multiple comparisons were employed for comparisons among the different groups. The Kruskal-Wallis test was employed for the analysis of the behavior scores. $p < 0.05$ was considered statistically significant.

3. Results

3.1. Time Course of Endogenous P-MST1 and Phosphorylated-MST1 Expressions in Mice after SAH Injury. There were 6 mice (2 in the 12 h group, 1 in the 24 h group, 1 in the 48 h group, and 2 in the 5 d group); those with a score < 8 or no obvious neurological deficits were excluded from further analysis. And 12 mice (3 in the 12 h group, 2 in the 24 h group, 3 in the 48 h group, 2 in the 72 h group, and 2 in the 5 d group) that underwent SAH died due to severe hemorrhagic volume within 24 h

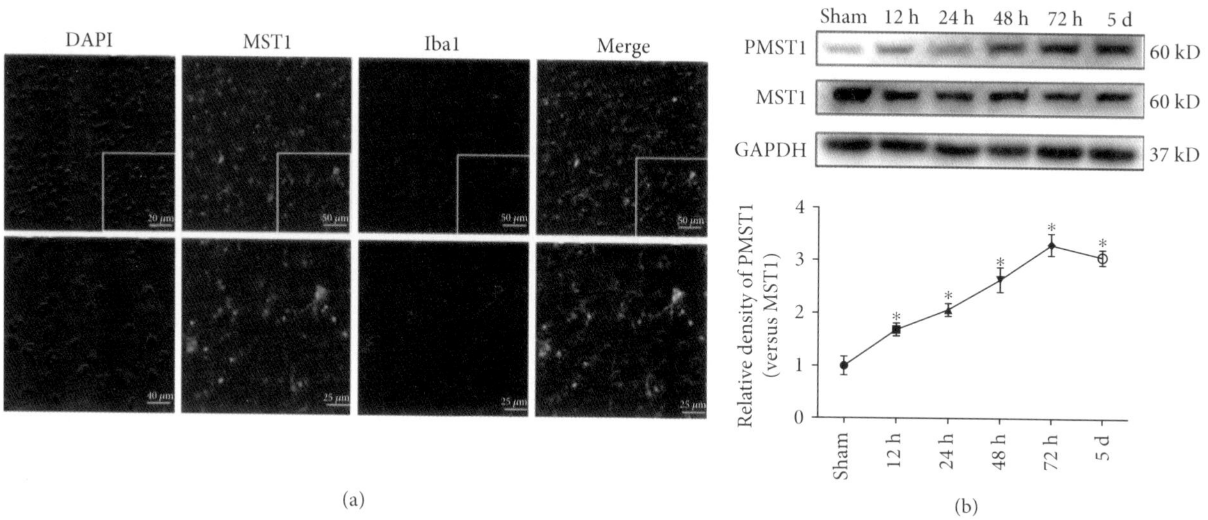

FIGURE 2: Time course of P-MST1 and MST1 expressions after SAH. (a) Representative images and Western blot analyses of P-MST1 and MST1 in the ipsilateral hemisphere in sham and SAH mice at 12 h, 24 h, 48 h, 72 h, and 5 days after SAH; $n = 6$ mice per group per time point. Relative densities were normalized against the densities in the sham group. $^*p < 0.05$ versus the sham group. (b) Representative immunofluorescence staining slices of MST1 and Iba1 in the ipsilateral cortex at 72 h after SAH. Scale bar = 50 μm (up) and 25 μm (down).

of SAH. There is no significant difference in the mortality of each group ($p > 0.05$).

The Western blot results indicated that the total protein expression of MST1 in the right/ipsilateral hemisphere decreased at 12 h after SAH and was subsequently maintained at a low level. Moreover, the phosphorylated MST1 increased at 12 h after SAH compared to the sham group, with a peak at 72 h (Figure 2(a)). Therefore, the tendency of the phosphorylation level of MST1 is the same as that of phosphorylated MST1. Furthermore, immunofluorescence images demonstrated that MST1 colocalized with microglia cells (Iba1) in the right cortex at 72 h after SAH (Figure 2(b)).

3.2. XMU-MP-1 Treatment Relieved Early Brain Injury after SAH. No toxic effect of MST1 inhibition was identified in this study. The SAH grading score results showed that there were no significant differences among the experimental SAH groups at 24 h or 72 h (Figure 3). 4 mice (2 in the SAH group, 1 in the 3 mg/kg group, and 1 in the 10 mg/kg group) with a score < 8 as well as no obvious neurological deficits were excluded from further analysis, and 8 mice (1 in the SAH group, 2 in the vehicle group, 1 in the 3 mg/kg group, 2 in the 10 mg/kg group, and 2 in the 15 mg/kg group) that underwent SAH died due to severe hemorrhagic volume within 24 h of SAH. There is no significant difference in the mortality of each group ($p > 0.05$).

Both neurobehavioral scores were significantly lower in the SAH mouse model group than in the sham group at 24 h and 72 h after SAH. Compared with the vehicle treatment after SAH, MST1 inhibition improved the SAH-impaired neurological function on the modified Garcia test; both the 10 mg/kg dosage and the 15 mg/kg dosage of XMU-MP-1 treatments significantly improved the neurobehavioral outcomes at 72 h after SAH, whereas only the 15 mg/kg dosage exerted neuroprotective effects at 24 h after SAH (Figures 4(a) and 4(b)). Furthermore, the beam balance score indicated that the SAH mice exhibited substantially worse neurological deficits at 24 h and 72 h after SAH compared to the sham group, and the high dosage (15 mg/kg) XMU-MP-1 treatment remarkably improved neurological function (Figures 4(c) and 4(d)).

In addition, there was significantly greater brain edema in both hemispheres of the SAH mice than in the hemispheres of the sham-operated mice at 24 h and 72 h after SAH. Low concentrations (3 mg/kg) of XMU-MP-1 showed a tendency to alleviate this SAH-induced brain edema, whereas high concentrations (10 and 15 mg/kg) of XMU-MP-1 significantly decreased the SAH-induced brain edema compared to the vehicle treatment (Figures 4(c) and 4(d)).

Compared with the brains of the sham-treated mice, the extravasated content of Evans blue was substantially higher in both hemispheres of the mouse model of SAH, and XMU-MP-1 (15 mg/kg) significantly alleviated the leakage (Figure 5(a)). Furthermore, Evans blue fluorescence in the ipsilateral cortex showed more dye leakage around the arteriole in the SAH mice than in the sham-treated mice, which was reduced by XMU-MP-1 treatment (Figure 5(b)). At 72 h after SAH, the continuous endothelial cells indicated by vWF-positive cells and the tight junctions indicated by ZO-1 structures were damaged. However, XMU-MP-1 treatment effectively reduced these disruptions (Figure 5(c)).

3.3. MST1 In Vivo Knockdown Improved Neurobehavioral Outcomes, Alleviated Neuroinflammation, and Reduced Evans Blue Extravasation at 72 h after SAH. The result of the SAH grading score showed that there was no significant difference among these experimental SAH (Figure 3(c)). 3 mice (2 in the SAH group and 1 in the shRNA group) with a score < 8 as well as no obvious neurological deficits were excluded from further analysis. And 4 mice (2 in the SAH group, 1 in the scramble RNA group, and 1 in the shRNA group) that underwent SAH died due to severe hemorrhagic

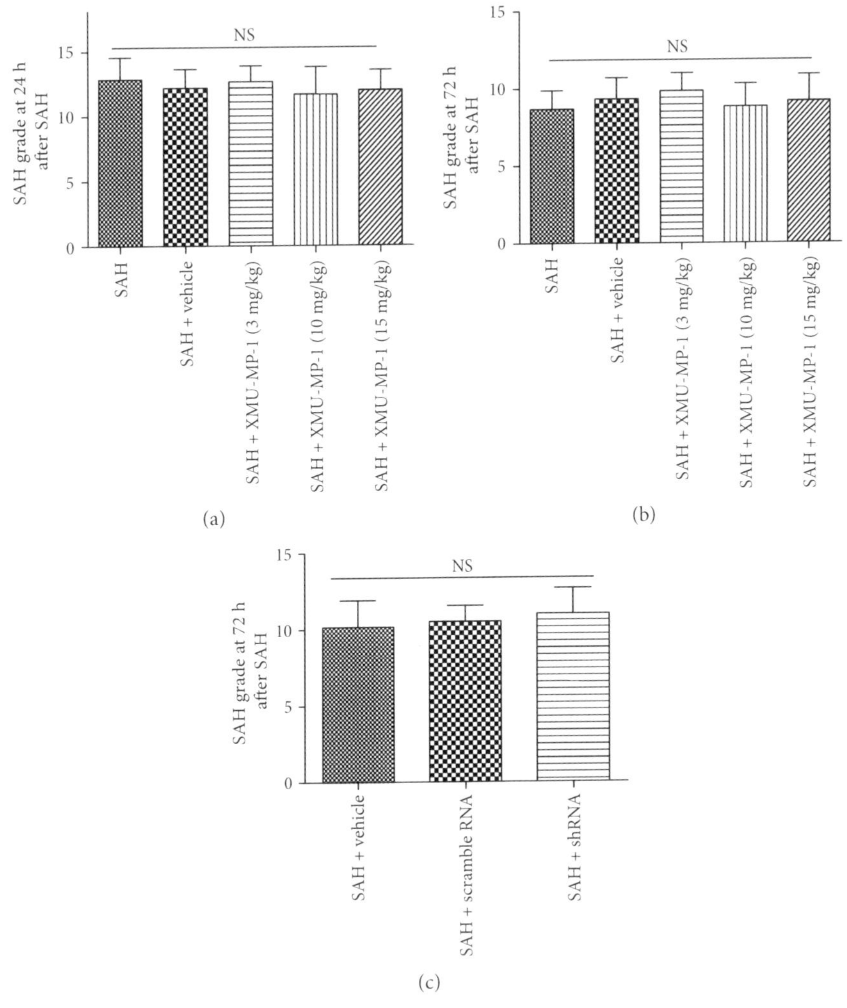

FIGURE 3: SAH grading scores of SAH mouse models in each group. The SAH grading scores of the SAH mouse models in experiment II at (a) 24 h and (b) 72 h after SAH, as well as in experiment III at 72 h after SAH.

volume within 24 h of SAH. There is no significant difference in the mortality of each group ($p > 0.05$).

To knock down MST1 protein expression, we used AAV to infect the whole brain (Figure 6(a)) and Western blotting to measure the infection and knockdown efficiency (Figures 6(b) and 6(c)). At 72 h after SAH, both the vehicle- and scrambled shRNA-pretreated SAH mice showed remarkable neurological deficits compared to the sham group; however, there was no significant difference between the two groups ($p > 0.05$). In the MST1 shRNA-pretreated group, the modified Garcia score was significantly improved (Figure 7(a)). In addition, compared with the sham group, there are much more TUNEL-positive cells in the cortex at 72 h after SAH (Figure 7(b)). In MST1 shRNA pretreatment group, the number of TUNEL-positive cells in the cortex was less than half of the vehicle group's (Figure 7(b)). Meanwhile, the MST1 shRNA-pretreated mice showed less Evans blue dye extravasation than both the vehicle- and scrambled shRNA-pretreated groups (Figure 7(c)). Based on the proteome profiler mouse cytokine array, the SAH groups exhibited 13 upregulated target proteins compared to the sham group. Among these upregulated proteins, cytokines (TNF-α) and chemokines (I-309, ICAM-1, MCP-1, M-CSF, CCL3, CXCL12, CXCL2, CXCL9, and CXCL10) were significantly downregulated by MST1 suppression compared with the expression in the negative control animals (Figure 7(d)).

3.4. Effects of MST1 Knockdown on p65 NF-κB, MMP-9, and Tight Junction Protein Expression at 72 h after SAH. To evaluate the p65 NF-κB activity, the cytoplasmic expressions and nuclear expressions of p65 NF-κB were detected in each group. In the vehicle- and scrambled shRNA-pretreated SAH mice, the cytoplasmic expressions of p65 NF-κB were significantly decreased and the nuclear expressions of p65 NF-κB were significantly increased compared to the sham mice (Figures 8(a) and 8(b)). In addition, the MMP-2 and MMP-9 protein expressions were elevated in the two groups. However, compared to the SAH + vehicle group, MST1 shRNA pretreatment preserved the expression of p65 NF-κB in the cytoplasm and decreased the nuclear expression of p65 NF-κB ($p < 0.05$). Furthermore, MST1 shRNA downregulated the expression of MMP-9 but not MMP-2 (Figures 8(c) and 8(d)). The

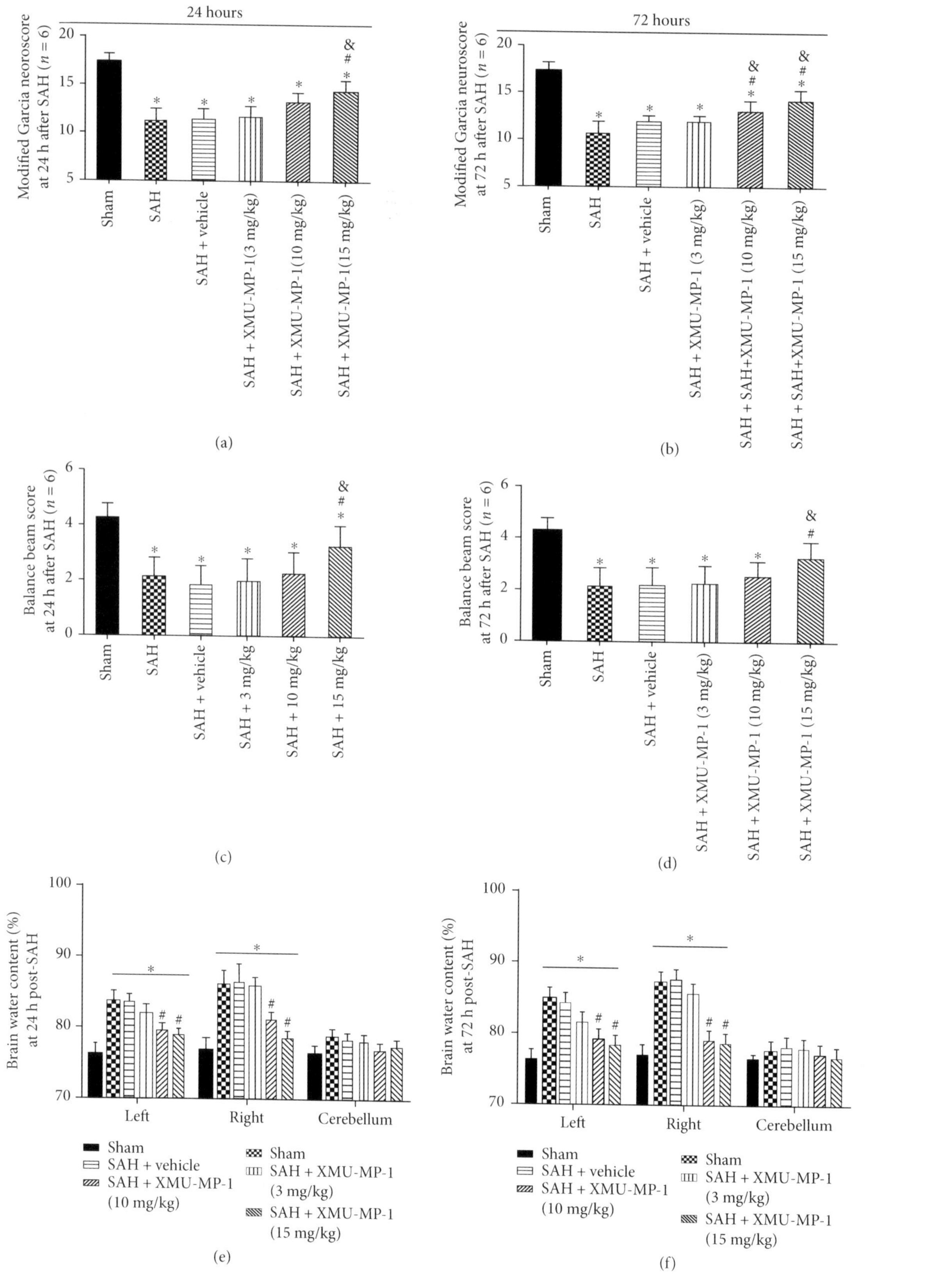

FIGURE 4: Effects of XMU-MP-1 treatment on early brain injury after SAH. Modified Garcia scores at (a) 24 h and (b) 72 h in each group after SAH. Beam balance scores at (c) 24 h and (d) 72 h in each group after SAH. Brain edema at (e) 24 h and (f) 72 h in each group after SAH ($n = 6$). $^{*}p < 0.05$ versus the sham group; $^{\#}p < 0.05$ versus the SAH group; $^{\&}p < 0.05$ versus the SAH + vehicle group.

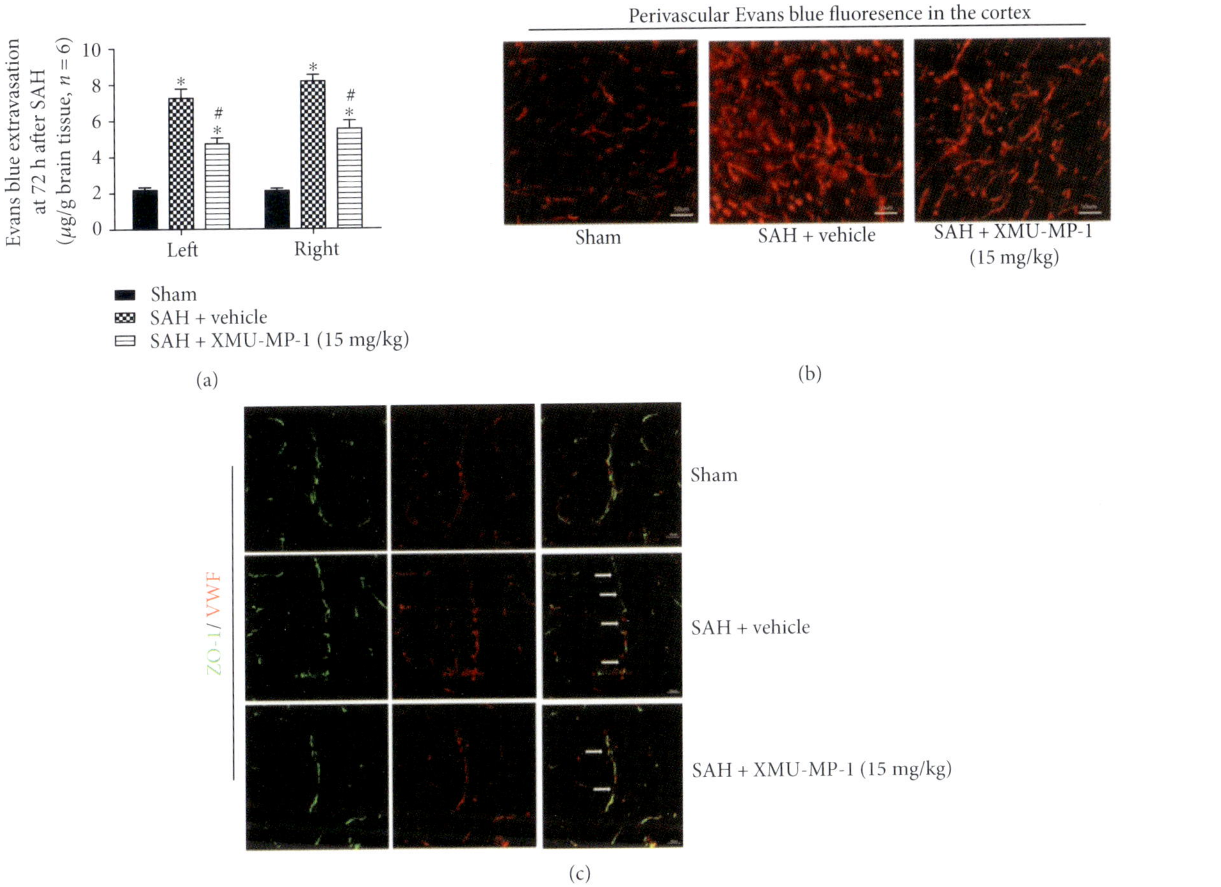

Figure 5: Effects of XMU-MP-1 administration on BBB integrity at 72 h after SAH. (a) Content of Evans blue extravasation at 72 h after SAH. (b) Representative Evans blue fluorescence images in the right/ipsilateral cortex at 72 h after SAH. (c) Representative immunohistochemistry images of ZO-1 and vWF at 72 h after SAH. White arrows indicate the disruption in continuous endothelial cells. $^{*}p < 0.05$ versus the sham group; $^{\#}p < 0.05$ versus SAH + vehicle. $n = 6$ per group. Scale bar = 50 μm.

vehicle- and scrambled RNA-treated SAH mice also expressed significantly less ZO-1, occludin, and claudin-5 than did the sham mice. However, MST1 shRNA pretreatment upregulated the expressions of ZO-1, occludin, and claudin-5 (Figures 8(e)–8(g)).

3.5. MST1 Knockdown Reduces White Matter Fiber Damage at 72 h after SAH. To evaluate the white matter damage after SAH, immunofluorescent staining was used to detect the protein marker of white matter injury. Both the vehicle- and scrambled shRNA-pretreated SAH mice expressed significantly less myelin basic protein (MBP) than did the sham mice, and MST1 shRNA preserved the expression of MBP (Figure 9(a)) at 72 h after SAH. In addition, the amyloid precursor protein (APP) expression, a classic marker of axonal injury indicative of cytoskeletal damage, was significantly increased after SAH; however, MST1 shRNA pretreatment alleviated the APP expression (Figure 9(b)).

4. Discussion

In our study, we explored the time course of the MST1 phosphorylation level and cellular localization, as well as the function and mechanism of MST1 in the early brain injury during SAH. We determined that the phosphorylated MST1 expression was increased at 12 h after SAH compared to the sham group, with a peak at 72 h. It was colocalized with the microglia marker Iba1 in the cortex. A high dose of XMU-MP-1 (15 mg/kg), identified as an inhibitor of MST1/2, alleviated the neurological deficits, brain edema, and BBB disruption caused by SAH. In addition, to rule out nonspecific effects of the MST1 inhibitor, we also used shRNA (packaged by AAV) to in vivo knock down MST1; the downregulation of MST1 increased the neurological score and reduced the neuroinflammation, BBB disruption, and white matter injury. MST1 knockdown suppressed the NF-κB-MMP-9 pathway, thus preserving the reduced tight junction proteins. In summary, these results supported our hypothesis that MST1 suppression could alleviate early brain injury in SAH mice by inhibiting the NF-κB/MMP-9 pathway.

After subarachnoid hemorrhage, BBB disruption contributes to brain edema, followed by brain swelling, increased intracranial pressure, neuronal death, and neurologic deficits [3]. Previous studies have demonstrated that the inflammatory response may increase BBB permeability after SAH [16, 18, 19]. However, the involvement of MST1 and its associated pathological process is unknown. MST1, the mammalian Hippo ortholog, is the central component of the Hippo

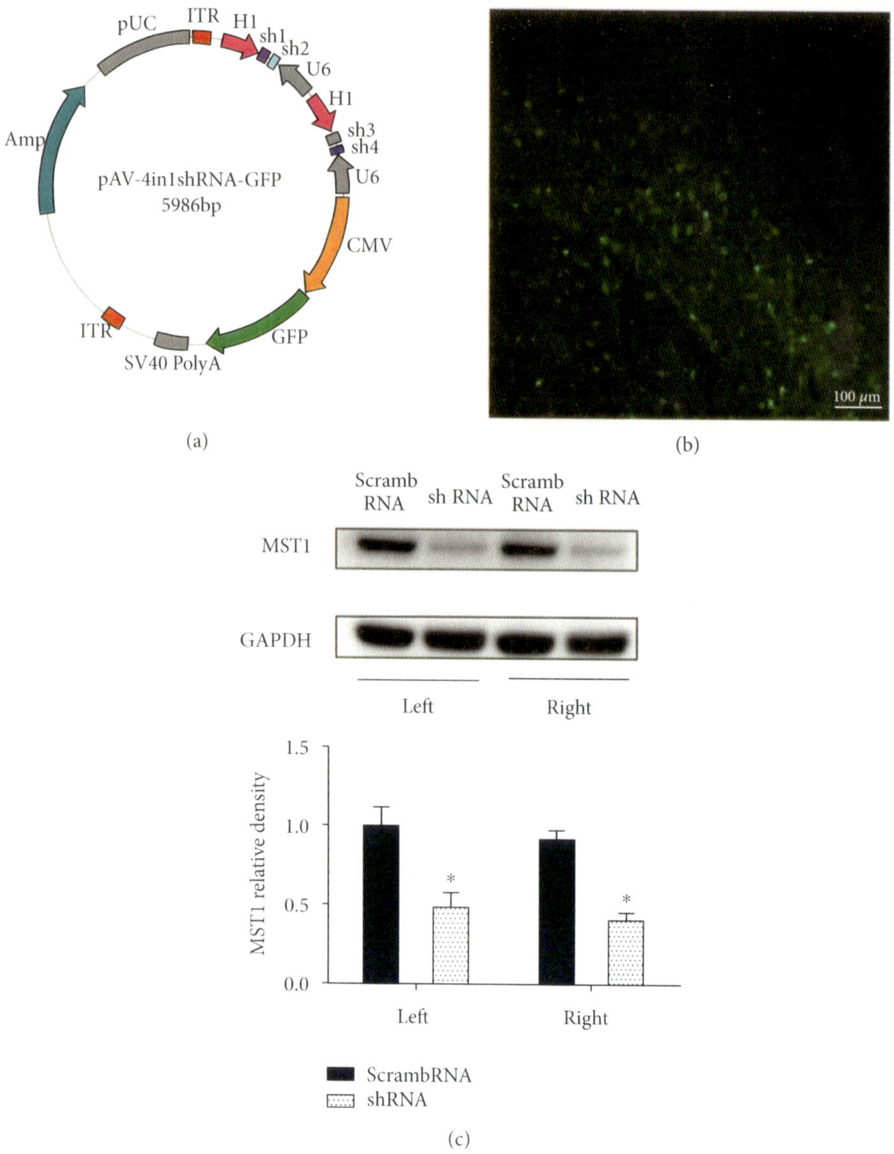

FIGURE 6: Infection and inhibition efficacy of the AAV. (a) The shRNA-containing vector. (b) Representative photo of the fluorescent tags (GFP). (c) Representative images and analysis by Western blot for the MST1 shRNA inhibitory effect. $n = 6$; $^{*}p < 0.05$ versus scrambled shRNA. Scale bar = 100 μm.

pathway [4]. Previous studies have suggested that MST1 activation contributes to neuronal apoptosis and inflammation. Genetic deletion of MST1 may reduce the inflammation and microglial activation after spinal cord injury and ischemic stroke [13, 14]. Consistent with these reports, we determined that pharmacological inhibition of MST1 or its knockdown alleviated the neurological deficits, brain edema, and BBB disruption induced by SAH. Furthermore, the expression of several proinflammatory cytokines was suppressed by MST1 inhibition, which is associated with NF-κB inhibition. The activation of MMPs, particularly MMP-9, may contribute to the disruption of the BBB via degradation of tight junction proteins after SAH [16]. Our current results suggested that MST1 suppression repressed the MMP-9 expression, alleviated the degradation of tight junction proteins, and reduced the leakage of Evans blue dye. Moreover, we determined that the cytoplasm-nuclear translocation of p65 NF-κB was substantially decreased by MST1 suppression.

MST1 has been associated with the immunological response in various systems. Our results demonstrated that increased MST1 contributes to the higher expressions of cytokines (TNF-α) and chemokines (I-309, ICAM-1, M-CSF, MCP-1, CCL3, CXCL12, CXCL2, CXCL9, and CXCL10), which play vital roles in neuroinflammation and early brain injury after SAH. Salojin et al. knocked out MST1 to alleviate experimental autoimmune encephalomyelitis and improve collagen-induced arthritis [20]. In addition, MST1-mediated dendritic cell- (DC-) dependent Th17 differentiation has been shown to regulate experimental autoimmune encephalomyelitis and antifungal immunity [21]. Kurz et al. reported that MST1-deficient ($Mst1^{-/-}$)

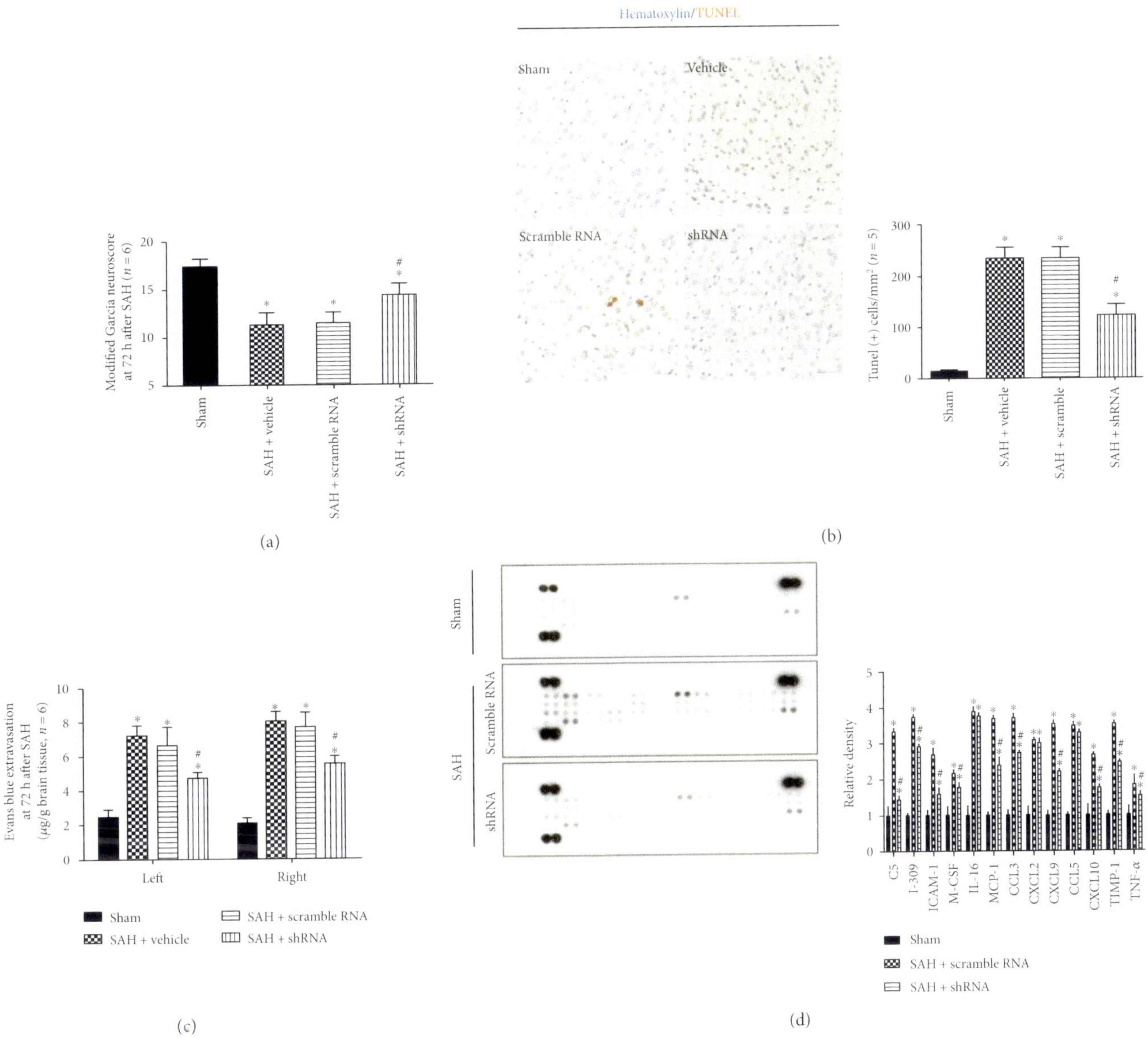

FIGURE 7: Effects of MST1 shRNA on neurobehavioral score, neural cell injury, Evans blue extravasation, and neuroinflammation. (a) Statistical analysis of the modified Garcia scores at 72 h after SAH. (b) Representative figures and statistical analysis of the cell counting of the TUNEL-positive cells at 72 h after SAH. (c) Statistical analysis of the Evans blue extravasation of each group at 72 h after SAH. (d) Representative bands and quantitative analyses of the proteome profiler mouse cytokine array in the indicated groups. Relative densities were normalized against the density in the sham group. $n = 3$; $^{*}p < 0.05$ versus the sham group; $^{\#}p < 0.05$ versus SAH + scramble RNA. Scale bar = 50 μm.

neutrophils were unable to migrate into inflamed tissues [22]. However, to date, the mechanisms by which MST1 and its downstream pathways affect neuroinflammation in acute central neural system injuries remain unknown and require further investigation.

After SAH, acute white matter injury is an important pathological process during early brain injury [23, 24]. Several recent studies have indicated that the activation of MMP-9 contributed to SAH-induced white matter injury. Genetic deletion of MMP-9 may alleviate the white matter damage observed after SAH [25]. Our studies also indicated a role of MST1 in activating MMP-9; therefore, we evaluated the effect of MST1 suppression on white matter after SAH. Consistent with previous studies, pretreatment with MST1 shRNA partially rescued the reduction in MBP (marker of myelin degradation) expression caused by SAH, whereas the elevated expression of β-APP (maker of axonal damage) induced by SAH was moderately inhibited by MST1 shRNA pretreatment. These results suggested that MST1 suppression protects nerve fibers and reduces brain edema after SAH.

The present study has several limitations. First, we investigated the short-term neuroprotective effects of MST1 suppression within 3 days after SAH. The long-term effects of MST1 suppression should also be examined in the future to

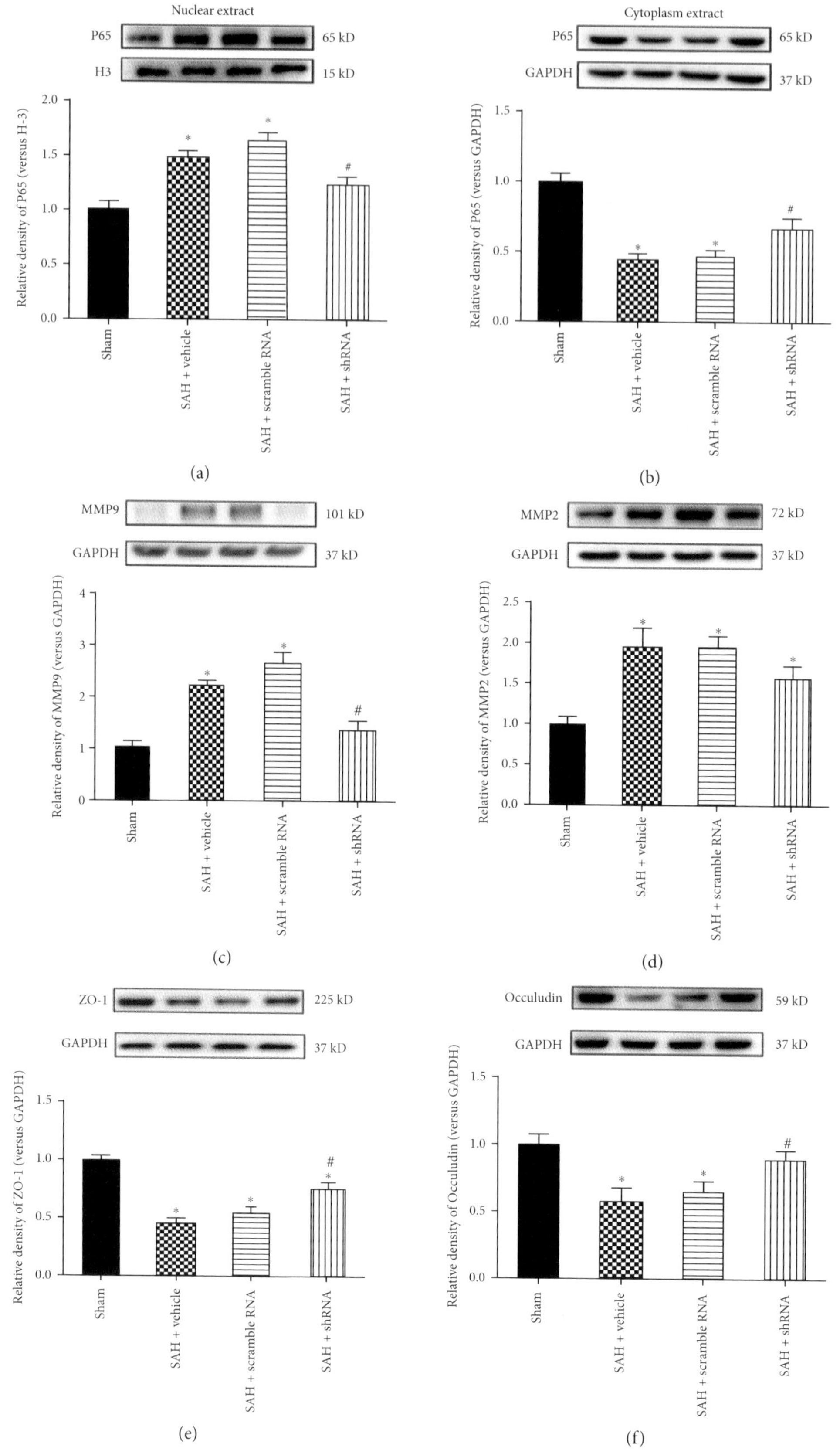

Figure 8: Continued.

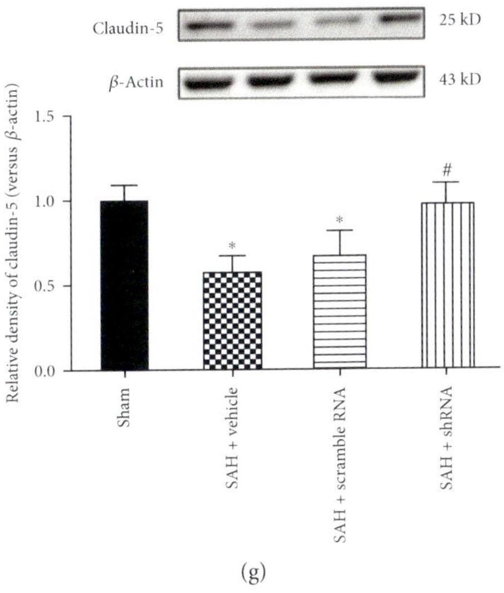

FIGURE 8: Western blot analysis of the effects of MST1 shRNA. Representative images and analysis of p65 NF-κB protein expression in the (a) cytoplasm and (b) nucleus at 72 h after SAH. Representative images and analysis of (c) MMP-9 and (d) MMP-2 protein expressions at 72 h after SAH. (e–g) Representative images and analysis of ZO-1, occludin, and claudin-5 at 72 h after SAH. The band density values were normalized to the sham group. $^{*}p < 0.05$ versus sham; $^{\#}p < 0.05$ versus SAH + vehicle.

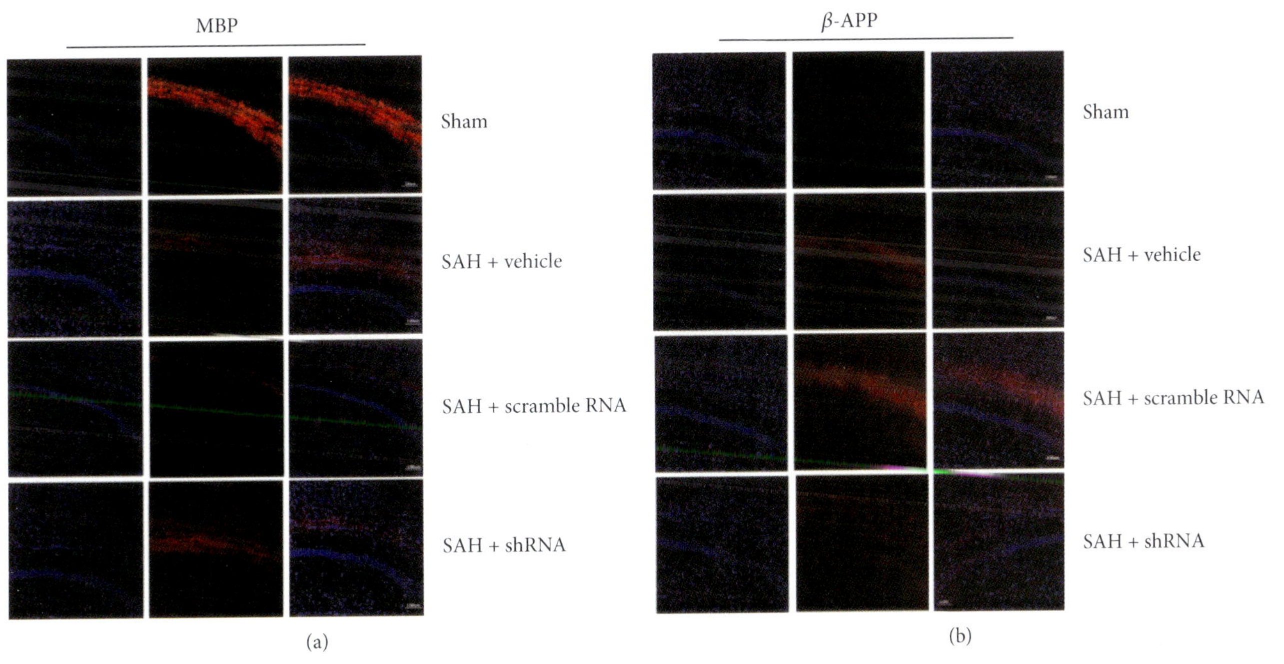

FIGURE 9: Effects of MST1 shRNA pretreatment on the white matter fiber damage induced by SAH. Representative immunofluorescence staining of MBP (a) and β-APP (b) in each group. Scale bar = 100 μm.

further understand the MST1 involvement after SAH. In addition, XMU-MP-1 is an inhibitor of MST1/2 [26]. Although MST1 and MST2 have been shown to have the same effects in many studies [4, 27–29], they may not be equivalent in SAH. Thus, we cannot eliminate the possibility that MST2 suppression provided the neuroprotective effects for the early brain injury post-SAH. Finally, we explored the relation between MST1 and NF-κB-MMP-9; however, how MST1 influences NF-κB remains unknown. Thus, future studies should explore downstream of MST1.

5. Conclusions

In summary, our findings suggested that the serine/threonine kinase MST1 plays a pivotal role in the pathophysiological process of early brain injury after SAH. Inhibition of MST1 alleviated the neurological deficits, preserved the BBB integrity, reduced brain edema, and prevented white matter damage by inhibiting the downstream NF-κB/MMP-9 signal after SAH. Therefore, MST1 suppression treatment may represent a promising therapeutic strategy for the future management of SAH patients.

Acknowledgments

This work was supported by the National Natural Science Foundation of China (Grant nos. 81501002 and 81220108009), the Incubation Foundation of Interdisciplinary Laboratory of Physics and Biomedicine (Grant no. WSS-2015-08), and the Major Innovation Project of Southwest Hospital (no. SWH2016ZDCX1011).

References

[1] S. Chen, H. Feng, P. Sherchan et al., "Controversies and evolving new mechanisms in subarachnoid hemorrhage," *Progress in Neurobiology*, vol. 115, pp. 64–91, 2014.

[2] J. H. Zhang, J. Badaut, J. Tang, A. Obenaus, R. Hartman, and W. J. Pearce, "The vascular neural network–a new paradigm in stroke pathophysiology," *Nature Reviews Neurology*, vol. 8, no. 12, pp. 711–716, 2012.

[3] M. Fujii, J. Yan, W. B. Rolland, Y. Soejima, B. Caner, and J. H. Zhang, "Early brain injury, an evolving frontier in subarachnoid hemorrhage research," *Translational Stroke Research*, vol. 4, no. 4, pp. 432–446, 2013.

[4] J. A. Galan and J. Avruch, "MST1/MST2 protein kinases: regulation and physiologic roles," *Biochemistry*, vol. 55, no. 39, pp. 5507–5519, 2016.

[5] S. Ikeda and J. Sadoshima, "Regulation of myocardial cell growth and death by the hippo pathway," *Circulation Journal*, vol. 80, no. 7, pp. 1511–1519, 2016.

[6] H. J. Yun, J. H. Yoon, J. K. Lee et al., "Daxx mediates activation-induced cell death in microglia by triggering MST1 signalling," *The EMBO Journal*, vol. 30, no. 12, pp. 2465–2476, 2011.

[7] S. J. Lee, B. R. Seo, E. J. Choi, and J. Y. Koh, "The role of reciprocal activation of cAbl and Mst1 in the oxidative death of cultured astrocytes," *Glia*, vol. 62, no. 4, pp. 639–648, 2014.

[8] L. Xiao, D. Chen, P. Hu et al., "The c-Abl-MST1 signaling pathway mediates oxidative stress-induced neuronal cell death," *Journal of Neuroscience*, vol. 31, no. 26, pp. 9611–9619, 2011.

[9] X. Zheng, C. Xu, A. Di Lorenzo et al., "CCM3 signaling through sterile 20-like kinases plays an essential role during zebrafish cardiovascular development and cerebral cavernous malformations," *Journal of Clinical Investigation*, vol. 120, no. 8, pp. 2795–2804, 2010.

[10] I. A. Tavares, D. Touma, S. Lynham et al., "Prostate-derived sterile 20-like kinases (PSKs/TAOKs) phosphorylate tau protein and are activated in tangle-bearing neurons in Alzheimer disease," *Journal of Biological Chemistry*, vol. 288, no. 21, pp. 15418–15429, 2013.

[11] J. K. Lee, J. H. Shin, S. G. Hwang et al., "MST1 functions as a key modulator of neurodegeneration in a mouse model of ALS," *Proceedings of the National Academy of Sciences*, vol. 110, no. 29, pp. 12066–12071, 2013.

[12] Y. Yang, L. Wang, Y. Wu et al., "Tanshinol suppresses inflammatory factors in a rat model of vascular dementia and protects LPS-treated neurons via the MST1-FOXO3 signaling pathway," *Brain Research*, vol. 1646, pp. 304–314, 2016.

[13] P. F. Wang, D. Y. Xu, Y. Zhang et al., "Deletion of mammalian sterile 20-like kinase 1 attenuates neuronal loss and improves locomotor function in a mouse model of spinal cord trauma," *Molecular and Cellular Biochemistry*, vol. 431, no. 1-2, pp. 11–20, 2017.

[14] S. Zhao, J. Yin, L. Zhou et al., "Hippo/MST1 signaling mediates microglial activation following acute cerebral ischemia-reperfusion injury," *Brain, Behavior, and Immunity*, vol. 55, pp. 236–248, 2016.

[15] Y. Chen, Y. Zhang, J. Tang et al., "Norrin protected blood–brain barrier via frizzled-4/β-catenin pathway after subarachnoid hemorrhage in rats," *Stroke*, vol. 46, no. 2, pp. 529–536, 2015.

[16] P. Pan, X. Zhang, Q. Li et al., "Cyclosporine A alleviated matrix metalloproteinase 9 associated blood-brain barrier disruption after subarachnoid hemorrhage in mice," *Neuroscience Letters*, vol. 649, pp. 7–13, 2017.

[17] J. H. Garcia, S. Wagner, K. F. Liu, and X. J. Hu, "Neurological deficit and extent of neuronal necrosis attributable to middle cerebral artery occlusion in rats: statistical Validation," *Stroke*, vol. 26, no. 4, pp. 627–635, 1995.

[18] S. Park, M. Yamaguchi, C. Zhou, J. W. Calvert, J. Tang, and J. H. Zhang, "Neurovascular protection reduces early brain injury after subarachnoid hemorrhage," *Stroke*, vol. 35, no. 10, pp. 2412–2417, 2004.

[19] B. Enkhjargal, D. W. McBride, A. Manaenko et al., "Intranasal administration of vitamin D attenuates blood-brain barrier disruption through endogenous upregulation of osteopontin and activation of CD44/P-gp glycosylation signaling after subarachnoid hemorrhage in rats," *Journal of Cerebral Blood Flow & Metabolism*, vol. 37, no. 7, pp. 2555–2566, 2017.

[20] K. V. Salojin, B. D. Hamman, W. C. Chang et al., "Genetic deletion of Mst1 alters T cell function and protects against autoimmunity," *PLoS One*, vol. 9, no. 5, article e98151, 2014.

[21] C. Li, Y. Bi, Y. Li et al., "Dendritic cell MST1 inhibits Th17 differentiation," *Nature Communications*, vol. 8, article 14275, 2017.

[22] A. R. M. Kurz, M. Pruenster, I. Rohwedder et al., "MST1-dependent vesicle trafficking regulates neutrophil transmigration through the vascular basement membrane," *Journal of Clinical Investigation*, vol. 126, no. 11, pp. 4125–4139, 2016.

[23] Y. Wu, J. Peng, J. Pang, X. Sun, and Y. Jiang, "Potential mechanisms of white matter injury in the acute phase of experimental subarachnoid haemorrhage," *Brain*, vol. 140, no. 6, article e36, 2017.

[24] T. T. Kummer, S. Magnoni, C. L. MacDonald et al., "Experimental subarachnoid haemorrhage results in multifocal axonal injury," *Brain*, vol. 138, no. 9, pp. 2608–2618, 2015.

[25] Y. Egashira, H. Zhao, Y. Hua, R. F. Keep, and G. Xi, "White matter injury after subarachnoid hemorrhage: role of blood-brain barrier disruption and matrix metalloproteinase-9," *Stroke*, vol. 46, no. 10, pp. 2909–2915, 2015.

[26] F. Fan, Z. He, L. L. Kong et al., "Pharmacological targeting of kinases MST1 and MST2 augments tissue repair and regeneration," *Science Translational Medicine*, vol. 8, no. 352, article 352ra108, 2016.

[27] X. Du, H. Shi, J. Li et al., "Mst1/Mst2 regulate development and function of regulatory T cells through modulation of Foxo1/Foxo3 stability in autoimmune disease," *The Journal of Immunology*, vol. 192, no. 4, pp. 1525–1535, 2014.

[28] J. Geng, X. Sun, P. Wang et al., "Kinases Mst1 and Mst2 positively regulate phagocytic induction of reactive oxygen species and bactericidal activity," *Nature Immunology*, vol. 16, no. 11, pp. 1142–1152, 2015.

[29] S. J. Rawat, D. Araiza-Olivera, L. E. Arias-Romero et al., "H-ras inhibits the hippo pathway by promoting Mst1/Mst2 heterodimerization," *Current Biology*, vol. 26, no. 12, pp. 1556–1563, 2016.

Permissions

All chapters in this book were first published in BN, by Hindawi Publishing Corporation; hereby published with permission under the Creative Commons Attribution License or equivalent. Every chapter published in this book has been scrutinized by our experts. Their significance has been extensively debated. The topics covered herein carry significant findings which will fuel the growth of the discipline. They may even be implemented as practical applications or may be referred to as a beginning point for another development.

The contributors of this book come from diverse backgrounds, making this book a truly international effort. This book will bring forth new frontiers with its revolutionizing research information and detailed analysis of the nascent developments around the world.

We would like to thank all the contributing authors for lending their expertise to make the book truly unique. They have played a crucial role in the development of this book. Without their invaluable contributions this book wouldn't have been possible. They have made vital efforts to compile up to date information on the varied aspects of this subject to make this book a valuable addition to the collection of many professionals and students.

This book was conceptualized with the vision of imparting up-to-date information and advanced data in this field. To ensure the same, a matchless editorial board was set up. Every individual on the board went through rigorous rounds of assessment to prove their worth. After which they invested a large part of their time researching and compiling the most relevant data for our readers.

The editorial board has been involved in producing this book since its inception. They have spent rigorous hours researching and exploring the diverse topics which have resulted in the successful publishing of this book. They have passed on their knowledge of decades through this book. To expedite this challenging task, the publisher supported the team at every step. A small team of assistant editors was also appointed to further simplify the editing procedure and attain best results for the readers.

Apart from the editorial board, the designing team has also invested a significant amount of their time in understanding the subject and creating the most relevant covers. They scrutinized every image to scout for the most suitable representation of the subject and create an appropriate cover for the book.

The publishing team has been an ardent support to the editorial, designing and production team. Their endless efforts to recruit the best for this project, has resulted in the accomplishment of this book. They are a veteran in the field of academics and their pool of knowledge is as vast as their experience in printing. Their expertise and guidance has proved useful at every step. Their uncompromising quality standards have made this book an exceptional effort. Their encouragement from time to time has been an inspiration for everyone.

The publisher and the editorial board hope that this book will prove to be a valuable piece of knowledge for researchers, students, practitioners and scholars across the globe.

List of Contributors

Theresa M. Smith
Department of Occupational Therapy, Texas Woman's University, 6700 Fannin Street, Houston, TX 77030, USA

Monique R. Pappadis
Division of Rehabilitation Sciences, School of Health Professions, University of Texas Medical Branch, 301 University Blvd, Galveston, TX 77555, USA
Sealy Center on Aging, University of Texas Medical Branch, 301 University Blvd, Galveston, TX 77555, USA

Timothy A. Reistetter
Division of Rehabilitation Sciences, School of Health Professions, University of Texas Medical Branch, 301 University Blvd,
Sealy Center on Aging, University of Texas Medical Branch, 301 University Blvd, Galveston, TX 77555, USA
Department of Occupational Therapy, School of Health Professions, University of Texas Medical Branch, Galveston, 301 University Blvd, Galveston, TX 77555, USA

Shilpa Krishnan
Department of Rehabilitation Medicine, Division of Physical Therapy, Emory University, School of Medicine, 1462 Clifton Road, Atlanta, GA 30322, USA

Batya Engel-Yeger and Naomi Josman
Department of Occupational Therapy, Faculty of Social Welfare and Health Sciences, University of Haifa, Haifa, Israel

Leeanne M. Carey
Occupational Therapy, Department of Community and Clinical Allied Health, School of Allied Health, La Trobe University, Melbourne, VIC, Australia
Neurorehabilitation and Recovery, Stroke Division, The Florey Institute of Neuroscience and Mental Health, Heidelberg, VIC, Australia

Tamara Tse
Occupational Therapy, Department of Community and Clinical Allied Health, School of Allied Health, La Trobe University, Melbourne, VIC, Australia
Neurorehabilitation and Recovery, Stroke Division, The Florey Institute of Neuroscience and Mental Health, Heidelberg, VIC, Australia
Occupational Therapy Department, St Vincent's Hospital Melbourne, Fitzroy, VIC, Australia

Carolyn Baum
Program in Occupational Therapy, Washington University School of Medicine, St Louis, MO, USA

Elias Koutsoukos and Elias Angelopoulos
Medical School, 1st Psychiatric Department, Eginition Hospital, Athens University, 72-74 Vas. Sofias Ave., 115 28 Athens, Greece
Signal Processing Laboratory, University Mental Health Research Institute, 2 Soranou Efessiou, 115 27 Athens, Greece

Alkinoos Athanasiou,Nikos Terzopoulos, Maria Karagianni, Charis Styliadis and Panagiotis D. Bamidis
Lab of Medical Physics, School of Medicine, Faculty of Health Sciences, Aristotle University of Thessaloniki (AUTH), 54124 Thessaloniki, Greece

Niki Pandria and Evangelos Paraskevopoulos
Lab of Medical Physics, School of Medicine, Faculty of Health Sciences, Aristotle University of Thessaloniki (AUTH), 54124 Thessaloniki, Greece
Northern Greece Neurofeedback Center, Thessaloniki, Greece

Chrysoula Kourtidou-Papadeli
Aeromedical Center of Thessaloniki, Thessaloniki, Greece

Athanasia Pataka
Pulmonary Department, Oncology Unit, "G. Papanikolaou" General Hospital, Aristotle University of Thessaloniki,Thessaloniki, Greece

Evgenia Lymperaki
Department of Medical Laboratories, Alexander Technological Educational Institute of Thessaloniki, Sindos, Greece

Masao Omori, Hideto Sano, Kazutaka Igarashi and Shoichi Ichimura
Department of Orthopaedic Surgery, Kyorin University School of Medicine, 6-20-2 Shinkawa, Mitaka, Tokyo 181-8611, Japan

Satoshi Shibuya, Tsuyoshi Nakajima, Shun Irie, Ryohei Ariyasu and Yukari Ohki
Department of Integrative Physiology, Kyorin University School of Medicine, 6-20-2 Shinkawa, Mitaka, Tokyo 181-8611, Japan

Takashi Endoh
Faculty of Human Development and Education, Uekusa Gakuen University, 1639-3 Ogura-cho, Wakaba-ku, Chiba 264-0007, Japan

Shinya Suzuki
Department of Physical Therapy, School of Rehabilitation, Health Sciences University of Hokkaido, 1757 Kanazawa, Tobetsucho, Ishikari-gun, Hokkaido 061-0293, Japan

Satoshi Unenaka
Department of Sports Education, School of Lifelong Sport, Hokusho University, 23 Bunkyodai, Ebetsu, Hokkaido 069-0833, Japan

Mohammed S. Jilani, Dexter Tagwireyi, Louis L. Gadaga and Cosmas Mutsimhu
Drug and Toxicology Information Service (DaTIS), School of Pharmacy and Department of Clinical Pharmacology, College of Health Sciences, University of Zimbabwe, Avondale, Harare, Zimbabwe

Charles C. Maponga
School of Pharmacy, University of Zimbabwe, Mount Pleasant, Harare, Zimbabwe

C. Guijarro-Castro, I. Gómez-Moreno and L. Gómez-Romero
Sección de Neurología, Hospital Virgen de la Luz, Cuenca, Spain

Y. Aladro-Benito, M. J. Laredo and M. Cerezo-García
Sección de Neurología, Hospital Universitario de Getafe de Madrid, Madrid, Spain

A. Sánchez-Musulim
Hospital Santa Bárbara de Puertollano, Ciudad Real, Spain

A. Belen-Caminero
Sección de Neurología, Hospital Ntra. Sra. de Sonsoles de Ávila, Ávila, Spain

I. Pérez Molina
Hospital Universitario Virgen de la Salud de Toledo, Toledo, Spain

J. Millán-Pascual
Sección de Neurología, Hospital La Mancha Centro de Alcazar de San Juan, Ciudad Real, Spain

Yanhua Qin
Department of Psychiatry, Sir Run Run Shaw Hospital, Zhejiang University School of Medicine, Hangzhou, China

Weiming Hu
Department of Psychiatry, The Third Hospital of Quzhou, Quzhou, China

Yang Yang, Weiyun Li and Marong Fang
3Institute of Neuroscience, Zhejiang University School of Medicine, Hangzhou, China

Zhiying Hu
Department of Obstetrics and Gynecology, Hangzhou Red Cross Hospital, Hangzhou, China

Yannick Ezo'o Ezo'o and Hervé Hervé Pafroumi Fachagbo
Department of Life and Earth Sciences, Higher Teachers' Training College, University of Maroua, Maroua, Cameroon
Department of Animal Biology and Physiology, Faculty of Science, University of Yaoundé 1, Yaoundé, Cameroon

Stéphane Zingue
Department of Life and Earth Sciences, Higher Teachers' Training College, University of Maroua, Maroua, Cameroon
Department of Animal Biology and Physiology, Faculty of Science, University of Yaoundé 1, Yaoundé, Cameroon

Ngatanko Abaïssou and Sefirin Djiogue
Department of Animal Biology and Physiology, Faculty of Science, University of Yaoundé 1, Yaoundé, Cameroon

Dieudonné Njamen
Department of Animal Biology and Physiology, Faculty of Science, University of Yaoundé 1, Yaoundé, Cameroon

Harquin Simplice Foyet
Department of Biological Sciences, Faculty of Science, University of Maroua, Maroua, Cameroon

Rui Lan, Tao Wu, Yun-Zhi Ma, Ya-Na Li, Yan Wang, Chun-Qing Gu and Ji-Tao Wu
Encephalopathy Hospital, The First Affiliated Hospital of Henan University of Chinese Medicine, Henan 450000, China

Yong Zhang
Cerebral Palsy Rehabilitation Department, The Third Affiliated Hospital of Zhengzhou University, Henan 450000, China

Bao-Qi Wang and Hai-Zhong Zheng
Henan University of Chinese Medicine, Henan 450000, China

Ozgul Ekmekci
Department of Neurology, Faculty of Medicine, Ege University, Izmir, Turkey

Tivadar Lucza and Kázmér Karádi
Institute of Behavioral Sciences, University of Pécs, Pécs, Hungary

Sámuel Komoly and Zsuzsanna Ascherman
Department of Neurology, University of Pécs, Pécs, Hungary

Márton Kovács, Attila Makkos and Márk Harmat
Department of Neurology, University of Pécs, Pécs, Hungary
Doctoral School of Clinical Neuroscience, University of Pécs, Pécs, Hungary

Annamária Juhász, József Janszky and Norbert Kovács
Department of Neurology, University of Pécs, Pécs, Hungary
MTA-PTE Clinical Neuroscience MR Research Group, Pécs, Hungary

Krisztina Dorn
Pediatric Clinic, University of Pécs, Pécs, Hungary

Ying-Jui Ho and Mei-Shiuan Shen
Department of Psychology, Chung Shan Medical University Hospital, Chung Shan Medical University, Taichung 402, Taiwan

Jun-Cheng Weng
Department of Medical Imaging and Radiological Sciences, Chang Gung University, Taoyuan 33302, Taiwan
Department of Psychiatry, Chang Gung Memorial Hospital, Chiayi 613, Taiwan

Chih-Li Lin and Hsin-Hua Li
Institute of Medicine, Chung Shan Medical University, Taichung 402, Taiwan

Wen-Chieh Liao
Department of Anatomy, Faculty of Medicine, Chung Shan Medical University, Chung Shan Medical University Hospital,Taichung 402, Taiwan
Department of Pediatrics, Chung Shan Medical University Hospital, Taichung 402, Taiwan

Nu-Man Tsai
School of Medical Laboratory and Biotechnology, Chung Shan Medical University, Taichung 402, Taiwan

Ching-Sui Hung
Occupational Safety and Health Office, Taipei City Hospital, Taipei 10341, Taiwan

Te-Jen Lai
Department of Psychiatry, Chung Shan Medical University Hospital, Chung Shan Medical University, Taichung 402, Taiwan
Institute of Medicine, Chung Shan Medical University, Taichung 402, Taiwan

I-Yen Lee
Division of Urology, Department of Surgery, Tungs' Taichung Metroharbor Hospital, Taichung 43503, Taiwan

Zongya Zhao Zhenxin Li and Yi Yu
School of Biomedical Engineering, Xinxiang Medical University, Xinxiang 453003, China
Key Lab of Neurosense and Control, Xinxiang Medical University, Xinxiang 453003, China

Yaqing Cheng
Department of Computer Technology, Henan Information Engineering School, Zhengzhou 450000, China

Yao-Chin Wang
Graduate Institute of Biomedical Informatics, College of Medical Science and Technology, Taipei Medical University, Taipei, Taiwan
Department of Emergency, Min-Sheng General Hospital, Taoyuan City, Taiwan
International Center for Health Information Technology (ICHIT), Taipei Medical University, Taipei, Taiwan

Tahmina Nasrin Poly, Chieh-Chen Wu and Md Mohaimenul Islam
Graduate Institute of Biomedical Informatics, College of Medical Science and Technology, Taipei Medical University, Taipei, Taiwan
International Center for Health Information Technology (ICHIT), Taipei Medical University, Taipei, Taiwan

Yu-Chuan (Jack) Li
Graduate Institute of Biomedical Informatics, College of Medical Science and Technology, Taipei Medical University, Taipei, Taiwan
International Center for Health Information Technology (ICHIT), Taipei Medical University, Taipei, Taiwan
Department of Dermatology, Wan Fang Hospital, Taipei, Taiwan
TMU Research Center of Cancer Translational Medicine, Taipei, Taiwan

Hsuan-Chia Yang
Graduate Institute of Biomedical Informatics, College of Medical Science and Technology, Taipei Medical University, Taipei, Taiwan
Department of Surgery, School of Medicine, Buddhist Tzu Chi University, Hualien, Taiwan

Po-An Tai
Department of Surgery, School of Medicine, Buddhist Tzu Chi University, Hualien, Taiwan

Cinzia Femiano, Francesca Trojsi, Giuseppina Caiazzo, Antonio Russo, Alvino Bisecco, Mario Cirillo,Maria Rosaria Monsurrò and Gioacchino Tedeschi
Department of Medical, Surgical, Neurological, Metabolic and Aging Sciences; MRI Research Center SUN-FISM Università degli Studi della Campania "Luigi Vanvitelli", Naples, Italy

Mattia Siciliano
Department of Medical, Surgical, Neurological, Metabolic and Aging Sciences; MRI Research Center SUN-FISM Università degli Studi della Campania "Luigi Vanvitelli", Naples, Italy
Department of Psychology, Università degli Studi della Campania "Luigi Vanvitelli", Naples, Italy

Gabriella Santangelo and Carla Passaniti
Department of Psychology, Università degli Studi della Campania "Luigi Vanvitelli", Naples, Italy

Fabrizio Esposito,
Department of Medicine, Surgery and Dentistry, Scuola Medica Salernitana, University of Salerno, Baronissi, Salerno, Italy

Peyton Teutsch and Mara E. Kaiser
VA Portland Health Care System, Portland, OR, USA

Carolyn E. Jones
VA Portland Health Care System, Portland, OR, USA
Department of Behavioral Neuroscience, Oregon Health and Science University, Portland, OR, USA

Natasha Avalon Gardner
VA Portland Health Care System, Portland, OR, USA
Portland State University, Portland, OR, USA

Miranda M. Lim
VA Portland Health Care System, Portland, OR, USA
Department of Behavioral Neuroscience, Oregon Health and Science University, Portland, OR, USA
Department of Neurology, Department of Medicine, Division of Pulmonary and Critical Care Medicine, Oregon Institute of Occupational Health Sciences, Oregon Health and Science University, Portland, OR, USA

Hui-Chi Lin
Department of Neurology, Mackay Memorial Hospital, Taipei, Taiwan

Chuo-Yu Lee
Department of Neurology, Mackay Memorial Hospital, Taipei, Taiwan
Graduate Institute of Chemistry, Tamkang University, New Taipei City, Taiwan

Department of Medicine, Mackay Medical College, New Taipei City, Taiwan

Shih-Jung Cheng
Department of Neurology, Mackay Memorial Hospital, Taipei, Taiwan
Department of Medicine, Mackay Medical College, New Taipei City, Taiwan
Department of Physical Therapy and Assistive Technology, National Yang-Ming University, Taipei, Taiwan

Pei-Hao Chen
Department of Neurology, Mackay Memorial Hospital, Taipei, Taiwan
Department of Medicine, Mackay Medical College, New Taipei City, Taiwan
Graduate Institute of Mechanical and Electrical Engineering, National Taipei University of Technology, Taipei, Taiwan

Yu-Lu Liao
Department of Accounting Information, Takming University of Science and Technology, Taipei, Taiwan

Qingqing Huang, Xiping Liang, Shiqiang Wang and Xiaosong Mu
Chongqing University Cancer Hospital and Chongqing Cancer Institute and Chongqing Cancer Hospital, Chongqing, China

Rosario Iodice
Catholic University of Pereira, Risaralda, Colombia
Institute of Neurosciences of Castilla y León, University of Salamanca, Salamanca, Spain

Juan José García Meilán and Juan Carro Ramos
Institute of Neurosciences of Castilla y León, University of Salamanca, Salamanca, Spain
Department of Psychology, University of Salamanca, Salamanca, Spain

Jeff A. Small
School of Audiology and Speech Sciences, The University of British Columbia, Vancouver, BC, Canada

Tong Li, Shu-na Duan and Liang Dong
Department of Neurology, Shánxi Medical University, 56 Xinjian S Rd., Yingze, Taiyuan, Shanxi 030001, China
Department of Neurology, The Second Hospital, Shanxi Medical University, 382 WuYi St., Taiyuan, Shanxi 030001, China

Gaiqing Wang
Department of Neurology, Shanxi Medical University, 56 Xinjian S Rd., Yingze, Taiyuan, Shanxi 030001, China
Department of Neurology, The Second Hospital, Shanxi Medical University, 382 WuYi St., Taiyuan, Shanxi 030001, China

Xin-gang Sun and Fang Xue
Department of Neurology, The Second Hospital, Shanxi Medical University, 382 WuYi St., Taiyuan, Shanxi 030001, China

Heng Yang, Wei Ni, Hanqiang Jiang, Yu Lei, Jiabin Su, Yuxiang Gu and Liangfu Zhou
Department of Neurosurgery, Huashan Hospital, Fudan University, Shanghai, China

Songyun Zhang, Lingling Yuan, Lihui Zhang, Caige Li and Jie Li
The Second Hospital of Hebei Medical University, No. 215 Heping Road (West), Shijiazhuang City, Hebei Province, China

Sheng-Kung Yang
Department of Neurology, Chang Bing Show Chwan Memorial Hospital, Changhua County, Taiwan

Weishan Chen
Management Office for Health Data, China Medical University Hospital, Taichung, Taiwan
College of Medicine, China Medical University, Taichung, Taiwan

Chun-Hsien Su
Department of Exercise and Health Promotion, College of Education, Chinese Culture University, Taipei, Taiwan

Chung-Hsiang Liu
Department of Neurology, China Medical University Hospital, Taichung, Taiwan

Po-Chi Chan
Department of Neurology, Show Chwan Memorial Hospital, Changhua, Taiwan

Chien-Tai Hong
Department of Neurology, Taipei Medical University Shuang Ho Hospital, New Taipei City, Taiwan
Department of Neurology, School of Medicine, College of Medicine, Taipei Medical University, Taipei, Taiwan

Dean Wu
Department of Neurology, Taipei Medical University Shuang Ho Hospital, New Taipei City, Taiwan
Department of Neurology, School of Medicine, College of Medicine, Taipei Medical University, Taipei, Taiwan
Sleep Center, Taipei Medical University Shuang Ho Hospital, New Taipei City, Taiwan

Chaur-Jong Hu
Department of Neurology, Taipei Medical University Shuang Ho Hospital, New Taipei City, Taiwan
Department of Neurology, School of Medicine, College of Medicine, Taipei Medical University, Taipei, Taiwan
Vertigo and Balance Impairment Center, Taipei Medical University Shuang Ho Hospital, New Taipei City, Taiwan

Hsun-Hua Lee
Department of Neurology, Taipei Medical University Shuang Ho Hospital, New Taipei City, Taiwan
Department of Neurology, School of Medicine, College of Medicine, Taipei Medical University, Taipei, Taiwan
Sleep Center, Taipei Medical University Shuang Ho Hospital, New Taipei City, Taiwan
Vertigo and Balance Impairment Center, Taipei Medical University Shuang Ho Hospital, New Taipei City, Taiwan

Ji Zhang, Lingsong Ma, Shoucai Zhao, Shizun Li, Tingting Huang and Zhaohu Chu
Department of Neurology, First Affiliated Hospital of Wannan Medical College, No. 2, ZheShanXi Road, Wuhu 241001, China

Yang Xu
Department of Neurology, First Affiliated Hospital of Wannan Medical College, No. 2, ZheShanXi Road, Wuhu 241001, China
Non-Coding RNA of Major Diseases Research Center, Central Laboratory, First Affiliated Hospital of Wannan Medical College, No. 2, ZheShanXi Road, Wuhu 241001, China

Jie Qu, Hengli Zhao, Qiang Li, Pengyu Pan, Kang Ma, Xin Liu, Hua Feng and Yujie Chen
Department of Neurosurgery, Southwest Hospital, Third Military Medical University, Chongqing, China

Index